Management and Welfare
of Farm Animals

The Universities Federation for Animal Welfare

UFAW, founded 1926, is an internationally recognized, independent, scientific and educational animal welfare charity concerned with promoting high standards of welfare for farm, companion, laboratory and captive wild animals, and for those animals with which we interact in the wild. It works to improve animals' lives by:

- Promoting and supporting developments in the science and technology that underpin advances in animal welfare;

- Promoting education in animal care and welfare;

- Providing information, organizing meetings, and publishing books, videos, articles, technical reports and the journal *Animal Welfare*;

- Providing expert advice to government departments and other bodies and helping to draft and amend laws and guidelines;

- Enlisting the energies of animal keepers, scientists, veterinarians, lawyers and others who care about animals.

"Improvements in the care of animals are not now likely to come of their own accord, merely by wishing them: there must be research ... and it is in sponsoring research of this kind, and making its results widely known, that UFAW performs one of its most valuable services."

Sir Peter Medawar CBE FRS, 8 May 1957
Nobel Laureate (1960), Chairman of the UFAW Scientific Advisory Committee (1951–1962)

UFAW relies on the generosity of the public through legacies and donations to carry out its work improving the welfare of animals now and in the future. For further information about UFAW and how you can help promote and support its work, please contact us at the address below.

Universities Federation for Animal Welfare
The Old School, Brewhouse Hill, Wheathampstead, Herts AL4 8AN, UK
Tel: 01582 831818 Fax: 01582 831414 Website:www.ufaw.org.uk
Email:ufaw@ufaw.org.uk

UFAW's aim regarding the UFAW/Wiley-Blackwell Animal Welfare book series is to promote interest and debate in the subject and to disseminate information relevant to improving the welfare of kept animals and of those harmed in the wild through human agency. The books in this series are the works of their authors and the views they express do not necessarily reflect the views of UFAW.

Management and Welfare of Farm Animals

UFAW FARM HANDBOOK
5th edition

Edited by John Webster,
MA Vet MB PhD MRCVS

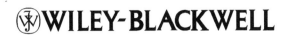

A John Wiley & Sons, Inc., Publication

This edition first published 2011. © 2011 by Universities Federation for Animal Welfare
Series editors: James K. Kirkwood and Robert C. Hubrecht

Fourth edition published 1999 by Universities Federation for Animal Welfare
Third edition published 1988 by Baillière Tindall
Second edition published 1978 by Baillière Tindall
First edition published 1971 by Churchill Livingstone

Blackwell Publishing was acquired by John Wiley & Sons in February 2007. Blackwell's publishing program has been merged with Wiley's global Scientific, Technical and Medical business to form Wiley-Blackwell.

Registered office: John Wiley & Sons Ltd, The Atrium, Southern Gate, Chichester, West Sussex,
PO19 8SQ, UK

Editorial offices: 9600 Garsington Road, Oxford, OX4 2DQ, UK
The Atrium, Southern Gate, Chichester, West Sussex, PO19 8SQ, UK
2121 State Avenue, Ames, Iowa 50014-8300, USA

For details of our global editorial offices, for customer services and for information about how to apply for permission to reuse the copyright material in this book please see our website at www.wiley.com/wiley-blackwell.

Library of Congress Cataloging-in-Publication Data

Management and welfare of farm animals: UFAW farm handbook / edited by
John Webster. – 5th ed. p. cm.
Includes bibliographical references and index.
ISBN 978-1-4051-8174-7 (pbk. : alk. paper)
1. Livestock–Great Britain–Management. 2. Livestock–Great Britain–Handbooks, manuals, etc.
I. Webster, John. II. Title: UFAW farm handbook.
SF61.M23 2011
636–dc22

2010040974

A catalogue record for this book is available from the British Library.

Set in 10/12.5 pt Sabon by Thomson Digital, Noida, India
Printed and bound in Malaysia by Vivar Printing Sdn Bhd

1   2011

Contents

Contributors

Fiona Benson
14 St. Joseph's Court
Tedder Road
York YO24 3FE

Cristian Bonacic MV, MSc, DPhil
School of Agriculture and Forestry Sciences
Pontificia Universidad Catolica de Chile
Casilla, 306
Correo 22, Santiago
Chile

Bernadette Earley BSc, PhD
Teagasc, Animal Bioscience Department
Grange Research Centre
Dunsany
Co. Meath
Ireland

Sandra Edwards MA, PhD
School of Agriculture, Food and Rural Development
Newcastle University
Newcastle on Tyne NE1 7RU

Pete Goddard BVetMed, PhD, MRCVS
Macaulay Land Use Research Institute
Craigiebuckler
Aberdeen AB15 8QH

Keith Gooderham BVSc, DPMP, MRCVS
38 Marsh Lane
Hemmingford Grey
Huntingdon
Cambridgeshire PE28 9EM

Alison Hanlon BSc, MSc, PhD
UCD School of Agriculture, Food Science and Veterinary Medicine
University College
Dublin
Ireland

Susan Haslam BVSc, PhD, DWEL, MRCVS (deceased)

Stephen Lister BSc, BVetMed, CertPMP, DiplECPVS, MRCVS
Crowshall Veterinary Services
1 Crowshall Lane
Attleborough
Norfolk

David Main BVetMed, PhD, CertVR, DWEL, MRCVS
Department of Clinical Veterinary Science
University of Bristol
Langford
Bristol BS40 5DU

Jean Margerison BSc, PhD
Institute of Food, Nutrition and Human Health
Massey University
Palmerston North
New Zealand

Alan Mowlem CBiol, MSB
Water Farm, Stogursey
Bridgwater
Somerset TA5 1PS

Christine Nicol MA, DPhil
Department of Clinical Veterinary Science
University of Bristol
Langford
Bristol BS40 5DU

Graham Scott BSc, PhD
Harper Adams University College
Edgmond
Newport
Shropshire TF10 8NB

Tony Wall BVM&S, CertVOphthal, MSc, MRCVS
Fish Vet Group
22 Carsegate Road
Inverness IV3 8EX

John Webster MA, VetMB, PhD, MRCVS
Old Sock Cottage
Mudford Sock
Yeovil
Somerset BA22 8EA

David Welchman MA, VetMB, PhD, MRCVS
VLA – Winchester
Itchen Abbas
Winchester SO21 1BX

Helen (Becky) Whay BSc, PhD
Department of Clinical Veterinary Science
University of Bristol
Langford
Bristol BS40 5DU

Foreword

The first edition of the UFAW *Handbook on the Care and Management of Farm Animals* was published forty years ago (UFAW, 1971*). Some aspects of farm animal production have changed considerably since those days. Global economic pressures (including the fact that the human population has roughly doubled and eats much more meat per head) have driven a tendency for greater intensification: the pursuit of more product per unit cost. This has led to changes not just to animals' environments – feeding, housing and disease control – but also to dramatic genetic changes in some species and strains. Since the first edition was published, the time taken by broilers to reach slaughter weight has roughly halved, and the milk production of high-yielding dairy has approximately doubled.

Forty years ago, concerns about the environmental impacts of farm animal production had yet to gather much momentum and, although the 'Brambell' Report of the Technical Committee to Enquire into the Welfare of Animals kept under Intensive Livestock Husbandry Systems had been published in 1965, neither had animal welfare acquired the profile that it has now. However, attitudes to animal welfare and to protecting biodiversity were changing rapidly and both are now increasingly major factors in the shaping of farm animal management practices. As Pete Goddard says, in his chapter on sheep, regarding just the last 10 years: 'there has been a significant shift in the public view of how we treat farmed livestock and assess their welfare. With much more emphasis being placed on quality of life aspects there is a pressing need and responsibility to critically examine how diligent livestock management can deliver the greatest welfare benefit'.

In short, there are a multitude of ongoing changes to farming practices driven by economics, animal and veterinary science, and attitudes to food production and animal welfare, and changes also in the regulatory environment and in the animals and strains farmed. In view of this, the task of drawing together an up-to-date

---

* UFAW (1971) *The UFAW Handbook on the Care and Management of Farm Animals.* Churchill Livingstone, Edinburgh.

practical handbook for all those involved in, or aspiring to be involved in, livestock farming was clearly going to be a very demanding and challenging one.

It has been our great good fortune that John Webster – whose energy, very extensive knowledge and experience of farm animal husbandry and welfare, rare literary skills and organisational abilities, fatefully conspired to place him right at the centre of the danger zone when we were seeking an editor – was prepared to take this on. (And nice to note, incidentally, that he took over the Chair of Animal Husbandry at Bristol University Veterinary School from T. K. Ewer who was Chair of the Editorial Committee of the first edition.) It is our great good fortune also that he was able to assemble such a very excellent and eminent team of contributors.

The aim of this book, as with previous editions, is to put the case for good welfare in as rational a way as possible. UFAW does not necessarily support all the procedures described and hopes that welfare improvements will continue to be made as knowledge develops but, as UFAW's founder, Charles Hume, noted in his foreword to the first edition, 'It is acknowledged, however, that farming is a business and that, in the face of intensive competition, improved and more humane techniques can be brought about only if consumers will pay more for the food they buy'.

We are most grateful to John Webster and all the chapter authors: Fiona Benson, Cristian Bonacic, Bernadette Earley, Sandra Edwards, Pete Goddard, Keith Gooderham, Alison Hanlon, Susan Haslam, Stephen Lister, David Main, Jean Margerison, Alan Mowlem, Christine Nicol, Graham Scott, Tony Wall, David Welchman and Helen (Becky) Whay, for this book.

James K Kirkwood
UFAW

December 2010

Preface

The Universities Federation for Animal Welfare (UFAW), founded in 1926, is an internationally recognized animal welfare charity concerned with promoting high standards of welfare for farm, companion, laboratory and captive wild animals. One of the most important ways by which it works to improve animals' lives is through the promotion of education in animal care and welfare. This includes the publication of books, videos, articles, technical reports and the journal *Animal Welfare*.

Through successive editions, *Management and Welfare of Farm Animals* has become internationally recognized as a classic introductory textbook for university and college students of agriculture and veterinary science. Each edition has adhered firmly to the principles originally put forward by Charles Hume, UFAW's founder, in his forward to the first edition, namely: '*This book . . . seeks to put forward the case for the humane treatment of farm animals in as rational a way as possible. UFAW does not necessarily support all the procedures that are described. However, it is acknowledged that farming is a business and that in the face of intensive competition improved and more humane techniques can be brought about only if consumers will pay more for the food that they buy.*'

Recent years have seen many changes in what is deemed acceptable practice in regard to the husbandry and welfare of animals. The European Union has passed a series of laws to prohibit, now or in the near future, practices such as the confinement of laying hens and pregnant sows in, respectively, barren cages and individual stalls. Although, to date, there have been no such changes in USA federal law, an increasing number of individual states are passing state laws to ban these and other practices that arouse public concern. Thus the legal definitions of acceptable practice are in a state of continuous flux. Moreover there has been an upsurge of consumer demand for alternative methods and improved standards in the production of food from animals, which has, in the more than ten years since the publication of the fourth edition, had a far greater impact than that which has been achieved through legislation.

This, the fifth edition, maintains the primary aim of its predecessors, namely to provide a comprehensive introductory textbook for young people requiring professional, technical or vocational education in the management and welfare of farm animals. However, we have, in many ways, sought to broaden our remit. Although much of the book deals, as before, with the large-scale commercial rearing of animals for food (rightly so, since this affects the welfare of the overwhelming majority of farm animals) authors have been asked to give special attention to alternative farming systems. One example is the commercial farm that seeks to meet the market for added-value products from consumers seeking higher standards of animal welfare. Another is the small-scale, non-industrialized farm in which animals are likely to be cared for on an individual basis, whether these are traditional family farms in the developing world, or 'hobby farmers' in the Western world who wish to practise good husbandry and ensure welfare on a more intimate scale. In all circumstances: the industrial farm mass-producing a commodity, the specialist 'high welfare' farm producing added-value food for discerning consumers, or the family farm producing food whether as a rewarding hobby or as the only realistic alternative to starvation, the health and welfare needs of the animal are the same.

Most of the chapters in this edition deal, as before, with management and welfare on a species by species basis or group by group (e.g. camelids, game birds) basis. Three animal groups appear for the first time: game birds, South American camelids and ostrich, and a chapter on horses has been reinstated. There are also three conceptually new chapters that reflect new understanding of animal welfare science, ethics and the role of society in helping to ensure and improve standards of animal welfare. These cover general principles of good husbandry and its impact on animal welfare, animal behaviour as an indicator of welfare, and the assessment, implementation and promotion of high standards of animal welfare in practice, on the farm. Each chapter concludes with a brief list of suggestions for further reading. In the case of online references we give you the website and expect you to follow the links, in recognition of the fact that this approach is quicker and less subject to error than attempting to type long sequences of inconsequential letters and symbols.

Writing as editor, I must express my thanks to all the authors who have found time within their busy careers to write these comprehensive and authoritative chapters. Your reward will, I hope, be found in the knowledge that you have contributed to the production of something of real value to a lot of sentient and sapient creatures. These include, of course, students doing courses in agriculture, veterinary science, animal nursing, companion and equine studies, animals and the environment. I hope that these chapters will prove especially valuable as a basis for courses in English-speaking countries within the developing world, because of the breadth of information they convey within a single book. I also suggest that they may prove useful to those wishing to learn the elements of animal welfare and good husbandry on a more informal basis, perhaps as a prelude to keeping farm animals for themselves. Finally, and critically, our book is addressed to the animals themselves. There is an international groundswell of public concern for farm animal welfare and, in principle, this has to be a good thing. However, caring *about* animals is not enough. Caring *for* them is what matters. This requires compassion, understanding and a great deal of skill. These things cannot be gathered from any single source, but what we offer here is, I hope, a useful beginning.

John Webster

Acronyms and Abbreviations

ACNV	automatically controlled natural ventilation
ACOS	Advisory Committee on Organic Standards (UK)
ACP	Assured Chicken Production (UK)
ADF	acid-detergent fibre
AE	avian encephalomyelitis
AI	artificial insemination
AV	artificial vagina
BCS	body condition score
BKD	bacterial kidney disease (in fish)
BLUP	best linear unbiased prediction (of genetic merit)
BRD	bovine respiratory disease
BSE	bovine spongiform encephalopathy
BT	bluetongue
BVD-MD	bovine virus diarrhoea–mucosal disease
CAP	Common Agricultural Policy of the European Union
CIDR®	controlled internal drug release (device)
CLA	caseous lymphadenitis
CLA	conjugated linoleic acid
CNS	central nervous system
COD	cystic ovarian disease
CODD	contagious ovine digital dermatitis
CP	crude protein
CR	conception rate
CS	[body] condition score
CT	computed tomography
DA	displaced abomasum

DCAB	dietary cation: anion balance
DD	digital dermatitis
DEFRA	Department for Environment, Food and Rural Affairs (UK)
DIC	disseminated intravascular coagulation
DM	dry matter concentration in animal feeds
DMI	dry matter intake
DoA	dead on arrival
DUP	digestible undegradable protein
DVE	duck viral enteritis
DVH	duck viral hepatitis-1
EAE	enzootic abortion of ewes
EBV	estimated breeding value
EC	Commission of the European Union
EE	electro-ejaculation
EFSA	European Food Safety Authority
EID	electronic identification
EP	enzootic pneumonia
ERDP	effective rumen degradable protein
ET	embryo transfer
EU	European Union
EUROP	beef classification scheme in the European Union
FAO	Food and Agriculture Organisation of the United Nations
FAWC	Farm Animal Welfare Council (UK)
FCE	feed conversion efficiency (output/input)
FCR	feed conversion ration (input/output)
FME	fermentable metabolizable energy
FPD	foot pad dermatitis
FSH	follicle-stimulating hormone
GE	gross energy
GFA	Game Farmers' Association (UK)
HACCP	hazard analysis and critical control points
HDF	highly digestible fibre
HMSO	Her Majesty's Stationery Office
IBD	infectious bursal disease
IBR	infective bovine rhinotracheitis
ICC	improved contemporary comparisons (of traits in dairy cows)
IDD	interdigital dermatitis
idL	ileal digestible lysine

IPN	infectious pancreatic necrosis (in fish)
KKCF	kidney, knob and channel fat
LT	laryngotrachieitis
M/D	metabolizable energy concentration in feed DM (MJ/kg)
MAFF	Ministry of Agriculture, Fisheries and Food (UK)
MCF	malignant catarrhal fever
MCP	microbial crude protein
ME	metabolizable energy
MJ	megajoules
MOET	multiple ovulation and embryo transfer
MP	metabolizable protein
ND	Newcastle disease
NDF	neutral-detergent fibre
NE	net energy
NIPH	National Institute for Poultry Husbandry (UK)
NPN	non-protein nitrogen
NSA	National Sheep Association (UK)
NSAID	non-steroidal anti-inflammatory drug
OCDS	Older Cattle Disposal Scheme
OID	ovine interdigital dermatitis
OP	organophosphorus compounds
OTMS	Over Thirty-Month Scheme (cattle)
PCV	packed cell volume
PHS	pulmonary hypertension syndrome
PI-3	parainfluenza-3
PMSG	pregnant mares' serum gonadotrophin
PMWS	post-weaning multisystemic wasting syndrome (pigs)
PR	pregnancy rate
PRID	progesterone-releasing intravaginal device
PRRS	porcine respiratory and reproductive syndrome
PTA	potential transmitting ability (of genetic traits)
PUFA	polyunsaturated fatty acid
QA	quality assurance
QBT	Quality British Turkey
QTL	(gene) quantitative trait loci
REL	reliability

RH	relative humidity
RSCPA	Royal Society for the Prevention of Cruelty to Animals
RSV	respiratory syncytial virus
SAC	South American camelid
SARA	subacute rumen acidosis
SCC	somatic cell count
SCOPS	Sustainable Control of Parasites in Sheep (programme)
SEW	segregated early weaning
SFA	saturated fatty acid
SMT	special marketing term
SPF	specific pathogen free
TB	tuberculosis
TBC	total bacteria count (in milk)
TMR	total mixed rations
TSE	transmissible spongiform encephalopathy
UDN	undegraded dietary nitrogen/protein
UFAW	Universities Federation for Animal Welfare
UKROFS	United Kingdom Register of Organic Standards
USDA	United States Department of Agriculture
VFA	volatile fatty acids

Husbandry and Animal Welfare

JOHN WEBSTER

Management and Welfare of Farm Animals: The UFAW Farm Handbook, 5th edition. John Webster
© 2011 by Universities Federation for Animal Welfare (UFAW)

1.1 Introduction

The broad aim of this book, as in earlier editions, is to provide an introduction to the management and welfare of farm animals through the practice of good husbandry within the context of an efficient, sustainable agriculture. Successive chapters outline these principles and practices for the major farmed species within a range of production systems, both intensive and extensive. This chapter is an introduction to this introduction. It opens with concepts in animal welfare that may be applied to any sentient farm animal, then progresses to general principles that may be applied to their management. These general principles are illustrated by specific examples relating to animal species and production systems (e.g. broiler chickens, dairy cows). For those of you who are new to the study of animal management and animal welfare, some of these examples may only make sense when you have read the chapter on the species to which they refer. I also suggest that, when you have read, learned and inwardly digested a chapter on a particular species, you could refer back to this opening chapter and consider how well (or not) current management practices for that species meet the general criteria for good husbandry and welfare within the categories outlined here.

The purpose of farming is to use the resources of the land to provide the people with food and other goods. The successful farmers are those who have the best idea of what it is the people want and need. Successful livestock farmers are those who also have the best understanding of what it is their animals want and need. Successive chapters will consider the special needs of different farmed species and provide practical advice as to how to meet these needs within the context of viable production systems. The aim of this opening chapter is to introduce principles of husbandry and welfare as they apply to the feeding, breeding, management and care of animals throughout their lives on farms large and small, and in times of special need such as during transport and at the point of slaughter. Most of the meat, milk and eggs for sale to the public in the developed world comes from highly intensive systems in which very large numbers of animals are confined and 'managed' by very few people. However, most of the people who actually work with farm animals in most of the world do so within traditional communities where animals are more likely to be cared for on an individual basis. Within the developed world, there is a growing movement to reject industrialized farming methods and return to systems that appear to afford more care and respect to farm animals as individuals. This applies both to those who seek organic, high-welfare or trusted local produce in the shops and to those who wish to farm, whether full- or part-time, to such standards. Of course the fundamental welfare needs of an animal such as a chicken are the same, whether it is scavenging for food in an African village or confined in a controlled environment building containing 100,000 birds. The ethical challenge in either circumstance is how to reconcile the welfare needs of the animals, the needs of the farmers to obtain a fair return for their investment and labour, the needs of the people for safe, high-quality, affordable food and last (but not least) the need to preserve the quality of the living environment.

1.1.1 Traditional agriculture

Agriculture, past, present and future, can be defined by four eras, traditional, industrial, value-led and one-planet. Traditional agriculture, as practised for most of history, and still practised in much of the world today, was low output but sustainable, not least because most of the animals looked after themselves. Sheep and goats consumed fibrous food, unavailable to humans, commonly grazing land the farmer did not own. Chickens and pigs (where culturally acceptable) were fed or scavenged leftovers, and food that humans failed to harvest or elected not to eat. In many traditional communities chickens also fulfilled a valuable community service, consuming ticks and other pests of humans and animals. A dairy cow justified more attention from the farmer (or more likely his wife) who would cut, cart and conserve her feed since she (the cow) was a source of real income through sale of milk. The system seldom generated great riches but it was usually sustainable, partly because it imposed a minimal drain on capital reserves such as fossil fuels, but mainly because nothing was wasted. The use of food and other resources by humans and farm animals was complementary rather than competitive.

1.1.2 Industrial agriculture

It is easy for the well-educated, well-fed citizen of the developed world to paint a rosy picture of traditional agriculture. However, it provided little more than subsistence for most farmers, most of the time, and could not meet our modern expectations for a wide variety of good, safe, cheap food in all seasons. This has been achieved through an industrial revolution in farming that began only about 70 years ago, and only in the industrialized world. In undeveloped countries, it has hardly started. The key distinction between the traditional and the factory livestock or poultry farm is that most or all of the inputs to the latter system – power, machinery and other resources (e.g. food and fertilizers) – are bought in. Thus output is constrained only by the amount that the producer can afford to invest in capital and other resources and the capacity of the system to process them.

The key objectives of industrialized livestock production can be summed up in a single phrase: to control the environment. Feeding involves provision of a nutritionally balanced ration in optimal quantities and at least cost. Housing is designed partly to provide animals with comfort and security, but mainly to maximize income relative to the costs of building and labour. Control of health is achieved through attention to biosecurity and hygiene. These general principles will be developed below and applied to the various species of farm animals in successive chapters.

Figure 1.1 outlines the genealogy of the intensive livestock farm, as typified by modern intensively housed pig and poultry units (Webster, 2005). Some feed for pigs and poultry (e.g. cereals) may be grown within the farm enterprise, but this, along with purchased feed supplements to ensure a balanced diet, is trucked onto the unit and dispensed to animals in controlled environment houses by mechanical feeding systems. Mechanical and electrical power is used to control temperature and

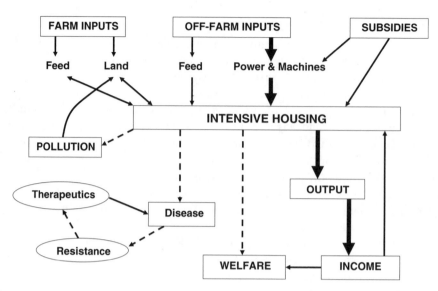

Figure 1.1 Factors influencing the development of industrialization in livestock farming. Potentially adverse effects are indicated with broken lines (from Webster, 2005).

ventilation, to dispense feed and to remove and disperse the manure. Factory farming was born when it became cheaper, faster and more efficient to process feed through animals using machines than to let the animals do the work for themselves. Once the high set-up costs had been met, the input of cheap energy and other resources from off-farm was able to increase output and reduce running costs. In consequence, poultry meat from chickens and turkeys, once the food of family feasts, is now the cheapest meat on the market.

Potential (although avoidable) harmful outputs from intensive livestock systems (hatched lines in Figure 1.1) include increased pollution, infectious disease and abuse of animal welfare. Bringing animals off the land and into close confinement inevitably increases the risks of infectious disease. To combat this increased risk it has been necessary to introduce strict new strategies to eliminate, or at least reduce, exposure to infection. The key to elimination in an intensive pig or poultry unit is biosecurity. This requires strict controls on the movement of animals and stock-keepers who shower and don protective clothing before entering the unit. This will normally ensure the health of the animals (one essential element of welfare) but there are obvious limits to the expression of natural behaviour in a large isolation hospital. The key element of hygiene is to minimize contact between animals and their excreta.

Where exposure to infection cannot be eliminated through exclusion or hygiene, it is necessary to develop routine disease control measures through the use of vaccines, antibiotics and antiparasitic drugs. If access to cheap power had been all that was necessary for the success of intensive livestock farming, then this industrial revolution would have happened in the 1920s. In fact the greatest rate of expansion only occurred in the 1950s when antibiotics effective against the major endemic bacterial diseases of housed livestock became cheap and freely available. Alternative, subtler approaches to disease control, such as the development of specific vaccines and strains of animals genetically resistant to specific diseases, have also contributed to the commercial success of intensive systems, especially in the case of poultry. However, it is fair to claim that industrialized farming of pigs and poultry has, for the last 50 years, been sustained by the routine use of antibiotics, coccidiostats and other chemotherapeutics to control endemic diseases. In some cases these diseases could be life threatening. In most cases, however, chemotherapeutics have been used routinely to increase productivity by reducing the effects of chronic, low-grade infection.

In Europe there is now a ban on the routine use of antibiotics and many other chemotherapeutic 'growth promoters', mainly on the basis of concern that the development of microbial resistance to antibiotics used as growth promoters will pose an increasing risk to human health. The scientific evidence in support of this legislation is inconsistent. However, on balance, and in time, it has to be a good thing, both for the animals and ourselves, to restrict the routine use of antibiotics in livestock agriculture. It is an unequivocal insult to the principle of good husbandry to keep animals in conditions of such intensity, inappropriate feeding or squalor that their health can only be ensured by the routine administration of chemotherapeutics.

Although the industrial farming of livestock and poultry does present opportunities, assessed in terms of animal health and welfare, it also presents inherent threats. It is obviously impossible to care for each chicken as an individual within a poultry house containing over 100,000 animals. Any individual that falls behind the average by virtue of ill health, impaired development or reluctance to compete at the feed trough has little chance of being nursed back to normality through sympathetic stockmanship.

1.1.3 Value-led agriculture

The main impact of industrial agriculture has been to provide an ample supply and wide, year-round choice of food that is reliable, safe and cheap, and looks and tastes good. This is what most of the people have wanted most of the time. However, in recent years and within societies that can afford such morals, consumers have begun to display an increasingly compassionate concern for other, less tangible, elements of food quality, especially animal welfare and the quality of the environment. Farmers and retailers involved in livestock production have responded to this demand by developing alternative husbandry systems that give increased attention to animal welfare and environmental sustainability through developments and improvements to husbandry. The development of such alternative systems will be a feature of this book. It is however, necessary to point out at the outset that the amount of care that farmers can give to the welfare of both their animals and the land is constrained by what they can afford. If society wishes to give added value to such things as animal welfare and the environment, then society must pay for it.

1.1.4 One-planet agriculture

The aim of good husbandry has always been twofold: to provide a good food and other goods for humans, while at the same time sustaining the quality of the land and the life of the land. In the future, the pressure on agriculture throughout the world, intensive and extensive, will increasingly be driven by the need to sustain the living environment. This may challenge our current, comfortable feelings of compassion for other sentient creatures, farm animals, wildlife and poor people. The challenge will be to sustain improvements in animal welfare within the context of animal production systems that are efficient in use of resources, do not pollute the soil and waterways, and restrict the production of greenhouse gases, especially from ruminants. This book outlines the basic principles that define our duty of care to farm animals and the practices that contribute to their management. However, these principles and practice can never be divorced from the primary need to ensure the economically competitive production of food and other goods, while sustaining the productivity and quality of the living environment. This being so, compromise is inevitable. An ethical approach to such compromise is presented in the closing section of this chapter.

1.2 Concepts in Animal Welfare

The expression 'animal welfare' has two distinct meanings. The first is a description of the physical and mental state of an animal as it seeks to meet its physiological and behavioural needs. It is a measure of welfare as perceived by the animal itself and something that we can study through careful observations of animal behaviour and the disciplines of welfare science. The second concept of animal welfare is as an expression of moral concern. It arises from the belief that animals can experience feelings that we would interpret as pain and suffering, thus we have duty to protect animals in our care from these things. A concern for animal welfare is obviously a virtue. It is good that we should care about animals. Caring *for* animals, however, involves more than virtue; it requires a sound understanding of the principles of husbandry and welfare and these things can only be acquired through education and practical experience. This book is aimed mainly at those who will have direct responsibility for the care of farm animals. However, the moral responsibility to provide a duty of care does not apply only to those directly involved with animals on the farm, in transport and at the place of slaughter. The responsibility must be shared by all who, directly or indirectly, derive any value from the exploitation of animals to suit their ends, whether for food, clothing, sport or companionship. These responsibilities may be outlined as follows:

1. to acknowledge and understand the concepts of welfare, sentience and suffering in farm animals;
2. to breed and manage farm animals so as to promote good welfare and avoid suffering throughout their working lives;

3. to increase public awareness of the welfare needs of farm animals, within a context that also recognizes the needs of farmers to produce good food and maintain a decent living through the practice of good husbandry: the competent and caring management of the land and the life of the land;

4. to work towards improved standards of farm animal welfare through the parallel development of improved husbandry systems and increased public demand for food and other goods produced to these higher standards.

1.2.1 Sentience, welfare and wellbeing

Animal welfare has been defined as 'the state of an animal as it attempts to cope with its environment' (Fraser and Broom, 1990). The definition may be applied to any animal from an ant to an ape. Farm animals, however, have been classified, at least within the European Union, as 'sentient creatures', a definition that acknowledges that their welfare is defined by their success in meeting both their physiological and behavioural needs. For farm animals therefore the definition of welfare becomes 'the state of body and mind of a sentient animal as it attempts to cope with its environment'. This definition covers the full spectrum of welfare from healthy to sick, pain to pleasure. The aim of the sentient animal is to achieve a state of good welfare, or *wellbeing*, defined simply as *'fit and happy'* or *'fit and feeling good'* (Webster, 2005). This, too, is a state of body and mind. For the body it implies sustained health; for the mind it implies, at least, an absence of suffering from such things as pain, fear and exhaustion. Ideally it should embrace a sense of positive wellbeing (*feeling good*) achieved by such things as comfort, companionship and security.

Animal sentience involves feelings. It also implies that these feelings matter. Marian Dawkins (1990) has pioneered the study of motivation in animals by seeking to measure how hard animals will work to achieve (or avoid) a resource or stimulus that makes them feel good (or bad) (see Chapter 2). So far as animals are concerned, sentience may therefore best be defined as *'feelings that matter'* (Webster, 2005). This definition recognizes that the behaviour of animals is motivated by the emotional need to seek satisfaction and avoid suffering. Many of these emotions are associated with primitive sensations such as hunger, pain and anxiety. Some species may also experience 'higher feelings' such as friendship and grief at the loss of a relative, and this may expand the nature of their sentience. However, we should not assume that the distress caused to animals by the emotions of hunger, pain and anxiety is any less intense because they are primitive.

Figure 1.2 illustrates how sentient animals perceive their environment and how this motivates their behaviour (Webster, 2005). The 'control centres' in the central nervous system (CNS) constantly receive information from the external and internal environment. Much information, e.g. the perception of how an animal stands and moves in space, is processed at a subconscious level. However, any stimulus that calls for a conscious decision as to action must involve some degree of interpretation. Motivation scientists observing the response of sentient animals may define

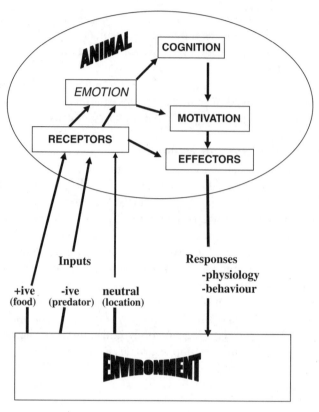

Figure 1.2 Animal sentience; pathways involved in the conscious perception of sensations and information, motivation and behavioural response.

a stimulus as positive, aversive or neutral. In simpler words, the animal, when presented with the stimulus, will experience feelings that are good, bad or indifferent. This is an emotional (i.e. sentient) response to the stimulus. The sentient animal (within which category we must include *Homo sapiens*) may or may not also interpret the incoming information in a cognitive fashion, i.e. apply reason. However they, and we, are usually and most powerfully motivated by how we feel.

This psychological concept of mind makes a clear distinction between the reception, categorization and interpretation of incoming stimuli. Although it may appear abstract it is soundly based in neurobiology. Kendrick (1998) has made recordings from nerve centres involved in these processes. When a sheep is presented with grain or hay (or photographic images of these things) this triggers signals in a family of neurones that convey the generic information 'food'. A second set of stimuli or images, e.g. dogs and men, form another generic category of information that we may call 'predator'. The information 'food' then proceeds to a second processing centre where it stimulates a family of neurones that transmit a positive emotion (good). The information 'predator' passes to another centre that transmits the negative emotion (bad). However, if the sheep is now presented with a picture of a human carrying a sack of food, two categories of information (food and predator) are passed to the emotion centre, evaluated together and in this case passed on as a single, unconfused emotional message, namely 'good'.

The sentient animal is then motivated to respond according to how it feels (good, bad or indifferent) about the information it has received. Moreover, the interpretation is not a simple yes/no decision. The intensity of its feelings will vary. It will, for example, feel more or less hungry, more or less afraid, and this will determine the strength of its motivation to respond in positive or negative fashion. By studying the strength of motivation of an animal to seek or avoid the feelings it associates with certain sensations and experiences, we can measure not only what an animal sense as good and bad but also how much these feelings matter.

Having behaved in a way designed to achieve a satisfactory emotional state, the sentient animal will then review the consequences of its action. If it has been effective, it will feel better and it will gain the assurance that it knows what to do next time. If its action fails, either because the stress was too great, or because it was constrained in such a way that it was unable to do what it felt necessary in order to cope, then it is likely to feel worse and be more anxious for the future. Thus a sentient animal does not live only in the present: its mood and understanding are modified in the light of experience.

1.2.2 Stress and suffering

The fact that the emotional response of an animal to stimuli is governed by its past experience carries obvious survival advantages in a challenging environment, and forms an essential contribution to the survival of the fittest. The interpretation of past experience is equally important to a domestic animal since it is a key indicator of the animal's success, or otherwise, in coping with stress. To illustrate this point, consider the difference between fear and anxiety (Figure 1.3). Fear is an emotional response to a perceived threat that acts as a powerful motivator to action designed, where possible, to evade that threat. It is also an educational experience since the memory of previous threats, the action taken in response to those threats and the consequences thereof ('was it less bad than I feared or worse?') will obviously affect how the animal feels next time around. Thus fear, like pain, is an essential part of sentience. These emotions have evolved as key elements for survival. An animal that has no sense of pain or fear, for itself or its offspring, is at a profound disadvantage in the struggle for existence. So too is an animal that cannot remember what gave rise to pain or fear in the past and how well or badly it coped.

Stress and suffering are not the same. Animals are equipped to respond and adapt to challenges in circumstances that permit them to make an effective response. If so, then they learn that they can cope. An animal is likely to suffer when it fails to cope (or has extreme difficulty in coping) with stress:

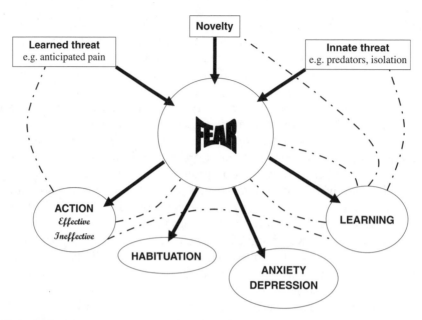

Figure 1.3   Causes and consequences of fear (from Webster, 2005; for further explanation see text).

- because the stress itself is too severe, too complex or too prolonged (e.g. a dairy cow worn out by the sustained complex stresses of metabolic overload and chronic pain from lameness); or
- because the animal is prevented from taking the constructive action it feels necessary to relieve the stress (e.g. a sow in the extreme confinement of an individual pregnancy stall).

1.3 Principles of Husbandry and Welfare

1.3.1 The five freedoms and provisions

The essence of good farm animal husbandry is to provide the resources and management necessary to ensure the economic production of food and other goods in a way that does not compromise the health and welfare of the animals (and the environment). Since wellbeing has been defined as 'fit and happy', provision must be made to promote both the physical and psychological elements of good welfare. These aims have been expressed according to the principles of the 'five freedoms and provisions' (Farm Animal Welfare Council, 1993) as set out in Table 1.1. The 'five freedoms' identify the elements that define an ideal state of wellbeing as perceived by the animals. The 'five provisions' define the husbandry and resources required to

Table 1.1 The five freedoms and provisions. Source: Farm Animal Welfare Council (1993).

1 *Freedom from thirst, hunger and malnutrition* – by ready access to fresh water and a diet to maintain full health and vigour
2 *Freedom from discomfort* – by providing a suitable environment including shelter and a comfortable resting area
3 *Freedom from pain, injury and disease* – by prevention or rapid diagnosis and treatment
4 *Freedom from fear and distress* – by ensuring conditions which avoid mental suffering
5 *Freedom to express normal behaviour* – by providing sufficient space, proper facilities and company of the animal's own kind

promote, though possibly never achieve, this ideal state. This requires proper attention to physiological needs through good nutrition, good housing, and attention to health and hygiene. It also requires attention to the psychological needs of sentient animals to avoid fear and stress and achieve satisfaction through the freedom to express normal, socially acceptable behaviour. The five freedoms should not be interpreted as a counsel of perfection but as a set of standards for compliance with acceptable principles of good welfare and a practical, comprehensive checklist from which to assess the strengths and weaknesses of any husbandry system, whether within the context of international standards for production systems or at the level of the individual farm.

Application of the five freedoms to the evaluation of standards for production systems is illustrated by Table 1.2, which considers alternative husbandry systems for laying hens: the conventional barren battery cage that constitutes the environment for most hens worldwide, the 'enriched' cage, that will become the minimum standard for Europe in 2012, and the 'free range' system. These systems are reviewed in detail in Chapter 7. Here they are briefly compared using the evaluation structure provided by the five freedoms. Thus:

Table 1.2 An outline comparison of the welfare of laying hens in the conventional battery cage, in the enriched cage and on free range. Source: Webster (2005).

Factor	Conventional cage	Enriched cage	Free range
Hunger and thirst	Adequate	Adequate	Adequate
Comfort, thermal	Good	Good	Variable
Comfort, physical	Bad	Adequate	Adequate
Fitness, disease	Low risk	Low risk	Increased risk
pain	High risk (feet and legs)	Moderate risk	Variable risk (feather pecking)
Stress	Frustration	Less frustration	Aggression
Fear	Low risk	Low risk	Aggression, agoraphobia
Natural behaviour	Highly restricted	Restricted	Unrestricted

- Adequate freedom from hunger and thirst can be achieved in all systems.
- Thermal comfort can be maintained in all cage systems. On free range it will be variable. However, since hens can choose whether to be indoors or out, then thermal comfort is likely to be satisfactory most of the time.
- Physical comfort is unacceptably bad in the conventional barren battery cage when the floor space allowance for hens is only $450\,cm^2$. To give two examples only: the birds damage their feet on the wire floors and they are unable by virtue of restricted space and the barren environment to perform natural comfort behaviours such as wing flapping, grooming and dust bathing. In the enriched cage, which provides a perch, a scratching surface and more space, some of these comfort behaviours become possible. Outdoors, on free range, the bird has both the freedom and the resources necessary to perform comfort behaviour.
- Control of bacterial and parasitic infections is easier in cages, mainly because the birds are kept out of contact with their own excreta, and that of passing wild birds. This assumes great importance when there is a risk of their contracting a disease such as bird flu, especially strains that may also infect humans.
- Osteoporosis leading to chronic pain from bone fractures is likely to be a problem with all laying birds in the extreme confinement of the barren cage stocked at $450\,cm^2$ per bird. This is because one of the major predisposing factors to osteoporosis is extreme, enforced inactivity. The enriched cage permits more movement and some increase in bone strength. Active birds on free range have denser bones but are at greater risk of damage, e.g. to the sternum or keel bone as they fly to roost.
- There is good evidence that laying hens experience extreme frustration in the barren cage, most especially the frustration associated with their inability to select a suitable nesting site prior to laying their daily egg. The enriched cage and the free-range unit are both equipped with nest boxes.
- A laying hen may be less likely to experience fear when confined in a group of three or four birds within a caged system, than when in a group of 10,000 birds on a free-range unit. Fear in free-range birds may result from experience of aggression, or it may simply involve agarophobia, i.e. fear of open spaces. Note, however, that while fear may be a stress, it may lead to adaptation rather than suffering if the birds learn to cope. On free range, birds have greater freedom of action and opportunities for education. They can take action (e.g.) to avoid the consequences of aggression. They can also habituate to the experience of being outdoors, i.e. learn that it is not a cause for alarm but a source of satisfaction.
- According to the fifth of the freedoms, the freedom to express normal behaviour, the free-range unit wins by a distance.

Application of the five freedoms and provisions to the evaluation of animal welfare on an individual farm is illustrated in Table 1.3. In this example, the five provisions create a structure for the identification of risks and hazards, and thus the application of a programme for the monitoring and control of animal welfare at farm level

Table 1.3 Application of the 'five provisions' to the identification of risks and hazards to farm animal welfare.

Provision	Hazard	Risk	Examples
1. Nutrition	Under-feeding	Hunger	Out-wintered sheep
	Unbalanced diets	Metabolic disease	High-yielding dairy cows
2. Housing	Concrete floors	Discomfort	Lameness in cows and pigs
	Cages	Injury and pain	Bone fractures in hens
3. Health care	Poor hygiene	Infectious disease	Mastitis in cows
	No vaccination policy		Respiratory diseases in poultry
	Lack of foot care	Pain	Lameness in cattle, sheep
4. Security	Barren environment	Injury	Tail-biting in pigs
	Poor stockmanship	Anxiety	Rough handling
5. Choice	Extreme confinement	Frustration	Sow stalls
	Barren environment	Learned helplessness	Barren cages for hens

according to internationally recognized HACCP (hazard analysis and critical control point) principles. This approach is considered in more detail in Chapter 18. Hazards characterized as inadequate provision of nutrition include underfeeding, e.g. in out-wintered sheep, creating a risk of hunger, possibly amounting to starvation. The category also includes the feeding of nutritionally imbalanced diets creating a risk of metabolic disease, e.g. in high-yielding dairy cows. The other hazards and risks within the categories of housing, health care, security and choice should now be self-explanatory. As one further example, I would cite freedom from fear and stress, here expressed by the single word, security. Hazards include barren environments for growing pigs that can increase the risk of tail-biting and aggression, and poor stockmanship, especially rough handling, that can provoke increased anxiety in farm animals when in the presence of humans.

These examples are presented here in brief to illustrate the central logic of the five freedoms. The welfare of animals in any system must be assessed according to all the paradigms. It is not sufficient to claim that the free-range system is superior simply because the birds are free to express normal behaviour. If mortality, preceded by a period of malaise (i.e. feeling unwell) on a free-range unit is shown to be significantly greater than in a caged system, then this must be taken into account, not just on economic grounds, but also because it is an important measure of poor welfare. Different individuals and different societies rank the importance of the five freedoms differently when passing judgement in matters of animal welfare. For example, the long-term housing of pregnant sows in individual stalls is prohibited within the European Union but currently permitted in the USA by federal law.[1] The fact that legislators within the two communities reviewed the same scientific

---

[1] Individual states within the USA (e.g. California, Maine, Michigan) have passed state laws to ban pregnancy stalls for sows and barren cages for laying hens.

evidence but came to opposing conclusions reflects the fact that, while such decisions may claim to be based on science, they are in fact value judgements reflecting belief in the current will of society. However, whatever may be the overall judgement on animal welfare on an individual farm or within a production system; it must include reference to all the freedoms. The best judgement is likely to be that which assesses the importance of the different freedoms in a way that most closely approximates to the animal's own measure of these things. This requires a profound understanding of the nature of animal motivation and animal behaviour (Chapter 2).

1.3.2 Good feeding

So far as the animals are concerned, the first provision of good husbandry is to ensure freedom from hunger and thirst. Freedom from thirst is achieved by provision of water fit for drinking from natural sources, containers (e.g. water troughs) or dispensers (e.g. nipple drinkers) that allow each individual to satisfy its needs. Provision of food for farm animals is a much more complex affair. In most livestock production systems animal feed is the major cost to the farmer. Thus the first essential for economic production is to maximize the efficiency of conversion of animal feed into saleable animal produce (meat, milk or eggs). The terms 'food conversion efficiency' (FCE) and 'food conversion ratio' (FCR) are used both by farmers and throughout this book. FCE is the proper description of efficiency (i.e. output : input). However, FCR (input : output) is in more common use. A broiler production unit may report an FCR of 1.56. In this case it is the ratio of total of feed consumption by a flock of birds relative to the weight of birds sold for slaughter.

Figure 1.4 outlines the steps involved in the conversion of animal feed to animal product as seen by both the animal and the farmer. Consider the case of intensive pig and poultry systems where machines are used to mix and dispense a 'compound' ration usually based on a cereal such as barley combined with a protein source (e.g. soya bean meal) and other supplements to provide a balanced supply of nutrients. This feed mixture (illustrated for simplicity in Figure 1.4. by ingredients A, B and C) is broken down in the digestive tract to supply nutrients available for metabolism: energy, protein (as amino acids), minerals and vitamins to meet the animals' requirements for maintenance and production of saleable produce such as meat, milk or eggs. Feed required to sustain maintenance of body tissues generates no output (i.e. FCE at maintenance is zero). As output increases relative to maintenance FCE increases, although as nutrient supply approaches the genetic capacity of the animal to produce milk, meat or eggs, increasing amounts of energy will be stored as fat in adipose tissue. These fat reserves can, of course, be called on in times when nutrient demand exceeds supply. This can occur when supply of digestible nutrients is restricted, as is the case for grazing animals during the winter in higher latitudes or during the dry season in the tropics. It can also occur when the productive capacity of the animal exceeds its capacity to consume and digest feed, as is the case for many high-yielding dairy cows in early lactation.

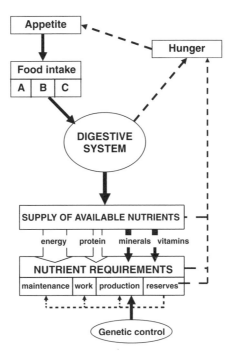

Figure 1.4 Factors affecting the supply and demand for digestible nutrients in animals.

An animal's motivation to eat is driven by hunger and appetite. These two things are not quite the same. The conscious appetite of an animal may be stimulated by the sight or smell of good food, or the foreknowledge that feeding time is approaching. If it has not eaten for some time its appetite will be increased by a sense of hunger. If it has recently eaten a large meal, it will be satiated and its appetite will be less. The internal sensations of hunger and satiety are determined partly by sensations from the digestive tract (e.g. a full stomach) and partly by a sense of 'metabolic hunger' stimulated (e.g.) by a low blood concentration of an essential substrate such as glucose. An animal that is unable to meet its dietary requirements for maintenance and production will experience metabolic hunger. As indicated above, this can occur in a sheep kept outside over winter where the quantity and quality of the food are insufficient to meet maintenance needs. It can also occur in a high-yielding dairy cow when her nutrient requirements for lactation exceed her capacity for digestion. In these circumstances she can be both 'hungry and full-up'. She experiences the simultaneous discomfort of metabolic hunger and digestive overload.

A 'good feed' for farm animals should meet four criteria:

• It should provide a balanced supply of nutrients for the needs of maintenance and production (work, growth, pregnancy and lactation).
• It should promote efficient, healthy digestion.

- It should provide oral satisfaction.
- It should do no harm.

The provision of a ration containing a balanced supply of nutrients has been introduced already. It is equally important that the feed should be provided in a form that matches the digestive function and digestive capacity of the animal. This is particularly important when feeds are prepared for natural grazers such as ruminants. The rumen of cattle and sheep has evolved to permit the anaerobic microbial digestion of cellulose and other fibres within a large well-stirred fermentation vat. Most compound rations for ruminants at high levels of production (e.g. the dairy cow) supply energy from a mixture of fibrous grasses, fresh or conserved as silage or hay, and starchy cereals. If the ratio of starch to digestible fibre is too high, fermentation may proceed too rapidly, leading to indigestion and acidosis within the rumen, with complications such as painful inflammatory laminitis within the feet. If the ratio of highly digestible starch to less digestible fibre is too low, the dairy cow will be unable to consume and digest enough feed to meet her nutrient requirements for lactation. She will then draw excessively on her body reserves, leading to loss of body condition, infertility and increased predisposition to injury and disease.

The feed should provide oral satisfaction. This is particularly important in housed adult animals such as horses and pregnant sows fed rations well below the limits of their appetite and given little to occupy their time. It is natural for a grazing animal such as the horse to nibble at food for 8–10 hours a day. It is natural for a pig to root in the ground for nuts, worms and other attractive food sources. Offered only a highly digestible, high-energy diet, a horse or pig may be able to consume enough nutrients to meet its needs within 10 minutes. It is then likely to become hungry and frustrated for the rest of the day. This frustration can lead to profoundly disturbed, stereotypic behaviour (Chapter 2) such as bar-chewing in sows, crib-biting and wind-sucking in horses. The oral satisfaction provided by a diet that includes hay or chaff for a horse, or by an environment that allows a sow to root in the earth, can prevent these behavioural disturbances and the frustration that they reveal.

The fourth essential of a good diet is that it should do no harm. It should not contain poisonous weeds or other toxic substances such as heavy minerals. Furthermore, it should be free from infectious agents, such as pathogenic bacteria or fungal toxins acquired during improper storage. Any feed of animal origin must be demonstrably free from prions responsible for the transmission of spongiform encephalopathies (TSEs), most notably responsible for 'mad cow disease'.

1.3.3 Housing and habitat

Farm animals are housed mainly for the convenience of the farmer. Pigs and poultry are confined in houses to save land and reduce the cost and labour involved in feeding and handling. Cattle are brought off pasture in the winter more to protect the pasture than to protect the animals. It is however good husbandry, and usually good economics, to design housing and other facilities so as to meet the environmental

Table 1.4 Major environmental requirements of farm animals (adapted from Webster, 1995).

Comfort, thermal	Neither too hot nor too cold
Comfort, physical	A suitable resting area
	Space for grooming, limb-stretching, exercise
Security	Of food and water supply
	From death or injury due to predation, aggression, floods etc.
	From fear of predation or aggression
Hygiene	To reduce the risk of disease
	To avoid the discomfort of squalor
Choice	To permit coping behaviours
	To allow animals to acquire security through experience and adaptation to the normal sights and sounds of farm activity

requirements of the confined animal. The four most important environmental requirements of farm animals are comfort, security, hygiene and freedom to perform behaviours intended to achieve these things. In Table 1.4, freedom of behaviour is described by the single word, 'choice'. Freedom from thermal discomfort is achieved by providing an environment that is neither too hot nor too cold, where hot and cold cannot be defined simply by air temperature but must take into account all factors that determine heat transfer between an animal and the environment; especially air movement, precipitation and solar radiation. Provision of an optimal thermal environment is dealt with on a species-by-species basis in subsequent chapters. As a general rule, most intensively farmed pigs and poultry are kept in controlled environment buildings, mainly to minimize feed energy requirement for maintenance and so maximize FCE. For most grazing animals, shelter from excessive sun, wind and rain is usually sufficient to ensure both adequate welfare and efficient production. For a fuller description of factors affecting the heat exchanges of farm animals, see Wathes and Charles (1994).

The most important requirement in terms of physical comfort, security and hygiene is a good resting area. The relative importance of the different criteria necessary to define a suitable resting area is summarized in Table 1.5. Poultry, for example, do not require a soft bed or a yielding mattress. They prefer to rest on perches. Chickens are motivated to perch at night by an innate fear of predators operating at ground level. This has been essential to their survival in the wild. Although there be may no real risk of predation in a controlled environment poultry house, the innate fear persists, so their selection of resting area is driven primarily by the need to experience a sense of security. The need to achieve a real (rather than imagined) degree of security is important for laying hens, who can and will injure one another, but not for young broilers, who do not.

The requirements of the large, bony, heavy dairy cow may be placed at the opposite end of the spectrum from those of the laying hen. Her greatest need is for a bed that is soft and yielding when she lies down, but does not impede her movement

Table 1.5 The relative importance of the different criteria necessary to define a suitable resting area for farm animals (adapted from Webster, 1995). Importance is ranked from 0 (unimportant) to *** (highly important).

	Hygiene	Dryness	Softness	Warmth	Security
Poultry, broilers	*	***	0	*	0
Poultry, layers	*	**	0	0	**
Pigs, weaners	**	**	*	**	*
Pigs, dry sows	*	**	**	**	***
Cattle, young calves	**	***	**	**	0
Cattle, dairy cows	**	**	***	0	**
Sheep, adult ewes	*	**	*	0	*
Horses, adult	**	**	**	0	*
Neonates, general	***	***	*/0	***	***

when in the act of standing up and lying down. Bare concrete fails on both counts. Rubber mats are barely adequate. Deep straw is comfortable but may fail on grounds of hygiene and increase the risk of mastitis. Deep, dry sand is close to ideal both in terms of comfort and hygiene (see Chapter 3). Most of the other rankings in Table 1.5 should now be self-explanatory and all will be considered in more depth in subsequent chapters. However, note all the reasons why it is important to provide a suitable resting area for neonates, especially when they have been removed from their mothers. Hygiene and warmth are particularly important, the former to reduce the risk of exposure to infection, the latter to reduce the risk of thermal stress leading to a loss of resistance to infection.

The last, but not the least, environmental requirement listed in Table 1.4 is defined as 'choice'. Sentient animals make decisions that enable them to cope with environmental challenges and improve the way they feel. As explained earlier, an animal such as a sow in the extreme confinement of an individual pregnancy stall may suffer because it is prevented from taking any constructive action it feels necessary to relieve its frustration. This is an extreme example (and in Europe, illegal). However, as a general rule, farm buildings and confinement areas should be designed and managed so as to allow the animals to acquire a sense of security through experience and adaptation to the normal sights and sounds of farm activity. This requirement is clearly stated in the UK *Codes of Welfare for Farm Animals* (http://www.defra.gov.uk/foodfarm/farmanimal/welfare/onfarm/index.htm#we) (DEFRA, 2003).

1.3.4 Fitness and health

The third of the five freedoms (Table 1.1) is 'freedom from pain, injury and disease, by prevention or rapid diagnosis and treatment'. The aim of good husbandry should go beyond this: it should be to breed, feed and manage farm animals so that they can sustain productivity and maintain physical fitness throughout a profitable working life. Since most animals reared for meat are killed at a very young age, this concern relates mostly to adults, breeding sows, laying hens and lactating cows. Here physical fitness implies more than just freedom from pain, injury and disease; it includes the maintenance of fertility and body condition. To give an extreme example, too many emaciated dairy cows are culled for infertility after a working life of less than three lactations. This is not only a measure of poor welfare for the cows, it also represents a loss to the farmer from animals that might have been highly productive at the start of their first lactation but failed to achieve an economically satisfactory lifetime performance.

Farm animals are susceptible to a wide range of diseases for which the primary cause is infection with pathogenic viruses or bacteria, or infestation with parasites. Farm animals may also act as carriers of infections that cause them little or no harm but can cause serious diseases in humans. The most important of these are bacterial infections with certain strains of *Campylobacter*, *Escherichia coli*, *Salmonella* and *Listeria* species. Thus control of infection and disease on farms is essential not only for the health and welfare of the animals but also for the protection of the general public. The strategies adopted for the prevention and control of farm animal diseases are outlined in Table 1.6. The surest way to protect farm animals from a specific pathogen is to adopt a strategy of total exclusion: i.e. ensure that the animals never come into contact with the infectious agent. This strategy can operate at national level, e.g. the UK policy to exclude and eliminate foot and mouth disease. It can also operate at farm level. Many pig farms are designated as carrying Minimal Disease, or Specific Pathogen Free (SPF) herds. In this case, the animals are protected from infection by a rigid programme of biosecurity. Animals live in controlled environment buildings protected from contact with possible disease carriers such as wild animals and birds. Stock-keepers have to wear protective clothing and shower in and out. Any new animals brought onto the site (e.g. breeding sows) must come from a farm operating to the same standards of SPF control. The exclusion approach is

Table 1.6 Strategies for the prevention and control of infectious diseases in farm animals.

Strategy	Examples
Exclusion	National exclusion and eradication: e.g. foot and mouth disease
	Biosecurity at farm level: e.g. swine pneumonia
Vaccination	Poultry: Newcastle disease, coccidiosis
	Sheep: clostridial diseases
Hygiene	Dairy cattle: contagious and environmental mastitis
	Sheep, horses: parasite control through pasture management
Drug therapy	Pigs: antibiotic control of post-weaning diarrhoea
	Sheep, horses: parasite control through routine worming
Natural immunity	Calves: controlled exposure to endemic infections
	Pigs: reducing weaning stresses

highly effective so long as it works. However, if there is a breach of biosecurity and disease enters the country, or the farm, the next step is draconian: slaughter all animals infected or exposed to infection, disinfect, leave the buildings unoccupied until safe to re-enter, then start again.

For many infectious diseases of farm animals, the most effective means of prevention is to promote a lasting immunity through vaccination. Poultry in controlled environment buildings are vaccinated *en masse* against Newcastle disease (fowl pest), an infection that would otherwise cause catastrophic losses in an environment where so many birds are confined in a small space. Vaccination is the only effective method for control of clostridial diseases (see Chapter 5) in sheep at pasture because the bacteria that cause these diseases can survive for many years in the soil. Unfortunately many diseases of farm animals are not controlled by vaccination, because the vaccine does not exist, is limited in its effect or is too expensive.

Prevention of infectious disease through exclusion or vaccination is highly effective but only for those diseases for which such a strategy is possible. Since these methods are effective, these diseases are usually under control. It follows that most of the infectious disease problems on modern commercial farms are those associated with endemic organisms that cannot be eliminated from the environment and where absolute immunological protection is unfeasible. Examples include parasitic infections in grazing cattle and sheep, mastitis in dairy cows, and many respiratory diseases. With this category of diseases, it is not possible to exclude the possibility of infection. Indeed, infection is the natural state: the aim of the farmer must be to create an environment wherein the balance between the challenge from the pathogens and the immune and other defence mechanisms of the animal is shifted in favour of the animal.

The three strategies for control of endemic diseases where vaccination is not an option are hygiene, use of chemotherapeutics (antibiotics and antiparasitic drugs) and promotion of natural immunity. In each case the aim is not to eliminate infection but to reduce the risk that infection will proceed to disease. Hygiene is designed to reduce the magnitude of the challenge. Examples presented in Table 1.6 include the control of mastitis in dairy cattle through good hygiene in the milking parlour, and the control of parasitic worm infestation through pasture management. These practices are admirable but not infallible. It is customary, and usually good husbandry, to reinforce the practice of good hygiene with the controlled use of chemotherapeutics (antibiotic or antiparasitic drugs) to keep the pathogen burden under control. However this approach can be abused. To take but one example: it has been common practice to dose growing pigs routinely and regularly with antibiotics. This was done initially to prevent catastrophic losses from diarrhoea and pneumonia. However, it was discovered that animals that were apparently healthy (to a casual eye) grew more efficiently (FCE was improved) when dosed regularly with antibiotics, which then acquired the name of 'growth promoters'. The reasons for this are complex but one of the reasons was a reduction in low-grade infection. This practice gave rise to public concern, mainly relating to the public health risks of increasing antibiotic resistance in bacteria pathogenic to humans. The use of antibiotics as growth promoters for farm animals is now banned in Europe. However, it is still possible for veterinarians to prescribe antibiotics for all the animals in a piggery when only a few appear to be sick. Thus the practice has not gone away. The use of chemotherapeutics for the prevention of disease in populations, rather than the treatment of individuals, is something that has to be considered on a case-by-case basis and in accordance with fundamental principles of good husbandry. It is, for example, good practice to incorporate regular worming of horses and sheep (especially the young animals) as part of an overall strategy for parasite control. It is good practice to control mastitis in dairy cows through dry cow therapy (Chapter 3). It is *not* good practice to rely on antibiotics as a strategy for keeping calves, pigs or poultry alive in conditions of squalor.

Last but not least among the strategies for prevention and control of infectious disease is to design systems that enhance natural immunity and so reduce the risk that exposure to infection will proceed to losses and ill thrift due to clinical disease. Natural immunity can cope with many infections when the challenge is not too severe and the immune mechanisms are not impaired by stress. Weaning is a particularly stressful time for young animals and can precipitate outbreaks of diarrhoea in pigs or pneumonia in calves. The aim should be to minimize weaning stresses and ensure that these do not coincide with increased exposure to infection (e.g. not moving weaned calves directly into a building containing older animals who are likely to be carriers of respiratory viruses).

Some of the most important diseases and disorders of farm animals are described as 'production diseases'. This description acknowledges that the prevalence and severity of these diseases are profoundly influenced by the standards of feeding, housing and hygiene imposed by the husbandry system. Table 1.7 lists some of the more common production diseases. These include infertility, mastitis and lameness in dairy cows, diarrhoea and wasting in weaner pigs, osteoporosis and bone fractures in laying hens, and lameness and hock burn in broiler chickens. Diarrhoea in weaner pigs, and mastitis and digital dermatitis in dairy cattle involve infectious agents but their cause and control are largely down to management. Other conditions such as lameness in broiler chickens and osteoporosis in laying hens can be attributed entirely to the way the animals are bred, fed and housed.

Table 1.7 Some common production diseases of farm animals.

Animal	Disease
Dairy cattle	Infertility, mastitis, claw lameness, digital dermatitis
Beef cattle, finishers	Rumen acidosis, liver abscess, laminitis
Pigs, weaners	Diarrhoea and wasting
Laying hens	Osteoporosis, bone fractures
Broiler chickens	Lameness, hock burn

Infectious diseases and injuries that cause pain and lameness compromise both the success of the farm enterprise and the welfare of the affected animals. The aim is to control these things, ideally by prevention, but when they occur, by early diagnosis and treatment. The first aim of treatment is to attack the causative agent, e.g. by administration of an appropriate antibiotic in the event of bacterial infection. It is also necessary to address the welfare of the sick or injured animal through symptomatic treatment and nursing. To give two examples: the welfare of a lame cow will be improved if she is not required to stand on concrete but can be moved to a box with a comfortable straw bed. The welfare of a calf or foal suffering the chills of a pneumonic fever will be improved if it is allowed to lie under a heat lamp.

1.3.5 Freedom from fear and distress: the art of stockmanship

The aim of good husbandry is to promote freedom from fear and distress by ensuring conditions which avoid mental suffering (Table 1.1). In all but the most extensive farming systems (e.g. hill sheep) the animals come into regular contact with humans. The essence of good stockmanship is therefore to do all that is possible to avoid causing fear and distress and to strive to instil in the animals a sense of security. The principles of good stockmanship as applied to the different farm species are excellently set out in the DEFRA *Codes of Recommendations for the Welfare of Livestock* (http://www.defra.gov.uk/foodfarm/farmanimal/welfare/onfarm/index. htm#we). Daily routines should be carried out calmly and consistently with the aim of accustoming the animals to the normal sights and sounds of farm activity. Farm animals, in common with most sentient creatures, are neophobic; they have an innate fear of novelty (Figure 1.3). Once the sights and sounds become routine, they habituate and acquire a sense of security.

There are, however, some occasions when the imposition of fear and distress is inevitable. These include procedures such as castration, de-horning, foot trimming, sheep dipping, transport and the routine administration of medicines. The use of anaesthetics is required by law for many painful procedures such as castration. Even procedures unlikely to cause pain (e.g. foot trimming, loading on to a lorry) can cause distress because they are novel, and because the animals are severely restrained, or forced in a direction they don't want to go. These procedures are likely to cause the most distress to extensively reared animals like sheep coming off the hill for the first time. The best way to minimize distress in animals that need to be moved or handled is through the design of facilities that permit the animals to move naturally with minimal disturbance and in the company of their own kind. The best exposition of the principles and practice of good livestock handling and management is that of Temple Grandin (1993).

1.4 Breeding for Fitness

Evolution through natural selection involves the survival of the fittest. Those animals whose genetic make-up is better suited to a particular environment are those more likely to breed successfully and pass on their genetic superiority (in that environment) to their offspring. By domesticating animals and controlling their breeding to suit our own purposes, we have redesigned their phenotypes to produce more of the things we want and at greater efficiency: more milk per cow, more eggs per hen, faster growth and leaner carcasses in pigs and poultry, improved FCE. Controlled breeding of farm animals has been conspicuously successful at achieving these aims and, in the case of growth rates, milk yields and FCE, the evidence would suggest that the rate of progress can be sustained.

If a trait, such as growth rate, is heritable, then that trait can be 'improved' through genetic selection at a rate that is determined by its heritability. However, the consequences of selection are not limited to the trait or traits included in the selection programme, and some of these correlated responses to selection may compromise fitness and welfare. Thus, selection for increased milk yield in dairy cows has led to correlated increases in infertility (Simm, 1998); selection for increased growth rate in broiler chickens has led to an increase in the prevalence of limb disorders (Kestin *et al.*, 1992). The principles and practice of genetic selection in farm animals are too complex to consider here in any detail: for an excellent introduction see Simm (1998). There is, however, one general truth that needs emphasis. The traits that carry the highest heritability, such as coat colour, growth rate, and proportion of meat in the most expensive cuts, tend to be those which carry little or no benefit to the animals themselves within the Darwinian context of fitness. The traits that really matter to the animal, like mothering ability and viability of the offspring, carry a very low heritability.

The impact of genetic selection on production and production efficiency has been most conspicuous in the intensive poultry and pig industries. This does not automatically imply that these industries are more advanced. The first reason for the high response to selection is that these animals are kept securely in controlled environment houses with all the high-quality feed they need. The second reason is that selection has been directed almost entirely at 'improved' traits in animals destined directly for slaughter (e.g. growth rate, carcass quality, FCE) with little regard for traits that may affect the fitness of the breeding animals. Table 1.8 outlines some of the key factors that determine the efficiency of production in meat animals and their implications for genetic selection. The most important single factor is the prolificacy of the breeding female. A broiler breeder that produces 250 chicks/year, slaughtered for meat at an average weight of 1.5 kg, can produce 120 times her own weight in the form of saleable meat per annum. At the other extreme, a ewe that produces 1.6 lambs per year yielding on average 18 kg of saleable meat/lamb only yields 32% of her own weight. In the case of broilers, 96% of feed is eaten by the slaughter generation; in pigs it is 80%, in sheep only 32%, i.e. 68% of feed is eaten by the breeding generation. Thus the improvements in efficiency (output : input) achieved through genetic selection in the pig and poultry industries reflect the fact that the slaughter generation dominates both outputs and inputs. Where the requirements of the breeding generation are relatively high (e.g. suckler beef cattle and sheep) then

Table 1.8 Factors affecting the efficiency of meat production: allocation of food energy to the breeding and slaughter generations in broiler chickens, pigs, sheep and suckler beef cattle. Source: Webster (2005).

Inputs and outputs	Broilers	Pigs	Sheep	Beef cattle
Weight of breeding females (kg)	3	180	75	450
Progeny/year	240	22	1.6	0.9
Carcass yield from each meat animal (kg)	1.5	50	18	250
Total carcass yield/weight of dam	120	6.2	0.38	0.50
Proportion of feed energy/year				
to slaughter generation	0.96	0.80	0.32	0.48
to breeding generation	0.04	0.20	0.68	0.52

selection based on simply on growth rate, FCE, and so on can drive efficiency in the wrong direction. It would, for example be extremely unproductive to stock the hills of Scotland with Suffolk sheep. In these circumstances breeding policy is typically based on the principle of 'divergent selection'. In sheep this might involve selection for 'meaty' traits in the sire breeds (e.g. Suffolk or Texel) and hardy, low-maintenance traits in the breeding females (e.g. Scottish Blackface). A fuller explanation of breeding strategies in the sheep industry is given in Chapter 5.

Within the global poultry, pig and dairy industries, the phenotype of the ideal production animal is determined by a small number of international companies who constitute the nucleus breeders. They provide the 'superior' male genes (usually in the form of semen) and breeding females and market these products either direct to commercial farms or through 'multiplier' units (Chapter 6). The superior genotypes are developed on the basis of a 'selection index' that nominates multiple traits relating both to productivity and fitness and weights them with the aim of achieving the most efficient compromise, measured in strictly economic terms. This will inevitably put greatest weight on production traits such as growth rate in broilers, even if it leads to a deterioration in the leg strength of growers and the fitness of broiler breeders (Chapter 8). However, breeding companies have, in recent years, come to place increased emphasis on fitness traits, in response to criticism from both producers and consumers that so-called high genetic merit animals were becoming increasingly unable to sustain fitness throughout their productive lives. Thus dairy cow selection in the USA is now based on an 'index of lifetime merit' that still gives 62% weighting to milk fat and protein yield but now allocates 38% to fitness-related traits such as reduced somatic cell count in milk and increased productive life.

In summary, the overall aim of controlled breeding in farm animals is to produce a superior animal, measured mainly in terms of production and productive efficiency. However, genetic superiority is not an absolute concept: it can only be measured in the context of a specific environment and in relation to the criteria used to define superiority. The 'superior' lines of pig or broiler chicken generated from the nucleus breeders for intensive, controlled environment production systems all tend to be very similar because both the selection criteria and the environments for which they have been selected are all much the same. Moreover, traits that may be defined as superior in commercial terms may not be consistent with fitness, especially in breeding adults. One sees the most genetic diversity within extensive livestock systems, where animals have to fend for themselves in a wide range of environments. Where environmental control is not an option, it makes more sense to exploit natural selection and genetic diversity to match animals to the environment, rather than vice versa, and this inevitably implies giving added weight to fitness traits. Paragraph 29 in the Welfare of Farmed Animals (England) Regulations (2000) states: '*No animals shall be kept for farming purposes unless it can reasonably be expected, on the basis of their genotype or phenotype, that they can be kept without detrimental effect on their health or welfare.*' The intention of this regulation is admirable but it has yet to be tested in the form of a challenge as to whether any current breeding programme might be detrimental to animal health and welfare.

1.5 Transport and Slaughter

The procedures involved in the transport of farm animals and their handling in abattoirs up to the point of death will inevitably involve some degree of stress. Recent UK orders, the Welfare of Animals (Transport) Order 1997 and the Welfare of Animals (Slaughter or Killing) Regulations 1995, based on European Council Regulations, acknowledge that these procedures are inherently stressful and are designed to minimize the risk that animals will suffer physically as a direct consequence of any of these procedures, or suffer mentally in anticipation of them. The Transport Order sets out regulations concerning vehicle design, journey times and rest periods. The Slaughter Regulations state that 'No person engaged in the movement, lairaging, restraint, stunning, slaughter or killing of animals shall: (a) cause any avoidable excitement, pain or suffering to any animal; (b) permit any animal to sustain any avoidable excitement, pain or suffering. '

This legislation recognizes the range of potentially stressful experiences that an animal might encounter from the moment it is taken from the relative security of the farm environment to the point of death. The humanity of processes involved in the transport and slaughter will be determined by how well these principles are put into practice. Once again the five freedoms may be used as a comprehensive structure that can identify the major problems and point to solutions (Table 1.9).

Pigs and poultry are much more susceptible to thermal stress (especially heat stress) than cattle and sheep, mainly because of their limited ability to regulate heat loss by evaporation. Pig and poultry transporters are designed, ventilated and sometimes air-conditioned to minimize the risk of thermal stress for the sound commercial objective of preventing animals from arriving dead at the abattoir. Sheep and cattle are unlikely to be killed as a direct consequence of heat stress but it can

Table 1.9 Application of the `five freedoms' to identify welfare problems for farm animals in transport and at the place of slaughter. Source: Webster (2005).

	Poultry	Pigs	Cattle	Sheep
Hunger and thirst			Thirst	Thirst
Physical discomfort	Overcrowding **	Overcrowding*	Exhaustion	Exhaustion
	Shackling			
Thermal discomfort	Heat stress ***	Heat stress ***		
	Cold stress*			
Pain and injury	Bone fractures		Bruising	Smothering
Infection	Day-old chicks		Young calves **	
Fear and stress		Fighting	Fighting	Neophobia

exacerbate their suffering from severe thirst and physical exhaustion when they are transported long distances. European regulations state that journey times for cattle, sheep and goats should not exceed 14 hours and must be followed by a rest period of at least 1 hour (Council Regulation (EC) 1/2005 on the Protection of Animals during Transport). This recognizes that the main problem for these animals will be exhaustion because they are likely to remain standing throughout the journey for reasons of security. Journey times for pigs may be up to 24 hours provided they have continuous access to liquid. This is because they lie down. Fighting, and injuries caused by fighting, constitute one of the main sources of stress in pigs and cattle, especially in lairage. All farm animals are likely to experience the stress of neophobia when exposed for the first time to the procedures involved in loading and unloading from vehicles. This problem is likely to be greatest for animals such as hill sheep that have had little or no previous experience of contact with humans and hardware. I repeat, the most effective way to minimize stresses in transport and at the place of slaughter is to design facilities that minimize human contact and encourage animals to move naturally and with a sense of security (Grandin, 1993). This assumes particular importance when handling animals such as red deer (Chapter 10) where overexcitement and fear can also lead to serious injuries.

This is not the place to review in any detail the methods used for the stunning and slaughter of farm animals. For more information see Gregory (1998) and publications produced by the HSA (http://www.hsa.org.uk/). Regulations state that 'animals should be slaughtered instantaneously or rendered instantaneously insensible to pain until death supervenes'. In most cases animals are first stunned to render the animal insensible, then 'stuck' and bled to death. The most common stunning method for cattle involves concussion, using a captive bolt pistol or percussion bolt gun. Pigs and poultry have conventionally been stunned by application of electric currents to induce an epileptic seizure. However, in recent years there has been increasing use of the gases carbon dioxide, argon or mixtures thereof to create insensibility prior to bleeding out.

The 1995 Slaughter Regulations recognize two key stages essential to ensure the humanity of the slaughter process:

- The stunning process should ensure that animals are rendered (almost) instantaneously insensible to pain (and fear) until death ensues.
- All abattoir procedures from the time of the animals' arrival to the time of death should be designed and executed in such a way as to avoid excitement, pain or suffering to any animal.

Incorporation of these principles into abattoir design and management is a complex business but vital in terms of both animal welfare and meat quality, since the two are related (Gregory, 1998). The key principle must always be compassion. At an excellent abattoir in Scotland, there is written above the point of animal entry the words 'Quality control starts here. Treat all animals with care and kindness.' That says it nicely.

1.6 Ethics and Values in Farm Animal Welfare

Ethics, or moral philosophy, is a structured approach to examining and understanding the moral life: right thought and right action. There are two classic approaches to addressing moral issues, conveniently abbreviated as 'top-down' and 'bottom-up'. The classical 'top-down' approach asks the question: 'What general moral norms for the evaluation and guidance of conduct should we accept, and why?' The drawback to this approach is that practical issues tend to be given little emphasis or ignored. The alternative 'bottom-up' approach is first to identify a specific practical issue, then construct an analysis of relevant moral issues by a process of induction. Beauchamp and Childress (2001) have developed a powerful and widely adopted 'bottom-up' approach to addressing problems in biomedical ethics which builds upon well-established principles of 'common morality'; i.e. those principles and norms identified as relevant and important by reasonably minded people. These principles have been adapted by Mepham (1996) to livestock farming. The three pillars of common morality are all based on the central principle of respect:

- *beneficence*: – a utilitarian respect for the aim to promote the greatest good and least harm for the greatest number;
- *autonomy*: – respect for the rights of each individual, e.g. to freedom of choice;
- *justice*: – respect for the principle of fairness to all.

Any ethical evaluation of the use of animals by humans is complicated by the fact that the animals cannot contribute to the debate, and no benefit accrues to the individuals used in the process. This applies particularly to the principle of justice. Humans are moral agents and carry moral responsibilities. The animals are 'moral patients'.

In this context, therefore, the concept of justice demands that we should always seek a fair and humane compromise between the likely benefits to humans and our moral duty to respect the welfare and intrinsic value of any animal in our care. Respect for the general welfare of individuals and populations is a utilitarian principle; respect for the intrinsic value of every farm animal is in accord with the principle of autonomy. However, no moral judgement regarding animal welfare, nor any action consequent upon this moral judgement, can be made in isolation. It must also consider the farmers who produce our food, consumers, especially those with little money to spend on food, and the overall impact of any decision on the living environment.

The three principles of respect and the four parties commanding respect are brought together in Table 1.10 in the form of an ethical matrix (after Mepham, 1996). Farmers and all who work in the food chain have a duty to provide the public with safe, wholesome, affordable food. The utilitarian principle commands that we, the general public, have a duty to help farmers to promote the welfare of their animals and the living environment through our actions and our laws. This help may take the form of financial rewards for food produced to high welfare standards and subsidies for conservation of a living environment that can sustain biodiversity, wildlife and the beauty of the living countryside.

Our moral duties to farmers and their animals may be explained largely in utilitarian terms. They are also motivated by self-interest. Even the duty to sustain the living environment reflects not only our human respect for beauty but our long-term need to preserve the planet for our own ends. The matrix however recognizes that utilitarianism alone is not enough: our actions should also be motivated by the principles of autonomy and justice. The principle of autonomy commands respect for other living creatures and for the living environment by virtue of their very existence. It is most simply expressed by the maxim: 'Do as you would be done by.' In this context, the most important element of autonomy is equal freedom of choice, for us and for them. Individual consumers should have the right to select their food on the basis of knowledge (or at least trust) of those things that matter to them – price, quality, safety and maybe (if they wish) production methods. Farmers should have the freedom to adopt, or not adopt, production methods of which they may or may not approve, such as hormone implants in beef cattle, or genetically engineered crops.

Table 1.10 The ethical matrix as applied to the production of food from animals (adapted from Mepham, 1996).

Respect for	Beneficence Health and welfare	Autonomy Freedom/choice	Justice Fairness
Farm animals	Animal welfare	*Telos*	Duty of care
Producers	Farmer welfare	Choice of system	Fair trade and law
Consumers	Safe, wholesome food	Choice/labelling	Affordable food
Living environment	Conservation	Biodiversity	Sustainability of populations

Respect for the autonomy of the moral patients, farm animals and the living environment is a more difficult concept since it cannot be reciprocated (we may assume that animals feel no moral obligation to us). Nevertheless, the principle encourages us to recognize the '*telos*', i.e. the fundamental biological and psychological essence of any animal; in simple terms 'the pigness of a pig'. A pregnancy stall for sows that denies them the freedom to express normal behaviour is an insult to *telos*, even if we cannot produce evidence of physical or emotional stress. If you disagree with this concept (and many do), consider two more extreme possible manipulations of farm animals in the interests of more efficient production: breeding blind hens for battery cages, or genetically engineering pigs to knock out genes concerned with perception and cognitive awareness (in essence, to destroy sentience). A strictly utilitarian argument could be marshalled to defend both practices since it could be argued that blind hens would be less likely to damage one another, and less sentient pigs would be less likely to suffer the emotional effects of discomfort and frustration. I offer these examples in support of the argument that, even when considering non-human animals, utilitarianism is not enough.

The principle of justice implies fairness to all parties. In the context of farm animal welfare the principle of justice imposes on us the duty of care. All those who keep farm animals and all those who eat their products should accept that these animals are there to serve our interests. Their 'purpose' is to contribute to our own good. It is therefore only fair to do good to these animals in a way that is commensurate with the good they do for us. We owe them a duty of care.

This chapter has introduced the major elements of good farm animal husbandry and welfare. Successive chapters describe the practical application of these principles to the management of farm animals in the major production systems. Our understanding of good husbandry is founded on science, technology and, most important of all, generations of practical experience and it is these things that that make up most of this book. Nevertheless, our duty of care to farm animals and to the living, farmed countryside cannot be measured in scientific terms. It can, and should, be informed by science, but it is defined by our sense of *values*. Ethics has been defined as the 'science of values': it offers justification and guidance for right action. The ethical matrix (Table 1.10) has something in common with the 'five freedoms' in that it can operate in practice as a checklist of concerns and an aid to diagnosis in matters of value. I invite you to use both frameworks when evaluating the welfare of farm animals within different production systems. The five freedoms will help you to assess how the animals feel ('fit and happy?'); the ethical matrix will help you to assess how well we meet our duty of care.

References and Further Reading

Beauchamp, T.L. and Childress, J.F. (2001) *Principles of Biomedical Ethics*, 5th edn. Oxford University Press, Oxford.

Dawkins, M.S. (1990) From an animal's point of view: motivation, fitness and animal welfare. *Behavioural and Brain Sciences* **13**, 1–61.

DEFRA, (Department for Environment, Food and Rural Affairs) (2003) *Revised Codes for the Welfare of Pigs, Laying Hens, Meat Poultry and Dairy Cattle*, HMSO, London.

Farm Animal Welfare Council (1993) *Second report on priorities for research and development in farm animal welfare*. DEFRA Publications, London.

Fraser, D. and Broom, D.B. (1990) *Farm Animal Behaviour and Welfare*. CABI Publishing, Wallingford.

Grandin, T. (ed.) (1993) *Livestock Handling and Transport*. CABI Publishing, Wallingford.

Gregory, N. (1998) *Animal Welfare and Meat Science*. CABI Publishing, Wallingford.

Kendrick, K.M. (1998) Intelligent perception. *Applied Animal Behaviour Science* **57**, 213–31.

Kestin, S.C., Knowles, T.G., Tinch, A.E. and Gregory, N.G. (1992) Prevalence of leg weakness in broiler chickens and its relationship with genotype. *Veterinary Record* **131**, 191–4.

Mepham, B. (1996) *Ethical analysis of food biotechnologies: an evaluative framework*. In Food Ethics, Mepham, Ben (ed.), pp. 101–19. Routledge, London.

Simm, G. (1998) *The Genetic Improvement of Cattle and Sheep*. Farming Press, Ipswich.

Wathes, C.M. and Charles, D.R. (1994) *Livestock Housing*. CABI Publishing, Wallingford.

Webster, J. (1995) *Animal Welfare: a Cool Eye Towards Eden*. Blackwell Science, Oxford.

Webster, J. (2005) *Animal Welfare: Limping towards Eden*. Blackwell Science, Oxford.

Behaviour as an Indicator of Animal Welfare

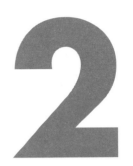

CHRISTINE NICOL

Management and Welfare of Farm Animals: The UFAW Farm Handbook, 5th edition. John Webster
© 2011 by Universities Federation for Animal Welfare (UFAW)

2.1 Introduction

The study of animal behaviour can contribute to the assessment of animal welfare in two main ways. First, farm animals need to perform many behaviours, but certain housing systems constrain or restrict them so that this performance is difficult or impossible. By identifying the behaviours that matter most to the animals, housing can be designed to accommodate these behavioural priorities. Second, a knowledge of animal behaviour can permit the identification of potential problems at a very early stage or, conversely, provide reassurance that animals are content and in good health. In many ways behaviour is an ideal indicator of welfare. It reflects both the internal physical and physiological state of the animal, and the animal's response to the external environment. However, the seemingly simple idea that normal behaviour can be used as a sign of good welfare and abnormal behaviour as a sign of poor welfare should be resisted. 'Normal' behaviour (in the sense of behaviour that evolved as an adaptation to a particular ancestral environment) no longer exists for some of our domesticated farm species. Moreover 'abnormal' behaviour can mean different things to different people. Behaviours that are performed by only a minority of animals, or behaviours that look odd to humans, are sometimes described as abnormal but can often be perfectly appropriate responses to captive environments. The goal for all who work with animals, from scientists to stock-people, is to work out which behaviours matter to the animals in the farm environment, and which behaviours are reliable indicators of good or bad welfare.

The chapter will consider four main themes:

1. Behaviours that matter in captive environments
   • studies of wild ancestors and domestic animals leading feral lives
   • the learning and mental abilities of farm animals
   • the study of animal motivation: preferences, aversions and behavioural priorities
   • animal adaptation, allostasis and flexibility: the role of learning and experience
2. Behaviours as welfare indicators
   • behavioural indices of poor welfare: signs of disease, pain, frustration and deprivation
   • redirected behaviours and stereotypies
   • behavioural indices of good welfare
3. Animals as individuals
   • social environments
   • predictability and control
4. Good husbandry
   • how to meet the behavioural needs of farm animals within large-scale agricultural systems
   • how animal behaviour can be used in the design of more humane living environments.

Box 2.1 contains definitions of the terms used in this chapter.

Box 2.1   Definitions

Allostasis – the process of achieving stability through physiological or behavioural change

Aversion – an observed tendency to avoid one resource or environment over another

Behavioural priority – a behaviour for which the animal shows a demonstrably high demand in a given housing environment

Behavioural substrate – an environmental material towards which an animal directs exploratory, foraging or comfort behaviour

Candidate behaviour – a behaviour that may be important for animal welfare in a given housing environment, but for which further evidence is required

Causal factor – an input to the brain's behavioural decision making centre, derived from changes to the environment (external cues) or from changes to the animal's physiological state (internal cues)

Conspecific – a member of the same species

Economic demand theory – a method of assessing animals' priorities by establishing how much energy, work or time they will allocate to obtain one resource or behavioural opportunity relative to another. The methods were derived from economists' studies of human consumer behaviour

Habituation – the gradual waning of a response to a repeated event, in the absence of any reward or punishment associated with that event

Motivation – the study of the proximate causes of behaviour; the constantly shifting internal and external factors that result in decisions to change from one behaviour to another at any given time

Preference – an observed tendency to choose one resource or environment over another

Rebound behaviour – a response that indicates that internal causal factors have risen above the level that would normally result in behavioural performance in an unconstrained environment. When the behaviour is permitted after a period of prevention or restriction it occurs more intensely, more frequently or for a longer duration than normal

Stereotypic behaviour – a repetitive and invariant response, that develops when other behavioural responses are frustrated, but eventually becomes emancipated from its original causal factors

---

2.2 Behaviours that Matter in Captive Environments

2.2.1 Identifying candidate behaviours

If a domestic animal is observed in a barren environment doing little other than feeding and resting it is difficult to know whether all is well, or whether something important is missing. The animal might be content, or it might be frustrated because the resources that would allow it do a wider range of activities are absent. Unless information is available about what the animal *should* perhaps be doing (its candidate behaviours) it is impossible to distinguish these possibilities. To identify these candidate behaviours we need to consider how behaviour evolved. Normal behaviour evolved in the wild ancestors of our domestic species, so it is inconvenient (and rather sad) that many of these wild ancestors and ancestral habitats no longer exist. Identifying the behaviours that matter for the welfare of domesticated animals living in artificial environments is therefore not straightforward. Where wild ancestors are still alive they can be studied, although it is important to remain aware that domestication for improved production may also have changed the behaviour of our modern farm breeds. Nonetheless, this is a good place to start.

2.2.1.1 Wild ancestors

The European wild boar (*Sus scrofa*) is the ancestor of the modern pig. Despite the fact that there are many different subspecies, wild boar can still be studied relatively easily in a natural environment (similar to that in which they evolved), and their behaviour highlights the busy and complex repertoire that we should expect to see today, in even our most intensely selected domestic pigs. Wild boars have varied and adaptable foraging behaviour patterns and complex social lives, with strong matrilineal bonds between mothers and daughters. Suckling activities and family life are guided by a range of vocal communications that lead to co-ordination and synchrony of group activities.

Finding the wild ancestors of the domestic chicken is a little more challenging. Wild members of the progenitor species, the red jungle-fowl (*Gallus gallus*), still survive in the jungles of Southeast Asia. But these jungle-fowl are not easy to study. They are shy birds that live in inaccessible places. It is therefore not surprising that most observations come from small groups of jungle-fowl living in zoos or laboratories, where they are easier to see. The downside is that these small groups behave dissimilarly in different zoos, suggesting that genetic drift or adaptation to the various captive environments has occurred. It is therefore not easy to decide which zoo population provides the most authentic picture of natural jungle-fowl behaviour. In addition, selection for production has been more intense in chickens than in any other species, so nowhere does the warning about making comparisons between wild ancestors and domestic breeds apply more strongly than with this species. From the limited information available, it seems that domestic hens differ from wild jungle-fowl by showing consistently lower fear levels, and reduced foraging, social and exploratory behaviour (reviewed in Jensen, 2006). All of this means it is difficult to take the behaviour of wild animals as some sort of 'gold standard' to which domestic breeds should adhere. For example, the observation that jungle-fowl kept in zoos spend 60% of their active day in ground pecking has been suggested as a baseline for the assessment of the welfare of domestic fowl, but it is also possible that domestic fowl don't *want* to spend 60% of their time foraging. Observations of wild ancestors therefore give us clues as to the sorts of behaviours we might expect to see and the issues we should examine, but we cannot automatically infer the behaviours that matter to a chicken, by observing a jungle-fowl.

If this approach is useful for pigs, and difficult for chickens, it is sadly impossible for many other species. There are no longer any aurochs (the extinct ancestor of modern cattle) alive today, or any direct ancestors of the domestic horse. Genetic evidence suggests that domestic horses arose from a large number of founder animals, but seemingly not from the only wild horse still in existence, the Przewalski's horse. So, there are no wild ancestors left to study. Even the Przewalski's horse survived only in zoos until a few years ago, when efforts were made to reintroduce them into Mongolia (http://www.treemail.nl/takh/).

2.2.1.2 Feral lives

While it may be impossible to find wild ancestors of our farm animals, or the genetic distance between them and our modern breeds may be too large, we can however observe populations of domestic animals that have escaped or been released from captivity, and now live and reproduce freely with little or no interference from humans. Such populations are described as feral and, usefully, they will have the same genetic composition as managed domestic breeds. Therefore they potentially provide very useful information about the candidate behaviours that may matter to modern domestic farm animals. In a classic study, Duncan *et al.* (1978) released domestic chickens onto a small Scottish island and observed how they formed small, stable groups, roosted at night and selected extremely well-hidden nest sites. In fact, at that time, there was no evidence that the capacity to perform any major behaviour pattern had been lost. However, since the time of that study, it appears that many modern strains of domestic hen have now lost the capacity to brood and raise their own offspring. It would be interesting to know how modern strains might fare on the same Scottish island today.

Scientists have sometimes deliberately released domestic animals into semi-natural or highly enriched environments in an attempt to examine their behaviour under 'ideal' conditions. The most famous study of this kind was conducted by Stolba and Wood-Gush (1989) on pigs. They observed the undisturbed social, foraging, reproductive and exploratory behaviour of the pigs. They found that the pigs spent more than 50% of their time rooting and grazing, even when their energy needs were met with concentrate feed rations. Piglets from the same litter formed close social bonds with each other, and subsequent studies have shown that these can be maintained throughout life. The maternal behaviour of many feral sows is complex and attentive. However, observations of domestic pigs show that piglet mortality can be high, even in unconstrained environments, as many individual sows have lost the vital tendency to respond appropriately to the squeals or distress calls of their piglets. Instead of standing up rapidly if they accidentally start to lie on a piglet, some sows just continue to lie down, with disastrous consequences for the crushed piglet.

Observations of animals living feral lives have thus revealed latent capacities to perform a wide range of reproductive, social and foraging behaviours in our domestic breeds, but have simultaneously uncovered stark evidence that some key adaptive behavioural patterns have been lost.

2.2.1.3 Ethology in the laboratory

In addition to studying wild animals, or domestic animals in wild or semi-natural environments, there is also a place for laboratory studies which can provide insights as to the flexibility of normal behaviour patterns, and especially the learning and cognitive abilities of farm animals. A significant proportion of the applied ethology literature comprises studies of this kind. Good welfare will be more likely if animals are able to exercise their mental abilities, so identifying candidate cognitive abilities may be just as important as identifying those behaviours concerned with satisfying more immediate physical requirements.

Sometimes this mental complexity and flexibility of farm animals is quite astounding, particularly when shown by animals that are often regarded as simple. In 2001, the journal *Nature* published a paper showing that individual sheep could remember 50 other different sheep faces for more than two years (Kendrick *et al.*, 2001; 2007).

The result itself was perhaps less surprising than *Nature*'s thoughtless headline 'sheep are not so stupid after all'. Careful studies have revealed complex patterns of sheep behaviour. For example, within most pastures preferred plant species are concentrated in certain areas and experiments reveal, not only that sheep use sophisticated spatial memory strategies to remember the location of these favoured foraging patches, but also that they integrate this knowledge with an assessment of their own position within the group social structure. Dominant sheep develop their own expectations of where preferred food might be found, and also monitor, use and exploit their subordinates' expectations about food. It should not be a surprise that sheep have developed behaviours appropriate to survival in sheep country; sheep are good at being sheep.

Chickens are another species that suffer from an ill-deserved 'bird-brained' reputation. Take the maternal behaviour of the hen. It is now known that hens discourage their very young chicks from pecking at attractive but inedible items and encourage them to peck at food, with a complex vocal and behavioural display. Hens give characteristic food calls, and demonstrate the edibility of an item by picking it up and dropping it again in front of their chicks. They increase the intensity of this display when the food is of particularly high quality, or when the chicks move away or fail to respond. Even more remarkably, hens seem to recognize when the chicks make mistakes. This has been investigated in experiments that ensure that the chicks' information about food palatability is different from the hen's. If the hen perceives that her chicks are wrong, then she increases the intensity of her food-calling display (Nicol and Pope, 1996).

Hens also respond in a variety of ways to warn their chicks of danger from predators. Again, however, the hen is not simply prompted to perform a suite of behaviours in a mindless way. On the contrary, hens discriminate between subtle differences in predator size and relate this to the growth rate and size of their chicks. Thus, specific alarm calls and defensive postures are given when relatively small birds of prey, which pose the greatest threat to the chicks, are spotted. A different pattern of response is shown towards larger, less dangerous hawks (see Figure 2.1).

These remarkable studies have provided evidence that farm animals have sophisticated spatial and social memories, and that their communications often convey subtle meaning. They are also able to infer information from indirect sources: chickens, for example, assess their own relative social position against a strange bird, once they have observed it in encounters with familiar dominant and subordinate companions. There is even preliminary evidence that farm animals gain some pleasure from solving problems. All of this suggests that the opportunity to use these candidate cognitive abilities should be considered as something that might be relevant for good welfare.

2.2.2 How much do these behaviours matter?

So far this chapter has considered how the range of candidate behaviours and mental abilities that might be shown by domestic animals can be deduced by studying wild ancestors, and by observations and experiments with domestic breeds in wild and semi-natural environments. The studies generally highlight a rather impressive complexity of behaviour and cognitive ability. Further information about the behaviour patterns of cattle, sheep, horses, pigs and poultry can be found in a variety of books (see Jensen, 2009; Mills and McConnell, 2005). The focus of this chapter now turns to the relationship between behaviour and welfare. It would be relatively easy to make a blanket assertion that, for good welfare, animals should be free to perform all of the candidate behaviour patterns that have been identified, but would this be justified and might there even be negative consequences of following this prescription?

It is possible that there are some advantages in simply making a decision and then sticking with it, rather than getting too mired in detail and complexity. The Brambell Committee, constituted in 1965 to investigate the effects of increasing intensification of animal production, concluded without too much deliberation that any animal should have 'sufficient freedom of movement to be able without difficulty to turn round, groom itself, get up, lie down and stretch its limbs' (Brambell Committee, 1965). These were the original 'five freedoms'.

With good intentions, this original ideal was broadened by the UK Farm Animal Welfare Council and one of the modern five freedoms currently states that 'Animals

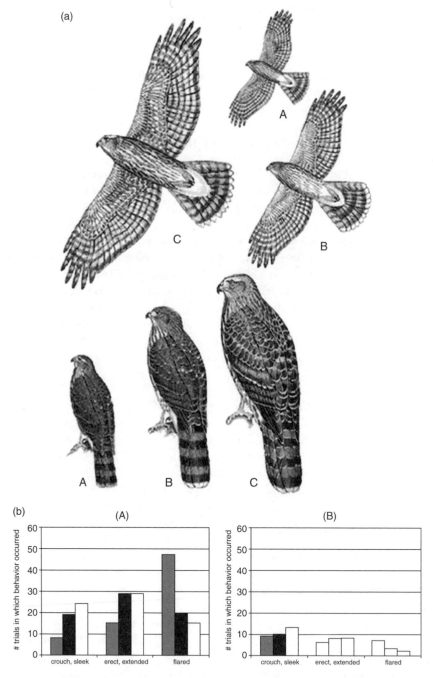

Figure 2.1 Fear responses of hens and chicks to predator birds (from Palleroni et al., 2005). Hawks of different sizes (A, B and C) were trained to fly over pairs of adult bantam chickens and their young. When chicks were young (graph A), the broody female chickens respond to the greatest threat of the smallest hawks (light grey columns) with a flared posture, while tending to shown crouching or an erect threat posture to the larger hawks (dark grey and white columns). As the chicks age and become less of a potential target for the hawks, the defensive behaviour of the hens reduces (graph B). With kind permission from Springer Science+Business Media.

should be free to express normal behaviour' (http://www.fawc.org.uk/freedoms .htm). This is a noble aspiration, but one that raises many questions, including that of realism. If the definition of normal behaviour is restricted to the types of simple body movements identified by the Brambell committee, then few would disagree that modern farming systems can, and should, be devised to allow this. However, we have already seen that the range of candidate behaviours is wide, and some behaviours may be virtually impossible to accommodate in captivity. The ordinary, wild house mouse, for example, has a home range that varies from 0.0002 to 8.024 hectares (mean 0.27 ha) (Chambers *et al.*, 2000) and yet no laboratory is going to be able to provide any such space allowance. As a second example, despite the ethological complexity of the hen–chick interaction, the vast majority of commercial chicks are reared in hatcheries without their mothers and it is difficult to see how this could change, given increasing worldwide demand for cheap food. Putting practicalities to one side, though, there is also the question of desirability. A whole set of normal anti-predator responses can be elicited in naïve European rabbits simply by presenting them with the odour of fox (*Vulpes vulpes*) faeces. Purists might argue that rabbits should on principle be given the chance to perfom anti-predator responses, whereas welfare scientists would first seek evidence that a lack of occasion to perform anti-predator behaviour was accompanied by any form of suffering.

To obtain such evidence we need to explore the question of desirability in more depth. If we are to maximize animal welfare within whatever economic or political constraints are operating, it is essential to know which behaviours it is *most important* for animals to perform in the captive environments in which they live. Simply comparing the behaviour of a captive animal with that of its wild or feral counterpart is not sufficient to draw conclusions about animal welfare. We need to know how much the mouse needs space, whether commercially hatched chicks miss hens, and whether there is anything missing from the rabbit's life if it doesn't have a chance to perform anti-predator behaviour. These are not easy questions but we need to know how much these activities *matter*.

2.2.3 The study of animal motivation

Animal behaviour can be studied from different viewpoints, all of which are simultaneously relevant. If we ask 'why does the pig forage?', a valid functional answer would be that foraging is a good method of finding food, and pigs that forage effectively are most likely to survive and reproduce. But the same question can be re-phrased slightly to ask 'why has the pig just stopped doing its current behaviour and switched to foraging?' This is a question about the more immediate causes of behaviour and, to answer it, the various current internal and external influences on foraging behaviour have to be identified. The study of animal *motivation* takes this causal viewpoint and is concerned with establishing the nature and strength of the cues for each behaviour. For foraging, these cues might include things like the concentration of glucose in the blood and the smell of the litter material on the floor. Studying motivation is highly relevant for animal welfare. First, if a given behaviour is elicited by known *causal factors*, those internal or external cues can potentially be manipulated to change the animal's desire to do something. Second, if the motivational strength for a particular behaviour is so strong that it outcompetes all others, then we know that the animal has a *behavioural priority* that must be accommodated within a farming system.

These ideas can be explored further by comparing the behaviour of a fictional group of sheep in an indoor lambing shed, with that of flock of feral sheep (of the same breed) on an exposed hillside. Careful quantification of the behaviour of each group might realistically show that the feral sheep frequently stand vigilantly in an alert posture, an activity not noted in the indoor sheep. A naïve interpretation (based on the idea that animals should perform all their candidate behaviours) would be that the welfare of the feral sheep is better because they are performing an activity that is not seen in the indoor sheep. In terms of the five freedoms they are doing a normal behaviour. Actually the indoor sheep will suffer only if they *want* to perform vigilance behaviour and are unable to do so. It is perfectly likely that the indoor sheep have no desire to perform vigilance behaviour at all. At the end of this fictional study it might plausibly be shown that members of this breed of sheep have a tendency to be vigilant only when predatory cues (such as odours, fleeting movements or noises) are present. If the stimuli that motivate vigilance behaviour are entirely absent in the indoor environment, then the indoor sheep will have no vigilance motivation. The general point is that, if a behaviour is motivated entirely by external causal factors, good welfare can be achieved either by allowing the animal to respond appropriately to those external cues, *or* by removing those cues completely.

The fictional example above suggests that it might be quite easy to work out the types of internal and external cues that cause particular behaviours. But in reality this can be quite difficult. Take wing-stretching, a comfort behaviour shown by jungle-fowl in the wild, and seen in feral and free-range domestic fowl, but an activity rarely observed when hens are housed in conventional battery cages. To assess the welfare of the caged hens, knowledge about whether they wanted to perform wing-stretching behaviour would be needed, and this would depend on which cues trigger stretching. One possibility might be that the behaviour is caused by an external cue such as the sight of a large open space. If so, then birds in cages would not be motivated to wing-stretch and there would be no welfare problem. Alternatively, wing-stretching might be caused by an internal cue such as inactivity of stretch receptors in the skin for a certain period of time. If so, then birds in cages would be highly motivated to do this activity and the lack of wing-stretching would indicate a significant welfare problem. But without a detailed understanding of the physiological mechanisms underpinning wing-stretching, how could these possibilities be distinguished?

One way around this conundrum is to examine the behaviour of animals after the physical constraint preventing the behaviour is removed, or after a missing physical substrate is supplied. If a significant *rebound* is observed on release to an unconstrained environment, this is reasonable evidence that the behaviour is motivated by internal causal factors. Thus, just as rebound feeding occurs after a fast because falling energy reserves results in increased feeding motivation, so rebound locomotion occurs after a period of inactivity, because the motivation to exercise has increased, even if we do not know exactly what physiological factors are involved. The observed rebound permits the inference that motivation to exercise will be present whatever environment the animal is in. Observing reduced movement in spatially confined animals therefore indicates a welfare problem, not an adaptation.

In chickens, many comfort behaviours such as wing-stretching, tail-wagging, leg-stretching and wing-flapping show a significant rebound when birds are moved from small to large cages after 4 weeks of confinement (Nicol, 1987). For some behaviours, the intensity of the rebound correlates positively with the duration of confinement, strongly suggesting that chickens do not acclimatize in any way to prolonged spatial restriction. Other examples of rebound behaviour include dust-bathing by chickens allowed access to litter after a period of deprivation, and the cantering, galloping and bucking shown by calves and horses when they are allowed to exercise after some weeks or months of confinement (Figure 2.2). The lying-down behaviour of cows and sheep also shows a rebound pattern, in that the longer the animals are prevented from lying, the more time they spend lying down once the opportunity is available. They are more tired after 48 h on their feet than after 24 h.

In contrast, there is little convincing evidence of a rebound in aggression or anti-predator activities. In the face of a threat, these activities occur at the same intensity, no matter how long ago the behaviour was last performed. Animals are not more aggressive after 48 h without a fight than after 24 h. In his 1963 book, *On Aggression*, Konrad Lorenz argued that the tendency to be aggressive built up over time (in human and non-human animals alike) until it was so overwhelming that the slightest excuse would trigger an aggressive outburst. Thankfully, there is little or no evidence to support this view. The performance of both aggressive and anti-predator

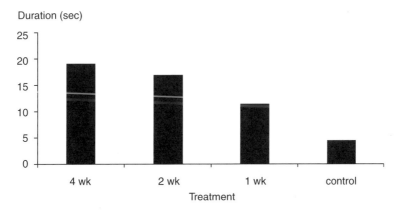

Figure 2.2 Rebound in galloping and bucking shown by calves on release after 1, 2 or 4 weeks' confinement. The increase in bucking and galloping with duration of confinement suggests that the motivation to exercise continues to increase during the confinement period (after Jensen, 1999). Used with permission from Elsevier.

activities depends almost entirely on the presence of the relevant external cues (the appearance of the stealthy fox, or the hated rival). Internal cues are not entirely irrelevant – the aggressive tendencies of sheep or deer, for example, increase in association with altered patterns of reproductive hormones during the breeding season – but these reflect a varying threshold rather than an actual trigger.

In summary, although the mechanisms are sometimes unclear or unknown, behaviours such as feeding, drinking, resting and exercising seem to be motivated by internal cues that increase in strength during periods when the behaviours are not performed. So animals get hungrier, thirstier, more tired and more cramped if they are housed in systems that prevent feeding, drinking, lying or exercise. Aggressive and anti-predator activities are motivated in a different way and animals should not need to do these behaviours in most farming systems, when the relevant environmental stimuli are absent. The causation of many other behaviours such as exploration, foraging, social and parental behaviour involves a complex interplay of both internal and external cues.

2.2.4 Preferences, aversions and behavioural priorities

We have seen that some behaviours are largely caused by internal cues and therefore animals will be motivated to perform these behaviours irrespective of the environment they are in. Other behaviours are primarily caused by external cues and so animals will be motivated to perform these behaviours only when the relevant environmental stimuli are present. In both cases, the next step in assessing how much these behaviours matter is to assess the strength of the animal's motivation.

Investigating behavioural priorities has been a particularly active area for animal welfare researchers because sometimes it is impossible both to allow animals to perform all of their candidate behaviours and simultaneously run an effective or profitable farming system. The aim, then, is to identify those behaviours that matter the most for good welfare – those where the animal has, at least some of the time, a very strong motivation – and to ensure that farming systems are designed to permit these priority activities. This has been attempted using a variety of methods and so this section will review some of the work conducted to assess, first, animals' preferences and aversions, and then work undertaken to establish their behavioural priorities.

2.2.4.1 Preferences

Early *preference* tests made little distinction between asking animals which of their *behaviour patterns* they most needed to perform, and asking which *substrates* they most preferred to use to enable a particular behaviour to take place. Simple preference tests are far more suited to the latter question, where they provide a useful tool for establishing how animals would most like to express a given behaviour. Thus, a large body of work has now established the preferred foods of most farm animal species, the dust-bathing materials of chickens, the lying and flooring material preferences of dairy cows and goats, the types of walls that are most preferred by sows to lean against when lying down, and the lighting types and

Table 2.1 Pig preference for foraging substrate. Pigs generally prefer the earth-like substrates (peat and mushroom compost) to those more commonly offered as enrichment substrates on farms. In this experiment preferences between each pair of substrates were tested using a different four groups of six pigs. Pigs could also spend time in the lengthy passage between the two preference chambers (Beattie et al., 1998). Reprinted with permission from UFAW.

Mean number of pigs in each group of six, observed in each substrate area over 144 h period	
Peat	Sawdust
3.03	0.97
Peat	Straw
3.51	1.17
Mushroom compost	Wood bark
2.26	0.87
Mushroom compost	Sand
3.14	1.09
Mushroom compost	Straw
2.94	0.76

regimes favoured by pigs, ducks and turkeys. One of the most important areas of preference testing has been the search for the most satisfying foraging and exploratory materials, as these have the potential to be included as environmental enrichment in a variety of housing systems. In general, animals seem to prefer substrates that can be manipulated in natural ways rather than things that are superficially exciting ('shiny toys') but give no lasting reward. The strong preferences of pigs for materials such as peat or compost (see Table 2.1) are related to their evolutionary history as animals that root with their snouts.

Many of these studies take as their measure of preference the amount of time the animal spends using the available resources, although this can result in confounding if some types of resources are easier to use than others. More recent studies use a technique whereby animals can work simultaneously for two different resources. The cross point of these double demand curves provides a measure of the relative attractiveness of the two resources (Figure 2.3).

2.2.4.2 Aversions

Just as animal behaviour experiments can be used to ask what sorts of stimuli or environments animals prefer, they can also be used as a tool to discover what animals find most aversive. Assessing *aversion* generally involves study of the learnt associations formed between stimuli that predict an aversive event and the onset of that same event. This means that animals do not have to be exposed repeatedly to potentially highly unpleasant events. Techniques for studying aversions depend therefore on associative learning.

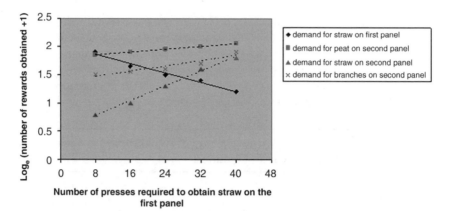

Figure 2.3 The double-demand approach assesses the relative preference of animals for two resources. Here, pigs worked to obtain straw on panel 1, and an alternative substitute (peat, straw or branches) on panel 2. The experiment was designed so that when straw on panel 1 required 8 presses, the alternative substrate required 40 presses; when straw on panel 1 required 16 presses, the alternative substrate required 32 presses, and so on. The pigs' preference for peat was stronger than their preference for the other substrates. Equal amounts of straw and peat were obtained when straw cost 9 presses and peat cost 39 presses (adapted from Pedersen *et al.*, 2005). Used with permission from Elsevier.

A technique that relies on classical conditioning is to teach a subject to perform a positively reinforced task, such as pecking a key to obtain food, until a regular baseline level of responding is achieved. An inescapable, potentially aversive, stimulus is then presented immediately after a warning signal. Later, the animal's key-pecking is examined before and after the warning signal is replayed. The extent to which the animal's baseline responding for food is reduced when it hears the warning signal for the second time is taken as a measure of its aversion to the stimulus that originally followed the signal. This procedure showed that pigeons found the distress of their companions aversive but it has not been used within the farm animal literature and its theoretical basis is rather obscure, as suppression of responding for food does nothing to prevent the onset of the warning signal. Active avoidance techniques have been used to assess the aversiveness of pollutant gases such as ammonia (Jones *et al.*, 2005) or gases used for stunning. In this important work, animals are generally allowed to enter or leave a feeding chamber at will. For example, a gas under test for its potential use as a humane stunning agent could be gradually introduced into a feeding chamber and the number of animals that choose to leave recorded. More animals will leave if the gas is perceived as pungent, irritant or painful. Turkeys, for example, avoid carbon dioxide in air to a much greater extent than either argon in air, or a mixture of carbon dioxide and argon (Raj, 1996). Sometimes, however, animals are unable to mount effective active avoidance behaviours in the presence of highly aversive or frightening stimuli. They can literally become too scared or confused to move. For this reason, passive avoidance

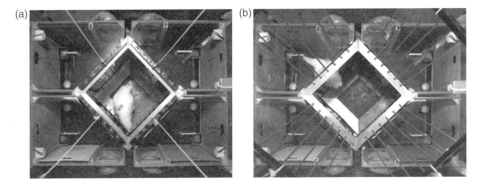

Figure 2.4 An apparatus to assess aversion of broiler chickens to conditions experienced during transport. Each of the four differently coloured chambers presented a different environment: heat, vibration, concurrent heat and vibration, or a control chamber. Chickens had to make 20 choices over 4 days to receive food rewards. Each choice resulted in confinement in the chosen chamber for 1 hour. Vibration was significantly avoided, but the heated environment was not avoided relative to the control (Abeyesinghe *et al.*, 2001). Reprinted with kind permission from Siobhan Abeyesinghe.

techniques are most often used to assess aversion in farm animals. In passive avoidance procedures, animals learn *not* to perform a response, such as walking down a runway, or pecking a key, if they want to avoid exposure to an aversive event. Thus, the measure of aversion fits much better with the animals' innate response to the event. Such methods have been used to demonstrate that particular handling methods are aversive (Pajor *et al.*, 2000). Some of the strongest reactions are shown by animals in response to the practice of electro-immobilization (illegal in the EU, but still practised in countries such as Australia), the isolation of sheep from each other during shearing, and in response to some of the types of motion experienced during transport (Abeyesinghe *et al.*, 2001) (Figure 2.4).

2.2.4.3 Behavioural priorities

Knowing something of animals' preferences and aversions is an important advance, but the question of how strong these preferences are still needs to be addressed, as does the importance of the underlying behaviours. It might be thought that a simple preference test could be done to establish whether one behaviour is more important than another. But because candidate behaviours are scheduled in complex patterns it makes little sense to ask an animal to choose directly between doing two very different behaviour patterns, particularly if the measure of 'preference' is something simplistic such as the time spent engaged in each. An animal may spend more time resting than engaging in social interaction, but this does not automatically mean that social interaction is of lesser importance.

So, to determine whether some behaviours matter more than others in particular captive environments it is useful to know whether animals are prepared to pay for the opportunity to perform them and whether they are willing to make trade-offs. This original economic approach outlined by Dawkins (1983) argued that motivational strength could be assessed using *economic demand* techniques. By applying economic models she argued that we could infer the value that animals place on particular behaviour patterns. This could be determined by reducing the animal's effective income (its energy or time budget) and seeing how it redistributed its activities. Activities that continued to be performed under these constraints were termed resilient. Alternatively, the price paid to perform a specific activity could be altered. For example, a pig wanting to engage in social behaviour might be required to press a panel. If the pig worked when the price was low (few presses required for each period of social contact) but stopped working when the price increased, then its demand for social contact would be described as elastic, and social activity categorized as a 'luxury'. If, however, the pig continued to work for social contact even when the workload became very high, then its demand would be described as inelastic, and social activity categorized as a 'necessity'. Dawkins (1983) argued that it might be useful to compare the price elasticity of different behaviours against a common yardstick, such as demand for food. A priority behaviour would thus be one that could be shown to be resilient and/or for which demand was inelastic. One advantage of the economic demand approach is that the importance of different behaviours can be compared independently of whether they occupy a large part of a daily time budget (sleeping) or a very small part (stretching). Subsequent authors have emphasized that other useful economic measures of behavioural priority, such as consumer surplus or maximum price paid, can also be derived from economic demand experiments (Mason *et al.*, 1998).

Despite generating a lot of theoretical interest, experimental work in this area has been slow to get off the ground, particularly for the larger farm animal species, and there is still little or no information available about the behavioural priorities of sheep and horses. However, there has been an upsurge in experimental activity in relation to establishing the behavioural priorities of poultry, pigs and cattle and the key findings from this work are described next.

2.2.4.4 Behavioural priorities of poultry

The behavioural priorities of poultry have been reviewed by Weeks and Nicol (2006). Hens have a demonstrably high motivation to access resources which allow nesting behaviour and they place a high value on access to discrete, enclosed nest sites. Their motivation to access a nest increases the closer they get to the time of egg-laying. They are prepared to pay high costs such as squeezing through narrow gaps or opening doors to gain access to nest boxes before egg-laying. Their demand for a nest site during the pre-laying period is as strong as that for food following deprivation of up to 8 h. Nesting is therefore a behavioural priority. There is also some evidence that hens will work to gain access to perches for roosting at night.

Both laying hens and broilers will work for food, although it is hardly surprising that feeding is a behavioural priority. For broiler breeders, subject to feed restriction, feeding motivation is not diminished by bulking the diet with additional fibre, suggesting that chronic hunger is a welfare problem for these birds. Some breeds of poultry prefer to forage for their food than to receive it too easily. Time spent pecking and scratching was relatively constant even when hens had to pay a 'cost' of squeezing through a narrow entrance to obtain this foraging opportunity (Weeks and Nicol, 2006).

Evidence that the types of comfort behaviours previously discussed are behavioural priorities comes from studies showing that hens will not just choose cages of a size that permits these behaviours but will work to obtain sufficient space to perform these activities. Early work in France showed that hens would work to achieve an increased cage size (above the 450 cm^2 per bird allowance current at the time) for some 60% of the tested time. Their intermittent need for this additional space was associated with the performance of behaviours that require more space for just a proportion of the day. In contrast, the evidence that hens will work for access to a dust-bathing substrate is inconsistent. There are real difficulties with knowing how important dust-bathing is for fowl, as even the subtlest of cues seem to trigger dust-bathing. If a good litter substrate is unavailable, birds may use food particles from their feeding dishes, or perform most of the sequences of dust-bathing on AstroTurf, or even on bare wire. This behaviour is often called sham dust-bathing, suggesting that it is somehow inadequate. So the real question is whether sham dust-bathing is sufficient to ensure good welfare (van Liere, 1992). The answer appears to be that it is a partial substitute and better than nothing. Sham dust-bathing reduces the birds' subsequent motivation to dust-bathe but does not return it to baseline levels. Although it is difficult to engineer an experiment that will test this definitively, it is quite possible that dust-bathing is a behaviour that birds may not miss doing, or may not seek out if no eliciting cues are present, but one that they enjoy if the opportunity arises (Widowski and Duncan, 2000).

2.2.4.5 Behavioural priorities of pigs

Pigs will work consistently to obtain food and appear to be constantly hungry when kept under commercial conditions of food restriction. As with hungry chickens, dietary dilution with fibre is only marginally successful as a means of reducing feeding motivation (Lawrence et al., 1989). Although formal economic demand experiments have not been conducted to look at the motivation to nest-build in sows, earlier work suggests that, for a short period of time prior to farrowing, it is an absolute behavioural priority. During the 24 h prior to farrowing, the motivation to nest approaches or outcompetes even the very strong motivation to obtain food in these feed-restricted animals. Sows will also work hard to obtain additional space prior to farrowing.

EU legislation requires that pigs have access to rooting materials, to permit exploratory and foraging activities. This seems justified since pigs show strong demand for rooting materials, particularly more complex ones such as peat, branches, silage and compost. Food reward is an important quality of the rooting material, showing that foraging, rather than abstract exploration, is the primary behavioural priority. Matthews and Ladewig (1994) examined the relative demand of eight male 12-week-old pigs for food, limited contact with a conspecific through a door, or a control condition where the door opened but no social contact was obtained. The pigs had to press a plate between 1 and 30 times to obtain each reward. They showed an inelastic demand for food over this range, but a much lower demand for social contact (although this was still demonstrably higher than for the control condition, and more responses were made). It is possible, but so far untested, that young pigs might work harder for full social contact. Kirkden and Pajor (2006) also found only a weak demand for social contact with subordinates, in stall-housed sows. These authors do caution, however, that the test sows were only deprived of access to companions for one day and suggest that their motivation might be higher after longer periods of social isolation. This, and the importance of many other pig behaviours, remains to be tested.

2.2.4.6 Behavioural priorities of cattle

The importance of social contact for calves has been demonstrated more clearly than for pigs. In a study comparing demand for periods of 3 minutes of partial social contact (head contact through metal bars) or full social contact, Holm *et al.* (2002) reported strong demand for both types of contact, particularly when account was taken of the amount of time actually spent engaged in social activity. Other work has investigated the lying requirements of heifers allowed either 6 h or 9 h per day free lying time. The price of access to lie down for additional periods was assessed using variations in the number of panel presses required, and variations in reward duration of between 20 and 80 min. The experiment gave consistent results. Heifers showed an inelastic demand to lie down for some 12–13 h per 24 h (Jensen *et al.*, 2005). The relative importance of lying behaviour is also revealed in a study that manipulated 'income' rather than 'expenditure' by progressively reducing the amount of time that cows could allocate between lying, eating and social contact. As the pressure on allocated time to these three activities intensified, the cows generally increased the proportion of time spent lying at the expense of other activities (Munksgaard *et al.*, 2005), although they were partially able to compensate for reduced feeding time by increasing their rate of eating.

2.2.4.7 Interim conclusions and unresolved issues

One of the interesting things about the growing body of work on farm animal motivation and behavioural priorities is that patterns are at last beginning to emerge. Behaviours that are concerned with essential body maintenance and function, such as eating, resting and stretching, are largely controlled by internal processes. The motivation to do these behaviours increases when performance is prevented by constraints of space or lack of resources. Rebounds in activity (or inactivity and rest) are observed when constraints are removed and animals will work hard and consistently for access to food, for places to rest and lie down, and for sufficient space to stretch and exercise. A few other behaviours, notably the nesting behaviour of hens and farrowing behaviour of sows, appear to share this general profile.

Despite this growing evidence base, in many countries farm animals are still kept under conditions of extreme spatial confinement where physical health is poor and behavioural priorities ignored. After decades of argument and scientific debate in Europe this situation is gradually changing. In 1999 Directive 1999/74/EC setting down minimum standards for the protection of laying hens required the phasing out of conventional cages by 2012. The scientific evidence base that led to this ground-breaking legislative change included evidence that severe spatial restriction caused disuse osteoporosis and increased susceptibility to fractures. But behavioural evidence that hens in conventional cages could not perform simple movements, that they preferred and would work for more space, and that nesting, foraging and perching behaviours were all priorities was also highly influential, as documented in reviews published by the European Food Safety Authority in 2005 and by the LayWel consortium (www.laywel.eu). Veal crates for calves were also banned throughout the EU in 2007, following a review by the standing veterinary committee which considered (among many other issues) the behavioural evidence that calves are strongly motivated to exercise and to form social contacts.

Assessing behavioural priorities using economic demand techniques cannot answer all questions about animal welfare. Behaviours such as dust-bathing, exploration and social interaction generally appear to be strongly influenced by the presence or absence of the appropriate external stimuli, and by factors such as animals' familiarity with the environment and each other. Where formal demand experiments have been conducted to try and assess the importance of these behaviours, it has not been easy to demonstrate that they are necessities or even that, in some cases, they matter very much at all. Before drawing this final conclusion we should, however, consider whether the methodology used in demand experiments is perhaps less suited to assessing the importance of some behaviours (social interaction, exploration) than others (feeding, stretching). In these experiments, rewards are usually allocated in bite-sized chunks. Repeated short periods of access to increased space may permit stretching behaviour, but not satisfactory social interaction, thereby inadvertently diminishing the value of a social reward. Indeed, if the importance of social relationships is assessed in the field, by examining how animals re-prioritize their time budgets as constraints increase, then we can see clear evidence that some primate species conserve time spent in social interactions at the expense of time spent resting (Dunbar and Dunbar, 1988). Another factor that has not yet been taken into sufficient account is consideration of the identity of the companion that the test animal works with. Humans will travel around the world to visit close friends and relations, but may cross the street to avoid unpleasant neighbours. Farmed mammals are no less discerning. They have preferred companions, their maternal–offspring and family relationships are particularly strong, they pay attention to, and learn from, some companions and not others, so their demand for social contact may be highly variable. Such social niceties must be considered.

Experimental designs should also take account of the animals' perceptual abilities and cognitive constraints. There is evidence, for example, that behavioural priorities can be influenced by whether or not the animal can see the resource it is working to obtain (Warburton and Mason, 2003) and it has long been debated whether farm animals are sufficiently 'clever' to weigh up the longer-term consequences of their choices. Encouragingly, recent research shows that most birds and mammals possess an object 'permanence' ability, a form of spatial memory which allows them to appreciate that an object still exists, even when it has moved out of sight (Freire *et al.*, 2004) (Figure 2.5).

Other recent work on the cognitive abilities of the domestic fowl provides evidence that they are able to make rational choices, at least under tightly controlled experimental conditions. Experiments have shown, for example, that chickens are able to 'plan ahead' and forego a small immediate food reward in order to obtain a delayed but larger reward (Abeyesinghe *et al.*, 2005). So they can consider the short-term future consequences of their actions. This background work gives us some confidence that choices in experimental situations involve integration of information about possible outcomes, and are not simply instinctive reactions to immediate stimuli, but much more work on the cognitive abilities of farm animals is needed to ensure that we ask them sensible questions in sensible ways. Work to establish the

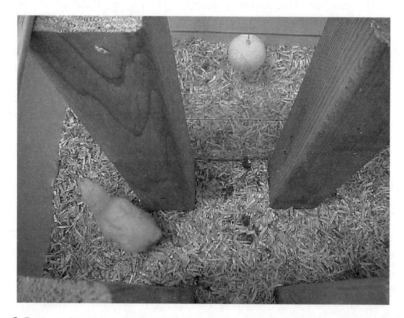

Figure 2.5 Spatial memory in chicks. In this experiment the chick desires to stand next to the yellow tennis ball on which it has been imprinted. The Perspex screen prevents the chick walking straight towards the ball, instead it must take a detour during which time the ball is momentarily out of sight. The ability to solve this task is influenced by the complexity of the rearing environment (Freire *et al.*, 2004).

importance placed by animals on using their cognitive abilities *per se* has not even begun.

The outcome of economic demand tests can vary depending on factors such as whether the animal pays the cost for a resource on entry or exit, its duration of access to a resource, whether it is interrupted during its use of the resource gained, whether it is tested individually or in a group, and its previous experiences. In preference tests, the precise choices on offer and the combination of alternatives that are available may also influence the animals' decisions. This is not an argument against using preference tests and demand procedures, as similar contextual variables almost certainly influence every other welfare indicator we can think of, but it does mean that the experimental design needs to be carefully considered. Even more importantly, new methods of assessing behavioural priorities in real and relevant farming or commercial environments need to be developed. Some aspects of formal experimental design may have to be sacrificed to establish behavioural priorities under on-farm conditions, but it will nonetheless be useful to know something about animals' cost–benefit trade-offs and decisions in the real world, to use alongside economic measures obtained in the laboratory.

Demand experiments cannot answer the difficult question of whether animals 'miss' resources that are currently out of sight (or out of the perceptual range of any other sense organs) or that have never been experienced, and so it could be argued that strong demand in an experiment may be an artefact of the experimental situation itself. Economic demand methodologies rely on the animal gaining some experience of the resource that they are working for, either during training or testing. Methods of assessing whether animals are deprived are considered later in this chapter.

A question that is more easily answered is whether farm animals need to perform goal-directed behaviours if they are simply provided with the end-goal itself. There is no one answer to this question, as it seems to vary between species and resource. Thus, hens and sows continue to build nests even if they are given a perfect pre-formed nest. Similarly, mice spend the same amount of time burrowing when provided with peat or with a previously constructed burrow, but gerbils show a notably reduced motivation to dig if a pre-formed burrow is provided. For these reasons, nest-building in sows is sometimes described as a behavioural need, unlike the digging behaviour of gerbils.

Despite our growing certainty that we can ask animals some questions in a way that they are able to answer, it is certainly not clear that chickens, or any other farm animal, would be capable of weighing up the longer-term implications of choosing, say, between living in a free-range system over an indoor system.

2.2.5 Adaptability, allostasis and learning

If we are to use behaviour as an indicator of welfare we have to acknowledge that animals that have been domesticated, and are by nature adaptable and flexible. There will be a range of environments that could potentially provide good welfare, not just one ideal system of housing. The degree of flexibility possessed by domestic animals is highlighted by a reconsideration of those individuals living feral lives. Occasionally, the environments in which feral populations live differ so profoundly from either the evolved environment or current farming systems that their adaptability seems truly amazing. Feral pigs have adapted so well to some tropical regions of Australia that they cause significant damage to native bird and reptile populations. They seem to specialize on a diet of turtles – not something that they would have encountered frequently during their evolution in European forests. From a different part of the world, come anecdotal reports that feral dogs in Moscow can negotiate the underground system and use traffic lights as cues to cross busy streets (Schoofs, 2008).

It is thus absolutely clear that our domestic animals may be able to thrive in a relatively wide range of environments. This is recognized in the concept of allostasis, the idea of 'stability through change' (Korte *et al.*, 2007). Good animal welfare is characterized within this framework as a broad capacity to anticipate and deal with environmental challenges, and it predicts that farm animals will be able to adapt within a relatively broad range of situations. Barnard (2007) similarly argued that so long as animals are free to make trade-offs and decisions on their own adaptive terms then even situations which superficially appear to be stressful will not cause suffering. If the animal has entered willingly into the situation and has the resources to deal with it, then all will be well. The capacity to adapt may be what is most crucial for animal welfare.

In behavioural terms, adaptability arises through developmental experiences and the capacity to learn. The degree to which initial reactions to stimuli can be modified by learning is a critical component in the animal's ability to cope with many modern housing systems, and learning can sometimes shift an animal's preferences and aversions. A novel noise, for example, may be initially experienced as frightening or unpleasant, but the animal may learn that there really is nothing to fear.

Habituation is a process whereby animals learn not to react with innate responses (such as flight or attack) to stimuli that are functionally irrelevant. Habituation is stimulus-specific (the animals will continue to react as before to new stimuli – they are not simply becoming fatigued) and occurs most rapidly if the animal is exposed to the irrelevant stimulus repeatedly with short intervals between exposures. Habituation to the presence of people is perhaps the most useful adaptation of farm animals, as well as for wild animals forced into ever-closer proximity with human visitors and tourists. It is crucial to appreciate that habituation takes place *only* to stimuli that are irrelevant. Animals will not habituate to aversive stimuli such as rough handling by humans, or excessive noise, such as encountered in some milking parlours. On the other hand, the effects of habituation can persist through generations. Quail raised by human-habituated mothers do not become generally less fearful, but they do show a specific reduction in fear of humans.

The converse of habituation is sensitization, a process whereby animals react more intensely to stimuli that they have encountered repeatedly. In most farming systems this is not a good thing, particularly if the reaction is one of fear or pain. It is well established that exposure to acute pain can result in later chronic sensitization or hyperalgesia. This requires recognition of the fact that early life experience can have a major effect on later reactivity thresholds. In mammals, the high turnover of neural connections during early growth of the brain allows a much greater degree of plasticity than is possible in later life, so early exposure to stress or pain can have profound effects on stress, pain and behavioural responses throughout life. Farm animals, such as sheep and pigs, are routinely subjected to painful husbandry procedures (e.g. tail-docking, castration) soon after birth, which can permanently alter their threshold responses to pain in later life. So, not only are such mutilations a cause for concern on welfare grounds at the time, but for many months or even years afterwards.

Habituation and sensitization generally involve innate responses that have not been established through any process of associative learning. But associative learning is the other major way in which animals can adapt to their environments. The learning abilities of farm animal species and horses have been well reviewed (e.g. Mendl and Nicol, 2009) and common examples of learning within farming systems abound – the use of electric fencing, electronic sow feeders and robotic milking systems all depend on the ability of animals to learn by trial and error. As always, the influence of mothers on their offspring is a crucial component of this type of learning. Lambs, for example, show a more prolonged tendency to avoid unsafe feeding sites avoided by their mothers, than if they rely purely on their own experience.

There will of course be limits on the adaptive abilities of farm animals. Animals have little flexibility in their need to perform priority behaviours so most farm animals will not be able to adapt to environments that provide no social contact or foraging materials. They may also struggle to adapt to practices such as early weaning, or even to environments that provide them with little opportunity to make choices and exert some degree of control over events. Failure to adapt may be immediately obvious or detectable only by subtle signs. To explore this further, the next section of the chapter considers how behaviour can be used as a general welfare indicator.

2.3 Behaviours as Welfare Indicators

Animal behaviour can provide a highly sensitive indicator of animal welfare. Against a background of constantly shifting internal state, and variable external environment, an animal must integrate all inputs and produce just one behavioural output at any given time. Very subtle shifts in internal state or external circumstances can therefore produce observable changes in the type of behaviour performed, or the overall structure or patterning of behaviours over time. This section will review the types of behavioural changes that may be diagnostic of the occurrence of pain or disease, and then those changes that seem to accompany situations where animals are severely or chronically frustrated in their attempts to adapt.

2.3.1 Behavioural signs of disease and pain

The most obvious way in which animal behaviour can contribute to our understanding of welfare is when behavioural signs of disease or pain are the first or most obvious manifestation of a problem. Expert veterinary clinical examination of an animal for signs of pain or disease is based on a combination of clinical signs (such as fever, inflammation and pain) and behavioural changes (such as lameness, apathy and loss of appetite).

Even early-stage infections or the initial onset of a progressive chronic condition will force a reallocation of physiological resources and reserves. In such situations, priority behaviours will be defended but behaviours that matter less (such as exploration) may be reduced or cease entirely. This has been shown in studies where mice developing early signs of Huntington's disease stopped using cage enrichments such as ropes and climbing equipment earlier than their cage-mates.

Careful experimental design can also identify which vocalizations are reliable signals of pain. For example, although restraint alone prompts a great deal of vocalization in piglets, calls occur more frequently when piglets are castrated, compared with uncastrated controls (Figure 2.6), or with piglets given analgesics. During the actual castration period, the mix of high frequency ($>1000\,\text{Hz}$) calls given in response to restraint changes to a less variable $3000\,\text{Hz}$ shriek (Figure 2.7).

Paradoxically, if a large number of farm animals are affected with chronically painful conditions, particularly inflammatory conditions such as mastitis in cows, or leg and foot disorders in cows, sheep and broiler chickens, farmers or others in daily contact with these animals may regard behaviours indicative of pain as almost normal. This can significantly hamper attempts to motivate farmers or veterinarians

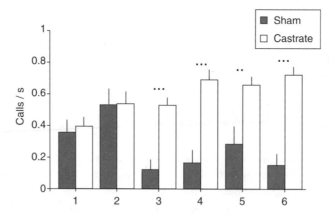

Figure 2.6 Effects of handling and castration on the frequency of vocalisation in piglets. The x-axis presents the different stages of the castration procedure. During stages 1 and 2, pigs from the castration and sham groups were restrained and the scrotal area was washed. During stages 3 to 6 the castration group of pigs experienced incision of the scrotum and severance of the spermatic cords (Taylor and Weary, 2000). Used with permission from Elsevier.

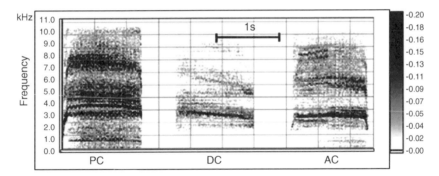

Figure 2.7 Calls during castration are purer than calls in the pre-handling and post-surgical phase. High-frequency calls given by a piglet during pre-castration handling (PC), during castration (DC) and after castration (PC). During the painful DC period, the frequency range of the call is reduced (Puppe *et al.*, 2005). Used with permission from Elsevier.

to change management or treatment practices (Whay, 2007). Studies have repeatedly shown that, despite rigorous culling practices designed to remove the worst affected birds, more than 25% of broiler chickens have difficulty walking (Knowles *et al.*, 2008), at least in the last few weeks of their lives, as they approach slaughter weight. This figure has changed little since the early 1990s, suggesting that eradicating the problem of lameness has not been a priority for the meat industry. It has even been argued that limping is not a reliable indicator of pain in birds, because they may not be capable of feeling pain. Under this view, limping is regarded as a nociceptive response (analogous with the human ability to remove a hand from a hot flame *before* feeling any sensation). In humans, the feeling of burning is experienced just moments later, but it is possible that bird brains are different. Although birds show protective avoidance responses, perhaps they never experience the subsequent *feeling* of pain. This may sound unlikely, but it is a view held by some distinguished scientists and philosophers, and experiments that show that decerebrate chickens are quite capable of limping, only add to the controversy. So it is important to know what sort of evidence might be required to show that an animal is able to feel pain. A promising approach is to see whether animals such as chickens can learn to control their own pain by self-administering analgesics (pain-killing drugs). Initial work suggests that chickens may be able to do this, showing that some aspects of their pain experience must be experienced by central parts of the brain, but there is much more to do in this area and, meanwhile, the problem of endemic lameness in meat chickens persists.

2.3.2 Behavioural signs of frustration and deprivation

An emotional state of frustration can arise when animals are highly motivated to perform a specific behaviour but are unable to do so because of the presence of physical barriers or other constraints blocking access to key resources. One of the earliest aims of applied animal ethology was to identify and characterize behavioural signs of frustration or thwarting in experimental situations, and then to see whether animals in commercial housing conditions showed the same signs. If they did, it was argued, then this would provide evidence of poor welfare. Early experiments showed that birds thwarted from accessing food, by covering food with a clear plastic cover, increased their pacing and preening behaviour. And indeed, increased pacing is typically observed in hens that lack a nest-site, indicating that they are frustrated prior to egg-laying. One problem, though, is that some of the most restrictive housing systems (conventional cages for hens, veal crates for calves) will prevent not just priority behaviours, but also behaviours indicative of frustration. The battery hen cannot fly, and she cannot pace to indicate her frustration.

Animals may also experience an emotional state in response to deprivation, the total absence of key resources. Examining whether animals are deprived presents a difficult conundrum as the resource of interest has to remain absent during the experiment. Attempts have been made to assess how hard deprived animals will work to perform searching behaviour, as this could provide evidence that animals 'miss' things that are absent from their environments. There is, for example, some evidence that voluntary wheel-running in caged rodents occurs more frequently in animals deprived of key resources, as if the rodents were searching for the missing resource. Similar experiments show that hens deprived of food or a litter substrate also appear to perform more exploratory behaviour, but it is difficult to demonstrate unequivocally that the animals have a specific representation of a resource goal. Recent work showing that devaluation procedures can be adapted to examine whether rats expect specific or general rewards provide a possible way forward for animal welfare researchers (Burke *et al.*, 2008).

2.3.3 Stereotypies and redirected behaviours

Stereotypies and redirected behaviours are often regarded as reliable indicators of poor welfare. They are often described as abnormal, although this rather vague term is used to describe a real hotch-potch of different behaviours. Not all abnormal behaviours do in fact indicate welfare problems. The rapid preening or grooming that can suddenly occur during an aggressive encounter, and which can look inappropriate to a human onlooker, are fleeting indications that the animal is some form of motivational conflict, unsure whether to approach or retreat. But this indecision is temporary and the problem soon resolved. This section will therefore focus on two categories of behaviour that are highly relevant when considering farm animal welfare – first, redirected behaviours which are normal activities redirected towards an unusual or inappropriate substrates, and second, stereotypic behaviours, which are repetitive, and highly invariant patterns of behaviour that develop in response to severe frustration.

2.3.3.1 Redirected behaviours

Redirected behaviours are not necessarily indicators of poor welfare for the animals performing them – it probably does not matter for the welfare of a horse whether it

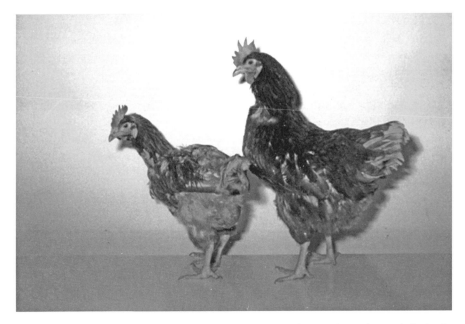

Figure 2.8 The consequences of normal foraging behaviour that is redirected towards the feathers of a conspecific. The pecked bird experiences pain as feathers are removed, and a subsequent increased risk of disease. Thermal insulation is also lost, reducing overall production performance.

ingests fibre from a rotting branch of a tree, or from an expensive wooden fence (although clearly it may matter to the owner of the horse). However, if animals redirect their normal foraging behaviour towards their companions then severe welfare problems can arise for the recipients, which are all too often other pigs or chickens. Redirected pecking in hens (Figure 2.8) results in the loss of feathers from the recipient birds, skin injuries and even cannibalism, and this is a surprisingly prevalent problem with over 55% of UK farmers reporting pecking in their free-range flocks. The behaviour has not been observed in red jungle-fowl, indicating that it arises in captive environments that do not provide a full range of foraging materials, or where access to areas to forage is restricted or difficult. It is possible to selectively breed for and against the behaviour, although a systematic approach to this has not yet been taken. Steps to reduce the problem therefore depend on improving the birds' management and husbandry, with studies showing that the problem can be significantly reduced if free-range hens are encouraged to make more use of the outdoor range.

Outbreaks of tail-biting on pig farms can similarly result in severe welfare problems including infections, abscesses, paralysis and even death. Many farmers tail-dock newborn piglets in an attempt to prevent tail-biting but this is a painful and rather ineffective strategy. Again, management strategies that permit piglets greater foraging opportunities provide a better solution on all counts.

2.3.3.2 *Stereotypies*

More has been written about stereotypies than any other type of putative behavioural indicator of welfare, but interpretation of these behaviour patterns is far from
straightforward. Stereotypic behaviour patterns have been described as repetitive,
invariant and apparently functionless (Mason 1991), and classic examples include
pacing in confined zoo animals, bar-biting in sows or weaning and crib-biting in
stabled horses. Most stereotypies develop under conditions of frustrated motivation.
An animal may wish to escape from a cage or other enclosure but be unable to do so.
The original source behaviour pattern, a perfectly normal action that might lead to
escape in a natural environment, becomes repeated over and over again, developing
an increasingly fixed or unvarying appearance and pattern. This general developmental story has been verified by many different experiments, including innovative
work showing that mice direct most of their bar-biting at cage doors which have
previously provided exit opportunities (Nevison *et al.*, 1999) (Figure 2.9).

It is usually obvious that the source behaviour pattern of locomotor stereotypies is
an attempt to escape from an enclosure, but the causation of mouth-based or oral
stereotypies has remained much more obscure. A clearer picture of the factors
involved in the development of oral stereotypies is gradually emerging, and tends to
support the idea that the source behaviour pattern for these stereotypies also
represents an attempt to cope with adversity. Previous suggestions that crib-biting
in horses is caused either by boredom or by stress are not well supported by recent
evidence, which strongly implicates feeding practices instead. The risk of crib-biting
is increased by feeding a low forage or high-grain diet, such that the onset of crib-
biting may be an adaptive attempt to deal with the uncomfortable digestive consequences of the wrong diet (Nicol *et al.*, 2002). Crib-biting could be performed

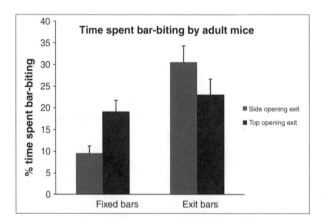

Figure 2.9 Demonstration of stereotypic behaviour in mice. Mice, given the opportunity to exit
their cage through side or top openings when young, subsequently directed more of their stereotypic
bar-biting towards these areas of the cage as adults. The effect was most marked with side-opening
cage doors, with top-opening doors being more difficult to access (Nevison *et al.*, 1999). Used with
permission from Elsevier.

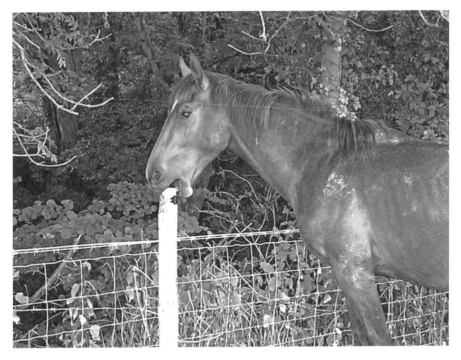

Figure 2.10 Stereotypic behaviour in a young horse. This horse was kept with other horses and cattle in a 10 ha field. It has never been confined in a stable and so it is difficult to argue that it is bored. It is, however, regularly fed large amounts of grain-based rations by its well-intentioned owner.

initially as a response to pain, as it results in a small release of saliva which may partially alleviate gut acidity problems. However, crib-biting (Figure 2.10), like other stereotypic behaviours, develops its repetitive and invariant nature precisely because the animal's reasonable response to the consequences of the wrong diet does *not* fully succeed in resolving the problem.

The initial frustration of the animal that leads to stereotypy development is itself a serious source of poor welfare, but most debate has centred on whether established stereotypies can be regarded as reliable indicators of welfare (Mason and Latham, 2004). The arguments hinge on two issues: (1) whether the development of an established stereotypy allows the animal to cope better with a suboptimal environment than do its non-stereotypic companions; and (2) whether established stereotypies reflect current welfare state at all, or are simply persistent behavioural 'scars' of previous frustration.

Whether or not stereotypies help animals cope with the adversity of the eliciting environment has been a controversial question in applied ethology. Some researchers have found that stereotypies in laboratory animals reduce stress or aversion to a barren environment, but others have failed to find such stress-reducing effects. Oral stereotypies in horses show a rebound in performance after a period of prevention, indicating that these stereotypies may have a functional role, but stereotypic wire-gnawing in mice shows no such rebound. To make sense of this conflicting evidence there is a great need for longitudinal studies that examine baseline differences in stress responding in animals before they do, or do not, develop stereotypies. Without this background it is impossible to know whether stereotypic animals were more or less stressed than their companions even before they developed the abnormal behaviour.

Mason and Latham (2004) suggest that, for stereotypy to be used as an indicator of welfare, it will be important to check that non-stereotypic animals are not faring worse than stereotypic animals housed in the same environment. An environment that gives rise to stereotypic animals can be regarded with great suspicion, as it is likely to be causing severe frustration in some way, and therefore resulting in poor animal welfare. But we cannot assume, without checking using other measures, that it is the stereotypic animals in that environment that are suffering most. The performance of the stereotypy may actually have some benefits, if only in increasing exercise levels. Moreover, steps taken to prevent the appearance of the stereotypy (including surgical operations, electric shock collars) can result in worse welfare outcomes than allowing the stereotypy to persist.

2.3.4 Behavioural signs of good health and contentment

Good welfare is more than simply the absence of negative feelings that may accompany states of pain, fear or frustration, and so scientists have begun to look

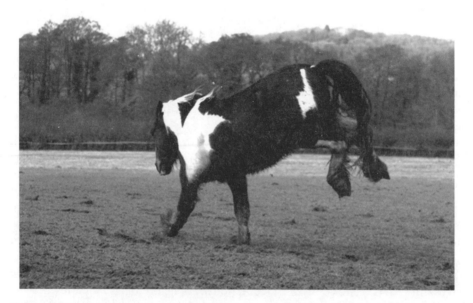

Figure 2.11   Positive welfare. Luxury behaviour in an unconfined animal.

for the presence of behaviours that indicate contentment and pleasure (Figure 2.11). In some ways this may be a question of semantics. Because we can never fully experience the subjective feelings of another species we cannot know, for example, at what point something we label contentment might be experienced as something we might label boredom. However, there are good reasons to suppose that animals show signs of pleasure in anticipation of reward or if the reward that arrives is larger or more appetising than expected, with such signs including increased activity and, in pigs at least, frequent behavioural transitions between different play activities.

In general, behaviours that are thought to be associated with pleasurable feelings include play behaviour, affiliative behaviour, allo-grooming (reciprocal grooming between companions) and exploration. All of these behaviours are, in a sense, luxury activities. They demand time and energy and yet do not result in immediate practical benefit. Their benefits are longer-term and they are often the first activities to be lost from the repertoire when conditions get difficult. Correspondingly, their appearance in the animals' repertoire may be a reliable indicator that conditions are not too tough.

Other possible indicators of good welfare include certain vocalizations produced in rewarding situations. The scientific study of this possibility has so far mostly involved rats, where short ultrasonic chirps are shown during play, sex or even tickling by a human (Panksepp and Burgdorf, 2003). However the notion cannot have escaped the mind of any cat owner when stroking their purring pet.

2.4 Animals as Individuals

Much of the literature on farm animal behaviour and welfare considers animals as if they were identical group members. Solutions to housing or management problems are proposed that are based on a hypothetical average animal. In reality, it is quite obvious that even genetically similar animals are individuals, possibly with different coping styles or personalities, but certainly with their own unique social and environmental preferences. Solutions that work for the average animal may therefore fail dismally to cater for the individual. Nowhere is this more apparent than when the *social* environment suits some individuals but not others.

2.4.1 Social environment

Many animals benefit from group living. In the right circumstances, the benefits can include protection from predators as group members share the costs of vigilance, insulation from extremes of weather as group members huddle or crowd together, and greatly increased chances of finding food or killing prey. To live in a group the advantages must, on average, outweigh the disadvantages of increased competition, conspicuousness and risks of disease transmission. Simply living in an aggregation, where no social relationships are formed between group members (imagine a fly within a cloud of other flies, or a jellyfish within a large drifting shoal) can confer these benefits. But, in mammals especially, group living involves the formation of social relationships and preferential interactions with certain companions.

Social factors are powerful modulators of both stress response and immune functions and so an animal's social position within a group may be one of the most important determinants of its welfare. In humans, social stress is one of the strongest risk factors for depression and anxiety, and in animals social stress leads to related changes in anxiety, brain structure and survival. Social stress is a recurring factor in the lives of almost all mammals, and conflict in particular can *profoundly* reduce the animal's ability to cope with a variety of environmental challenges. There may be almost nothing worse than being in a bad social situation and being unable to get away.

A striking example of the social difficulties faced by a minority of individuals is the presence of 'pariah' birds within flocks of hens. These birds are repeatedly attacked by other birds and tend to shelter under any cover they can find for prolonged periods of time, foregoing food and water intake until the last possible moment. These pariah birds have significantly reduced welfare by almost any measure. Thus, although a non-cage barn or free-range system provides better welfare than a cage for the majority of birds, the welfare of the pariah birds is severely compromised.

Even in less extreme situations, different individuals will have divergent social needs. It has not been easy to demonstrate experimentally that animals value social contact, and yet this may be because the nature of the social contact (who one spends time with) may be more important than the quantity of social contact *per se*. Although it is quite clear that animals can discriminate amongst familiar individuals, experiments on the value of social contact tend not to consider whether animals prefer some individuals over others, just whether they prefer social contact over no social contact. Good social relationships with preferred partners can provide social support, increasing adaptive capacity, reducing anxiety and probably producing feelings of great pleasure. Perhaps the strongest social bond of all is that between the mother and her offspring. Again, this is highly selective – the mother essentially falls in love with her own offspring and not just young animals in general. In mammals, this strong attachment is formed during parturition and lactation, processes associated with the release of high concentrations of oxytocin. Indeed, in some species it has been shown that individual differences in the density of oxytocin receptors in the brain's reward areas are correlated with differences in the level of maternal care shown. When the mother and infant are close then stress levels are low, but separation results in extreme anxiety. Despite this, early weaning is a very common, and often unquestioned, practice in Western agricultural systems. Many studies have documented the severe effects of weaning on infants, but the effects on the mothers are also now beginning to be appreciated. It may seem a distant goal, but systems that allow mothers and infants to stay together are now being developed (Hepola *et al.*, 2007).

2.4.2 Predictability and control

Different animals may have divergent preferences and individual animals may not want the same thing all of the time. In our recent work, it has been shown that apparently identical commercial laying hens chose different living environments. Birds with consistently worse feather damage, longer latencies to approach novel objects and higher corticosterone concentrations were more likely to choose wire-floored environments than other types of birds, which tended to prefer wood shavings. Because different individuals, even of genetically similar commercial strains, may have quite different environmental preferences, it may be difficult to provide a uniform housing environment that suits all animals. One possible solution is to consider providing more opportunities for animals to exercise control and to make their own choices. In natural conditions animals have a high degree of control over their diet selection, social companions and degree of activity. A controllable event is, by nature, also predictable, and both these features are important for good welfare. In captivity much of the capacity for control is removed. A lack of control over the timing or termination of an aversive event is accompanied by increased levels of physiological stress, reduced general activity, interference with learning and higher fear levels. This is demonstrated by experiments that give a treatment group control over the arrival or termination of an aversive stimulus, while a second group is linked or 'yoked' to the treatment group. Both groups receive physically identical reinforcement, but individuals within the treatment group retain control over events, while the yoked individuals have no control. The stress responses of animals with control can be lower than both yoked animals *and* animals that never even experience the aversive stimulus. The benefits of control can also be demonstrated by observing the effects of its removal: chickens trained to control their own food delivery react with frustration calls when that control is removed (Zimmerman and Koene, 1998), and pigs become aggressive when previously reliable signals of food arrival become unreliable.

Stimuli do not have to be inherently aversive for similar effects to occur. Greiveldinger *et al.* (2007) examined the effects of dropping a patterned panel suddenly into a pen of lambs. Lambs able to predict the arrival of the panel, by the use of a light cue signalling its arrival, showed lowered startle and cardiac responses and spent more time feeding than lambs given no prior signals. The use of classical conditioning to reduce stress responses in farm animals is used routinely, for example, when stockpersons knock on the door of a chicken shed before entering to avoid startling them, but the benefits of providing predictability and control should be more widely considered.

The benefits of control do not have to be provided with complex pieces of operant apparatus. Providing varied environments, with gradations in temperature, light, substrate type and areas where animals can congregate or avoid social contact will provide for the varied preferences and needs of different individuals, and will provide the benefits of control *per se*. Such environments may also present opportunities for problem-solving, thereby allowing animals to make better use of their cognitive abilities.

2.5 Good Husbandry

The ground covered in this chapter has shown that farm animal housing should adhere to the following principles:

1. The performance of all behaviours that are motivated largely by internal cues should be permitted. Behaviours such as feeding, simple comfort movements and self-grooming need to be performed in any environment. The desire to do these behaviours cannot be alleviated simply by altering the environment.

2. The performance of behaviours that can be shown to be priorities in the captive environment of interest should be permitted. These may be behaviours that are triggered by the external cues prevailing in that environment, or behaviours that are motivated by a complex interaction of internal and external cues. The point is that performance of the priority behaviour is important to the animal – it is willing to expend time and energy or to forgo other opportunities to do these behaviours. Foraging and nesting behaviours are good examples.

3. Sounds, smells or other stimuli that are highly aversive should be avoided, unless they are truly harmless, in which case the animals can realistically be expected to adapt after repeated exposure.

4. An appropriate social environment should be provided, ensuring that strong social attachments are not disrupted.

5. Animals should be observed frequently and carefully by attentive and well-trained stockpeople. If the behavioural repertoire of the animals narrows at any point, so that only the highest priority behaviours are observed, it will be worth checking for signs of pain or disease. Conversely, a broad behavioural repertoire that includes lower-priority behaviours such as play and exploration is a reasonably good indicator that the animals are essentially healthy and that they are adapting to the environment provided.

6. Finally, it should be recognized both that animals are individuals and that they are, within limits, adaptable and flexible. It is a mistake to think that good welfare will therefore be provided by just one type of housing. Opportunities for animals to make choices and exert some degree of control over their environment will therefore be of great importance.

Growing numbers of farmers are embracing the idea that good welfare is more than just good health. Many farmers provide much higher welfare standards for their animals than are required under current legislation. Consumers benefit from knowing that the produce they purchase has been assured by independent inspectors such as, in the UK, those employed by the RSPCA Freedom Food assurance scheme (www .rspca.org.uk). Groups such as the Farm Animal Initiative (www.modelfarmproject .org) are going one step further and have established productive model farms that explicitly and systematically avoid the need for practices such as early weaning, while providing opportunities for the animals to perform priority behaviours. At the same time, supermarkets and other retailers are responding to public demand by offering improved contracts and premium prices to farming systems more sympathetic to these broad concepts of animal welfare. This is discussed in more detail in Chapter 18.

References and Further Reading

Abeyesinghe, S.M., Wathes, C.M., Nicol, C.J. and Randall, J.M. (2001) The aversion of broiler chickens to concurrent vibrational and thermal stressors. *Applied Animal Behaviour Science* 73, 199–215.

Abeyesinghe, S.M., Nicol, C.J., Hartnell, S.J. and Wathes, C.M. (2005) Can domestic fowl show self-control? *Animal Behaviour* 70, 1–11.

Barnard, C. (2007) Ethical regulation and animal science: why animal behaviour is special. *Animal Behaviour* 74, 5–13.

Beattie, V.E., Walker, N. and Sneddon, I.A. (1998) Preference testing of substrates by growing pigs. *Animal Welfare* 7, 27–34.

Brambell Committee (1965) *Report of the Technical Committee to Enquire into the Welfare of Animals Kept Under Intensive Livestock Husbandry.* HMSO, London.

Burke, K.A., Franz, T.M., Miller, D.N. and Schoenbaum, G. (2008) The role of the orbitofrontal cortex in the pursuit of happiness and more specific rewards. *Nature* 454, 340–4.

Chambers, L.K., Singleton, G.R. and Krebs, C.J. (2000) Movements and social organization of wild house mice (*Mus domesticus*) in the wheatlands of northwestern Victoria, Australia. *Journal of Mammalogy,* 81, 59–69.

Dawkins, M.S. (1983) Battery hens name their price: consumer demand theory and the measurement of ethological needs. *Animal Behaviour* 31, 1195–205.

Dunbar, R.I.M. and Dunbar, P. (1988) Maternal time budgets of Gelada baboons. *Animal Behaviour* 36, 970–80.

Duncan, I.J.H., Savory, C.J. and Wood-Gush, D.G.M. (1978) Observations on the reproductive behaviour of domestic fowl in the wild. *Applied Animal Ethology* 4, 29–42.

Freire, R., Cheng, H.W. and Nicol, C.J. (2004) Development of spatial memory in occlusion-experienced domestic chicks. *Animal Behaviour* 67, 141–50.

Greiveldinger, L., Veissier, I. and Boissy, A. (2007) Emotional experience in sheep: predictability of a sudden event lowers subsequent emotional responses. *Physiology & Behaviour* 92, 675–83.

Hepola, H., Raussi, S., Veissier, I., Pursiainen, P., Ikkelajarvi, K., Saloniemi, H. and Syrjala-Qvist, L. (2007) Five or eight weeks of restricted suckling: influence on dairy calves' feed intake, growth and suckling behaviour. *Acta Agriculturae Scandinavica (Animal Science)* 57, 121–8.

Holm, L., Jensen, M.B. and Jeppesen, L.L. (2002) Calves' motivation for access to two different types of social contact measured by operant conditioning. *Applied Animal Behaviour Science* 79, 175–94.

Jensen, M.B. (1999) Effects of confinement on rebounds of locomotor behaviour of calves and heifers, and the spatial preferences of calves. *Applied Animal Behaviour Science* 62, 43–56.

Jensen, M.B., Pedersen, L.J. and Munksgaard, L. (2005) The effect of reward duration on demand functions for rest in dairy heifers and lying requirements as measured by demand functions. *Applied Animal Behaviour Science* 90, 207–17.

Jensen, P. (2006) Domestication: from behaviour to genes and back again. *Applied Animal Behaviour Science* 97, 3–15.

Jensen, P. (ed.) (2009) *The Ethology of Domestic Animals: An Introductory Text*, 2nd edn. CABI Publishing, Wallingford.

Jones, E.K.M., Wathes, C.A. and Webster, A.J.F. (2005) Avoidance of atmospheric ammonia by domestic fowl and the effect of early experience. *Applied Animal Behaviour Science* **90**, 293–308.

Kendrick, K.M., da Costa, A.P., Leigh, A.E., Hinton, M.R. and Peirce, J.W. (2001) Sheep don't forget a face. *Nature* **414**, 165–6.

Kendrick, K.M., da Costa, A.P., Leigh, A.E., Hinton, M.R. and Peirce, J.W. (2007) Sheep don't forget a face (correction to Nature **414**, 165, 2001). *Nature* **447**, 346.

Kirkden, R.D. and Pajor, E.A. (2006) Motivation for group housing in gestating sows. *Animal Welfare* **15**, 119–30.

Knowles, T.G., Kestin, S.C., Haslam, S.M., Brown, S.N., Green, L.E., Butterworth, A., Pope, S.J., Pfeiffer, D. and Nicol, C.J. (2008) Leg disorders in broiler chickens: prevalence, risk factors and prevention. *PloS One* **3** (2), e1545.

Korte, S.M., Olivier, B. and Koolhaas, J.M. (2007) A new animal welfare concept based on allostasis. *Physiology & Behavior* **92**, 422–8.

Lawrence, A.B., Appleby, M.C., Illius, A.W. and Macleod, H.A. (1989) Measuring hunger in the pig using operant-conditioning: the effect of dietary bulk. *Animal Production* **48**, 213–20.

Mason, G.J. (1991) Stereotypies: – a critical review. *Animal Behaviour* **41**, 1015–37.

Mason, G.J., McFarland, D. and Garner, J. (1998) A demanding task: using economic techniques to assess animal priorities. *Animal Behaviour* **55**, 1071–5.

Mason, G.J. and Latham, N.R. (2004) Can't stop, won't stop: is stereotypy a reliable animal welfare indicator? *Animal Welfare* **13**, S57–S69.

Matthews, L.R. and Ladewig, J. (1994) Environmental requirements of pigs measured by behavioral demand-functions. *Animal Behaviour* **47**, 713–19.

Mendl, M. and Nicol, C.J. (2009) Learning and cognition. In *The Ethology of Domestic Animals: An Introductory Text*, 2nd edn, Jensen, R. (ed.). CABI Publishing, Wallingford.

Mills, D.S. and McConnell, S.M. (2005) *The Domestic Horse: The Evolution, Development and Management of its Behaviour*. Cambridge University Press, Cambridge.

Munksgaard, L., Jensen, M.B., Pedersen, L.J., Hansen, S.W. and Matthews, L. (2005) Quantifying behavioural priorities: effects of time constraints on behaviour of dairy cows, *Bos taurus*. *Applied Animal Behaviour Science* **92**, 3–14.

Nevison, C.M., Hurst, J.L. and Barnard, C.J. (1999) Why do male ICR(CD-1) mice perform bar-related stereotypic behaviour? *Behavioural Processes* **47**, 95–111.

Nicol, C.J. (1987) Behavioural responses of laying hens following a period of spatial restriction. *Animal Behaviour* **35**, 1709–19.

Nicol, C.J. and Pope, S.J. (1996) The maternal feeding display of domestic hens is sensitive to perceived chick error. *Animal Behaviour* **52**, 767–74.

Nicol, C.J., Davidson, H.P.B., Harris, P.A., Waters, A.J. and Wilson, A.D. (2002) Study of crib-biting and gastric inflammation and ulceration in young horses. *Veterinary Record* **151**, 658–62.

Pajor, E.A., Rushen, J. and de Passille, A.M.B. (2000) Aversion learning techniques to evaluate dairy cattle handling practices. *Applied Animal Behaviour Science* **69**, 89–102.

Palleroni, A., Hauser, M. and Marler, P. (2005) Do responses of galliform birds vary adaptively with predator size? *Animal Cognition* **8**, 200–10.

Panksepp, J. and Burgdorf, J. (2003) 'Laughing' rats and the evolutionary antecedents of human joy? *Physiology & Behavior* **79**, 533–47.

Pedersen, L.J., Holm, L., Jensen, M.B. and Jorgensen, E. (2005) The strength of pigs' preferences for different rooting materials using concurrent schedules of reinforcement. *Applied Animal Behaviour Science* **94**, 31–48.

Puppe, B., Schon, P.C., Tuchscherer, A. and Manteuffel, G. (2005) Castration-induced vocalisation in domestic piglets, *Sus scrofa*: complex and specific alterations of the vocal quality. *Applied Animal Behaviour Science* **95**, 67–78.

Raj, A.B.M. (1996) Aversive reactions of turkeys to argon, carbon dioxide and a mixture of carbon dioxide and argon. *Veterinary Record* **138**, 592–3.

Schoofs, M. (2008) In Moscow's metro, a stray dog's life is pretty cushy, and zoologists notice. *Wall Street Journal* 20 May 2008; p. A1. Available at: http://online.wsj.com/.

Stolba, A. and Woodgush, D.G.M. (1989) The behavior of pigs in a semi-natural environment. *Animal Production* **48**, 419–25.

Taylor, A.A. and Weary, D.M. (2000) Vocal responses of piglets to castration: identifying procedural sources of pain. *Applied Animal Behaviour Science* **70**, 17–26.

Van Liere, D.W. (1992) Dustbathing as related to proximal and distal feather lipids in laying hens. *Behavioural Processes* **26**, 177–88.

Warburton, H. and Mason, G. (2003) Is out of sight out of mind? The effects of resource cues on motivation in mink, *Mustela vison*. *Animal Behaviour* **65**, 755–62.

Weeks, C.A. and Nicol, C.J. (2006) Preferences of laying hens. *World's Poultry Science Journal* **62** (2), 296–307.

Whay, H.R. (2007) The journey to animal welfare improvement. *Animal Welfare* **16**, 117–22.

Widowski, T.M. and Duncan, I.J.H. (2000) Working for a dustbath: are hens increasing pleasure rather than reducing suffering? *Applied Animal Behaviour Science* **68**, 39–53.

Zimmerman, P.H. and Koene, P. (1998) The effect of frustrative nonreward on vocalisations and behaviour in the laying hen, *Gallus gallus domesticus*. *Behavioural Processes* **44**, 73–9.

Dairy Cattle

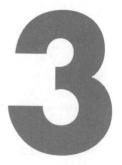

JEAN MARGERISON

Key Concepts

Management and Welfare of Farm Animals: The UFAW Farm Handbook, 5th edition. John Webster
© 2011 by Universities Federation for Animal Welfare (UFAW)

3.1 Introduction

The regions that produce the greatest quantities of milk from dairy cattle are the European Union (EU), Asia and North America (Table 3.1). The majority of milk is produced from specialized dairy cattle breeds, predominantly the Holstein Friesian, followed by a relatively small percentage of Jersey and even fewer numbers of Brown Swiss, Guernsey and traditional breeds such as Ayrshire and Dairy Shorthorn. The Holstein Friesian represents over 90% of dairy cattle in North America and the EU, with relatively low levels (5%) of Jersey. The Holstein breed has been actively selected as a specialist, single-purpose milk-producing animal capable of high volumes of milk production, managed in automated milking systems. The milk yield per cow continues to increase mainly due to improved genetic merit, nutrition and disease prevention. However, infertility has also increased and as a consequence in recent years fertility problems have led to the crossbreeding of Holstein and Jersey, which has been popular in New Zealand pasture-based systems for a number of years and is being adopted more widely in Europe and the USA. The other main dynamic of dairy production has been the general continued trend towards fewer larger dairy herds, with many dairy units now including thousands of cows. This leads to new challenges in herd and personnel management in the dairy industry. Other advances have been the successful application of on-farm quality assurance schemes that ensure the quality and safety of milk production for humans and give an increasing emphasis to animal welfare and protection of the environment.

3.1.1 Milk production for human consumption

The production of milk is monitored through on-farm assurance schemes, which are based on recording and regular assessment of the production system. The areas

Table 3.1 World cow milk production, 1997 to 2006. Source: amended from FAO data.

Country	Cow milk production (`000 tonnes)			
	1997	2000	2003	2006
Europe EU-25	144.1	144.9	144.1	142.0
Extra EU-25	68.8	64.8	67.7	67.5
Northern America	78.9	84.1	85.3	90.5
Latin America	54.3	58.6	62.3	66.0
Asia	83.3	93.6	110.1	134.8
Oceania	20.4	23.4	24.4	24.8
Africa	17.14	19.2	23.8	24.0
World (total)	467.0	488.9	518.1	549.9
± % on the previous year		+1.66	+2.22	+2.96

ExtraEU-25: Albania, Bosnia and Herzegovina, Bulgaria, Croatia, Iceland, Liechtenstein, Macedonia, Moldova, Norway, Romania, Russian Federation, Serbia and Montenegro, Switzerland and Ukraine.

assessed include staff training, animal welfare using the five freedoms, food safety using the principles of hazard identification, risk assessment and control, management of animal health through forward planning and disease prevention, the adequacy and appropriateness of animal nutrition and protection of the environment. These are independently assessed by qualified inspectors using accredited systems to monitor dairy farms at regular intervals.

3.1.2 Milk consumption and human health

The main constituents of milk are water, fats, proteins and lactose (Figure 3.1). It can be consumed as liquid milk or converted by different processes (traditional or modern) into a variety of dairy products and food ingredients, and has some industrial uses. The concept of nutrition of humans in developed countries has progressed from the simple provision of adequate nutrition to include longer-term health benefits and risks. Although obesity and diabetes are major modern concerns in the developed, over-fed world, the high nutritive value of dairy products mean that they can make a valuable contribution to the daily human diet. Increasing wealth has allowed the consumption of dairy products in many countries. The greatest increases in production and consumption of milk are occurring in Asia (Table 3.1).

Milk plays a significant role in the human diet and the consumption of three portions of dairy products daily has been recommended for a well-balanced human diet. In addition, milk and dairy products are known to contain a number of components with potential functional properties in the promotion of good health. These include natural antioxidants and anti-carcinogenic agents, in particular conjugated linoleic acid (CLA). Fatty acid profiles in milk can be affected by the cow's diet and milk from cows consuming fresh forages tends to contain higher levels of CLA compared with cows consuming conserved forages. The issue of functional foods has received much research attention but it is too soon to come to definitive conclusions.

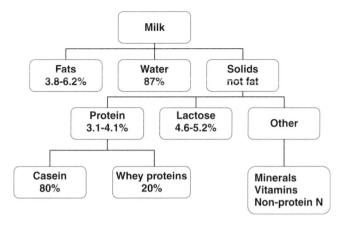

Figure 3.1 Components in whole milk from differing breeds of dairy cattle.

In developing countries, dairy products can make a great contribution to the improvement of human health although they may be scarce or prohibitively expensive. Milk and dairy products are particularly important in the development of dense bones, strong teeth and mental ability, especially in children. Milk products are an excellent source of amino acids, essential fatty acids, minerals (e.g. calcium, phosphorus) and vitamins. As a consequence, the development of dairy production in countries such as Thailand and China has been supported greatly by the government. These counties in general consume all home-produced milk and continue to be net dairy product importers, mainly in the form of milk powder.

The consumption of cow's milk is not considered suitable as a direct replacement in young infants and currently breast feeding is recommended, where possible, for at least the first 6 months of age.

3.2 The Global Dairy Industry

Globally the main milk-producing countries, in descending order of milk production are India, USA, China, Russia, Pakistan, Germany, France, Brazil, UK and New Zealand. The EU as a whole has been a large contributor to the world trade in milk products, as is New Zealand. The milk production from India differs from most of the other countries, in that more than half of the milk is produced from buffaloes, followed by indigenous cows and crossbred cows, with a small amount coming from goats.

3.2.1 Specialized dairy production

Milk production in the USA is dominated by dairy cows, in particular the Holstein Friesian breed. In New Zealand the domination of the Holstein Friesian is less pronounced, as smaller, lighter breeds are better suited to pasture-based systems. The Holstein Friesian represents less than 50% of the dairy cow population, along with an estimated 32% of cows being New Zealand Holstein Friesian cross Jersey and 14% Jersey. This reflects the dominance of pasture-based systems for low-cost milk production, which is facilitated by mild winters, high winter light intensity and sunshine, and relatively consistent rainfall in many areas or irrigation of pastures in others. However, increasing land prices, especially in the North Island, access to cost-effective by-products and the increased use of forage maize (especially in times of drought) have led to more farmers offering supplementary feeds to dairy cattle. The milk production is still largely concentrated in the North Island, but the conversion of land previously not used for dairy production into dairy production has continued apace since 2007.

The production of milk in countries with established dairy industries has continued to be characterized by declining numbers of milk producers, with larger herd sizes (mean > 350 cows) and increasing milk production per cow. The improvements made through genetic selection and breeding have increased the genetic potential of the dairy herds; in particular there has been a dominance of the Holstein Friesian dairy breed. Improved genetics, along with improvements in feed resources, conservation techniques, diet formulation and subsequent nutrition of dairy cattle, has led to substantial increases in milk yield per cow in the last 10 years. Unfortunately, this increase in milk yield has all too often been concurrent with increases in infertility. As a consequence in recent years, crossbreeding of differing dairy breeds, mainly Holstein Friesian and Jersey, has become more popular, as has the extension of the grazing season, where possible, in order to reduce feed costs. The most recent change has been the adoption of feed conversion efficiency as a measure of genetic merit. This has been characteristic of the pig and poultry industry, and it will be interesting to see the potential for success in the more complicated ruminant nutrition arena.

3.2.2 Developing milk-producing countries

In China and Thailand the importation of the Holstein Friesian has been central to the development of the dairy industry. However, in countries with more tropical climates, the use of imported dairy cattle genetics has been less successful, mainly due to their lack of heat tolerance and resistance to endemic disease. These genetics are often referred to as European, although they are likely to be American or Canadian Holstein in reality, but did originate from the original cows bred in Northern Europe. Holstein Friesian, Jersey and Brown Swiss breeds have been used to crossbreed with the 'local' breeds of cattle and this has been a much more successful method of improving milk yield, while retaining some of the desirable characteristics of the local breeds. However, the main problem is the maintenance of the advantages of the crossbreeding and segregation of the phenotype in the following generations. In this crossbreeding the Holstein Friesian tends to dominate as the preferred cross. In the long term, recording and selective breeding within the local population of dairy cattle offers the opportunity to retain the genetic biodiversity as a future resource. The extraction of milk for human consumption from many of the 'local' breeds and crosses with local breeds often requires the presence of the calf in order to aid milk letdown. These systems may also allow the calf to suckle from the cow on a restricted basis, rather than artificially rear the calf (see section 3.9.3.7).

3.2.3 Main milk product-exporting countries

The main milk product-exporting countries, where milk production exceeds the need of the local population, include the EU, Northern America, New Zealand and to a lesser extent Australia. The production of milk within the EU, with its expanding number of member states (33 in 2010), has been declining, while Australia's milk production has continued to be hampered by drought conditions and water shortages. New Zealand continues to expand its dairy industry, which now has one dairy cow (average yield 3,800 L) per member of population. This creates a large export market for milk products, mainly milk powder, cheese and butter. The emphasis is therefore on the production of milk solids (fat plus protein, measured in kg).

In general within countries, dairying is better suited, but not totally limited, to wetter areas, where animals can graze grass or consume a range of fodder crops or conserved forages. However, the dairy cow is a ruminant and is well able to utilize a range of forages and feed resources. A range of cereals, maize, straw and co-products from the food, beverage and biofuel industries also provide feed for dairy cattle. The cost, nutrient composition, fibre content and anti-nutritional factors of feeds are used as the basis of formulating a cost-effective diet to fulfil the nutrient requirements of dairy cattle. In many countries dairy cattle are housed for 6 to 8 months of the year, during the winter periods when pasture growth is low. In warmer regions of temperate countries where winter temperatures and sunlight levels are higher, such as New Zealand, some areas of Ireland, UK, South America and USA, cows can graze pasture or other forage crops all year around. However, during periods of low rainfall and drought, when fresh forage growth is limited, the use of conserved forage and/or supplements is required to ensure sufficient feed is available to maintain milk production, or milk output will be reduced.

3.2.4 Milk sale and purchase

3.2.4.1 Milk marketing and levy boards

The production, transport, processing and storage of milk and milk products need to be carefully managed to ensure quality and hygiene. As a consequence, many countries have or historically had milk marketing boards that regulate the continual production, collection, quality, processing and marketing of milk. In some countries milk is purchased by a number of cooperatives or purchasers. These individual contracts have enabled the milk purchasers to control milk supply, closely matching the level of production and milk composition to the specific processing and market needs. This has led to farmers calving cows all year round, thus providing a relatively consistent level of milk supply which allows the maximum use of the processing facilities and minimizes the need for investment in expensive processing infrastructure. In most countries the differing sectors of the agricultural industry have levy boards. The dairy levy boards collect money per litre of milk produced or kg of milk solids processed; the money is collected directly from the milk processor from farmers' payments and is used for the development of the industry through marketing, research and extension. The government of each country is also involved to a greater or lesser extent in the research, development, education and extension of technologies within the dairy industry.

3.2.4.2 Milk quotas and co-operative shares

Milk production in the 33 member states in the EU is controlled by milk quota. In the UK, quotas have been in place since the mid-1980s, while production quotas have been in place for much longer in other countries such as Canada. These quotas control the amount of milk farmers can produce, are milk fat linked and each EU country has a total quota. The quota is owned by the milk producer and can be bought, sold and leased in some countries. The European Commission is currently committed to phasing out milk quotas in 2015.

In New Zealand, while there is no quota system, the majority of farmers sell milk to a farmer-owned dairy cooperative and are required to own shares in order to supply milk to the cooperative, thus controlling the amount of milk supplied for processing. The milk production in New Zealand is highly seasonal, with the majority of milk being processed into commodity products such as butter, cheese and milk powder for export. The milk is produced cheaply to meet world market prices and producers block-calve their cows in spring (July to September) to coincide with the grass-growing season. The lactation length is approx 280 days and as a consequence many of the processing factories are closed for a period at the end of the season. There is a small population of milk producers that have cows calving in spring and autumn to allow continued production of liquid milk and for processing into dairy products for the relatively small internal population.

3.3 Animal Breeding

3.3.1 Animal selection and genetic improvement

The selection of dairy cows and sires to increase milk production, animal health and lifetime production potential is one of the main tools that has been used to increase milk production and economic efficiency. The selection process is based on the assessment of relatively heritable (25 to 50%) milk production and milk composition traits and body conformation (type) traits (7 to 54%), followed by less heritable but important traits such as longevity (8%), health (somatic cell counts – SCC: 12%) and fertility (4%). The use of computer-based linear production models (e.g. BLUP; best linear unbiased prediction) has allowed the calculation of relatively complicated indexes including economic weighting for milk components and for each sire and cow. The number of factors included in the index varies from country to country and these have changed considerably in the last 10 years. In some countries there are differing indexes according to the milk product to be produced, such as liquid milk or cheese, or overall 'net' genetic merit.

The traits selected can be described as production, durability and health including fertility (Table 3.2). In the past, many indexes gave the highest proportion (%) of weighting to production traits; however, this resulted in a relatively low number of lactations being completed by dairy cattle due to infertility, mastitis and lameness and reduced dairy margins. As a consequence, fertility, disease resistance, particularly to mastitis (e.g. low SCC), and traits related to increased herd life/durability of dairy cattle have increased in their importance in the breeding indexes of the majority of countries. The aim is to produce a more robust cow with an improved lifetime performance, reduced replacement cost and greater farm margins. In a breeding index selection traits are given weighting (numerical values) and positive values are given to 'desirable' traits, the higher the value the greater the selection intensity of

Table 3.2 Main production, longevity and health traits used in the breeding indexes for dairy cattle.

Category	Selection trait	Measurement criteria
Production	Milk protein	kg or %
	Milk fat	kg or %
	Milk yield	kg or litres
Health and fertility	SCC (mastitis)	Somatic cell count levels and/or incidence of mastitis
	Fertility	Fertility of the cow or her daughter
	Other diseases	Metabolic disease, lameness, etc
Durability	Longevity	Number of lactations completed, daughters lactations
	Feet/legs	Conformation score (legs mid range of scale), high/sharp foot angle
	Udder traits	High scores for attachment
	Calving ease	High scores (few calving problems or assistance)
	Temperament	High score (good temperament)
	Milking speed	Fast to average milking speed
Other factors	Live weight	Pasture-based systems aim to reduce this

that specific trait; negative weighting can be applied to reduce undesirable traits. The use of negative weightings (– values) on traits such as animal live weight or milk volume (l) would favour the selection of smaller cows or cows that produce a lower volume of milk. Positive weighting can be applied to increase desirable traits such as kg or % of milk fat or protein, fertility or animal conformation characteristics such as mammary system or foot and leg scores (see section 3.8.4.1). Overall, the majority of countries are applying a greater proportion (40 to 50%) of their breeding index (+ and highest numerical values) to durability, health and fertility traits and a lower proportion than previously to production traits (50 to 60%).

The pedigree societies in each country use professional personnel to assess dairy heifers in order to give the conformation scores, such as leg and foot, mammary, dairy type and many more. The use of breeding indexes can be used to compare the 'breed quality' of cows and sires within a herd, across herds and more importantly the reliability of a sire's potential transmitting ability (PTA) of traits in other countries, referred to as Interbull (international sire PTAs).

3.3.2 Improved contemporary comparisons and quantitative trait loci

The use of artificial insemination and the use of high-quality sires is a key factor in increasing the genetic merit of dairy herds. At present the performance of the daughters of sires in differing herds is defined in terms of 'improved contemporary comparisons' (ICC), accompanied by an expression of reliability (REL) which depends on the number of daughters across the number of herds and has been used to assess the potential transmitting ability of the sire. However, this process is inevitably slow. Sires need to be approximatetly 9 months of age to produce semen.

There follows 9 months of gestation and a 2-year growing period before the daughter produces milk and can begin to generate milk production data for the ICCs. In recent years genetic technology has identified an increasing array of gene quantitative trait loci (QTLs) that exert a positive effect on productivity traits. This creates the opportunity to increase the speed of genetic improvement by reducing the interval between generations.

3.3.3 Breeding herd replacements

In practical terms approximately 25% of the dairy herd requires replacement annually. In a commercial dairy herd, this can be provided at a sex ratio of 50:50, by mating half of the dairy herd to a selected dairy sire. A small selection of sires is generally used (to reduce the risk of inbreeding) at any one time to improve a few specifically selected production and conformation traits in daughters of the better-quality and more productive dairy cattle, based on milk production and conformation records. In this way each herd can increase its genetic merit over time. In pasture-based systems, with the added pressure of seasonal calving, the use of nominated sires for AI may take place at the beginning of the breeding season and this will be followed by the use of stock bulls, so that the calving season is limited to a short period to coincide with spring grass growth for the following season. Some pedigree herds with cows of high genetic merit may breed a larger proportion or the entire dairy herd to selected sires in order to produce high-quality dairy replacements for sale to other herds.

3.4 Lactation

The mammary gland of the dairy cow is made up of four separate quarters, with a single teat, orifice and streak canal for each of the four quarters. At birth the gland consists of the bud with few relatively poorly developed structures and starts to develop at a faster rate than the growth of the animal around puberty, which occurs at approximately 40% mature weight and at approx 4 to 6 months of age depending on the early growth rate of the animal. The gland continues to develop and a final rapid stage of development occurs during pregnancy, during which the milk-secreting epithelial cells within the alveoli develop and colostrum is produced.

Lactation and the secretion of milk are initiated by changes in hormone levels around parturition. The total milk yield per lactation is dependant on the genetic merit of the animal and level of feeding, with yields from 3,500 L being common in pasture/forage-based feeding systems and yields in excess of 10,000 L when cows are offered mixed rations based on concentrated feeds (e.g. cereals) and forage. The level of milk yield and composition of the milk is affected by the stage of lactation, breed and age of the cow. In early lactation the yield peaks and has a dilution effect on the milk composition, which declines as yield increases. Protein and fat concentration in milk can be manipulated by diet and genetic selection. Lactose, which acts as an osmotic

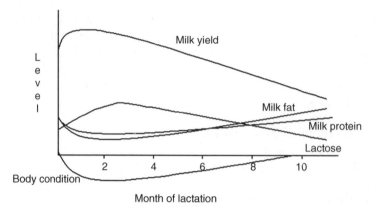

Figure 3.2 Lactation curve of dairy cattle including changes in milk yield, milk composition and body condition.

regulator in the mammary gland, follows the pattern of milk yield (Figure 3.2). The somatic cell count of the milk tends to be highest in early and late lactation.

3.5 Dairy Farm Infrastructure

The housing of dairy cattle is an important factor during cold winter conditions, both to promote the wellbeing of animals and to protect the pastures. Good levels of housing and hygiene are important in preventing disease and to ensure the production of high-quality milk for human consumption. The other main important requirements are the separation of calving cows into deep-bedded calving boxes or in calving paddocks, where they still have the sight and smell of other cattle. It is not good practice to allow cows to calve in cubicles.

3.5.1 Pasture-based systems

In pasture-based systems the majority of dairy units calve cows in spring to coincide with maximum pasture growth rates. These pasture-based systems are practised in New Zealand, areas of South America and some areas of Europe and the USA. The housing of dairy cattle is not regularly practised in New Zealand, but has become more common in recent years with cows housed for short periods of time on fully slatted floors. These systems require cattle to walk long distances and track (race) design and maintenance and the appropriate handling of cattle moving to and from the milking shed is of great importance to animal welfare and the prevention of lameness. In these systems there is less slurry stored, but leaching of nutrients and fertilizers into groundwater can be a considerable problem. Concreted areas (often without roofing, known as feedpads) may be used to offer feeds to dairy cattle and used to hold cattle ('stand offs') when pasture conditions are too wet to allow cattle to graze efficiently, thus reducing pasture and soil damage (poaching or pugging).

3.5.2 Cow housing systems

The majority of dairy cattle are housed during winter. There is an increasing trend towards housing cows throughout the year (or throughout lactation) in circumstances where fresh grass makes little or no contribution to the overall diet. The housing most commonly used is a building that provides a roof that acts as an umbrella over both the milking parlour and cow housing. The systems of housing are generally named after the type of cow accommodation for housing the animals.

3.5.2.1 Free stalls or cubicle systems

The most common form of housing is the 'free stall' or 'cubicle' system. In these systems the aim should be to maximize cow comfort, best assessed by lying time, which ideally should be over 10 hours. This has been associated with disease prevention and improved productivity. There should be at least one cubicle per cow and the design and size of the cubicle should be in accordance with the live weight and size of the cow (Table 3.3).

The cubicle size, design and bedding are the main important components of this system. The provision and maintenance of sufficient space in front of the cow, to allow her to lie down and rise (referred to as lunging space), is essential to prevent the cow becoming stuck in the cubicle. It is for this reason that stalls with a blind or 'closed' front need to be longer, to allow space for lunging. This space needs to be protected by a breast bar on the floor or a triangular construction in front of the cow, which prevents the cow moving too far forwards in the cubicle. The design of the division is also important, with divisions fixed above ground at the front, thus with no legs down to the floor being favoured, as these reduce leg damage. Finally, the provision of high levels of cow comfort and cleanliness are an important management factor and the use of rubber mats or mattresses, with regularly replaced clean bedding materials, is important in the maintenance of low levels of bacterial

Table 3.3 Area allocation for loose-bedded (UK) and free stall/cubicle bed length (UK and USA) for dairy cattle according to live-weight.

Live-weight (kg)	Straw-bedded yard area (m^2)			Cubicle/free stall bed length (m)			
				Open front		Closed front	
	Bedded	Loafing	Total	UK	USA	UK	USA
500	6.0	2.5	8.5	2.05	2.05	2.35	2.05
600	6.5	2.5	9.0	2.15	2.15	2.40	2.15
700	7.0	3.0	10.0	2.20	2.30	2.50	2.55
800	8.0	3.0	11.0	2.25	2.40	2.55	2.70

contamination and thus mastitis. Finally, increasing cow comfort increases cow lying time and reduces lameness in dairy cattle.

3.5.2.2 Deep bedding systems

In areas where cereal crops are grown, deep bedding systems may be used to house dairy cattle. These systems can provide a good level of cow comfort and are essential for calving cows. In deep bedding systems it is imperative that adequate amounts and regular provision of bedding material are applied, along with a separate feeding area that can be cleaned in order to reduce the risk of bacterial contamination and mastitis. The main criterion used to design and assess this system is the allocation of sufficient space per animal.

3.5.2.3 Tie barns

Some countries continue to use tie barns, where cows are tied by the neck. These mostly involve smaller herds in cooler climates. In some units cows are moved from the stalls to the milking parlour; in others they are permanently tethered and milked in the stalls. In both cases it takes a relatively long time to milk the cows, which limits the system to small herds. Moreover, the extreme restriction of cow movement and exercise can lead to hock swellings and lameness associated with abnormally low levels of hoof wear.

3.5.2.4 Herd homes

The introduction of herd homes in New Zealand has been increasing in recent years. These are low-cost polythene tunnel-type structures, with fully slatted floors. The impact of the introduction of these on dairy cattle has yet to be determined.

3.5.3 Milking management

The majority of dairy cattle are milked in parlours or milking sheds. In large herds these are typically of herringbone or rotary design. Smaller herds in Europe, Canada and developing countries may use abreast or tandem parlours, or even hand milking. Robotic milking has become more common in the last 10 years due to the reduced availability and increased cost of labour, along with technical innovation.

The herringbone parlour or shed (Figure 3.3) is the most common type, mainly due to its being one of the most cost-effective. The aim should be to ensure the throughput is sufficient to allow all the cows to be milked within about 2 hours of arriving at the site. Herringbones can have sufficient clusters to milk one side at once or all of the cows at one time and are described by the number of cows that can be held, followed by the number that can be milked at any one time, e.g. 48:48 or 24:48. Rotary sheds are described by the number of stalls or bales that they contain and these are one of the most popular for milking larger herds. Tandem milk parlours (Figure 3.4) allow greater access to the cows and allow individual cows to enter and leave the milking parlour or shed, but these have a slower throughput than herring bones and the operator needs to walk longer distances.

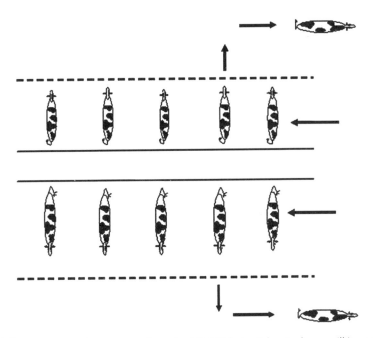

Figure 3.3 Diagrammatic representation of a (10:10) fast-exit herringbone milking parlour for dairy cattle.

3.5.4 Milking equipment and practice

The majority of cows are milked mechanically, by alternating between vacuum (approximately 38 to 50 kPa depending on the equipment) and non-vacuum (atmospheric pressure) phases, referred to as pulsations. The milk is removed from the cows by mimicking the suckling of the calf, where vacuum is used to reduce the pressure outside the teat end to below the pressure within the mammary gland, thus

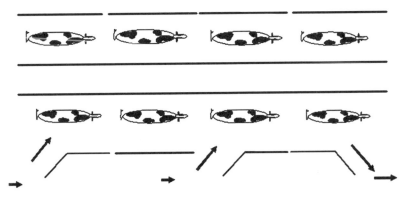

Figure 3.4 Diagrammatic representation of an (8 stall) tandem milking parlour for dairy cattle.

resulting in the milk flowing out through the teat canal. Maintenance of the correct and consistent vacuum level is one of the most important factors to ensure the health of the mammary gland. The regular checks required are:

- annual milking machine maintenance by professionally qualified and equipped personnel;
- daily checking of the vacuum gauge for the correct vacuum;
- daily checking of the vacuum regulator allowing air into the system;
- daily checking of all rubber wear for slits or cracks, which would allow air to leak into the system.

The correct vacuum level, along with the correct rate and ratio of pulsations, which prevent the build-up of tissue fluid and oedema within the teat, are important in efficient milking and to prevent teat damage. The final important factor is the effective function of the rubber liners, which should be changed approximately every 2,500 milkings or annually, whichever is the sooner, to ensure the function of these liners and prevent any cracking or splitting.

3.5.5 Milking frequency

3.5.5.1 Twice or thrice daily milking

The majority of cows are milked mechanically twice daily at relatively evenly spaced (14 and 10 h or 12 and 12 h) intervals. Milk yields can be increased by milking higher-yielding cows (>6,500 L/year) three times daily, which increases milk yield (15 to 25%) because of the enhancement of the longevity and function of the milk-secreting epithelial cells in the mammary gland mainly due to the removal of a small protein that acts as a feedback inhibitor, and increased frequency of oxytocin secretion. Increasing milking frequency increases the nutrient requirements of the animal, along with the labour and fixed costs associated with milking.

3.5.5.2 Once daily milking

Milking cows once daily has become a more popular option for some farm enterprises in recent years. Lower-yielding cows can be milked once daily, or three times in two days, particularly those producing milk of higher solids such as Jersey and Jersey cross in pasture-based systems, with a limited reduction in milk yield. This can be a useful management approach for dairy cattle managed in marginal areas where feed supplies may be limited and allows flexibility of working practices. Reducing milking frequency reduces labour and fixed costs, feed requirements and the distance walked by dairy cattle on a daily basis and has a relatively limited effect on somatic cell count levels in well-managed dairy herds with low levels of mastitis.

3.5.6 Milk quality and testing

Samples of milk are taken from farm vats prior to collection and from the bulk milk tanker on arrival at the factory. The milk samples from the bulk milk tanker are tested for temperature and the presence of antibiotics before the milk enters the factory processing area. The farm milk samples are subsequently further tested for milk fat, protein, bulk milk cell count, bacterial count and residues such as antibiotics. There are set standards and grades. Milk that fails any of the tests is unsuitable for producing quality products and the milk will be rejected. For most farmers, the milk price will depend on composition and hygiene, so it is extremely important that these samples are collected and stored correctly.

3.6 Dairy Cow Nutrition

3.6.1 Digestive anatomy and function

Dairy cattle are large ruminants. Their digestive system has evolved to enable the microbial fermentation of cellulose and other fibres in forage-based diets and consists of four main compartments – the rumen, reticulum, omasum and abomasum (Figure 3.5), which are followed by the duodenum, small and large intestine, caecum and colon.

3.6.1.1 The rumen

The rumen is a large organ (capacity 170 to 190 L), which allows large quantities of forages to be digested over a period of time. In the rumen there are bacteria, protozoa

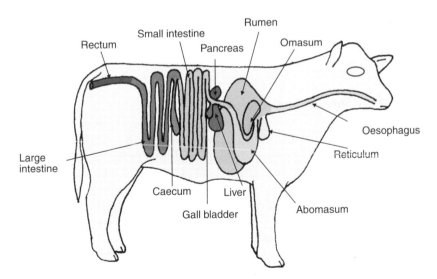

Figure 3.5 The digestive anatomy of the ruminant.

and fungi that ferment and break down the feeds consumed by the animal. These rumen-based microflora and -fauna grow and multiply while the fermentation of carbohydrates from dietary starch and cellulose produces volatile fatty acids (VFA) mainly consisting of acetic, propionic and butyric acids. The VFA are largely absorbed into the blood through the rumen wall whose surface area is greatly enlarged by tiny finger-like projections, the rumen papilli. Microflora and -fauna pass out of the rumen to be digested in the abomasum, thus providing a source of protein for the animal, which is referred to as microbial crude protein (MCP). This process allows ruminant animals to produce essential amino acids in addition to those provided by the feeds consumed. There are also bacteria in the rumen that produce B complex vitamins and some vitamin H or biotin.

3.6.1.2 Diet changes

The rumen microbial (flora and fauna) population develops in accordance with the composition of the diet offered to the cows and this occurs over approximately 2 weeks. In consequence, sudden changes in diet composition are inappropriate and the composition of the diet should be changed gradually to avoid potential indigestion and diarrhoea. The proportions of the microflora and -fauna within the rumen are directly affected by the composition of the diet, as are the proportions of the differing types of VFA produced. Diets high in structural fibre produce higher proportions of acetic acid to propionic acid, while diets lower in structural fibre produce higher proportions of propionic acid to acetic acid. These VFA proportions directly affect milk composition; high proportions of acetic acid result in higher fat composition in milk, while higher proportions of propionic acid favour higher milk protein levels. Moreover, the proportions of VFA affect plasma insulin and growth hormone levels and thus affect milk yield and body condition score. The production of high proportions of propionic acid to acetic acid not only tends to reduce milk fat concentration, it potentially reduces milk yield and increases the potential for live weight and body condition gain.

3.6.1.3 Dietary fibre and rumination

The rumen and the reticulum respond to the longer fibres that tend to accumulate on top of the rumen liquor and from here they are propelled up through the oesophagus into the mouth to be chewed and re-swallowed during rumination. The cow adds copious quantities of saliva to the ingesta, both on primary consumption and during rumination. Cows can produce up to 100 L of saliva per day, which contains phosphate and bicarbonates that help to maintain the rumen environment at an optimal pH of 6.0 to 6.5. As a consequence, dairy cows spend up to 6 to 8 h/d ruminating and the number of times they chew each cud depends on the amount of fibre and 'functionality' (length of fibre) of the diet. The amount of fibre in feeds is measured by chemical analysis (conventionally defined as neutral- or acid-detergent fibre (NDF or ADF). The functionality of the fibre is affected by the levels of chopping or processing. In recent years the physical assessment of fibre content has been applied to dairy cow diets, mainly due to a higher incidence of displaced abomasum (DA) in dairy cows offered mixed rations lacking long fibre. This involves a set of sieves with decreasing apertures, which allow the lengths of the fibres of the diet to be assessed. Other practical methods for assessing the adequacy of the diet include inspection of the dung and assessing the number of chews the cow applies to each cud, approximately between 45 and 70. The total of 45 is fairly low and would be common in a low-fibre, pasture-based system, while 50 to 70 chews would be more appropriate for mixed diets.

3.6.1.4 Water absorption and gastric digestion

The omasum can be identified as a small dark structure, relatively hard in structure, which contains many layers of tissue, which gives it an internal appearance similar to the leaves of a book. This organ is mainly responsible for the absorption of water.

The abomasum is relatively small compared to the rumen and has a relatively smooth texture and pale appearance. This is the equivalent of the simple stomach in the non-fermenting species and as such utilizes gastric juices at a low pH to aid digestion.

3.6.1.5 Dairy cow nutrition and the environment

The potential pollution of groundwater, rivers and lakes due to leaching of both nitrates and phosphates from agricultural practices has come under increasing levels of control in most countries. This includes the effective storage and application of manures, including potential restrictions to manure application to prevent damage to water quality and the environment. Moreover, rumen fermentation produces large amounts of methane which is a particularly powerful 'greenhouse' gas. The amounts of greenhouse gases produced by ruminants and their global population make them a significant contributor to global emissions. This problem may be addressed both at the level of the agricultural system and the individual cow. An example of the former approach is the capture and use of gases from manure using biodigesters. Production of gaseous methane direct from cows can be reduced through manipulation of diet and/or the population of ruminal microbes, mainly to increase propionate:acetate ratio in the end-products of fermentation.

3.6.2 Feeding the dairy cow

As for any animal, the aim of planned feeding is to match the supply of available nutrients to nutrient requirements. In the special case of the lactating dairy cow, nutrient requirement is high and supply is limited by the capacity of the animal to ingest and digest fibrous feeds that ferment slowly. Thus the process of dairy cow nutrition is based on two main elements – estimating the feed intake and nutrient requirements of the animal. In this process it is essential to consider the effects of stage of lactation, feed quality and feeding system when planning to provide nutrients in the diet in an adequate concentration to allow the animal to consume these within the constraints of its feed intake potential. Similarly when planning a diet it is important not to overestimate the dry matter intake and to ensure that there is sufficient energy in the diet, followed by protein and then minerals and vitamins.

3.6.3 Nutrient requirements

The nutrient requirements of dairy cattle are generally expressed in terms of energy and protein, along with minerals and vitamins. Lactating animals also require large quantities of water. The dairy cow requires these nutrients for maintenance and production (i.e. milk production, reproduction and pregnancy, growth and live weight gain). In early lactation the dairy cow will prioritize maintenance and milk production before reproduction, growth or live weight gain. This prioritizing of nutrients towards differing purposes is referred to as nutrient partitioning.

3.6.3.1 Energy

Energy is usually considered the first limiting factor in production. Dairy cows require energy for both maintenance and production. Energy is also essential for the function of the microbial population in the rumen. In most countries the energy requirements of dairy cattle are expressed as metabolizable energy (ME). Due to the importance of supplying energy for the rumen microbes, the ME terminology has been refined to include a measurement of the energy that can be fermented by the microbes in the rumen, which is fermentable metabolizable energy (FME). The USA and some other countries use net energy (NE), which is a measure of the energy directly available to the animal for production. The ME and NE are expressed in ruminant production in megajoules (MJ). The energy content can be calculated from the gross energy (GE) content, which is estimated using a bomb calorimeter, and the energy losses associated with the digestion and metabolism of differing feeds (Figure 3.6).

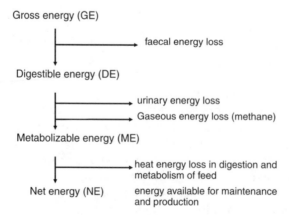

Figure 3.6 Schematic representation of the relationship between gross energy, metabolizable and net energy, and energy losses during digestion.

3.6.3.2 Protein

The requirements of dairy cows for protein are calculated in a similar way as for energy. The most common term presently used to describe proteins for ruminants is metabolizable protein (MP), which is that available for metabolism following digestion and absorption. The terminology used to describe the protein content of feeds directly reflects the areas of the digestive system in which it may be digested and the rate at which it may be degraded in the rumen. That fraction of the protein in the feed that is degraded in the rumen is referred to as effective rumen degradable protein (ERDP), while protein that is digestible but is not degraded in the rumen is digestible undegradable protein (DUP). The ERDP and DUP proportion of any feed is directly affected by the amount of time feed spends in the rumen. Feed that passes rapidly through the rumen will have a relatively lower ERDP and increased level of DUP.

The protein that is available to be digested by the dairy cow is that which arrives into the abomasum and this comes from two potential sources: microbial crude protein (MCP) and DUP. Both of these are digested in the abomasum to provide metabolizable protein. The amount of MCP delivered to the abomasum is a function of a combination of ERDP and fermentable metabolizable energy (FME) in the rumen. The level of DUP reaching the abomasum is affected by the degradability of the feed and the outflow rate of feed from the rumen.

3.6.4 Feed intake

As a ruminant animal, one of the main factors limiting the performance of the dairy cow is the voluntary feed intake, which is often referred as dry matter intake (DMI). The factors that affect DMI can be divided into those that are related to the animal or to the feed.

3.6.4.1 Animal factors

The main animal factors that affect DMI include weight or physical size, body condition, physiological state and health. In general, larger individuals or breeds tend to have greater DMI. Within a breed, animals with lower body condition (lower fat reserves) tend to have a higher DMI than those with greater body reserves. This is due to blood metabolites regulating intake, through chemostatic signals, and the physical limitation that internal fat places on space available for food within the rumen.

Physiological state is an important factor affecting both DMI and nutrient requirement. DMI becomes limited during the last trimester of pregnancy, due to the increasing size of the foetus reducing the physical space available for the rumen. This reduction in feed intake may persist, for up to 3 to 5 weeks following parturition. Thus stage of lactation should be taken into consideration when estimating DMI. This period of lowered nutrient intake coincides with high nutrient demands for milk production. This has been termed the 'energy gap' and over this period dairy cows tend to mobilize body fat and some protein to meet the nutrients required for milk production. This live weight and body condition loss should be

Table 3.4 Body condition scoring of dairy cattle.

5-point scale	10-point scale	Description/target
0	1	
1.0	2	Emaciated/too thin
1.5	3	Too thin
2.0	4	
2.5	5	Target body condition at calving
3.0	6	Target body condition at calving
3.5	7	
4.0	8	
4.5	9	Over-fat
5.0	10	Obese

managed by ensuring optimal body condition score (BCS) at parturition (3 to 3.5 on a scale of 1 to 5, or 5.5 on a scale of 1 to 10; see Table 3.4), to allow body reserves to be available, and cows should be offered sufficient nutrients to regain lost live weight prior to mating to optimize reproductive functions, such as regular oestrous cycling, follicle quality, increased oestrus behaviour and detection rates, thus improving conception and pregnancy rates.

3.6.4.2 Feed factors

The main feed factors that affect DMI include feed availability, type and quality. The DMI of the cow can be reduced when feed availability is limited or pasture availability (height) is low. This has the effect of under-utilizing the DMI capacity of the animal and thus reduces milk yield per cow, but may increase milk yield per hectare in grazed animals. The type of the feed affects the DMI mainly through the fibre content (conventionally described by NDF and ADF) and energy concentration (ME) or FME which is the major substrate required by the rumen microflora and -fauna. Thus the fibre content and energy density of the diet directly affect DMI through the degradation rate of feeds in the rumen. Feeds with higher fibre levels and lower energy concentration, which include straw, long pasture and late cut silage or hay, tend to degrade more slowly in the rumen, occupy the physical space of the rumen for longer, thus reducing DMI. Conversely feeds that have lower levels of fibre and higher levels of energy concentration, such as young leafy pasture, cereals and some co-products, degrade faster in the rumen and, when offered as an appropriate total diet, result in DMI closer to the animal's maximum potential. The main aim of feeding dairy cattle is to optimize feed intake by offering an appropriate combination of feeds and nutrients on a regular and unrestricted basis.

Other feed factors that affect DMI include the palatability of the feeds and the feeding system employed. A good example of feeds that are likely to have lower intake potentials are pasture with recently applied manure and poor-quality silages. Dairy cows should be offered high-quality silages, which mainly result from mowing pastures before 50% ear emergence, along with good ensiling and silage storage practices that minimize butyric acid production and microbial deterioration. Pasture silages with higher dry matter (DM) content (29 to 32% DM) tend to have a higher intake potential, compared with wetter silages (25% DM). The management of animal feeding can affect feed intake and this includes overstocking at feed troughs or at pasture and allowing feed quality to deteriorate due to poor clamp face management, feeding-out management and general hygiene.

3.6.5 Feeding and feeding systems

The main aims of dairy cow feeding are to optimize feed quality and feed intake through good pasture management, ensiling techniques, feed storage and feeding-out management. Most lactating dairy cows rely heavily on the consumption of high-quality forages in order to optimize milk yield potential. Dairy cattle can graze fresh grass or be offered conserved grass as silage or hay. These feeds can be complemented with a range of other feeds such as forage maize silage, cereal silages, cereals, co-products and pelleted compound feeds, along with minerals and vitamins. The use of a total mixed ration to provide both a balanced supply of nutrients and the correct substrates for stable fermentation through the day and night results in a more constant rumen pH, increased feed intake and higher milk yields, with less health problems associated with low rumen pH (see section 3.8.6.1).

3.6.6 Minerals and vitamins

Dairy cattle require a number of minerals and vitamins for healthy body function and to prevent deficiency diseases. Macronutrients include calcium (Ca), magnesium (Mg) and phosphorus (P) whose requirement is measured in g/kg feed. Micronutrients required in µg/kg include copper (Cu), cobalt (Co), selenium (Se) and zinc (Zn). The levels of macro-minerals will depend on the forage mineral levels, the requirements of the animal and the physiological stage, usually related to lactation or season.

3.6.6.1 Calcium deficiency (milk fever)

The most severe form of calcium deficiency is milk fever, which typically presents as extreme muscle weakness in a newly calved cow that can lead to collapse and death within hours, if untreated. Treatment involves administration of calcium salts subcutaneously, or intravenously in advanced cases. The risk of milk fever can be greatly reduced by attention to feeding practices during late pregnancy and transition from dry to lactating. Offering cows low levels of calcium and potassium during the late dry period enables cows to begin mobilizing body reserves of calcium from bone and thus prevent sudden plasma calcium deficiencies (hypocalcaemia) during early lactation. A more recent strategy for dry cows close to calving (3 to 4 weeks prepartum) may involve manipulating the dietary cation:anion balance (DCAB) to induce a mild metabolic acidosis and thereby encourage calcium and phosphorus mobilization during late pregnancy (see section 3.8.9).

3.6.6.2 Magnesium deficiency (grass staggers or hypomagnesaemia)

Magnesium deficiency in dairy cows is primarily associated with low levels of magnesium (Mg) in spring pasture. This can be exacerbated by the application of artificial fertilizers that can reduce magnesium availability. Early clinical signs of acute magnesium deficiency include hyperexcitability and a 'staggering' gait. The conditions can proceed to death within hours so prevention is critical. Supplementing the diet or water with magnesium is typically used as a preventive for magnesium deficiencies in spring.

3.6.6.3 Copper deficiency (clinical and subclinical)

The supplementation of cow diets with copper (Cu) is often required in areas where copper is deficient or high soil molybdenum or iron lead to reduced copper availability. This can be prevented by the implantation of long-acting copper boluses into the rumen. This can enhance oestrous behaviour and improve reproductive performance of dairy cattle.

3.6.6.4 Other important micronutrients for dairy cattle

The supplementation of zinc and selenium has become more popular, in the belief that these can improve hoof horn quality and immunity and reduce somatic cell count levels (see section 3.8.3). The vitamin H (biotin) has been seen in recent years to improve hoof horn quality, when offered for prolonged periods of up to 8 to 10 months, and reduce lameness (especially white line disease), and has been associated with increased milk yields. Finally, the availability of more complex (e.g. chelated or bioplex) forms of minerals has become more commonplace on the basis that they may be more bio-available so achieve similar effects on level animal performance at lower levels of inclusion and less risk of environmental pollution. The availability of minerals and micro-minerals can interact to reduce their availability, thus suboptimal levels can be created either by a lack in the diet or reduced availability due to an interaction with another mineral or micronutrient, resulting in suboptimal absorption by the animal. This can lead to a clinical or subclinical deficiency and suboptimal performance. The availability of copper, for example, is profoundly affected by interactions with other elements – sulfur, molybdenum, zinc and iron.

3.6.7 Grazing and pasture management

Grazed pasture is one of the cheapest forms of forage that can be offered to dairy cattle. Good management is essential to limit fibre content and optimize the nutrient concentration of the pasture. This is achieved by the use of pasture measurement techniques to assess pasture available for the month, by feed planning (monthly and annual), and by management of grazing frequency, grazing period and stocking rate to control pasture height. Pasture management also includes the incorporation of ensiling during periods of rapid pasture growth. The main aim is to maintain the grass plant in a vegetative stage through regular defoliation. This optimizes the nutrient density by minimizing the opportunity for the plant to enter the reproductive stage, thus limiting the fibre content of the pasture throughout the grazing season.

There are a number of grazing systems available, which allow varying levels of plant management and infrastructure requirements:

- *Paddock grazing*: – where the farm is divided into small paddocks according to herd size to allow one, two or three days of grazing. This allows the greatest control of pasture quality, but also has the greatest infrastructure requirements;
- *Set stocking*: – where pasture is controlled by the number of animals grazed on a set area;
- *Continuous grazing*: – where the area is continually grazed and the stocking rate is adjusted according to pasture availability;
- *Zero grazing*: – which is where pasture is not grazed but cut and carried to the cows;
- *Strip grazing*: – which can be used for pasture and forage crops, where there is a high volume of feed and there is a need to limit the area to which the animals have access within a paddock.

Finally, ensiling can be used to control plant growth, by cutting down the area to be grazed when pasture growth is rapid during spring, so that silage is available during periods of low pasture growth such as dry summer periods and in winter.

3.6.7.1 Forage crops

Forage crops include forage maize, fodder beet, kale and whole-crop cereals. The most popular of these is forage maize, which is used quite extensively due to the development of faster-maturing varieties that have allowed this crop to be grown in a wider range of environments. Forage maize makes an excellent complement to grass silage, due to its high level of starch, which increases the milk yield of dairy cattle when used at 30 to 75% of the forage in the diet. Other whole-crop cereal silages (e.g. wheat, barley) can be used in combination with grass silage, but seem not to be as effective as forage maize in increasing milk yield. Turnips and kale can be offered to dairy cattle and are generally strip-grazed to control intake levels to avoid scouring and milk taint.

3.6.7.2 Compound feeds, cereals and co-products

These are classified in the feed resource databases into energy and protein sources according to their chemical composition. A range of cereals and protein-rich oil seeds can be used, following some form of processing, for inclusion into dairy cow diets. The compound feeds are a combination of a number of products including, but not exclusively; cereals, oil seeds, minerals and vitamins that are formulated and processed into a pelleted feed containing a combination of energy and protein, with set levels of fat. The feed can be purchased as 'straights', which are single products that can be purchased in bulk loads, which require storage, and are used to combine with silages using mixer wagons. There are an increasing number and range of by-products from the food, beverage and more recently the biofuel industry. These include such products as bread and biscuit meal, vegetables, brewer's and distiller's grains, and maize co-products, to mention just a few.

3.6.8 Feed storage

Correct and appropriate feed storage is important in ensuring that the quality of the feed is maintained and risks to animal and human health are minimized. It is imperative that feed storage and feeding facilities are designed to ensure that cattle feed cannot be contaminated by bird, pest, rodent, cat or dog urine or faeces.

3.7 Diet Feeding and Management

3.7.1 Mixed rations

3.7.1.1 Feeder wagons and diet mixers

The use of total mixed rations (TMR) or complete diets (forages mixed with other concentrated feeds and minerals) has become increasingly popular as dairy cow yield potential has increased. The use of feeder wagons to dispense a pre-mixed complete diet has become very popular in both indoor and pasture-based systems. This machinery allows the maximum flexibility in the components that can be included in the diet, depending only on the ability of the mixer wagon to render the cow unable to select components from the mixture. These types of diet offer the opportunity to maximize the use of a range of feed resources and the consistency of the type of diet being offered throughout the day and thus optimize DMI and milk yield. This method increases the machinery and labour costs for diet mixing.

A mixed ration is typically formulated to provide sufficient nutrients for the maintenance requirement of the cow plus a specific level of milk production. These diets are described as 'maintenance plus'. This allows batches of diet to be made up and offered to groups of dairy cattle according to their milk yield or stage of lactation. Additional nutrient requirements can be offered through feeding systems that dispense feed to groups in the shed or to individuals in the parlour or via computerized dispensers. These mixed rations generally include a combination of forages, protein feeds and cereals with calcium carbonate for lactating cows. They may also contain some straw to ensure that the diet contains sufficient functional fibre to optimize salivation and rumen function and reduce the risk of abomasal displacement.

3.7.1.2 Offering forages (silages/cut forages and TMR)

Silages and TMR can be offered from feed bins or troughs. Silage can be offered from feed rings or eaten directly ('self feed') from the silage bunker. Straw is typically offered from feed rings. It is important to ensure that cows have sufficient eating space for all to eat at any one time. This should increase feed intake and milk production and reduce lameness. Cows that are required to use self-feed silage bunkers will have a lower DMI compared with cows offered feed freely.

3.7.1.3 Feed pads

These are common in pasture-based systems and are hard-floored areas or standing areas, often concreted, which are occasionally fitted with a roof structure. Here cows are offered feeds to supplement pasture, usually silage forage-based diets with other available cost-effective feeds such as cereals, co-products and plant-based food waste with diet balancers and minerals. Cows are given access to these feeds following milking, during periods of peak yield or when pasture supply is below that required by the animal (dry periods, cool spring, winter) or when high rainfall leads to wet soils and excessive damage to pasture (pugging or poaching) would be caused by cattle treading the ground.

3.7.2 Supplementing the forage diet with concentrated feed or compound feeds

The forage diet of dairy cattle can be supplemented with more concentrated sources of nutrients, thus increasing nutrient intake and subsequent milk yield. The dairy cow responds to a greater extent to these in early lactation and when the animal is genetically predisposed to higher milk yields. The allocation of concentrated feeds can be achieved on a group or individual cow basis. The feeding rates (kg DM/d) can be managed according to differing approaches:

- lead feeding where cows are fed high rates until peak lactation;
- stepped feeding rates, where differing rates are offered for set periods of the lactation;
- feeding to yield, where cows are offered a feed rate according to the milk yield of the cow, which can be adjusted on a weekly or monthly basis.

The choice of approach will depend on the resources available, and the allocation of concentrated feed to individual cows can be achieved using in-parlour/shed or out-of-parlour/shed automated cow feeders. In more simple systems, cows can be offered feed applied over the top of silage 'top dressed' as a midday supplement or offered liquid feeds from 'lick ball' feeders on an *ad libitum* basis.

3.7.3 Automated feeding systems

The use of automated equipment and electronic tags (or transponders) can be used to operate feeders that distribute feeds to individual cows according to preset levels held on a computer database system. These can be operated 'out of' or 'in' the milking shed/parlour.

3.7.3.1 In-parlour or shed feeding

This system, which can be electronic or manually operated, delivers concentrated feeds, usually pelleted or processed cereals, to cows while being milked. It can be used in addition to pasture or silage feeding and as a complement to mixer wagons. It allows individual cows to be offered feed levels according to their individual milk yield. Its limitation is the amount that can be offered at any one time. This should generally be restricted 3 to 5 kg DM at each milking, to avoid fluctuation in the pH of the rumen environment caused by cows being offered large quantities of rapidly degradable carbohydrates.

3.7.3.2 Out-of-parlour or shed feeding

These are electronic systems that deliver concentrated feeds, usually pelleted in nature, to cows throughout the day or night. They reduce the amount of compound feed that is required to be offered at one point in time, thus avoiding fluctuations in rumen pH, and thereby permit higher levels of concentrate feeding with consequent increases in milk yield.

3.7.4 Feeding management for dry cows (transition or lead feeding)

The advent of improved feeding management of dry (non-lactating) dairy cattle has been one of the major advances in cow husbandry in recent years. The main aim is to prevent metabolic disorders such as milk fever, ketosis and acidosis in early-lactation cows. This involves the management of calcium mobilization and body condition score and the introduction of a proportion of the lactation diet before calving to allow the rumen microflora and -fauna to adapt to the great increase in nutrient demand at the onset of lactation. To achieve this, specific dry cow supplements, limitations of pasture intake and the provision of straw are key components.

The prevention of milk fever requires the management of calcium and magnesium supplementation before calving. Low calcium and high magnesium before calving will encourage the cow to mobilize body reserves of calcium. Similarly, the management of dietary cation and anion balance (DCAB or DCAD), using negative (chloride) ions added to the diet, induce a mild metabolic acidosis and stimulate the cow to mobilize body calcium and phosphorus. Grass and silage are high in potassium, which will increase plasma pH and thus discourage cows to mobilize calcium; the levels of pasture silage should be restricted in dry cow diets, e.g. by inclusion of straw into dry cow diets to maintain intake levels and rumen capacity and to satiate the cow.

3.7.5 Feeding and management of cow body condition (body fat and protein)

The body condition of dairy cattle is evaluated using visual and/or manual palpation to estimate the level of body fat covering the tail head, ribs and spine. This is expressed using either a 5-point (with half points) or 10-point scale, with the lower numbers indicating lower fat reserves (thinner) and the higher numbers indicating greater levels of fat reserves (fatter, Table 3.4). The main aim is to allow cows to gain weight in late lactation and the dry period. Tthis will allow dairy cattle to calve in adequate body condition (3.5 on a 5-point scale) to enable them to have sufficient reserves to cope with the energy gap in early lactation. The provision of good quality feed and a nutrition plan in early lactation should then ensure that the dairy cow does not lose too much live weight during early lactation and is in a rising plane of nutrition and increasing body condition during the mating period in order to increase the conception rate and thus fertility.

3.8 Health

The main focus of dairy herd health management should be disease prevention. The majority of diseases of importance for dairy herds are often multifactorial in nature, with a number of factors that interact together to cause disease. In global terms, the three main reasons why cows leave (are culled from) the dairy herd are, in decreasing order:

- infertility;
- mastitis;
- lameness.

These diseases are of great importance in both economic and animal welfare terms and they will be discussed in detail because their control is central to good dairy herd management. Other major potential animal health issues include hypocalcaemia, hypomagnesaemia, acidosis, displaced abomasum, endometritis, acetonaemia (ketosis) and bloat.

3.8.1 Reproduction and fertility

On a global basis, poor reproduction or 'infertility' is the most common reason for dairy cows to be culled from the dairy herd. The loss of cows due to infertility and the subsequent need to provide herd replacement represents a considerable economic cost, while calving of cows on an approximately annual basis is a key factor in generating high levels of efficient milk production. As a consequence, the efficient management of reproduction in the dairy herd is one of the most important factors in dairy herd management. The annual management of reproduction is presented in Figure 3.7. (Further reading can be found in Peters and Ball, 2004, *Reproduction in Cattle.*)

3.8.1.1 Gestation

The gestation length of the dairy cow is a relatively fixed period of approximately 283 days, but varies slightly with the breed of the calf. The European or continental beef breeds tend to have longer gestation periods, as do male calves compared to female calves of dairy breeds. In New Zealand the Angus and Angus crossbreeds are favoured as terminal sires compared with the Hereford beef breeds due to the shorter gestation length and the need for a seasonal calving pattern. The use of hormones to induce calving and thus shorten the gestation period is not commonly used as a management practice for dairy cows, except when required in exceptional circumstances, due to the welfare implications for both the cow and calf.

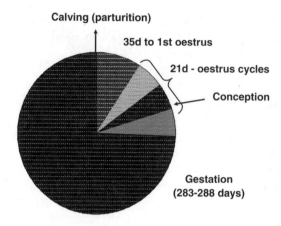

Figure 3.7 An example of the differing components (days) of an annual (365-day calving interval) reproductive cycle of the dairy cow.

3.8.1.2 Puberty and oestrous cycles

Dairy heifers reach puberty at around 40% of mature weight and this can be achieved as early as 4 month of age, where the plane of nutrition has been high in early life. The optimal age for heifers to calve is at approximately 2 years of age, at 85 to 90% mature weight and, as gestation length is relatively fixed, this can be achieved by heifers conceiving at 15 months of age at 55 to 60% mature weight.

3.8.1.3 Oestrous cycles and conception rate of lactating cows

The dairy cow has a natural period of non-ovulation (anoestrus) following calving, which is approximately 35 days long. This period can be minimized by ensuring adequate body condition at calving and providing adequate nutrition following calving. The aims should be to minimize live weight loss following calving and for the cows to be gaining weight by the time of insemination. First oestrus should occur between 20 to 40 days postpartum and this may be recorded in order to determine the return of 'normal' oestrous cycles in readiness for the next oestrus cycle. Dairy cows that have not shown oestrus behaviour following this period may have cystic ovarian disease (COD) and require treatment by the veterinarian. The uterus requires approximately 40 to 50 days following parturition to return to its normal size and function and, as a consequence, conception rate (CR) to inseminations before 50 days postpartum tends to be low. Due to this and the expense of high-quality semen, dairy cows are typically inseminated following standing heats (oestrus) from 50 days postpartum onwards and this may be delayed to 60 d postpartum in higher milk-yielding herds.

The CR to first insemination completed around 50 to 60 d postpartum tends to be lower compared to second and subsequent inseminations. In the assessment of conception rates, first, second and subsequent inseminations should be calculated and monitored separately. The conception rate of Holstein Friesian cows has tended to decline over the last 10 to 15 years. As a consequence fertility, despite its low heritability, has been included in the breed assessment index for animal selection and breeding purposes. Similarly, the use and evaluation of differing dairy breeds and the use of crossbreeding of dairy cattle breeds have become increasingly popular within the global dairy industry.

3.8.1.4 Oestrous behaviour

The length of the oestrous cycle ranges between 18 and 24 days, averaging around 21 days. The cow is 'on heat' or 'in oestrus' for an average of around 14 hours, but this can vary from as little as 1 hour to as long as 24 hours. Ovulation occurs around 10 to 12 hours following the onset of oestrus, but this timing will clearly be affected by the length of oestrus and the correct animal identification and timing of insemination following oestrus is critical in achieving high conception rates. The level and duration of oestrous behaviour can vary according to season, ambient temperature, housing environment, breed, body condition, social interaction and plane of nutrition. Oestrous behaviour tends to be lower in warmer climates or periods, during winter (reduced light), in housed conditions and for cows that have lower social status within the herd. The oestrous behaviour is likely to be higher for cows in good body condition, with adequate and appropriate nutrition including mineral supplementation, which are housed or grazed in compliance with the welfare regulations, housing codes of practice and conformance to the relevant farm assurance guidelines.

3.8.2 Factors affecting fertility

3.8.2.1 Oestrus detection

The use of cow observation by well-trained staff, supported by accurate recording and a good communications system, is the most commonly used approach to oestrus detection. This system relies on observation of cows expressing oestrous behaviour, identification of the correct cow and insemination at the appropriate time to coincide with ovulation. In an ideal situation the cows could be observed continually, but in reality cows are observed during period of 'natural' behaviour at regular intervals through the day and in the evening. For this approach to succeed, cows should be observed four times daily. It is important to be sure that the correct cow is accurately identified and recorded. This requires cows to be individually identified at a distance and that the cow standing to be mounted is identified as the cow in oestrus. There are some exceptions: a cow in oestrus may mount the front end of another cow, possibly due to frustration at not having been mounted herself. It is important that the cow 'stands' to be mounted. Should she move away she may not yet be in oestrus, but may be coming into oestrus. These observation periods should allow adequate time for the activities of the cows to be watched. A team effort from farm staff along with a good communication system is more likely to increase cow observation time and cows seen in oestrus.

3.8.2.2 Aids to oestrus detection

The trend to larger herds and to all-year-round calving has led to the development of several aids to the detection of oestrus to ensure timely insemination, high levels of conception and pregnancy rates (PR).

3.8.2.3 Tail paint and pads

Purpose-specific paint or pads of paint can be applied to the 'tail head' on the spine. Cows that have been 'mounted' by other cows can be observed and recorded at milking time and submitted for insemination.

3.8.2.4 Electronic monitors

During the oestrous period the activity level of cows on heat tends to increase beyond the normal levels. Meters that measure the number of steps or activity of the cow can be used to assess cow activity and the possible occurrence of oestrus. Similarly the body temperature of the cow tends to be higher during oestrus and this can also be monitored and interpreted in a similar way. However these technologies can give 'false positives' in cows with high activity or body temperature for reasons other than oestrus.

3.8.2.5 Hormone tests

Kits are available to measure milk progesterone levels on-farm. Progesterone is secreted from the corpus luteum. Thus it is high during the dioestrous period after ovulation and increases further in pregnancy. In a non-pregnant cows, milk progesterone levels fall sharply about 19 days after the previous oestrus and remain low for about 4 days, then start to rise at the time of ovulation. Analysis of milk samples for progesterone on days 7, 19 and 21 after previous oestrus can either predict optimal time for insemination or give a good early indication of the success of a previous insemination.

3.8.2.6 Vasectomized or 'teaser' bulls

The intermittent use of vasectomized or 'teaser' bulls can also increase oestrous behaviour levels. Undoubtedly the most successful way to achieve high fertility is through natural service. However, this is inconsistent with the need for genetic improvement of the herd that can be gained from the access to nationally and internationally ranked sires through the use of artificial insemination.

3.8.3 Mastitis

Mastitis is the second most common reason for culling cows from the dairy herd, affecting approximately 35% of cows annually (the range for 95% of herds being between 5 and 60%). It is caused by a bacterial infection of the mammary gland via the teat canal. The bacteria involved are classified as *contagious* (e.g. *Staphylococcus*, *Streptococcus*) because they are typically transmitted between cows through poor hygiene at milking, and *environmental* (e.g. *Escherichia coli*). Clinical mastitis results in inflammation of the affected quarter and can cause considerable pain and

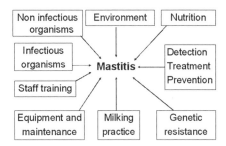

Figure 3.8 Main factors associated with mastitis of dairy cattle.

discomfort. As a consequence, mastitis represents a considerable challenge to the welfare of the dairy cow. Factors that affect the incidence of mastitis are shown in Figure 3.8.

3.8.3.1 Economic effect of mastitis

Mastitis reduces the economic efficiently of the dairy herd by causing losses and increasing costs. The losses associated with mastitis include:

- liquid milk sales (antibiotic milk discarded or offered to calves);
- milk price (lower price for milk with higher somatic cell counts;
- milk component levels (reduced due to mastitis);
- milk production (long-term reduction).
- Increasing costs associated with mastitis include:
- treatment (antibiotic or other);
- labour (treatment, dry cow therapy, separation from main herd);
- herd replacements (cows culled due to high SCC or clinical mastitis).

3.8.3.2 Management of mastitis

The level of mastitis in the dairy herd can be monitored using the somatic cell count (SCC) levels in the milk. This is essentially a measure of white blood cells recruited to combat chronic (typically non-clinical) infection with organisms of contagious mastitis (e.g. *Staphylococcus*). The maximum SCC allowed in bulk milk vary considerably in differing countries; within the EU and New Zealand a level of 400,000 (cells/mL) is applied, while in Australia (600 to 700,000 (cells/mL) and the USA (750,000 cells/mL) higher levels are applied. Milk that exceeds these levels will not be collected by milk purchasers or will attract demerit points and much reduced milk price (Table 3.5). In practice, there are moves in the USA to reduce the maximum levels to 400,000 cells/mL. In all countries the annual mean SCC levels achieved for milk are well below the maximum levels and in New Zealand, where a demerit system is used, few demerit points are generally applied.

Table 3.5 Examples of bacterial quality and somatic cell count levels used in milk purchase in differing counties (000/mL).

Country	Maximum bacterial count	Maximum somatic cell count
Denmark	100	400
France	100	400
Germany	100	400
UK	100	400
Australia	600	750
New Zealand	500	400
Canada	100	500
USA*	400	700–750

* Varies with county.

Milk purchasers use milk quality payment schemes to maintain and increase the quality of milk supplied by milk producers, and in some schemes SCC levels below 50, 100 and 150,000 cells/mL can attract additional payment for good milk quality. The bulk milk SCC levels are monitored by milk purchasers and used to calculate milk price in payment schemes, apply demerit points or refuse to collect milk considered not to be suitable for human consumption. On the farm the management of mastitis is best described as proactive, where a positive approach is used to prevent, rapidly diagnose and treat mastitis in order to maintain low SCC levels. The main potential for cows to be infected with mastitis is during mechanical milking. A key issue is the need to maintain low levels of SCC throughout the herd in order to minimize the risk of cross-contamination between cows with mastitis (high SCC >250,000) and cows without mastitis (low SCC <250,000). Milking heifers (with low SCC) before cows with higher SCC can prevent herd SCC from increasing, milking individual cows with high SCC following lower SCC cows and the use of pre-milking teat dip and wearing gloves during milking can reduce the risk of spreading the mastitis bacteria. The application of teat dips following milking is a key point at which mastitis-causing bacteria can be prevented from gaining access into the mammary gland, by protecting the teat canal from contamination while the sphincter muscle, that typically closes the teat canal, remains open following milking. The sooner cows with clinical mastitis are diagnosed and treated the less likely that the cows will have a prolonged infection and will directly reduce the opportunity for other cows to be contaminated (Table 3.6).

3.8.3.3 Mastitis in organic dairy herds
In organic herds, antibiotics are not used as first line of treatment for mastitis, unless withholding this treatment is likely to compromise the welfare of the animal. These greater restrictions to use antibiotics make the prevention of mastitis a key management strategy for organic herds. As a consequence, organic milk producers

Table 3.6 Prevention and treatment of mastitis using the 5-point plan or seasonal mastitis management (SAMM) plan.

Measure	Action
1. Teat dip or spray	Post-milking teat treatment – always
	Pre-milking teat treatment – problems with contagious bacteria spread at milking
2. Clinical cases	Prompt diagnosis and treatment
3. Dry cow therapy	Long-acting antibiotics
	Teat sealant for cows that have not had mastitis
4. Culling	Persistent and recurring cases
	Individuals with consistently high SCC (>250,000)
5. Equipment testing and maintenance	Observation of teats for normality of colour following milking and to ensure no damage to teat sphincters
	Daily checks of rubber wear for cracks and splits
	Daily check on vacuum level, pulsator and vacuum function Regular replacement of rubber cup liners Professional annual check of milking machine

emphasize the importance of good milking equipment design and maintenance, and hygienic milking practices, particularly the wearing of gloves for milking. The use of non-antibiotic treatments for the treatment of mastitis are also considered to be important and some of these include vaccination, drenching with vinegar and the use of arnica, peppermint udder creams and cold water applications to minimize inflammation, which is typical to this disease. The efficacy of these is unproven.

3.8.4 Lameness

Lameness is the third most common reason for cows to be culled from the dairy herd. The incidence of lameness in dairy cattle is approximately 35% of cows annually, but ranges from as low as 5% to as high as 60% on differing farms. Lameness is a multifactorial disease and the main factors involved in the cause and prevention of lameness include environment, especially housing and cow tracks, animal management and handling, genetic conformation, nutrition, and hoof trimming and bathing.

Nearly all lameness in dairy cattle is foot lameness (Figure 3.9). It can take many forms, but these may broadly be considered within two categories:

- disorders of the sole and hoof horn – these are usually non-infectious in origin and include sole bruising and ulceration, white line disease, toe ulcers and foot rot (as a secondary infection);
- infectious conditions of the skin adjacent to the hoof – e.g. digital and interdigital dermatitis, necrobacillosis ('foul').

Table 3.7 A five-point locomotion scoring method for dairy cattle.

Score	Locomotion	Head and back
1	Not lame	Flat back
	Good walking conformation	No head bobbing
2	Not lame	Slight arch
	Poorer walking conformation	(poorer conformation)
		No head bobbing
3	Becoming lame	Slight arch (poorer conformation)
	Tender feet	Some head bobbing
	Slightly lame on one or more limbs	
4	Lame	Arched back
	Not bearing weight evenly on one or more limbs	Head bobbing
5	Non-weight-bearing on one or more limbs	Arched back
		Severe head bobbing

3.8.4.1 Locomotion scoring

Locomotion scoring (Table 3.7) and the identification and accurate recording of claw horn disorders (Figure 3.9) are essential to the prevention and treatment of lameness. Locomotion scoring involves observing cows walking to assess how evenly cows bear weight in each foot, the evenness of the strides they take and the arch of the back and movement of the head. Table 3.7 describes how these are used to score lameness on a five-point scale. Lameness scores are used to record the prevalence (number of cows lame on any one day) and severity of lameness. The main aim of locomotion scoring is to identify and diagnose individual lame cows (score 3) as soon as possible, so that appropriate treatment can be applied, thus reducing both the

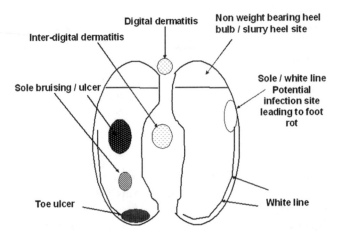

Figure 3.9 Diagram of the cow's weight-bearing claws and main types of lameness.

number of animals that progress to severe lameness (scores of 4 and 5) and length of time the cows spend lame. Correct identification of lesions (e.g. claw horn haemorrhage, digital dermatitis; Figure 3.9) will also help to identify hazards, risks and corrective measures at the herd level. This type of approach reduces the potential number of lame cows, associated labour costs, the treatment of secondary infections with antibiotics and the potential for lameness to contribute to other health issues through reduced feed intake, live weight loss, milk yield reduction and potential infertility.

3.8.4.2 Types of lameness
Sole and white line damage account for the majority of lameness in dairy cows. However the infectious conditions, digital dermatitis (DD) and interdigital dermatitis (IDD), are an increasing problem in the UK, EU and USA and have become endemic on many farms. DD and IDD are not common in New Zealand and other pasture-based systems.

3.8.4.3 Sole bruising and ulceration
This is a common problem and is typically at its greatest level at around 120 days following calving. It results from damage that occurs to the corium when it is trapped between the bone tissue within the hoof. Prolonged standing on concrete and walking on hard surfaces such as cow tracks is a major predisposing factor, as is inadequate (or improper) foot trimming. The resilience of the foot structures is also compromised around the time of calving and early lactation. This can be seen by the greater intensity of bruising and potential ulceration in Figure 3.9.

3.8.4.4 White line disease, disorders and toe ulcers
The white line, indicated in Figure 3.9, is where the wall horn is cemented to the sole horn. This is weaker than other parts of the claw. In consequence, this area of the claw horn is more subject to physical damage due to wear and damage from twisting and walking, while bruising in this area also occurs. Problems associated with this area of the claw are referred to as white line disease, disorders, erosion and bruising and ulceration. This area is particularly prone to damage in systems where cows walk long distances. The rotation of the last pharynx (P3) can similarly trap the horn-producing lamellae at the toe and lead to toe bruising and ulceration.

3.8.4.5 Foot rot
This seems to be quite common in New Zealand. It is most frequently a secondary infection and is often associated with ingressions of infectious organism through the white line/sole area (Figure 3.9), which is in contrast to lameness seen in other dairy cow systems of management. It is most apparent during wet conditions and when cows are confined on concrete pads (feed pads) to be offered feed and where cow tracks and lane ways have wet and poorly maintained areas. Feed pads and tracks or lane ways are commonly used in the pasture-based systems of New Zealand and

Australia. Good construction and maintenance of tracks and lane ways are imperative in reducing foot rot, and wet conditions in general tend to reduce claw horn strength and resilience to cow housing and management.

3.8.4.6 Digital and interdigital dermatitis

The primary cause of this infectious disease is a spirochete, which is very resilient, survives in manure and as such is more common in housed animals. This infection is spread through manure and can be reduced by attention to floor hygiene (e.g. twice-daily scraping and/or flushing with water). It can however be spread by frequent (inadequate) scraping with automated scrapers. Regular use of clean footbaths becomes essential where the disease is endemic. Some farms incorporate foot bathing as a daily routine. The appropriate use of medications and/or copper sulfate can be used to treat DD when there are lesions. This is not presently a common problem in pasture-based systems.

3.8.5 Environment and lameness

3.8.5.1 Pasture-based systems

In pasture-based systems, which are common to New Zealand, Australia and some areas of Europe and the USA, the cows are managed in large herds, often using paddocks which are grazed in rotation and, as a consequence, cows in these systems walk long distances. In these circumstances the most common types of lameness are white line disease and foot rot, which is a secondary infection that has often resulted from an infection of the white line at the heel area of the outer (lateral) claw, which tends to wear faster than the toe in these systems. The other types of lameness include sole bruising and ulceration, interdigital damage and swelling due to high stocking rates (paddock pressure). There is little infectious skin disease (e.g. DD).

In pasture-based systems the careful handing of dairy cattle and the infrastructure used to convey cattle to and from pasture are key areas of management in the prevention of lameness. The provision and maintenance of good-quality cow tracks, the steady movement of cattle (at their own speed) along tracks, the prevention of manure build-up and occurrence of wet muddy conditions and the accumulation of small stones or the development of rough surfaces where cows are required to walk, are key areas in the prevention of lameness.

3.8.5.2 Housed systems

In many countries cattle are housed, either permanently or, more commonly for 4 to 6 months of the year, when pasture growth is low due to cold wet conditions. Dairy cattle confined in housing or feed areas with concrete flooring may have more feet and leg problems. Due to increasing herd sizes the free stall or cubicle housing systems have become the most common. In these systems sole bruising and ulceration, white line disease and digital and interdigital dermatitis are the most common types of lameness. Provision of at least one stall or cubicle available for each cow, preferably with 5 to 10% additional (empty) stalls, will increase lying time and reduce sole and white line-related lameness. These stalls or cubicles should be of an appropriate size (Table 3.3) and construction to allow the cow to lie comfortably and have sufficient 'lunge space' to allow the cows to rise and reduce hock damage. These cubicles/stalls should provide a comfortable bed. Cow mats are common but not ideal. The best material would appear to be sand, which provides comfort when lying at rest and purchase for the feet when the cow is changing position (standing up and lying down).

Loose housing systems should have a bedding area and separate loafing/feeding area, which can be cleaned regularly to minimize bedding use and incidence of mastitis and milk SCC levels (Table 3.6) Tie barn systems, where cows are tethered, are much less common overall, but are still popular in some parts of Europe and Canada, where smaller herds are housed. In these systems, sole bruising along with claw overgrowth and hock swelling are more common types of lameness due to lack of exercise.

The exact details of housing requirements for dairy cattle, such as space allocation and appropriate cubicle/stall dimensions according to animal live weight, can be found in the building standards of each country along with reference to welfare codes of practice and farm assurance guidance notes.

3.8.6 Nutrition and lameness

3.8.6.1 Acidosis and subacute rumen acidosis

Laminitis, which should not be confused with sole haemorrhages arising from mechanical damage to the suspensory apparatus of the foot, arises from disturbances to the blood and oxygen supply to the corium, the area of horn production. This particular type of lameness is associated with nutritional disorders, especially acute (pH < 5.0), or intermittent or chronic subclinical rumen acidosis (pH < 5.5). A reliable indicator of subclinical acidosis is low milk fat composition. This has become more common in recent years; the use of diets with high levels of rapidly digestible carbohydrates or sugars and potentially low levels of dietary fibre and short forage chopping can result in low pH due to higher rate of fatty acid production in the rumen fluid (especially lactic and propionic acids). A low rumen fluid pH can result in the death of some rumen bacterial populations leading to the release of endotoxins that mediate an inflammatory response and cause the constriction of blood, oxygen and nutrient supply to the corium, where the hoof horn-producing lamellae are located. This causes a disturbance to horn formation, which can be sufficiently severe to result in a break or crack appearing on the outer wall of the hoof wall of the outer (lateral) claw, which typically occurs at the heel of the foot.

3.8.6.2 Vitamins and minerals

The structural integrity of the hoof horn depends on the effectiveness of the keratinization of epidermal cells and this can be affected by diet, e.g. vitamins A, D, E and H (biotin); minerals calcium, phosphorus and magnesium; trace elements zinc and selenium. Dietary deficiencies of minerals, vitamins and trace elements lead to disturbances in the keratinization process. This can result in decreased horn quality and development of secondary infection. Calcium, phosphorus and manganese are involved in the development and maintenance of bone and collagen formation. The addition of biotin and zinc sulfate have been found to reduce the levels of lameness, especially white line disease, and improve the rate of healing of hoof horn. Copper and cobalt supplementation may also affect hoof and foot health. However such dietary supplementation will not compensate for poor genetics, environment and/or management.

3.8.7 Genetic selection

The selection process favours cows with steeper hoof and mid range leg angles, which allow the cow to wear the toe of the claws and this has also been related to stronger hoof horn quality. This selection of dairy cows and sires for good 'conformation traits' such as leg and foot angle has been successfully practised to reduce the number of cows with low hoof angles and 'sickle' shaped hocks that tend to develop overgrown claws at the toe area. A slight overgrowth is indicated when the outer (lateral) claw is slightly longer than the inner (medial) claw and this should be corrected by hoof trimming before the cow develops an inability to wear the hoof wall at the toe.

3.8.8 Hoof trimming

The trimming of cows' claws is practised as a routine in some countries such as the UK, USA and Canada and is typically completed at drying off from lactation. This

Table 3.8 Preventing and reducing the incidence of lameness of dairy cattle.

Area	Factors to prevent/reduce lameness
Environment	Adequate housing, stalls (size and design), flooring and maintenance, good layout, collecting yard (adequate design and size)
	Appropriate backing gate operation
	Good cow tracks or race design, maintenance and management
Hygiene	To reduce occurrence of slurry heel, spread of digital dermatitis
Genetics	Good conformation; foot, leg and hoof angle
	Breeds and breeding
Nutrition	Avoid rumen acidosis and sub-acute rumen acidosis
	Adequate macronutrient (Ca, P), micronutrient (Zn, Cu, Se) and vitamin nutrition (Biotin, B vitamins)
Management	Appropriate foot trimming and foot bathing
	Appropriate cow handling and moving, backing gate operation

should be carried out by a qualified hoof trimmer or by a veterinarian or farmer who has completed an accredited hoof-trimming course. While good hoof-trimming is a major contributor to the control of lameness in dairy cattle, poor, overzealous trimming can make matters worse.

Table 3.8 summarizes methods of preventing lameness in dairy cattle.

3.8.9 Other potential health problems

3.8.9.1 Hypocalcaemia

Lactating dairy cattle produce large amount of milk, which contains calcium. This requires them to mobilize body reserves of calcium from their bones. However, during early lactation the requirement for calcium for milk production can result in a shortage of calcium in the blood plasma (hypocalcaemia). Acute calcium deficiency can result in lack of muscle function that is sufficient to cause paralysis and rapid death. Affected cows can be treated with calcium borogluconate injections, but the main aim is to prevent the occurrence of this calcium deficiency in the blood (see Section 3.6.6.1).

3.8.9.2 Hypomagnesaemia (grass staggers)

During periods of rapid pasture growth, typically in spring or following late autumn applications of nitrogen fertilizer, the magnesium levels of pasture can be low and result in a deficiency of magnesium in the plasma. Magnesium is required for muscle function. In acute deficiency, animals will initially show signs of 'staggers' and this can rapidly proceed to convulsions and death. Prevention involves giving magnesium supplements, which are typically added to water or included in concentrated diets offered at milking time. Since magnesium is unpalatable the most effective method of supplementation is by addition to water troughs. However this will not succeed if cows have access to an alternative source of fresh water.

3.8.9.3 Acidosis and subacute rumen acidosis

This disease has become more common in recent years (see section 3.8.4) and is classified as acidosis with a rumen pH <5.0 and subacute rumen acidosis (SARA) with a rumen liquor pH <5.5. These have become common due to the use of high levels of rapidly digestible carbohydrates or sugars and potentially low levels of dietary fibre and forage chopping, which has resulted in low pH due to higher rate of acid production leading to death of protozoa and some bacterial species in the rumen with increased production of lactic acid. The low rumen fluid pH results in low milk fat composition (below 2.9%) and potentially lowered dry matter intake. Attempts to prevent rumen acidosis in cows given diets high in starch and low in functional fibre include the dietary inclusion of bicarbonate of soda, the use of yeast preparations (live or dead) which utilize lactic acid, or the inclusion of highly digestible fibre (HDF) into the diet, usually as part of the compound feed offered at milking. The inclusion of some chopped straw in the diet may be an option, since this will stimulate salivation and thus increase the supply of endogenous sodium bicarbonate. However, this may cause an overall reduction in nutrient intake and thus an undesirable reduction in milk yield.

3.8.9.4 Bloat

Bloat is caused by the gas from rumen fermentation becoming trapped in a foam of air bubbles. The problem typically arises when cows graze pasture legumes that contain a protein that creates a 'strong' coating on the air bubble, making it resistant to being broken down. This build-up of gas bubbles results in the rumen crushing the lungs and large abdominal blood vessels of the animal, leading to death. This disease can be prevented by treating cows with bloat oil and or piercing of the rumen to let out the froth. However, the use of anti-bloat pasture species is much more practical than dosing animals with oils or other techniques. The main prevention is controlling access by cows to pastures likely to cause bloat, and the use of plant varieties that have low bloat potential.

3.8.9.5 Acetonaemia (ketosis)

Ketone bodies are produced as a result of the excessive mobilization and incomplete oxidation of fat, in cows that are too fat at the time of parturition (Table 3.4). The main prevention is to control live weight and condition score through proper nutrition in the transition period and early lactation.

3.9 Heifer Rearing and Transition into the Dairy Herd

3.9.1 Strategies

The overall replacement rate is typically around 20% to 25% of the dairy herd annually. Dairy heifers are typically provided from the dairy herd by selective breeding from the cattle in the herd that are the most productive, fertile and have the desired conformation and mating these to high genetic-merit sires, with desired dairy characteristics. The alternative is to buy heifers, but this introduces increased risk from disease and variability in cost and suitability to the dairy herd.

In herds where non-sexed semen is used, a 25% replacement rate will require mating a minimum of 50% of the highest-merit cows in the herd, using high genetic-merit semen from artificial insemination or possibly natural breeding in order to provide sufficient herd replacements on an annual basis. The optimal economic performance of dairy heifers will be achieved by calving dairy heifers at 85 to 90% mature weight at 22 to 24 months of age. This requires heifers to be served at 13 to 15 months of age, when for optimal herd performance they need to be 55 to 60% of their mature weight. Mature weight is highly heritable and thus can be predicted from the parents and breed of dairy heifer, but farmers must be realistic about the true mature weight of the adult animals as genetic improvement and breed will affect adult weight. Further reading for this section can be found in Garnsworthy (2005).

The application of higher feeding rates, increased protein intake and thus higher growth rates for dairy heifers between 0 and 3 months of age has been found to increase mammary development and subsequent milk yield, while higher growth rates around puberty (40% mature weight) predispose to fat deposition in mammary tissue and this can negatively affect subsequent milk yield potential. As a consequence, the rearing and nutrition of dairy heifers differs from that of beef cattle and will have a direct impact on the yield potential of the dairy herd. The effective provision of dairy herd replacements can be achieved through a specific and planned approach using target maturity for age and achieving appropriate growth rates for each phase of development.

3.9.2 Options for the provision of dairy replacements

Table 3.9 presents a range of options for the provision of dairy replacements, which include rearing calves from the dairy herd on the home farm, rearing calves to milk weaning and later transferring them to a 'contract grazier' or purchasing in calf heifers or freshly calved heifers as replacements. There are advantages and disadvantages to each of these options. If contract rearing is practised, all contracts should be legally binding documents, drawn up by a suitably qualified and experienced person. These must clearly state targets for growth rates and live weight/ maturity according to animal age and penalty clauses if targets are not met. They should include regular monitoring and reporting of heifer development. There should be a health plan and a contingency feeding plan, which should be developed with a veterinarian and nutritionist, documented and monitored.

3.9.3 Dairy heifer rearing programmes

3.9.3.1 Rearing young calves

The majority of dairy calves are removed from their mothers shortly after birth, once they have received adequate colostrum, and then reared artificially. Milk is offered by training calves to drink from a pail or suckle from a teat or from a mechanical calf-feeding machine. Suckling systems, where calves are suckled on a cow on a restricted basis or where multiple calves suckle a nurse cow, are less common in developed countries, but are used regularly in developing environments. Calves are offered either whole milk, milk replacer or colostrum. In addition, calves are offered specialized calf starter feeds and forages in order to encourage rumen development. The main objectives are to achieve low mortality and produce healthy calves that have few disease problems, grow rapidly (750 to 950 g/d) and achieve high levels of maturity particularly in the first 0 to 3 months of age. The single most important factor in ensuring good calf-rearing practice is the adequate provision of high-quality (high immunoglobulin content) colostrum from the first two milkings postpartum,

Table 3.9 Optional methods of providing dairy herd replacements and the effect on requirements, cost and risk.

	Home rearing	Full contract rearing	Contract grazing to calving	Purchased
Genetic improvement	Full control	Full control	Full control	Very limited control
Growth rate and maturity	Full control	Need contracts and monitoring	Need contracts and monitoring	Very limited control
Feeds	Full control	Limited control	Limited control	No control
Contracts	Not required	Contract required	Contract required	Not required
Infrastructure	Full requirement	Limited needs	Limited needs	None required
Labour	Labour, training and peaks	Limited requirement	Limited requirement	Only required for selection of animals
Finance	Low	Outward flow of cash	Outward flow of cash	Outward flow of cash
Land use	Requirement, but can use land not suited to dairy	Not required	Not required	Not required
Transport	Limited requirements	Required	Required	Required
Biosecurity	Full control	Limited control	Limited control	No control
Cost	Full control	Some control	Some control	No control
Risk	Low	Medium	Medium	High
Flexibility	Low	High	High	High

quickly (within the first 6 to 12 h of age) and to offer adequate quantity (10% of live weight).

3.9.3.2 Whole milk feeding

The use of whole milk offered at approx 4 to 5 litres/day (L/d) (or 10% of live weight) is popular in many countries and will achieve growth rates of 630 to 650 g/d, which are below the growth rates recommended for dairy heifers. Whole milk is deficient in nutrients, vitamins D and E and trace elements – iron, manganese, zinc, copper, iodine, cobalt and selenium. To achieve optimal growth rates for dairy calves, whole milk requires the nutrient concentration (fat, lactose and protein) to be increased along with additional vitamin A. These need to be achieved without substantial increase to feeding volume (L), with the addition of high-quality milk replacer, with additional lactose and high protein level (26 to 28%) or preferably with a specifically designed milk supplements. Increasing the feeding level of whole milk above 5 L/d is not recommended; this will reduce solid feed intake, delay rumen development and weaning from milk, which will increase rearing costs. Milk from cows being treated with antibiotics is not recommended for feeding to dairy heifers.

3.9.3.3 Colostrum feeding systems

Colostrum feeding is more popular in some counties than others, depending on calving pattern and other marketing opportunities for colostrum. Colostrum feeding at 4 to 5 L/d results in high growth rates (700 to 750 g/d) and healthy calves. The main point to remember is that continuing to feed colostrum will delay the development of an active immune system in the calf and a period of 'low' immunity, the 'weak' period between passive immunity from colostrum and active immunity in the calf, will occur within 1 to 2 weeks post-weaning or following the removal of colostrum from the diet. Changing the diet to whole milk 3 weeks prior to milk weaning will help avoiding a clash between milk weaning and low immune function.

3.9.3.4 Milk replacers

Milk replacers are typically either skimmed milk or whey-based milk powder. Skim milk powders and whole milk contain caseins, which coagulate in the abomasum and increase retention time, while whey-based milk powders do not form clots. The available comparisons of skim milk versus whey protein concentrate indicate that calves offered skim milk-based milk replacer do not seem to perform better than those offered whey protein concentrate. Heat damage, which can be estimated by testing the lysine content, can severely affect the digestibility of milk replacers and subsequent calf growth rates. The best performance will be achieved from highly digestible milk replacers that contain fractionated milk proteins (skim base) and natural antibodies, which increase disease resistance in the digestive tract and provide good-quality proteins. Milk replacer powders recommended for dairy heifers contain 20 to 21% fat along with additional lactose and 26 to 28% crude protein. When offered at 600 g/d they should promote growth rates of 750 to 950 g/d.

3.9.3.5 Ad libitum milk feeding

Ad libitum feeding of milk is not recommended for dairy heifers, due to this practice resulting in slow rumen development and inadequate balance of nutrients in milk.

3.9.3.6 Multiple suckling systems

Some farmers operate multiple suckling systems which involve running a number of calves with one or more 'nurse' cows. This system can be effective provided that calves receive sufficient milk (10% birth weight) to achieve adequate growth rates. Farmers sometimes use high somatic cell count cows for this purpose to prevent damage to milk quality supplied to the milk product manufacturer.

3.9.3.7 Restricted suckling

The use of restricted suckling of dairy calves in developing countries where the infrastructure to ensure hygiene and support factors are limited can be more successful than artificial rearing and feeding calves from buckets, pails or artificial teats. These systems allow the calf to suckle the dairy cow before milking to encourage milk letdown in crossbred cattle, and again after milking (by hand or mechanically) to remove the residual milk remaining. Depending on the milk yield of the cows, the calf may be allowed one or two full quarters or the residual milk of all quarters. The main factor is to ensure that the calf is allowed sufficient milk to ensure adequate growth, health and development. Calves are typically offered milk up until 10 to 12 weeks of age, up to a maximum of 4 to 5 L/d.

The advantages of restricted suckling systems are the lack of potential infection (enteric disorders or scours) of the calf due to poor feeding utensil hygiene, prolonged passive immunity for the calf and satiation of suckling behaviour. The cow will produce a greater quantity of milk and be less likely to have mastitis. The disadvantages are the potential to prolong the anoestrous period in the dam with twice daily suckling of the calf, which can be alleviated by reducing the suckling frequency to once daily to initiate ovarian activity.

3.9.4 Age at weaning from milk

Early weaning systems allow calves to be weaned from milk at 5 to 6 weeks of age when intake of the dry, cereal-based starter feed is 1 to 2 kg/d. In pasture-based systems calves are typically offered milk for longer, until 8 to 12 weeks of age. In New Zealand calves are generally weaned according to live weight and breed – approximately 80 kg for Jersey, 85 kg for Friesian Jersey cross and 90 kg for Friesian calves, which is achieved from 8 to 12 weeks of age.

3.9.5 Organic dairy systems

Organic systems have specific requirements for calf rearing and at present most specify feeding of whole milk till 12 weeks of age. Milk feeding level will be a minimum of 10% birth weight, but maximum milk feeding level will depend on the cost of organic calf starter diets and forage quality and availability. In these cases individual country and milk company guidelines should be followed.

3.9.6 Solid feeds and feeding

3.9.6.1 Calf 'starter' feeds

Young calves should be offered calf starter and will consume small amounts (200 g per head per day) of palatable cereal-based feeds within the second week of life. These cereal-based feeds are key to the development of the rumen and ruminal papillae, which respond well to volatile fatty acids produced from rumen fermentation. Specialist calf supplement feeds and meals need to be highly palatable, should be offered in small amounts initially and replaced daily, to encourage early and increasing consumption levels. Any leftovers can be collected and given directly to older (weaned) calves.

Good-quality calf supplements for dairy calves should be made from highly digestible components, 22% crude protein (CP) with a good amino acid profile (e.g. soya bean meal). Dairy heifer growth and mammary development are increased by higher levels of utilizable proteins (amino acids) in the diet. The levels of sugar (50 g/kg and fat (35 g/kg) need to be limited in barley-based diets, as calves have a limited capacity to digest these.

3.9.6.2 Calf starter and feeding levels

Calf starter feeds should be offered *ad libitum* prior to the time of weaning from milk but restricted thereafter according to the availability and quality of pasture or forage. The body condition of heifers can fluctuate: low body condition can be used to indicate the need to increase feeding levels. However, short-term increases in body condition should not be a reason to decrease feeding levels.

3.9.6.3 Hay and cereal straw

Ad libitum access to clean, dust-free fibrous feeds, preferably straw, should be offered to satisfy the investigative need of young calves for oral activity. Insufficient access (level offered or feeding space) to forage will result in calves sucking and chewing other objects in their surroundings, such as each other, building fences and anything they can reach, included string used to fix up gates or fences. Grazing calves will be consuming some pasture, but will benefit from being offered straws or hay with a high stem component, which needs to be kept dry and covered from rain, to prevent subsequent mould and aflatoxin development. The consumption of these forages will aid rumen development, although the main contributor to this is the consumption of cereal-based calf starter diets.

3.9.6.4 Water

All livestock are entitled to access to clean fresh water at all times; calves should be offered good-quality, fresh clean water that should be changed twice daily. The exception is a small proportion of calves that drink water as if it was milk, and these should have their access limited to feeding periods twice daily for the first week or so.

3.9.6.5 Bedding

Housed calves, unless housed on slatted floors, will require bedding materials. Calves will eat bedding and will eat this to a much greater extent when cereal straws or stalk hay is not provided separately. Wood shavings, sawdust, straw, wood chip and sand all make suitable bedding materials and can be used in combination. Calves prefer the softer, more comfortable, bedding types and straw has the added advantage of developing layers, increasing the opportunity for the top layer to remain dry for longer. Bedding choice generally will depend on availability. The cost needs to be considered according to ability to keep the bedding dry and subsequent amount required, and suitability to maintain the relative humidity in the building below 75% (see section 3.9.8.3).

3.9.7 Calf housing/management systems

3.9.7.1 Pasture-based management

In pasture-based systems, such as found in New Zealand, calves can be housed but are frequently reared at pasture in groups (mobs) of 20 to 40. They are housed briefly and, once they have learned to suck from an artificial teat, are offered milk at pasture from either from a machine or a calfertier (mobile milk vat with many teats, at least one per calf), which delivers colostrum, whole milk or milk replacer at approximately 4 to 5 L per head, each day. Unfortunately, drinking speed varies greatly between calves and unless the system can regulate milk on an individual calf basis this will result in calves drinking very differing levels of milk.

3.9.7.2 Housed calves

The main aims should be to provide a warm clean environment and prevent the development of pneumonia. This can be achieved by the provision of buildings with adequate air space and natural ventilation. Calf buildings should be built to allow the prevailing wind to pass directly through the top portion of the building to remove moist air, while avoiding any direct draught onto the animals. Conditions of high relative humidity in the building can be avoided through attention to good ventilation, regular (daily) addition of bedding and minimizing accumulation of water, through daily cleaning of any water, good drainage and limited addition of water through washing down.

In between groups or batches of calves, the buildings should be cleaned out, washed down thoroughly and rested (1 month) or disinfected between each batch of calves. This includes water troughs and bowls, as these harbour disease organisms. This is referred to as an 'all in, all out system' and can be applied to sections of buildings if required, as in pasture-based systems, where multiple groups of calves may use the building for short periods of time.

3.9.7.3 Calf hutches and tethering

Calf hutches, wherein calves can be kept outdoors in physical isolation but in social contact, have become popular in recent years. In some countries calves can be tethered without a hutch (not within the EU). Hutches should be moved onto new areas for each new calf to prevent disease build-up. Hutches should be placed on well-drained areas, cleaned using a similar approach that described above (section 3.9.7.2). These systems are labour intensive.

3.9.7.4 Individual pens and group housing

An individual pen for calves allows individual monitoring of feed intake and is favoured in early weaning systems. The calf should have sight of and contact with other calves. These systems are labour intensive and as a result group rearing has become more popular as herd sizes increase. Cleaning is essential using a similar approach to that described above (section 3.9.7.2).

3.9.7.5 Mechanical feeding

Due to skilled labour shortages and increased herd sizes, the use of machines for feeding dairy heifer calves is becoming more popular. The level of control and information provided varies greatly between machines. They can be used at pasture or in housing systems and the success relies greatly on skilled labour, but they do remove much of the work involved in calf feeding.

3.9.8 Disease prevention and minimizing mortality

One of the main factors in preventing disease and mortality is the adequate provision of good-quality colostrum, soon after calves are born. The main diseases that calves are likely to suffer include enteric disease (scours), clostridial diseases (see sections 3.9.3.3 and 3.9.9.3), joint ill and pneumonia. A disease prevention and treatment plan for dairy calves should be put in place with the advice of a veterinarian.

3.9.8.1 Enteric disease (scours)

Enteric diseases should be prevented through high levels of building management ('all in, all out' system for pens, with resting or disinfection), personnel and equipment cleaning and hygiene. This includes effective biosecurity measures that prevent visitors bringing disease onto the calf unit and into contact with the calves. On units where Rotavirus has been a problem, cows may be vaccinated before calving, so that they provide colostrum with specific antibodies against this organism. The treatment of scours (enteric disease) should include the prompt management of dehydration, which tends to kill more calves than the disease, by offering good-quality electrolyte solutions to scouring calves rather than milk for up to a maximum of 3 days (or according to manufacturer's recommendations). The identification of the pathogen involved and suitable treatment can be identified through faecal sampling. Scouring calves should be isolated from unaffected calves to prevent disease transfer and kept warm and dry to maximize their opportunity for survival. Pens that have held sick calves should be thoroughly cleaned and disinfected before further use. On the reintroduction of food, colostrum can be useful to promote healing.

A planned approach to calf health management is essential. All calves should be closely observed twice daily for signs of health or incipient disease. The unit should have a store of electrolyte preparations and suitable calf scour treatment products. Colostrum can be stored frozen for emergency use, and should be thawed in hot water, not in the microwave. There should be a herd health plan for the calf unit, which may incorporate (e.g.) a cow vaccination programme when Rotavirus is endemic.

3.9.8.2 Joint ill

Joint ill is a serious disease that can be fatal. Prevention is the key, followed by checking and prompt treatment (antibiotics) of any infected navels (umbilical cords). As soon after birth as possible, the umbilical cord should be treated with a suitable iodine-based solution, in the calving paddock or calving box. Further applications of iodine-based liquid until the cord has dried, and regular checking for a navel swelling, will allow the opportunity to identify and treat any infections quickly using suitable antibiotic therapy as advised by the veterinarian. The regular cleaning and replacement of bedding of calving boxes and calf transport equipment will help prevent infection, in addition to navel treatment. This should be added to the farm's herd health plan.

3.9.8.3 Pneumonia

Pneumonia is most likely to occur in housed calves and is best prevented by attention to building design and management (avoid overstocking, provide adequate air space and good ventilation; see section 3.9.7.2). Any calves, whether housed or kept at pasture, that develop coughing should be examined by the veterinarian, a suitable diagnosis and treatment should be sought immediately, the cause identified and prevention strategies put in place. Older heifers should not be housed within the same air space as younger calves, to prevent the transfer of pneumonia.

3.9.9 Stock tasks

The main stock tasks will include animal identification, de-horning, supernumerary (extra) teat removal and vaccination.

3.9.9.1 Animal identification

Accurate identification of dairy heifers is essential, not only for traceability, but also for herd improvement and practical management of dairy cattle. Legislation requires the accurate identification of individual animals and this is achieved through ear-tagging with an individual animal and herd number. These tags will be placed into the ears soon after birth. In many countries this is linked to a national animal identification scheme and animal passport system. It is regularly supplemented with electronic tagging soon after birth. Heifers are typically freeze-branded on entry to the dairy herd to present a large, easily visible number on the hindquarters. This facilitates individual management (e.g. feeding, oestrus detection, condition and locomotion scoring).

3.9.9.2 De-horning and supernumerary teat removal
Dairy calves will require de-horning and possibly the removal of any supernumerary teats at approximately 5 to 6 weeks of age. It is also important that local anaesthetic be used during these processes to maximize animal welfare, minimize growth checks and comply with local legislation. It is essential that these tasks are not carried out at the same time as any other changes such as vaccination, weaning, or changes in housing.

3.9.9.3 Vaccination
Vaccination against clostridial infections and/or lungworm may be necessary where dairy calves are likely to be infected by these. An appropriate vaccination programme should be applied according to the recommendations of the veterinarian and added to the farm's herd health plan.

3.9.10 Growing dairy heifers
Following the calf rearing point, dairy heifers will be managed at pasture and potentially housed during winter periods in countries where weather conditions are inclement. During period of grazing and following housing, the control of parasitic infections, provision of pasture and supplementary feeds, and regular monitoring of growth rate are the main tasks required to ensure that heifers are well grown and

Table 3.10 Energy and protein requirement and targets for live weight gain and wither height in growing Holstein Friesian heifers.

Age (months)	Weight gain (g/d)	Live weight (kg)	Wither height (cm)	Metabolizable energy (MJ/kg)	Crude protein (%/kg)
2	900	95	86	12	18
3	900	123	90	12	18
6	850	200	104	11	16
14	800	392	128	10	14
20	750	527	135	10	14
22	750	572	139	11	15
23	750	595	140	11	15

ready for service at 13–16 months to create a pregnancy and transfer to the dairy herd (Table 3.10).

3.9.10.1 De-worming

Young animals are susceptible to parasitic infection; as a consequence the control of parasitic worms of the intestine and potentially the lungs needs to be applied according to the requirements of the system. This will depend on the age of the animal, access to pasture and the infection that exists on the pasture. Pasture used by older animals will be infected with parasites and necessitate the more frequent control of parasitic infections in younger animals. Parasite infection can be controlled by the use of clean pastures that have not been infected by older animals, and reducing the potential infection by mixed grazing with other animal species not susceptible to the same species of parasites. This will usually need to be backed up with regular use of anthelmintics to control worm infestation levels both at pasture and during housing. This programme will typically involve two treatments – the initial treatment to kill adult worms, and the second to prevent reinfestation from the developing larvae.

3.9.10.2 Service (insemination)

The natural service or insemination of dairy heifer needs to take place at 13 to 15 months of age and the heifer will need to be 60 to 65% mature weight. This first service should be with a sire that has an 'easy' calving or 'low calving difficulty' rating for first-calving heifers. This rating can be taken from the 'sire' details for bull semen. Alternatively one can use an easy calving breed such as Jersey or Angus for AI or natural service. Many dairy heifers are synchronized using intrauterine devices and then inseminated to ensure they come into the dairy herd at 22 to 24 months at 85 to 90% mature weight. The body condition of heifers should not be a problem, but calving condition scores of 3 to 3.5 (on a 1 to 5 scale) and 5 to 5.5 (on a 1 to 10) New Zealand scale are recommended. There is a range, because breed and genetic merit within breed tends to affect actual condition scores for dairy cattle.

3.9.11 Transition of the heifer into the dairy herd

Increasing the longevity of the dairy cow through careful heifer management will reduce the cost of rearing replacement, and maximize herd breeding worth and productivity, thus increasing the profitability of the dairy herd. Introducing heifers to the dry cows and the milking parlour or shed before calving will reduce the number of stresses experienced by heifers around calving.

3.9.11.1 Heifer (first lactation) infertility

Infertility is potentially the greatest problem faced in first-lactation dairy cattle. Calving heifers at adequate mature weight (85 to 90%) is the main opportunity to reduce growth required in first lactation, competition for feed and aggressive social interaction, which results in higher feed intake, reduced live weight loss, time to weight gain, increased conception rates and reduced empty rate and potential culling. This will also reduced levels of a range of postpartum disorders such as ketosis and risk of displaced abomasum.

3.9.11.2 Lameness

Heifers are particularly susceptible to developing sole bruising and lameness that will lead to lameness in subsequent lactations, thus careful heifer transition and management can reduce the incidence of lameness through the whole herd.

3.9.11.3 Mastitis

The management of heifers in separate groups, and milking heifers before adult cows, will reduce the risk of transmission of infectious mastitis from adult cows. Teat sealants may also be carefully administered to dairy heifers before first calving to reduce the risk of mastitis-causing pathogens entering the mammary gland during late pregnancy and causing mastitis during first lactation.

References and Further Reading

Books

Garnsworthy, P.C. (2005) *Calf and Heifer Rearing: Principles of rearing the modern dairy heifer from calf to calving*. Nottingham University Press, Nottingham.
Gordon, I. (1996) *Controlled Reproduction in Cattle and Buffaloes*. CABI Publishing, Wallingford.
Holmes, C.W., Brookes, I.M., Garrick, D.J., MacKenzie, D.D.S., Parkinson, T.J. and Wilson, G.F. (1998) *Milk Production from Pasture*. Butterworth-Heinemann, Wellington, NZ.
Mcdonald, P., Edwards, R.A. and Greenhalgh, J.F.D. (2002) *Animal Nutrition*, 6th edn. Prentice Hall, Harlow, UK.
Peters, A.R. and Ball, P.J.H. (2004) *Reproduction in Cattle*, 3rd edn. Wiley-Blackwell, Oxford.
Phillips, C.J.C. (2002) *Cattle Behaviour and Welfare*, 2nd edn. Wiley-Blackwell, Oxford.
Pond, W.G., Church, D.C., Pond, K.R. and Schoknecht, P.A. (2004) *Basic Animal Nutrition and Feeding*, 5th edn. Wiley, Hoboken, NJ.
Roy, J.H.B. (1990) *The Calf: Management of Health*, 5th edn. Butterworth, London.
Wathes, C.M. and Charles, D.R. (1994) *Livestock Housing*. CABI Publishing, Wallingford.

Leaflets

BSI (2005) *Buildings and structures for agriculture – Part 40: Code of practice for design and construction of cattle buildings*. BS 5502-40:2005.
DEFRA (2004) *Reducing Injuries to Dairy Cows* (CD-ROM).
DEFRA (2006) *Housing the Modern Dairy Cow*.
MDC (2005) *Minimising Slurry Pooling in Dairy Housing*.
MDC (2006) *Effective Foot-bathing of Dairy Cows*.
MDC (2006) *Housing the 21st Century Cow*.

Beef Cattle and Veal Calves

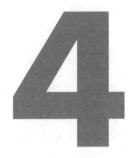

BERNADETTE EARLEY

Key Concepts

Management and Welfare of Farm Animals: The UFAW Farm Handbook, 5th edition. John Webster
© 2011 by Universities Federation for Animal Welfare (UFAW)

4.1 The Beef Industry

4.1.1 Suckler cow herds

Herds of suckler beef cows constitute a very important farming sector in the grassland areas of Europe. A total of over 12 million suckler cows are found in all EU countries (Figure 4.1) and the main suckler beef-producing countries are France, Spain, the UK and Ireland. Suckler beef production is a sustainable system producing high-quality meat with low inputs. In suckler herds, calves remain with the dam at pasture until they are 5 to 9 months old when they are separated from the dam. Many of the weaned animals are transported away from the suckler farms to fattening units. The industry (suckler farms and fattening units) produce a very high-quality meat.

In Europe cow-calf farms are located in three areas:

- the grasslands of Britain, Ireland, France and northern Europe (27%);
- the Mediterranean areas of Italy, Spain, Greece and Portugal (20%);
- the mountain areas of France, Spain and Eastern Europe (16%).

An estimated 65,000 cow-calf producers finish the majority of the progeny as suckler calves, bulls, heifers or steers on their farms. With a rather greater size than the pure cow-calf beef farms in herd and acreage, they manage land more intensively and produce forage crops: 23% operate at a stocking rate higher than 1.8 livestock unit/ha. This system represents 7% of the farms and 8% of the European bovine herd. Their contribution in the finishing phase is important, especially for bull and steer production. They are mainly located in the grasslands of Ireland and the UK and in the forage crops areas of France and northern Europe (Sarzeaud *et al.*, 2008).

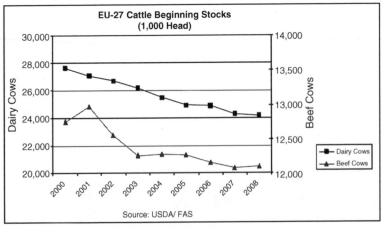

Source: USDA Foreign Agricultural Service (FAS)

Figure 4.1 Cow numbers in the European Union, 2000–2008. Source: USDA Foreign Agricultural Service (FAS).

Table 4.1 EU bovine population: cattle numbers in thousand head (per category). EU totals are given together with numbers for the six most populous countries that contribute 75% of the total population. Source: Eurostat.

	Total	<1 year	1–2 years	>2 years	Cows	Dairy cows	Other cows
France	19124	5070	3611	10443	7921	3759	4163
Germany	12609	3950	2950	5709	4789	4064	725
Ireland	5902	1633	1311	2957	2205	1088	1117
Italy	6577	1929	1436	2918	2280	1839	441
Poland	5406	1344	1053	3008	2739	2677	61
Spain	6410	2402	767	3240	2862	903	1959
United Kingdom	10078	2846	2455	4777	3643	1978	1665
Others	22646	6955	4159	11502	9996	7846	2183
Totals	88751	26130	17742	44554	36435	24154	12314

4.1.2 Beef from dairy farms

Within the European Union, 123,800 enterprises are involved simultaneously in dairy and beef production. These systems represent one-quarter of the beef producers and use 17% of the beef farming land. In most cases, beef production has been developed on farms with small milk quotas. According to land and labour availabilities, different types of production can be found, like bull fattening of dairy calves on the French or German farms, or like steer and heifer production on pastures in Great Britain and Ireland (Table 4.1). Their overall contribution to EU beef production is 20%.

Except in Ireland, the supply of beef animals in the EU is largely sourced from the dairy herd; two-thirds of the cows in the EU are dairy cows. The EU dairy herd is itself in decline due to the constraints enforced by the milk quota and increased milk yields per cow, and this decline in dairy cow numbers has led to a reduction in EU beef production. There has also been a decline of approximately 3% in the EU suckler cow herd between 2000 and 2008 (Figure 4.1).

The EU beef and veal sector (which is predominantly beef) has a total production of about 8 million tonnes. This contributes 10% to the total value of agricultural production in the EU, is the second biggest contributor after the dairy sector and represents about 13% of the total production of beef and veal in the world. Since the 1990s beef production in the EU has been gradually declining (total drop of 7.6% in 2003 compared with 1993). In the same period, global beef production increased by 6.3 million tonnes (16.8%) due to the substantial increase in other continents, particularly South America (increase of 2.6 million tonnes or 26%).

Figures for 2007 show that there are over 1,389 million cattle in the world, an increase of 0.6% (7.8 million) when compared with 2006. Over 58% of the total world cattle population were held by just 10 countries in 2007, with Brazil holding the most cattle – 207.2 million. The USA, which is the largest milk-producing country in the world, held 7.0% of world cattle in 2007. Figures show that the US cattle population has increased 0.3% (301,500) between 2006 and 2007 to over 97 million cattle. In 2007, Brazil held 207.2 million cattle, an increase of 0.6% when compared to 2006, and now accounts for 14.9% of the world cattle population. Other countries saw cattle population fall between 2006 and 2007 with India and China seeing falls of 0.5% and 2.0% respectively. In 2007 India held 12.8% of the world cattle population, while China accounted for 8.4%.

4.1.3 Trends in the UK beef industry

UK beef production fell by 11% from 1980 to 1995. This was entirely due to a decline in beef from the dairy herd. Following the bovine spongiform encephalopathy (BSE) outbreak, and the associated closure of the export market, a high proportion of dairy and dairy-cross calves were disposed of on-farm in the light of the poor returns achievable (particularly true of pure dairy male calves). Another consequence of BSE was a ban on the consumption of beef from animals aged over 30 months (the Over-Thirty Month Scheme; OTMS), which took more potential cattle for beef production out of the human supply chain. For example, in the UK in 1999 around 902,000 cows and 72,000 head of prime cattle entered the OTMS. By 2001 these figures had reduced to 56,000 cows and 62,000 head of UK prime cattle and the OTMS was finally withdrawn in January 2006. Following a change to the OTM rule, OTM cattle born after July 1996 were allowed into the food chain, subject to BSE testing. With effect from 23 January 2006, the Older Cattle Disposal Scheme (OCDS) replaced the OTMS for pre-August 1996 cattle. The OCDS disposed of older bovine animals, which were permanently excluded from the food chain, and provided farmers with compensation for their stock for a limited period. The OCDS was a voluntary scheme which lasted until 31 December 2008.

In contrast, suckler cow numbers almost trebled in Ireland during the past 25 years and they now comprise approximately half of the national cow population of 2.2 million. In the UK, the decline in beef and veal production in 2008 was a direct result of a reduction in prime cattle slaughterings of 130,000 head to 2 million head in 2008 from 2.2 million head in 2007 (6% fall). While prime cattle slaughterings were down, there was a 25% increase in cow slaughterings to nearly 560,000 head. Throughout the UK, cow beef accounted for 20% of total beef and veal production in 2008 compared with 16% in 2007. In Northern Ireland, a similar pattern exists with cows accounting for 19% of total cattle slaughtered in 2008, but only 14% in 2007.

4.2 Quality Beef Production

Success in beef production is dependent on:

1. breeding from high-quality animals;
2. achieving high animal performance;

3. achieving optimal carcass conformation and fatness at slaughter;
4. having a clearly defined grassland management programme;
5. low production costs;
6. detailed records of breeding, performance and health.

4.2.1 The product

Carcass quality is a major determinant of price. Conformation and fatness determine the value of a beef carcass. Conformation describes the shape of the carcass in terms of muscle to bone ratio and the proportion of meat in the expensive cuts. The value of a cut of beef depends on attributes of quality such as taste, tenderness and juiciness. Age at slaughter, position on the carcass (e.g. rump, shoulder) and fat concentration determine these qualities. Generally, meat from cows contains more mature connective tissue (gristle) than meat from prime beef carcasses, and is therefore tougher. Prime cuts such as fillet, sirloin and rump fetch higher prices because they contain little or no gristle or visible strips of intermuscular fat.

The proportion of meat in the hindquarter is highest for the progeny of Limousin cows (Table 4.2). Progeny of Limousin (L) and Charolais (C) cows have a similar proportion of fat in the hindquarter and are lower than Limousin × Friesian (LF), Limousin × Holstein-Friesian (LLF) and Simmental × (Limousin × Holstein-Friesian) (SLF). Bone proportion in the hindquarter is highest for progeny of Charolais cows and lowest for Limousin progeny. The meat to bone ratio is highest for progeny of Limousin cows (Drennan and McGee, 2009).

Under the EU beef carcass classification (EUROP) scheme, each carcass is assessed and classified at the weighing point on the slaughter line. Five conformation classes, represented by the letters E, U, R, O, and P, define an incremental scale ranging from P (poor), which denotes the worst conformation, to E (excellent), denoting the best.

Table 4.2 Carcass composition for progeny of five beef cow breed types. Source: Drennan and McGee (2009).

	Cow breed types				
	Limousin	Charolais	Limousin × Holstein-Friesian (LF)	Limousin × (Limousin × Holstein-Friesian) (LLF)	Simmental × (Limousin × Holstein-Friesian) (SLF)
Hindquarter (%)	50	50.1	49	49.7	48.8
Carcass meat (%)	76.5	74.6	74.3	74.4	74.2
Carcass fat (%)	5.9	6.3	7.2	7.4	7.6
Carcass bone (%)	17.5	19.1	18.5	18.4	18.2
Meat to bone ratio	4.4	3.9	4	4.1	4.1

Table 4.3 Percentage of beef carcasses in the different conformation (EUROP) classes and fat classes (1, 2, 3, 4 and 5) in 2007. Source: Department of Agriculture, Fisheries & Food (DAFF 2007, Ireland).

Animal type	Conformation class					Carcass weight (kg)	Fat class				
	E	U	R	O	P		1	2	3	4	5
Steers	—	7	45	42	7	358	1	11	53	34	1
Young bulls	1	43	42	13	1	368	4	40	51	5	—
Heifers	—	6	55	36	3	291	2	9	41	44	5
Cows	—	1	11	44	44	305	9	13	33	36	10

European Union regulations allow for three subdivisions of each conformation and fat class. In Ireland, conformation class P is subdivided into P+, P, and P−, describing declining conformation. The carcass fat classes describe the amount of fat on the outside of the carcass and in the thoracic cavity. Five classes are defined, represented by the numbers 1 to 5 where 1 denotes the least fat and 5 the most. Fat class 4 may be further subdivided into low (4L) and high fat (4H) (Table 4.3).

Beef carcass classification data in Ireland for 2007 shows that 87% of steers and 91% of heifers fall into the combined conformation classes of O and R (Table 4.3). A better differentiation would be achieved by classifying carcasses on a 15-point scale (e.g. R−, R, R+) rather than on a 5-point scale (Drennan and McGee, 2009). For the same reason it would be more informative to have carcass fat class also classified on a 15-point scale as 87% of steers and 85% of heifers were in fat class 3 and 4 in 2007. The mechanical carcass classification system currently in operation at Irish meat processing plants facilitates this expanded system (Drennan and McGee, 2009).

The decision when to slaughter a prime beef animal depends on its conformation and fatness. In practice, this occurs when the fat concentration in the carcass is 15–20%. A butcher will trim off about half this fat before the beef reaches the consumer. This appears wasteful but it is because quality beef requires a sufficient quantity of intramuscular fat (i.e. marbling). This only occurs when the animal has deposited substantial amounts of 'waste' fat in the subcutaneous tissues and within the abdomen (i.e. kidney, knob and channel fat; KKCF). However, one objective of selective breeding in all meat animals is to reduce the deposition of unsaleable subcutaneous and intra-abdominal fat while preserving a tasty amount of marbling fat. In general, young bulls are leaner than steers at slaughter and a greater proportion are grade E or U (24.2% in comparison with 10.1%). Heifers are usually fatter than steers at the same conformation class. Cull cows, especially from the dairy breeds, have poorer conformation than steers but carry more intra-abdominal KKCF at slaughter.

The following key points may be identified in relation to the feeding and breeding of cattle for quality beef production (Molony, 1999).

1. When cattle are fed *ad libitum*, increasing the metabolizable energy (ME) concentration of the feed (e.g. by feeding cereal concentrates) will increase both growth rate and the relative rate at which they fatten.
2. Fed the same ration, early maturing breeds (Hereford, Aberdeen Angus) animals will be fatter than late maturing animals (Charolais, Simmental) when slaughtered at the same carcass weight.
3. Grass silage or grazed grass produces yellower fat than concentrate feeds.
4. Type of feed can influence the fatty acid composition of beef intramuscular fat.

4.2.2 Eating quality

Eating quality is a very subjective term in the meat industry. Consumer studies show that tenderness and flavour are the most important characteristics determining the acceptability of meat. Juiciness, smell, colour and texture are next in importance, while leanness and absence of gristle tend to be least important. In the United States and Asian markets, 'marbling' (deposition of fat within the muscle bundles) is highly valued. In contrast, beef for EU markets is required to have little visible marbling. In recent years red meat has been perceived to be 'less healthy' relative to competing white meat products and other foods. This perception has contributed to red meat losing market share. Perceived 'healthiness' of beef is a significant long-term issue for the beef industry.

4.2.3 Beef consumption and human health

Beef fat contains a high proportion of saturated fatty acids which, when eaten to excess, are known to be a risk to health. However, it also contains a proportion of fat molecules that may have beneficial effects. These include monounsaturated fatty acids, some long-chain polyunsaturated fatty acids, with the first double bond at the omega-3 position, such as those found in oily fish, and conjugated linoleic acid. It is of major importance to determine how on-farm factors such as diet may affect the fatty acid profile of beef and so influence its positive and negative health attributes. Some recent observations are summarized below.

- Including grass in the finishing diet can enhance key 'health attributes' of beef by increasing conjugated linoleic acid (CLA) concentration and increasing the ratio of polyunsaturated fatty acids (PUFA) to saturated fatty acid (SFA).
- Beef from grass silage had a 'healthier' fatty acid profile than beef from maize silage.
- It is possible to raise beef CLA content and increase PUFA concentrations by manipulating the finishing diet, e.g. by inclusion of sunflower oil.
- Muscle from cattle finished on a grass or clover sward had higher PUFA but lower CLA concentrations than animals finished on grass.

4.3 Production Systems

4.3.1 Beef from the suckler herd

Beef suckler cows are kept in a wide range of grazing habitats. These range from herds kept at high stocking densities on improved pastures with high inputs of nitrogenous (N) fertilizer to herds raised extensively in habitats ranging from the European Alps to the great plains of North and South America. Calves born to beef cows stay with their mothers until weaning in late summer or autumn. In Europe, producers sell them into yards for winter feeding before they are finished out of yards in the spring or at pasture the following summer. In North America, weaned calves are typically finished (reared to slaughter weight) in large feedlots.

In Europe, calving is usually concentrated either in early spring, normally before turnout to grass, or at pasture in autumn. When calves are born in the spring, the peak period for lactation in the cows coincides with the peak period for production of grass. This reduces the cost of feeding concentrates to cow and calf. It is common practice to house autumn-born calves with their mothers and provide them with access to a special creep area. Such an area provides a place where they may rest and receive concentrate feed without competition from the adult cows. Farmers then turn them out to pasture in spring and wean calves in midsummer at 9 to 10 months of age and weights of 250 to 350 kg (depending on breed). The Meat and Livestock Commission (www.mlc.org.uk) publishes annual summaries of the physical and economic performance of recorded beef herds.

The cow herd uses approximately 0.85 and 0.66 of the total energy requirement in calf-to-weanling and calf-to-beef systems, respectively, with about two-thirds and one half, respectively, of the total energy consumed going towards maintaining the cow herd (Montano-Bermudez et al., 1990). Feed is the main variable cost on suckler beef farms and cow winter feed costs are a major proportion of feed costs. In systems that sell calves at weaning, approximately two-thirds of total feed energy goes towards maintaining the cow herd. In systems that rear calves to slaughter, feed energy costs are split approximately 50 : 50.

4.3.2 Beef from the dairy herd

Dairy beef production systems typically involve crossbreeding between dairy cows and semen from beef bulls. Male dairy/beef crosses (e.g. Charolais Holstein) will all be reared for prime beef. In the UK and Ireland, a substantial proportion of the crossbred females will be retained for use as dams in suckler beef systems. In Brazil, females from local adapted breeds are commonly mated to temperate, high genetic-merit dairy breed males to generate adapted, yet productive F1 females for the dairy herd and the males are reared for beef. The F1 females generally become either terminal females (defined as females whose immediate progeny are slaughtered) or are backcrossed to dairy breed males to generate terminal females.

Farmers producing prime beef from calves born to dairy cows remove them shortly after birth and rear them artificially. This involves providing them with a liquid milk replacer diet until they are eating sufficient digestible dry food to support maintenance and growth. This usually occurs at about 35 to 42 days old. The rearing system employed thereafter will be determined by a variety of factors such as phenotype, the cost and availability of feed, season of birth and seasonal variations in selling price.

4.3.2.1 Semi-intensive beef systems

The expression 'semi-intensive' describes systems in which young cattle live out at grass for one or two summers. Table 4.4 outlines two options, where farmers either finish cattle in yards during their second winter, or after a second summer at grass at 20 to 24 months of age. Beef producers normally castrate and rear male calves as steers.

4.3.2.2 Finishing in yards

Finishing in yards is the most common system for calves born from September to December. Despite financial incentives for earlier (summer) calving, this is still the peak calving period for dairy cows. The calves can grow at 0.7–0.9 kg/day over the first winter so that they weigh 200 to 220 kg when the spring comes and they go out to grass. At this stage of growth, the ruminant digestive system is sufficiently mature to enable them to thrive on a diet of grass alone (without milk or cereals). Such calves achieve weight gains close to 1 kg/day and reach 340 to 360 kg by October or November when they return to the yard. If they are to finish before the following spring, they will then need to receive a highly digestible diet *ad libitum*. This is primarily a mixture of forage (grass or maize silage) with a cereal-based concentrate ration supplement if necessary. An early maturing Hereford × Friesian steer may finish by January at a slaughter weight of 420 kg. Heifers will finish even younger and

Table 4.4 Semi-intensive beef production systems for calves from the dairy herd.

	Finishing in yards			Finishing at grass
	He × Fr	**Ch × Fr**	**Holstein**	**Ch × Fr**
Live bodyweight (kg)				
Weaning (5 weeks)	65	70	65	70
Turnout (year 1)	200	220	220	200
Yarding	340	360	340	360
Turnout (year 2)	—	—	—	480
Slaughter	420	520	510	600
Age at slaughter (months)	12–14	14–16	18–24	20–24
Carcass weight (kg)	205	277	260	318
Killing out (%)	51.0	53.2	51.3	53.0
Saleable meat: bone ratio	3.8	4.0	3.4	4.0

He, Hereford; Fr, Friesian; Ch, Charolais. (Cattle finished in yards are not turned out to grass in year 2.)

lighter. A Charolais × Friesian steer will grow faster but finish a little later at a much greater weight. A Holstein-type male calf may achieve a similar slaughter weight to the Charolais × Friesian, but will take much longer to finish.

4.3.2.3 Summer finishing

Traditionally farmers used the summer finishing system for calves that were born in mid- to late winter. This is because such animals are sufficiently mature to obtain the maximum benefit from grass during their first summer. Farmers also summer-finish calves from big, late maturing bulls, like the Charolais, that are difficult to fatten in yards over their second winter. If there is no intention of finishing cattle out of yards during their second winter, producers will put them through a 'store' period. During this time the animals receive only silage and supplements of essential minerals and vitamins. They may continue to gain weight at 0.5 to 0.8 kg/day but lose body fat, so that they end the winter bigger but leaner than when they entered it. When such lean and hungry animals return to pasture for their second summer, their appetite for good grass is initially high because they sense that they are thin (or underweight for age). In these circumstances they can achieve growth rates in excess of 1 kg/day on low-cost summer pasture. However, cattle in good to fat condition, moving to spring grass, initially lose weight which they may not recover for several weeks. For the same reason, it is important not to turn out cattle that are nearly finished at the end of winter on to grass; they will need feeding on in yards until they are ready for slaughter. In June 2003, EU farm ministers adopted a fundamental reform of the Common Agricultural Policy (CAP). The reform completely changed the way the EU supports its farm sector. These new 'single farm payments' are linked to respect for environmental, food safety and animal welfare standards.

4.3.3 Intensive systems for beef and veal

Intensive calf-rearing systems are those that involve rearing calves from the dairy herd in confinement from birth to slaughter. This is expensive in terms of housing, machinery, labour and, especially, feed which can account for up to 80% of total costs. Intensive high-input, high-output systems depend on achieving high daily gains. As cattle approach their natural mature weight, the rate of fat deposition increases and since each kg of fat takes about 2.25 times the energy of each kg of muscle (lean meat), feed efficiency declines. It is now recommended that cattle should be slaughtered at fat score 3 rather than 4L. Indeed, this is a trend that has occurred over the past few years. Almost 55% of steers were slaughtered at fat score 3.

It is most common to rear male dairy-type (Holstein-Friesian) calves that have a poorer conformation, so are cheaper to buy than beef × dairy calves, in intensive systems. The strategy in these systems is to offer the highest quality feed available at an economic price and finish the calves as quickly as possible. Inevitably this reduces both the age and weight, and therefore the price, of the animal at slaughter. For a good Charolais × Friesian calf, worth double, it pays to rear it semi-intensively to a greater slaughter weight even though it takes longer. The main feeding options for intensive

Table 4.5 Intensive systems for beef and veal production for Holstein/Friesian bull calves from the dairy herd (values from Meat and Livestock Commission, 1994).

	Grass silage concentrates	Maize silage concentrates	Barley beef	White veal	Pink veal
Daily live-weight gain (kg)	1.00	1.15	1.30	1.60	1.40
Slaughter weight (kg)	510	490	460	220	300
Slaughter age (months)	16	14	11	4	7
Concentrates feed (tonnes)	1.3	0.8	1.8	—	0.8
Milk powder (tonnes)	—	—	—	1.2	0.4
Target gross margin (£/head)	160	140	115	30	70
Equivalent sale price (pence/kg carcass)	209	204	214	380	240

beef are based on grass silage plus concentrates, maize silage plus (less) concentrates of 'barley beef' (Table 4.5). In the barley beef system, the main feed is cereal with small amounts of protein, minerals and vitamins plus a little straw to encourage rumination. Since barley is more energy-rich than grass or maize silage, this system finishes calves most quickly. It is, however, less profitable than silage-based systems, except where the barley is home-grown and more likely to provoke digestive disorders.

Intensive beef production systems require the confinement of animals throughout their lives at a high stocking density. This increases the risk of infectious diseases, such as pneumonia, relative to systems that permit the animals to spend half the year at pasture. These problems are particularly acute for calves in the first 3 months of life. In the early days of intensive beef systems, calves moved to the rearing accommodation and were exposed to carriers of infection directly after weaning at 5–6 weeks of age. This created serious losses from respiratory disease. Specialist contract-rearing units have developed which provide 12-week-old calves at a weight of 110 to 130 kg and, ideally, an acquired immunity to the major respiratory pathogens of intensive beef units.

4.3.3.1 Cereal and baby beef
Cereal-based diets are often used for bull beef production. Beef cattle that are finished indoors are offered concentrate feedstuffs at rates that range from modest inputs through to *ad libitum* access. Such concentrates frequently contain high levels of cereals such as barley or wheat. In addition to this, a certain amount of roughage may also be required in the diet to prevent metabolic disorders from hindering production. This is often supplied in the form of cereal straw. These cereals are generally between 14% to 18% moisture content and tend to be rolled shortly before being included in coarse rations or are more finely processed prior to pelleting. Farmers thinking of using 'high-moisture grain' techniques for preserving and processing cereal grains destined for feeding to beef cattle need to know how the yield, conservation efficiency

and feeding value of such grains compares with grains conserved using more conventional techniques. The animals on this system achieve a live-weight gain of 1.25 kg per day from 3 months of age and are slaughtered at 450 kg live-weight.

4.3.3.2 Veal

Veal is the pale meat (white veal) of calves maintained at the pre-ruminant stage on a liquid diet of milk or milk replacer. Formerly the diet was fed entirely in liquid form. However, it is now compulsory within the European Union to feed some solid feed in the form of digestible fibre to promote rumen development. Traditionally veal was produced by calves of dual-purpose breeds that were fed whole milk after milking, and by suckling calves of multipurpose or beef (Limousin, etc.) breeds. With the introduction of milk substitutes in the early 1960s the production of veal expanded. The carcass weight of veal calves may range from 105 to 140 kg.

Veal production is mainly prevalent in the EU, where it was highly stimulated by subsidized milk powder used for calf rearing (as one of the ways of using up the huge milk surpluses in the EU). Veal calves are exclusively given milk or milk substitutes in order to keep them at the pre-ruminant stage, thus avoiding the development of the forestomachs. Slaughtered at 2 to 5 months of age, at a live-weight varying from 100 to 250 kg, they must grow rapidly (over 1 kg per day) and provide a high dressing percentage (about 60%), well-conformed and sufficiently fat-covered carcass with pale pinkish meat. This last-mentioned characteristic is very important from a commercial point of view (high premiums are paid by consumers for this type of meat) and can only be obtained from pre-ruminant animals on an iron-deficient diet. Two main types of veal production can be distinguished.

4.3.3.3 Nursed veal calves

This system is limited to two areas in France and includes less than 12% of veal calves slaughtered in France. The calves are mainly offspring of French beef breeds and crosses with dairy cattle. Almost all calves are born on the farm where they are reared, but sometimes a few additional calves are bought. The price of this top-quality product is high (around 18% higher than calves reared on milk substitutes). This system is decreasing because it gives a lower income than suckling calves at pasture which are sold at weaning for further fattening and red meat production.

4.3.3.4 Veal calves reared on milk substitutes

The production of milk substitute-fed veal calves is mainly localized in western and southwestern France, northern Italy and central Netherlands. Friesians with an increasing proportion of Holstein blood predominate. Most of the calves are born outside the farms where they are reared. They are usually bought from various sources at 1 to 3 weeks of age; Italy imports calves for rearing from the Netherlands and France. A significant number is imported into mainland Europe from the UK. Over 85% of the production is organized under contract by dairy and non-dairy companies manufacturing milk substitutes as well as slaughterhouse companies.

4.3.3.5 Feeding and growth

Milk substitute fed to veal calves mainly contains milk ingredients (milk and whey powder; 70 to 90% of total). Starch derivates, fat substitutes (e.g. tallow, lard and saturated vegetable oils), minerals and vitamins are added in various proportions. Growth rates of an average 1.2 kg per day are common (0.7 to 0.8 kg during the first month, increasing to 1.4 to 1.6 kg during the last part of the fattening period) with an average daily consumption of 1.8 to 2.0 kg milk substitute powder.

4.4 Breeding and Genetics

The beef herds in the UK and Ireland consist of some pure bred breeds, e.g. Angus, Hereford, French breeds, but more crossbred cows (British breeds × dairy breeds) mated to the late-maturing beef breeds. The beef breeds in extensive grazing areas such as in France and Spain are predominantly local (rustic) breeds. The ideal characteristics for a suckler cow are as follows:

- *Fertility*: – calve at 2 years (early puberty), then a calf per year. Herd fertility 90%;
- *Conformation*: – produce a top grade carcass (E.U.R.) when bred to a good-quality sire;
- *Milk yield*: – sufficient to grow one calf well (but not excessive);
- *Ease of calving*;
- *Docility*: – cow should be manageable and safe to work with;
- *Feed efficiency*: – low maintenance requirement;
- *Cull value*: – replacement cost is lower where cull value is higher;
- *Uniformity*: – the herd should be reasonably uniform in type so that the progeny will be likewise.

4.4.1 The Holstein/Friesian dams

In areas such as the UK, where most beef comes from the dairy herd, most beef calves have Holstein/Friesian mothers. Until recently the Holstein and British Friesian were two different breeds in the UK but the two breed societies have now amalgamated. There remains, however, a profound difference in the conformation. The typical British Friesian has a superior muscle to bone ratio and proportion of meat in the expensive cuts relative to the long-legged, bony American Holstein. There is steady, and probably unchangeable, trend towards the extreme Holstein type of dairy cow that gives more milk but has a considerably inferior beef shape. One of the reasons for the UK increasing the number of calves it exports into white veal units in continental Europe is the rise in the number of poor-quality Holstein-type male calves. These calves are unsatisfactory for beef production, but are so cheap that it is profitable to rear them quickly for veal.

Table 4.6 Performance of principal beef breeds (pedigree recordings).

	No. recorded	Bulls 400-day weights (kg)			Backfat (mm)	
		Range	Mean	1975–1990	Range	Mean
Aberdeen Angus	1134	434–670	417	+86	1.6–8.5	4.6
Belgian Blue	508	511–655	519	—	—	—
Charolais	3315	453–831	617	+49	1.5–4.1	2.6
Hereford	1683	361–635	469	+35	1.3–9.3	4.2
Limousin	3404	410–669	525	+94	1.0–5.3	2.6
Simmental	3560	445–810	600	+73	1.5–5.2	3.3
South Devon	1228	424–730	546	+21	1.5–5.5	3.1

4.4.2 The beef breeds

The most desirable traits for a beef bull are: rapid growth rate, especially lean tissue; excellent carcass conformation, without excess subcutaneous and KKC fat; and good appetite, especially for grass and forages to achieve early finishing. These traits are somewhat incompatible and the relative importance of each depends on the nutrition and environment within the rearing system. Table 4.6 shows the variation in growth rate and fatness of different breeds of pedigree bulls (i.e. weights and backfat thickness at 400 days of age). There is no such thing as a perfect breed; different types suit different circumstances.

4.4.2.1 Hereford

The Hereford was, for many years, the most popular sire for beef production from the dairy herd. It is a relatively small animal, with an average 400-day weight of approximately 470 kg and a mature weight of 900 kg. The breed has an excellent conformation and finishes quickly due to a large appetite for forages relative to its energy requirement for maintenance. The bulls carry a low risk of dystocia (Table 4.8). The gene for a white face is dominant and therefore the beef producer, seeing a white-faced calf at market, knows that it was sired by a Hereford bull. The bulls are relatively gentle natured. For all these reasons they remain a popular breeding animal for dairy farmers to keep and run with their heifers. They also remain excellent sires of crossbred suckler cows. However, Charolais and Simmental have largely overtaken their role as a first-choice sire of prime beef calves. The beef trade has for many years favoured larger carcasses, although the largest carcasses are now about as big as men and current machinery can reasonably handle. Also the quality of feed for beef cattle has generally improved. The facility of the Hereford to finish early on poor forage has become something of a disadvantage. When forage quality is good, Herefords fatten too soon.

4.4.2.2 Aberdeen Angus

Aberdeen Angus cattle are black and polled and both these characteristics are dominant. Breeders developed the Angus to produce high-quality beef, with conspicuous marbling, on good land but in the short growing season of northeast Scotland. The traditional Angus is a small, early finishing animal suitable as a mate for heifers but fattens too quickly. There has been a move to increase size in this breed, mainly through importation of bulls from North America. Table 4.6 illustrates that average 400-day live-weights for Angus bulls are now higher than for Herefords and the top of the range is as heavy as any breed other than Charolais and Simmental.

4.4.2.3 Limousin

The Limousin is a red-coloured breed originating from central France. It is, on average, intermediate in weight between the British beef breeds and the very large Charolais and Simmental. It is lean and has excellent carcass conformation with a high killing-out percentage, and a high proportion of meat in the expensive cuts (Table 4.7). This makes it very popular with butchers. Calving problems are lower than for Charolais and Simmental; this makes it a suitable bull for mating with dairy cows to produce beef. Selection for leanness and high killing-out percentage (which implies a small gut) inevitably tends to select against appetite, especially for highly fibrous forages. Limousin crosses are therefore difficult to finish without expensive concentrate feeds. Intensive systems, which house animals in yards and slaughter them by 18 months of age, are most suitable for Limousins. Limousin × Friesian male calves in these systems are usually entire and can be difficult to handle.

4.4.2.4 Charolais and Simmental

It is possible to consider these popular large breeds together with other, less numerous large breeds, such as the Blonde d'Aquitaine and the South Devon. Pure-bred Charolais and Blonde d'Aquitaine have rather similar cream-coloured coats. The Simmental is very like the Hereford in colour. At best, these bulls and their calves grow fast and have the ability to reach a large size and excellent carcass conformation without getting too fat. Since the prime factor determining the price of a beef animal is its slaughter weight, these breeds, especially the Charolais, have become increasingly popular as sires for both dairy cows and suckler beef cows. The dairy farmer who sells male calves at 10 days of age can get much more money for a Charolais cross that may finish at 580 kg than for a Hereford cross that may finish at 450 kg. However, the dairy farmer cannot afford obstetric problems since they compromise the prime source of income, namely subsequent lactation performance. The suckler beef industry can only generate income from the sale of calves (and ultimately the cow) so, inevitably therefore, they often use very large bulls and carry the greater risk of dystocia (Table 4.8). To maximize slaughter weights, calves from these large bulls, whether out of dairy or beef cows, are best suited to 20–24-month systems. Most calves have the capacity to finish well (if slowly) off grass. Table 4.6

Table 4.7 Carcass composition of calves from sire breeds crossed with Friesian/Holstein cows. Source: Southgate in More O'Ferrall, 1982.

| | Sire breeds | | | |
	Angus	Charolais	Hereford	Limousin
Weight at slaughter (kg)	393.0	494.0	410.0	454.0
Feed conversion ratio (g gained/kg of feed)	86.0	82.0	88.0	85.0
Killing out (%)	52.5	54.8	52.3	54.7
Saleable meat in carcass (%)	72.5	72.7	71.9	73.3
Saleable meat in expensive cuts (%)	44.1	44.8	44.1	45.4
Fat trim in carcass (%)	9.6	9.0	9.7	9.2

shows that the Charolais and Simmental breeds are continuing to increase in size and growth rate to 400 days. The rate of improvement in these traits has been less impressive in the native red South Devon breed.

4.4.2.5 Belgian Blue
Breeders have developed the modern Belgian Blue from a breed similar in appearance to the traditional blue-roan beef shorthorn. They have selected for 'double muscling' (i.e. heavy muscling), especially in the hindquarters. This leads to a very high muscle to bone ratio but abnormalities of skeletal development, especially a reduction in pelvic dimensions. Cows carrying the double muscling trait in the homozygous form are seldom able to give birth normally and will need a caesarean section. The

Table 4.8 Effects of sire breed on calving difficulties and calf mortality in suckler cows, dairy cows and heifers (from Allen, 1990).

Breed of sire	Suckler cows		Holstein/Friesian cows		Holstein/Friesian heifers	
	Dystocia (%)	Mortality (%)	Dystocia (%)	Mortality (%)	Dystocia (%)	Mortality (%)
Aberdeen Angus	3.1	1.3	—	—	2.3	5.8
Hereford	3.8	1.6	1.2	2.9	3.1	6.2
Friesian	—	—	2.5	5.0	7.4	7.9
Limousin	7.2	4.4	3.2	6.1	8.1	9.7
Charolais	9.6	4.8	4.2	5.2	—	—
Simmental	9.3	4.2	3.1	5.6	—	—
South Devon	7.4	4.1	2.4	5.6	—	—
Belgian Blue	—	—	4.3	5.4	—	—
Average	6.7	3.4	3.0	5.1	5.2	7.4

homozygous double-muscled animal also does not thrive, partly because of a poor appetite and partly because of a predisposition to infectious diseases, especially pneumonia. In the natural state, this trait is a lethal recessive. However, F1 hybrid calves from a double-muscled bull do grow rapidly (although they are difficult to finish) and have a good carcass quality. The incidence of dystocia when using a Belgian Blue bull on a Holstein/Friesian cow is no worse than for a Charolais bull. There are no special welfare problems in the crossbred calves. However, the breeder who elects to use Belgian Blue semen must accept the welfare problems involved in producing the pure-bred double-muscled bulls.

4.4.3 Suckler cow breeds

The beef herds in the UK and Ireland consist of some pure bred breeds, e.g. Angus, Hereford, French breeds but more crossbred cows (British breeds × dairy breeds) which are then mated to the late-maturing beef breeds to produce the generation of calves for slaughter as prime beef. Most suckler cows in the UK are not pure-bred but first crosses between two pure breeds. This is partly because genetic traits relating to maternal behaviour and calf survival are more likely to improve by heterosis (hybrid vigour) rather than by selection within breeds. It is also partly because dairy farms are regularly producing and selling suitable half-bred heifers for the suckler herd, such as Hereford × Friesian or Limousin × Friesian. Such animals, that have been reared artificially, with little or no contact with their own mothers, manage the responsibilities of motherhood very well.

Over the last 200 years the Hereford has become the most popular breed of suckler cow in the world outside the hottest areas of the tropics. The ability of the breed to thrive and fatten on poor-quality grasses and forage may now be a disadvantage in a bull intended as a sire of calves destined for slaughter as prime beef. It is, however, an excellent trait for a bull siring hardy beef cows able to subsist and regularly produce calves, at least cost, on range in the USA or on the hills of the UK. Other traditional hardy British beef breeds include the Aberdeen Angus, Beef Shorthorn, Galloway and Welsh Black.

4.5 Behaviour

4.5.1 Social behaviour

Cattle in the wild form large, stable herds whose size appears to be limited only by the availability of pasture. Being part of a herd contributes to a sense of security since it reduces the risk of capture for a large animal that cannot hide. On open range and given plenty of space, cattle form stable subgroups. A dominance hierarchy is established, whereby each cow knows its place. Cattle perceive a predator as a threat but not as a source of real alarm if they can maintain a satisfactory flight zone and can see (or think they can see) an escape route. It is possible to build these principles into handling systems for range cattle.

Removing an individual from a herd will cause it distress. One exception is the cow about to calve, who will isolate herself from the herd to give birth. Having licked her calf clean and suckled it she will then leave it to lie hidden and go back to the herd. She will only return to feed her calf 4 to 6 times during the first few days until it is strong enough to run with the herd.

4.5.2 Reproductive behaviour

The cow normally has one calf per year, after a pregnancy of 9 months. There are small genetic differences in the duration of pregnancy that are largely due to the genotype of the calf. A Holstein/Friesian cow carrying a calf to a bull of her own breed has a gestation period of 281 days. If (to use an extreme example) the sire had been a Limousin bull, gestation would take 287 days. Table 4.8 gives values for the incidence of dystocia (calving difficulties) and calf mortality in suckler cows and dairy cows (Holstein/Friesians) artificially inseminated to bulls from different breeds. The traditional British beef breeds, Hereford and Aberdeen Angus, carry a lower incidence of dystocia, which is one reason why farmers traditionally use them to inseminate heifers. Their relatively small size and equable temperament is another reason why they are suitable to have running with heifers.

The incidence of dystocia in Holstein/Friesian cows is less than in suckler cows although, for calf mortality within the first 2 days of life, the reverse is true. The incidence of dystocia is higher for the cows mated with very large beef bulls, Charolais and Simmental. However, the risk of dystocia is due at least as much to the pelvic dimensions of the cow as the size of the bull. Left to themselves, beef cows are more likely than dairy cows to ensure that their calf stays alive (Table 4.8). Breeders have selected Belgian Blues for very heavy muscling, to the extent that many pure-bred cows are unable to calve normally; such cows require repeated, premeditated caesarean section and this constitutes a major welfare problem. However, the incidence of dystocia in Holstein/Friesian cows mated to Belgian Blue bulls is no greater than for the Charolais. Artificial insemination (AI) studs, for dairy and beef cows, keep records of the performance and progeny tests of their individual bulls. These include records of calving difficulty. When selecting a bull for AI it is possible to take this into account, to avoid, for example, mating a bull that carries a high risk of dystocia to a cow with a history of calving difficulties.

Cattle have no discrete breeding season. A non-pregnant sexually mature female will show oestrus at intervals of about 21 days throughout the year. When beef cows are on pasture or open range, natural service by a bull running with the herd is practically obligatory. When cows are confined, it is possible to induce and synchronize oestrus and ovulation by the use of hormones. There are two approaches, both of which rely on controlling the end of dioestrus, which initiates the period of rapid follicular development. This involves either injection in dioestrus of prostaglandin to destroy the corpus luteum, or insertion and timed withdrawal of progesterone-releasing intravaginal devices (PRIDs). The probability of fertilization following synchronization of oestrus followed by AI is unlikely to exceed 65%, so most beef farmers need a 'sweeper' bull to serve those cows that do not conceive to AI. However, AI does make it possible to use bulls of much higher genetic merit than one is likely to find on the average commercial beef farm.

4.6 Nutrition and Feeding

4.6.1 Digestion

When a cow grazes at pasture, all plant material enters the large paunch, or reticulo-rumen, where it is mixed, diluted with saliva and subjected to microbial fermentation. The end-products of microbial fermentation of plant carbohydrates (sugars, starch, cellulose and hemicellulose) are absorbed, largely across the rumen wall, as the volatile fatty acids – acetic, propionic and butyric acid – which form the major source of dietary energy for ruminants. The digesta that leave the reticulo-rumen and pass into the abomasum (which corresponds to the true stomach in humans) contain large amounts of microbial protein. These are subjected to further digestion and form the ruminant's principal supply of amino acids. The adult ruminant derives most of its nutrients from reactions in the rumen. The small intestine (duodenum, jejunum) is the major source for absorption of amino acids and minerals. The large intestine (caecum and colon) acts as a second fermentation chamber, but normally contributes less than 8% to nutrient uptake.

4.6.2 Metabolizable energy

By far the greatest quantity of nutrients absorbed from the gut is used as a source of energy (i.e. metabolizable energy; ME) to fuel the work of maintenance, activity and production. ME requirement is expressed in megajoules per day (MJ/day) and the ME concentration in the feed is expressed in MJ ME/kg dry matter (DM), which abbreviates to M/D. The DM intake of a ruminant is stimulated by its requirements for nutrients, especially energy, but restricted by the rate it can digest the food it eats, principally the amount of unfermented matter it can carry within the rumen. A growing calf or lactating cow will have a greater hunger for nutrients per unit of body weight than an adult, non-pregnant, non-lactating animal. However, the less digestible the food (i.e. the lower the M/D) the more difficult it becomes to meet its energy requirements within the constraints of gut fill.

The M/D of pasture grass and the best silages should be greater than 10 MJ/kg DM and can sustain weight gains of 1 kg/day or more. Cereals, with an M/D close to 13 MJ/kg, can provide enough ME to sustain maximum weight gains. However, they are deficient in protein and other essential minerals and vitamins. Moreover, a diet based almost entirely on cereals will not provide enough long fibre to stimulate rumination and can lead to problems such as bloat and rumen acidosis.

4.6.3 Protein

Ruminants, like all animals, require amino acids as essential building blocks for growth, reproduction and lactation and as constituents of all the enzymes that drive the processes of metabolism. Most of the amino acid requirements of beef cattle are provided by acid digestion in the abomasum of proteins synthesized within the rumen. This may be termed effective rumen degradable protein (ERDP). Rumen microbes synthesize their own proteins, partly from true protein in the diet and partly from simple sources of non-protein nitrogen (NPN), such as urea. In the natural state this urea arises from the recycling of blood urea, via the saliva or by direct absorption across the rumen wall. Blood urea is an end-product of protein catabolism within the body and, in simple-stomached animals, almost entirely excreted in the urine. The ability of ruminants to recycle urea is an elegant adaptation to seasonal shortages of protein and water, e.g. during the dry season in the tropics. In areas (e.g. the USA) where cattle are finished in feedlots on high-cereal diets, it is possible to meet amino acid requirements in part by providing a dietary source of NPN. In some high-producing ruminants (e.g. dairy cattle) it is not possible to meet amino acid requirement from the 'natural' mixture of microbial and undegraded dietary protein (UDN) that enters the abomasum (see Chapter 3). In these circumstances the diet can be supplemented with a protein source that is resistant to microbial degradation. However, there are probably no circumstances where it would be cost-effective to provide supplementary UDN for beef animals.

4.6.4 Minerals and vitamins

Diets based wholly on fresh or conserved grass are likely to provide sufficient calcium, but phosphorus and magnesium may be marginal. In certain cases the diet may be deficient in copper, cobalt or selenium and all these deficiencies may stunt growth. It is possible to feed exact amounts of minerals by incorporating them into the concentrate ration. It is also possible to offer cattle free choice in mineral licks. However, intake is erratic and does not relate to requirement. Moreover, selenium (and possibly copper) is toxic in excess. Some cattle may therefore consume too little and some too much. One of the most popular ways of delivering copper, cobalt and selenium to beef cattle is within a bolus that lodges in the rumen and releases these minerals at a steady rate; this is usually effective, but sometimes the bolus is lost.

Cattle have no dietary requirement for vitamin C and are able to acquire B vitamins and vitamin K (biotin) as end-products of microbial synthesis in the rumen. Green grass and silage are good sources of carotenes, the precursors of vitamin A. Sun-cured hay is a good source of vitamin D, and whole cereals good sources of vitamin E. Generally, adult cattle are unlikely to suffer from deficiencies of the fat-soluble vitamins A, D and E, but body reserves of these drop during the winter. Calves are born with almost no fat-soluble vitamins in their body and normally acquire them by drinking colostrum. The colostrum of beef and dairy cows in late winter may contain very low concentrations of fat-soluble vitamins. This gives the calves a poor start and makes them particularly vulnerable to infectious diseases of epithelial surfaces, such as diarrhoea and pneumonia.

4.6.5 Water

The *Codes of Recommendations for the Welfare of Livestock: Cattle* (DEFRA, 2003) state that 'cattle should have access to sufficient fresh, clean water at least twice daily'. This is necessary to maintain the water content of the body tissues while sustaining inevitable and regulatory losses. Cattle also require water for milk production and to sustain the continuous culture of microbes in the rumen. Published figures for the water intake of cattle range between 50 and 150 g/kg bodyweight per day. It is greater during lactation and hot weather and less when the food is very wet (e.g. fresh grass or grass silage). The first response of cattle to a water shortage is usually to reduce food intake. Ideally, cattle should have access to clean water almost continually. If only allowed access to water twice daily they should be free to drink for as long as they want on each occasion.

4.6.6 Feedstuffs

4.6.6.1 Grass

Grass is almost the perfect food for beef cattle. The most nutritious part of the plant is the young leaf, so its digestibility (and M/D) is greatest before the emergence of the seed heads. Grazing management should aim to ensure that the grass is long enough (at least 7 cm) to ensure that the cattle can consume enough during daylight hours, but not so long that it becomes stemmy and fibrous. Well-managed grassland provides sufficient ME and protein for maintenance and lactation in beef cows and for maintenance and growth in calves receiving milk from their mothers. It also provides sufficient ERDP. It cannot, however, sustain economically acceptable weight gains in calves from the dairy herd that are receiving neither concentrates nor milk from their mothers before they reach 200 kg in the case of British breeds or 300 kg for the larger continental breeds. This is because of the constraints of gut fill in the immature rumen. Cattle that receive all or nearly all their food from fresh and conserved grass may, in certain areas, suffer debilitating deficiencies of copper, cobalt, selenium or phosphorus. Such animals may be more susceptible to an acutely fatal attack of hypomagnesaemia or grass staggers. Increasing grass crop yields by application of inorganic fertilizer (N, P and K) inevitably reduces concentrations in grass of the trace elements (Cu, Co and Se). The claim of organic farmers that their cattle are far less prone to mineral deficiency diseases has a basis in that they do not reduce the concentrations of trace elements because they grow less per hectare.

4.6.6.2 Conserved forages

It is possible to sun- or air-dry grass crops and conserve them as hay or compact them into an air-tight clamp or big, covered bale, and conserve them anaerobically as silage. Well-made grass silage has a greater nutritive value than hay because the crop is cut at an earlier, leafier stage. When making grass silage for dairy cows, it is important to cut the grass very young to maximize M/D. For beef cows, it is usual to leave the crop a little longer to achieve a greater yield but lower M/D (*c*. 10 MJ/kg). The anaerobic fermentation of grass sugars (ideally by lactobacilli) in the silage clamp increases the acidity of the crop and inhibits further microbial breakdown. In effect, the crop is pickled. However, appetite for grass silage when it is fed on its own can be disappointing, partly because it digests slowly in the rumen and partly because it can contain a relative excess of EDRP. Both fermentation rate and appetite can be improved by the addition of a more rapidly fermentable feed with a relative excess of ME. Such ingredients include cereals, a root crop (turnips or fodder beet) or maize silage.

Well-made hay is less nutritious than silage but extremely palatable. Soft meadow hay made from a range of grass species is particularly suitable for encouraging young calves to develop an appetite for roughages. Barley straw has little nutritional value but is a good dietary supplement for cattle eating large quantities of cereals. The long, hard, relatively indigestible fibre dilutes the quickly fermentable starchy cereals and provides the necessary stimulation for increased rumination and therefore more salivation. Both these factors reduce the risk of ruminal acidosis. It is possible to improve the nutritive value of straw by treating with alkali – sodium hydroxide or ammonia. Alkali causes the cell walls to open up and release more fermentable cellulose from its bonds to unfermentable lignin. Alkali-treated straws have an M/D close to that of hay. In any year, economics strictly determine the case for alkali treatment of straw; if the grass crop (hay or silage) is poor (in a wet summer) or in short supply (in a dry summer) then it pays to treat the straw crop.

4.6.6.3 Maize silage

Maize (corn) silage is an excellent feed for all beef cattle in areas where the crop can be grown successfully. Yields of ME per hectare can be very impressive. The M/D is excellent but it is slightly deficient in ERDP. Properly supplemented, maize silage can sustain growth rates in excess of 1.0 kg/day. It is particularly effective when fed in combination with grass silage, not least because DM intakes are usually better for maize silage than when feeding grass silage alone. A mixture of 75 parts maize silage and 25 parts grass silage on the forage wagon is ideal for finishing cattle.

4.6.6.4 Cereals

The main nutrient in barley, oats and wheat is starch, which makes these cereals highly concentrated forms of ME for cattle. They are marginal or slightly deficient in protein, both as ERDP for the rumen micro-organisms and as a source of essential amino acids for growing or lactating cattle. When they constitute the major part of the ration (e.g. in a barley beef system) they may promote very rapid growth, but this will cause early-maturing breeds (e.g. offspring of Hereford and Angus bulls) to fatten too soon. All cereals may predispose to ruminal acidosis through too-rapid fermentation, unless diluted with long fibre. Oats is the safest cereal in this respect, being the most fibrous, but it is more expensive per unit of ME than barley or wheat.

4.6.6.5 Root crops

Root crops such as fodder beet, swedes and turnips have a DM content of less than 200 g/kg but are rich in sugars and very palatable. They are deficient in protein and minerals. A small quantity of a root crop such as fodder beet (e.g. 5 kg/day) can make an excellent supplement to grass silage. In the north and east of England and Scotland it is possible to grow roots as the main energy feed for wintering beef cattle. However, such a diet will need supplementing with protein, minerals and fat-soluble vitamins.

4.6.6.6 By-Products and crop residues

Most pelleted compound rations for cattle contain large proportions of by-products or residues from crops grown primarily for direct human consumption. The most common by-products that farmers feed their cattle are the protein-rich residues from plants such as soya bean, rapeseed or groundnuts. These are grown primarily as sources of vegetable oil for human consumption. Others include sugarbeet pulp, a highly palatable source of digestible fibre, and maize gluten, the crop residue after extraction of most of the starch from maize. Both sugar beet and maize gluten are reasonably well balanced in the ratio of ERDP to ME and it is possible to feed them directly to cattle as 'straights'. In areas where it permitted, feed manufacturers may also incorporate small quantities of fishmeal into compound feeds as an excellent source of undegradable amino acids, minerals and vitamins. In the past, manufacturers used meat and bone meal from abattoirs. However, since the epidemic of BSE it is illegal, in Europe, to include feed of animal origin in diets for cattle. The total ban on the use of meat and bone meal was introduced in 2001. The BSE crisis led to the European Union banning exports of British beef with effect from March 1996; the ban lasted for 10 years before it was finally lifted on 1 May 2006.

4.7 Environment and Housing

The UK Department for the Environment, Food and Rural Affairs Welfare Codes outline legislation and provide guidelines based on the principles of the 'five freedoms' (Chapter 1). In essence, these animal welfare guidelines are the application of sensible animal husbandry practices to the livestock present on the farm. Moreover the five freedoms provide a structure for the evaluation of the welfare of an animal or group of animals in various environments (Chapter 18). The overall welfare of cattle is defined by their physiological and behavioural state as they seek to reconcile exogenous influences with their natural endogenous state. Exogenous factors include the physical environment (temperature, humidity, wind, photoperiod, and so on) and social environment (feeding, housing, stocking rate, area per animal). Endogenous state is influenced by (e.g.) breed, age, sex, weight and temperament and impacts on social order (competition, aggression, dominance order, leadership, and so on).

4.7.1 Housing design

Beef cattle are normally outdoor at pasture for a 7- to 8-month period each year. Housing of cattle is designed to provide shelter from winter climatic conditions and protect pastures from undue damage (poaching) in wet conditions, particularly in the months of December and January when grass is in short supply. Housing provides structured management (feeding, drinking, health check) under controlled conditions. It also aids effective slurry and effluent control.

Slatted floor and loose-bedded systems are two main house types used for accommodating beef animals. In many instances, hybrid house types have developed which are constructed using combinations of the above, particularly in the situation where facilities have evolved over time, e.g. the addition of a slatted feed passage to a loose straw-bedded house. Many of these houses utilize liquid manure storage systems. The move away from the traditional design layouts of open yards with self-feed silage has also been driven by the management problems associated with the high volumes of dirty water produced with these designs due to the high levels of annual rainfall.

Slatted floor housing is the most relevant housing system in areas such as Ireland where the availability of straw is low and the cost prohibitive. Alternatively, and preferably, each pen may be divided into a well-strawed bedding area and a concrete area behind the feed fence at either side of the central feeding passage. Each pen is separated from the next by a gate which can be swung across daily to enclose the cattle in the bedding area and permit the concrete standing area behind the feed fence to be scraped down using a tractor. The building should be designed to permit the maximum amount of air movement without incurring draughts. This is best achieved by installing space boarding to a depth of at least 1 m and preferably 2 m below the eaves, and an open ridge, with flashing upstands to either side over the central feed passage. The air, which has been warmed by the cattle, and which leaves the building by this open ridge, will prevent the entry of rain or snow in all but the most severe conditions. In addition, over the winter, the ridge will probably let out about 100 times more moisture (from the cattle) than it will let in.

4.7.1.1 Essential elements of good building design

Essential elements of good building design include the following:

- All houses should be adequately ventilated, allowing for an adequate supply of fresh air, thus facilitating heat dissipation and preventing the build-up of carbon dioxide, ammonia or slurry gases.
- Floor surfaces should be even and non-slip. All buildings should be adequately ventilated with sufficient air exchange to meet the animals' requirements.
- The accommodation should contain sufficient source of natural or artificial light so as not to cause discomfort to the animals. Artificial light should also be provided to enable adequate inspection of the animals, in particular, for inspection of cows in late pregnancy and of young calves.

- Each building accommodation should have a suitable smoke or fire alarm system installed in order to detect fire or smoke at an early stage.
  Special requirements for slatted floor housing include the following:
- Housed stock should have freedom of movement and ample floor space for lying, grooming and normal animal-to-animal interactions.
- A well-designed, properly constructed and fully maintained slatted floor unit for cattle provides the necessary comfort with minimum distress or injury to the cattle.
- Escapes/creeps should be provided, if young calves are housed with adults, i.e. sucklers.

4.7.1.2 Feed barrier

Design of the feed barrier should include the following:

- There should be sufficient space for all animals to feed comfortably at the same time.
- The feed trough should be sufficiently large so that animals have adequate access to food at all times.
- Avoid any sharp edges or projections on the feed barrier or on the pen divisions, which could cause injury to cattle.
- The feed should be kept within reach of the animal.

4.7.2 Bedding area

The goal of a reasonably clean, dry comfortable bed is easier to define than to achieve. Cattle are undoubtedly very comfortable when lying in deep, clean straw. However, straw is probably too expensive unless a farm produces its own straw, and prohibitively so in some areas of good beef country such as Ireland. The main problem is that cattle urinate and defaecate indiscriminately. This makes it more difficult to maintain the bedding reasonably dry and clean even when the feed is dry (e.g. barley and straw) and practically impossible when the main feed is low dry matter grass silage. It is possible to house adult, non-lactating beef cows and growing cattle over 6 months of age on slatted concrete floors. These are far from ideal as a mattress to lie on but they can be kept clean and dry if the gaps between the slats are 40 mm wide and the cattle are stocked densely enough to tread the dung between the slats. However, young calves below 6 months of age should not be kept on slatted floors because 40 mm gaps are too wide for their feet and the stocking density necessary to ensure that the slats stay clean increases the risk of provoking pneumonia in these young animals. It follows that while pregnant beef cows may be housed on slatted floors, it is no place for a beef cow to rear her calf, still less give birth.

Beef cows and fattening heifers can be accommodated in cubicles. They are obviously unsuitable for males, who urinate into the middle of the cubicle bed. The dimensions of the cubicle should be determined by the size of the largest animal that

Table 4.9 Space requirements for beef cattle. Source: DEFRA, 2007.

	Calves		Fattening cattle over 1 year	Beef cows
	0–6 weeks	6–12 weeks		
Floor space (m^2)				
straw bed	2	2	3–4	4
slatted floor	—	—	1.4–2.2	3.0–3.7
Air space (m^3)	6	10	12	12

they are likely to accommodate. Each animal should be able to lie down entirely within the cubicle without interference from its neighbours (e.g. being trampled upon), change position (stand up and lie down) without difficulty, yet, so far as possible, urinate and defaecate in the dunging passage. A cubicle for a Hereford × Friesian suckler cow should be at least 2 m by 1 m. Fine tuning of the standing position can be achieved by adjusting the neck rail or brisket board at the front of the cubicle.

4.7.3 Space allowance

Recommended space allowances for beef cattle are summarized in Table 4.9. The minimum space allowances for cattle used in livestock production are those for animals housed in slatted-floor pens. This is because more traditional, bedded systems require more space per animal to maintain the integrity of the bedding and because slatted-floored systems require a certain stocking density in order to tread the dung between the slats and stop it building up inside the pen.

When cows or fattening cattle are given restricted amounts of concentrate feed, it is essential that all the animals can feed at the same time. Recommended trough spaces for cows and growing cattle are 0.6–0.8 m, and 0.4–0.6 m respectively, depending on age and breed. A group of 10 yearling cattle on slats with 0.4 m trough space per head and a floor area of 1.6 m^2 per head would require a square pen 4 m long by 4 m deep. However, the recommended minimum air space is 12 m^3 per head. For pens 4 m by 4 m either side of a 4 m wide feeding passage, the average height of the building should be 5 m. Examples of housing designs accommodating these basic environmental requirements are given later.

The housing of adult cattle raises concerns about space and flooring. There is still inadequate evidence regarding the effects of concrete slatted floors on animal wellbeing, although the preferences exhibited by cattle for softer surfaces may prompt the development of systems which combine the waste control advantages of slats with a softer coating. Provision of adequate space allowances during the housing period for cattle determines their welfare status and control over labour costs. However, insufficient space allowance may induce a state of chronic stress by preventing animals from performing their natural behaviour, and this may impair

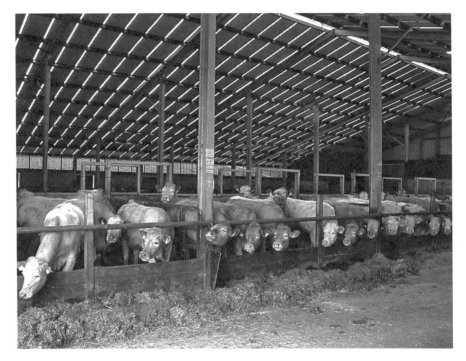

Figure 4.2   Beef cattle housing.

immune function and performance. Figure 4.2 provides an example of beef cattle housing.

4.7.4 Housing suckler cows and calves

Suckler housing should provide clean, comfortable, well-ventilated, draught-free accommodation for calves with suitable accommodation for cows. Housing should permit the accommodation of cows and calves in small groups according to calf age, to minimize the spread of disease from older to younger calves. A straw-bedded creep should always be provided for autumn/winter/early spring calves.

There are three types of housing for cows with suckling calves:

1. slatted housing with creep area;
2. cubicle housing with creep area;
3. loose housing with creep area.

The above systems can be combined. The most usual combination is slatted and loose housing, where cows are easy-fed along slatted passages. A kerb 200 mm to 250 mm high and 200 mm wide to retain bedding material should be provided between slats and bedded area. The floor area required per cow and calves is the same as for loose housing.

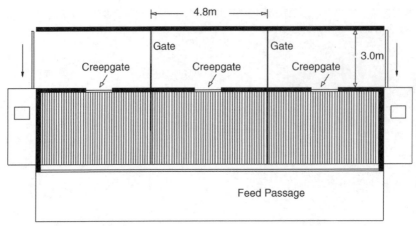

Figure 4.3   Slatted house and creep area. Source: Department of Agriculture, Fisheries & Food (DAFF 2007, Ireland).

Calving boxes should be provided if calving is indoors. In slatted units where the creep area is at the back of slats, part of the creep area may be partitioned to provide a suitable calving box. In larger herds a further box may be provided to keep cows with calves for a few days after calving; floor area should not be less than 14.5 m². Calving boxes may be provided in an adjoining building. It is recommended that a crush gate, set out 600 mm from the wall to facilitate handling, is provided in the calving box for suckler cows. Figures 4.3 and 4.4 show some suggested layouts for suckler housing.

4.7.5 Design of creep area

A creep area of at least 1 m² per calf should be provided for spring-born calves and up to 1.75 m² per calf for autumn-born calves.

A solid floor is preferred. The fall should be at least 1 in 30 (recommended 1 in 20) to a drainage channel discharging into the underground tank.

Slatted-floor pens normally used to house cattle may be covered with straw bedding for creep use. Underfloor draughts should, as far as possible, be excluded. It is recommended that slats are covered with a suitable material to prevent straw bedding entering the slurry tank.

The location of the creep area depends on:

- The preferred management system: autumn, winter, early spring or late spring calving. No creep area is required for late spring calving.
- Where part of the herd is early calving it is recommended that the creep area be located at the end of the house with calved cows accommodated in the adjoining pen.
- Where most of the herd is housed after calving the preferred location of the creep is at the back of the slatted area. The recommended minimum width is 3 m.

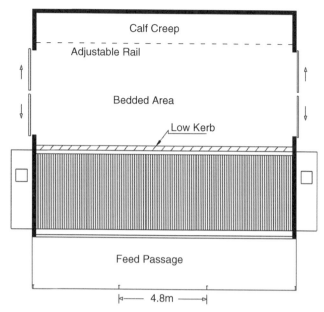

Source: Department of Agriculture, Fisheries & Food (Ireland).

Figure 4.4 Bedded/slatted house. Source: Department of Agriculture, Fisheries & Food (DAFF 2007, Ireland).

Separate external access to the internal divisions of the creep area, particularly in autumn and winter calving herds, is recommended to facilitate meal feeding and inspection of calves. It is recommended that the barrier between the cow area and the creep is a tubular steel gate framed with 50 mm tubular steel and incorporating a creep gate. To allow cows to see the calves the wall should be 1.1 m to 1.2 m high, and be installed with a horizontal top rail set at 1.5 m over floor level. One creep gate per pen should be provided.

4.7.6 Handling facilities

When cattle are brought into an indoor yard system, having been out at grass all summer, they are well adapted to a fibrous diet and reasonably immune to the viral and bacterial organisms that cause infectious pneumonia. Management, therefore, presents few problems. The objective is to feed the cattle so as to achieve pre-set targets for weight gain at the least possible cost. The most useful aid to management is, therefore, a good set of scales and an efficient arrangement for moving cattle in and out of their pens and over this weighbridge at intervals of about 4 weeks. Cattle may be driven fairly easily in groups into a collecting pen large enough to contain all the cattle from one pen in the beef-rearing unit. They may then be driven down a race with solid sides and a curved approach to a weighbridge and a crush, where individuals may be restrained for routine treatment or preventive medicine. The high, solid sides to the race prevent the cattle from being distracted or startled by the presence of handlers or other alarming objects in front of them, and the curve in the race encourages them to follow their leaders until it is too late to try to escape.

4.8 Management of the Suckler Herd

4.8.1 Breed selection

The ideal characteristics for a suckler cow (e.g. fertility, conformation, docility) were listed in the section on breeding and genetics. Strategies to achieve these targets include:

1. Continue to buy in some replacements as dairy cross heifers, and also breed from these to produce second cross (75% continental) replacements. The amount of dairy blood in the cow herd can be reduced to 30% to 35% on average, meaning that the majority of progeny will have minimal dairy genes.
2. Breed toward 100% continental beef cows, using careful selection and breeding programmes to maintain adequate milk output, and backcrossing two different continental breeds to secure hybrid vigour. In all but the very largest herds this system will involve the use of artificial insemination for replacement breeding.

Pure-breeding is seldom recommended for commercial herds, principally because the loss in hybrid vigour is too great, probably up to 22% less live-weight of calf weaned per cow bred. If replacement heifers are being bred from within the herd it is recommended that an AI sire be used, otherwise the stock bull will have to be replaced every 2 to 3 years to avoid inbreeding. Where second and third cross replacement heifers are being brought into a herd, it is recommended that sires with proven maternal traits be used to produce these heifers.

4.8.2 Management of fertility

Fertility targets for a suckler herd are:

- calving interval is 365 days;
- 90% of the herd calves within 10 weeks;
- 5% or less of the herd is culled for infertility.

The two major factors affecting reproductive efficiency in suckler herds using natural mating are the interval from calving to first heat (postpartum interval) and conception rate. When AI is the method of breeding, heat detection efficiency is a further significant factor.

One of the major causes of poor reproductive efficiency in beef cows is an extended interval from calving to first ovulation, or postpartum interval. This interval is considerably longer in beef than in dairy cows and is influenced by several factors including pre- and postpartum nutrition, suckling frequency, age of cow, season and the presence of a bull. Moreover the time from calving to first heat is very dependent on body condition. Thus condition scoring on a scale of 0 (very thin and emaciated) to 5 (grossly over-fat) is a practical aid to ensuring proper nutrition at this important time. Spring calving cows on good pasture are on a high plane of nutrition during the breeding season and a body condition score of 2 is satisfactory when breeding commences. The high nutrient intake from grass, assuming adequate leafy pasture is provided, offsets the adverse effects of low body condition on fertility. In contrast, autumn-calving cows fed silage are on a lower plane of nutrition during the breeding season and should have a body condition score of 2.5 at the start of breeding.

For autumn-calving cows, fertility can be a problem with cows bred indoors and it is essential during the breeding period to provide adequate feed either as good-quality silage or as a moderate-quality silage and about 2 kg of concentrates daily. With autumn-calving cows, the high summer weight gains at pasture will readily result in body condition scores of 3 or better at calving. In fact, there is a danger of cows becoming over-fat and pasture restriction may be necessary prior to calving. Following successful breeding, feed intake is not as important and a condition score of 2 is again adequate at turnout in spring.

4.8.3 Breeding seasons

Season of calving influences both the breeding management and the yearly feeding programme. The winter feed requirements of a cow rearing one calf are about 1.5 times those for a pregnant cow. Thus, autumn-calving cows lactating throughout the winter require about 1.8 tonnes more silage over a 5-month winter period than spring-calving cows. In the spring-calving suckling system there may be two target calving periods:

- early spring calving (January and February) where the intention is to produce a strong calf at turnout to grass, especially in the early grass growing areas, and a heavy weanling by the autumn;
- late spring calving (mid-February to mid-April) targeted at turnout to grass from mid- to late March.

4.8.4 Artificial insemination

The success of any AI programme depends on two factors:

- heat (oestrus) detection rate (shown to be 75% in good dairy herds);
- conception rate to AI (success of natural service shown to be 60%).

Heat detection in suckler herds is more difficult than in dairy herds. The intensity of heat is not as strong and does not last as long. The cow in heat is the one that stands to be mounted. However, cows that are most active at mounting are usually those cows which have either been recently in heat themselves or are about to come into heat shortly. Detecting the highest possible number of cows in heat each day during the breeding season presents a major challenge for suckler herd owners. In dairy herds it has been shown that early morning and late evening are the best times for observing the highest proportion of cows in heat. These data also indicate that three further checks at about 3–4 hours apart are required to detect 90% of cows in heat. Therefore, to achieve the highest possible number of cows in heat each day of the breeding season requires five regulated daily inspections.

4.8.5 Oestrus synchronization

Oestrus (heat) synchronization is a management practice that can help beef producers improve production efficiency and economic returns. It can help shorten the breeding and calving seasons and help increase calf weaning weights. Its purpose is to control oestrus and ovulation in cycling females, so that breeding can be completed in a short period of time. Instead of females being bred over a 21-day period, synchronization can shorten the breeding period to less than 5 days, depending on the programme selected. The use of synchronization has great potential for improving beef production, but it requires good management for success. Producers should understand the advantages of, as well as the requirements for, a successful oestrus synchronization programme. They should also know how the different oestrus synchronization products and programmes work, and the expected results and costs involved before initiating the practice.

4.8.5.1 Requirements for oestrus synchronization

1. Need a well-planned and implemented programme for successful results.
2. Need fertile heifers and cows on an adequate nutrition programme.
3. Need quality semen for AI, and experienced inseminators.
4. Need healthy, aggressive, fertile bulls for synchronized natural breeding.
5. Requires more concentrated labour at breeding and calving times.
6. May need facilities for bad weather during concentrated breeding and calving periods.
7. May result in lower pregnancy rates if procedures and requirements are not followed.

4.8.6 Management around calving

Management of the suckler cow in the final 2 months of pregnancy can have a major influence on cow health, calf survival and calf diseases. The increased use of highly muscled bulls has inevitably increased the risk of obstetric problems. However, this can be offset by attention to body condition of the cow and feeding over the final 2 months of pregnancy. The ideal condition score (CS) at calving is 2.50 to 3.25.

Above a CS of 3.5 there is definitely an increase in calving difficulty. Cows with a body condition score higher than 3 should be on a restricted diet with as much exercise as possible.

Cows whose CS is below 2 should be separated and given extra feed but care should be taken in the final month as the calf is now putting on about 0.5 kg per day. The weight gain of the calf over the final 4 to 6 weeks has a big influence on calving problems. The overall 'fitness' of the cow also has a bearing on calving process, so exercise is important too.

The interval from calving to first ovulation in beef cows is highly dependent on body condition. This is another reason to optimize body condition at calving. Increasing the level of postpartum nutrition for a thin cow, even to very high levels, has a negligible effect on the interval to first ovulation.

4.8.7 Management of cows and calves

Ideally, spring-calving herds should be turned out to grass before calving but, because of the fickle nature of the spring and the shortness of the summer in classic beef country, this is usually impracticable. This means indoor calving, which carries severe risks of infection.

The main problems of infectious disease for the newborn calf in a suckler herd are septicaemia, usually caused by *Escherichia coli*, and enteritis caused by viruses such as Rotavirus. Both organisms are inevitable inhabitants of winter accommodation for adult cattle. Calves born into such an environment can be infected with *E. coli* at birth and the resultant septicaemia may (at worst) kill them within 2 to 3 days. Rotavirus and other enteroviruses usually induce diarrhoea beginning in the second week of life, which can also be fatal or may severely stunt the calf's development.

Turnout to grass takes place as soon as possible. The main risk for the cows at this time is hypomagnesaemia, and magnesium supplements are essential. If the cows are not getting a concentrate ration, these minerals can be incorporated into a block, added to the water supply or delivered from an intra-ruminal bolus. The bulls are introduced to the cows in June, when the weather is good and the cows are on a high plane of nutrition and gaining condition. In these circumstances, fertility should be high.

4.8.8 Weaning suckled calves

In suckler herds, calves remain with the dam at pasture until they are 5 to 9 months old. Weaning of the suckled calf from its dam can be stressful for the calf. In addition to removal from the dam, the weaning procedure may be compounded by other stressors, e.g. change of diet (grass and milk to conserved feed with or without concentrates), change of environment (outdoors to indoors), transport/marketing, de-horning and castration. Weaning therefore is a multifactorial stressor, in which nutritional, social, physical and psychological stress are combined. Psychological stress is present in the form of maternal separation and social disruption, whereas physical and nutritional stressors are often present in the introduction and adaptation to a novel diet and novel environment.

Calves that are weaned abruptly in the autumn, housed and introduced to silage and concentrates have a low feed intake initially. All calves should be provided with a concentrate creep feed prior to weaning. While suckled calves may be slow to adapt to creep feeding, the stress that normally occurs following weaning will be reduced considerably if calves are consuming 1 kg of creep feed daily prior to weaning. The preferred option is to keep the herd in a properly fenced field with a good grass supply or with silage (or hay) fed and the cows removed gradually (up to one-quarter on any one occasion) to a location away from the calves. As the calves remain in the same herd, with adequate feed supplies, the upset caused is reduced considerably. During this period the concentrate creep can be increased gradually to about 1 kg per calf daily. Where calves are going to be castrated, they must be castrated at least 4 weeks prior to weaning date, or at least 2 weeks after the calf has been weaned. It is illegal to castrate an animal over 6 months of age without veterinary involvement. In Ireland, the Suckler Herds Welfare Scheme was introduced in 2008 in order to improve the standards of animal welfare and the breeding quality of animals in suckler herds. Details are given in Box 4.1.

Box 4.1   Appropriate weaning procedures: The Irish Suckler Welfare Scheme

Castration

Where male calves are to be castrated (not compulsory under the Scheme, e.g. where the farmer is involved in the production or sale of bulls), castration must be carried out at least 4 weeks prior to the weaning date, or at least 2 weeks after the weaning date. It is illegal to castrate an animal over 6 months of age without veterinary involvement. In the UK it is an offence to castrate without an anaesthetic calves older than 2 months. Devices to restrict blood flow to the scrotum are only permitted without an anaesthetic if they are used during the first week of life (DEFRA, 2003).

Age

8 weeks is the minimum age at which a calf can be weaned.

Meal (concentrates) feeding

Concentrates must be introduced to calves a minimum of 4 weeks before weaning. The daily allowance per animal must be increased over this period until all animals are eating, on average, 1.0 kg/head/day at weaning. Meal feeding must be continued through the weaning process for a minimum period of 2 weeks after weaning.

Graduated weaning

Abrupt weaning of all animals at one time is not permitted. For herds with more than 10 suckler cows, a gradual weaning procedure must be followed:

- At pasture – Calves must be weaned in at least two separate groups with each group being removed at a minimum interval of 5 days. The first group of cows must be removed, allowing their calves to stay with the remaining herd. After a few days the cows can be taken away to another area. Again the calves must be weaned in at least two separate groups.
- Indoors – Calves are housed in a pen adjacent to the cows with access to these cows. Calves must be weaned in at least two separate groups with each group being removed at a minimum interval of 5 days. The first group of cows must be removed, allowing their calves to stay with the remaining herd. Cows for culling and those in poor body condition (e.g. young cows or very old cows) should be weaned first and late calving cows in good body condition weaned towards the end.

Source: www.agriculture.gov.i.e./schemes/SucklerScheme.

4.8.9 Health and welfare problems

In general, the spring-calving suckler cow gets very little compound ration and therefore has no opportunity to obtain supplementary minerals in her regular diet. The energy and protein requirements of most suckler cows in late pregnancy can be supplied by silage. Normally, grass and good-quality silage are reasonably well balanced for the major minerals, but deficiencies of trace elements can occur. The most common trace mineral deficiencies in cattle on forage are copper, iodine, selenium and cobalt. Deficiencies can cause a range of health problems that affect growth, performance, disease resistance and reproduction. Some of the chemical signs of deficiencies in copper, iodine and selenium are common to each other. These are stillbirths, abortions, lowered immunity to diseases such as calf scours, pneumonia, mastitis and below normal survival rates in calves around the time of birth.

Getting a definitive diagnosis of trace mineral deficiencies can be tedious. Doing a large range of tests and/or giving a large selection of mineral supplements can be costly. Sometimes a blood test could show a deficiency but if there are no clinical signs and performance is satisfactory there is unlikely to be a response to extra mineral supplementation. Blood and feed tests do not give a full diagnosis and are best used to support a clinical diagnosis by the veterinarian.

Mineral supplements for suckler cows in late pregnancy can be fed loose at 100 g/day (sprinkled on the silage) or by way of mineral blocks or licks. Cows fed on poor hay or straw should receive supplementation of calcium, phosphorus, sodium and magnesium. However, excess calcium combined with low magnesium in the diet of pre-calving cows can result in milk fever immediately after calving. Therefore, pre-calver minerals should contain little or no calcium (depend on the forage) but up to 15% magnesium in the mineral mix.

4.8.9.1 Acute hypomagnesaemia (grass tetany)

Acute hypomagnesaemia, or grass tetany, is still the biggest killer of suckler cows each year. Cows need to be supplemented with 20 g of magnesium per day during the months of April and May. Mineral feeding options are:

- high magnesium bucket licks – not very expensive but some cows' intake can be very low;
- pasture dusting – again, not very expensive and is very effective but can be time consuming to apply;
- high magnesium compound feeds – effective but expensive;
- water medication – is effective and some products are relatively inexpensive but cows may not drink a lot in wet weather or if fresh water is available from streams;
- magnesium bolus – expensive compared to other methods but does provide reasonable control.

4.8.9.2 Mastitis

Autumn-calving cows immediately after weaning and during the 6 to 8 weeks of the dry period are at high risk of summer mastitis. Other high-risk groups are the fattening cull cows and in-calf heifers. Summer mastitis is an acute, infectious and painful disease of the udder that occurs mainly during the months of July, August and September. Research in the UK indicates that almost 70% of cases occur in August, with 25% split between July and September and the remainder at other times of the year including the winter months. It is believed that flies play a major role in the spread of the disease, first by causing damage to the teat orifice and second by transmitting the bacteria from infected udders to healthy ones. However, the evidence for this is mostly circumstantial, with the highest incidence of the disease coinciding with the month of highest fly populations. While the vast majority of cases occur in dry cows, in-calf heifers and milking cows are also susceptible. The disease has also been found in maiden heifers and even in male cattle, though this is rare.

4.8.9.3 Recognition and control of mastitis

Of the several causes of mastitis, only microbial infection is important. Although bacteria, fungi, yeasts and possibly virus can all cause udder infection, the main agents are bacteria. The most common pathogens are *Staphylococcus aureus*, *Streptococcus agalactiae*, *Str. dysgalactiae*, *Str. uberis* and *Escherichia coli*, though other pathogens can cause occasional herd outbreaks. Mastitis occurs when the teats of cows are exposed to pathogens which penetrate the teat duct and establish an infection in one or more quarters within the udder. The course of an infection varies; most commonly it persists for weeks or months in a mild form which is not detected by the stockperson (i.e. subclinical mastitis). With some pathogens, typically *E. coli*, the infection is frequently more acute and there is a general endotoxaemia with raised body temperature, loss of appetite and the cow may die unless supportive therapy is given. When clinical mastitis occurs the effective therapy is a course of antibiotic infusions through the teat duct.

The necessary steps to eliminate infections are:

• treat all quarters of all cows at drying off with antibiotic products specifically designed for dry cow therapy;
• cull chronically infected cows.

The necessary steps to control mastitis and lower somatic cell count are:

• teat dipping (see section 4.8.9.4 below);
• treat dry cows;
• practise proper milking procedure;
• use a properly functioning milking system;
• maintain a clean, dry environment for the cows.

4.8.9.4 Control of environmental mastitis

The key to controlling environmental mastitis is prevention, by reducing the number of bacteria to which the teat end is exposed.

Attention should be paid to the cows' environment:

• The cow environment should be as clean and dry as possible.
• Cows should not have access to manure, mud, or pools of stagnant water.
• The dry cow's environment is as important as the lactating cow's environment.
• The calving area must be clean.
• Stalls should be properly designed and maintained.

The following factors are important in considering cow bedding:

• The number of bacteria in bedding depends on available nutrients, amount of contamination, moisture, and temperature.
• Inorganic materials (such as crushed limestone or sand) are low in nutrients and moisture, and thus low in bacteria.
• Finely chopped organic bedding (such as sawdust, shavings, recycled manure, pelleted corn cobs, various seed hulls, chopped straw) are frequently high in bacteria numbers.

The facts about teat dipping include:

• Post milking teat dipping with a germicidal (germ-killing) dip is recommended.
• Dipping controls the spread of contagious mastitis.

- Teat dipping exerts no control over coliform infections.
- Barrier dips are reported to reduce new coliform infections; however, they do not appear to be as effective against environmental streptococci and the contagious pathogens.
- Attempts to control environmental mastitis during the dry period, using either germicidal or barrier dips, have been unsuccessful.

4.9 Management of Artificially Reared Calves

This section deals with the artificial rearing of calves born to dairy cows, for the first 6 months of life, whether destined as dairy replacements or for beef. Box 4.2 presents a brief summary of the most important aspects of the European Communities (Welfare of Calves) Regulation 1995 and 1998 amendments, which apply to calves less than 6 months of age (see DEFRA, 2009a, for legislation relating to farmed cattle). Many of them have particular relevance to calves reared for the production of white veal, and were designed to prevent the worst abuses of welfare involved in the practice of rearing these animals on all-liquid diets and in individual pens without bedding. Nevertheless the principles apply to all calves.

Box 4.2   Welfare of calves to 6 months

- Calves shall not be kept permanently in darkness. To meet their behavioural and physiological needs, the accommodation shall be well lit, by natural or artificial light, for at least 8 hours a day.
- All housed calves shall be inspected by the owner or the person responsible for the animals at least twice daily and calves kept outside shall be inspected at least once daily. Any calf which appears to be ill or injured shall be treated appropriately without delay and veterinary advice shall be obtained as soon as possible for any calf which is not responding to the stock-keeper's care. Where necessary, sick or injured calves shall be isolated in adequate accommodation with dry, comfortable bedding.
- The accommodation for calves must be constructed in such a way as to allow each calf to lie down, rest, stand up and groom itself without difficulty. No calf shall be confined in an individual pen after the age of 8 weeks, unless a veterinarian certifies that its health or behaviour requires it to be isolated in order to receive treatment. For calves kept in groups, the unrestricted space allowance available to each calf shall be at least equal to 1.5 m² for calves of less than 150 kg, at least 1.7 m² for calves from 150 to 220 kg and at least 1.8 m² for calves weighing 220 kg or more.
- Calves shall not be tethered, with the exception of group-housed calves which may be tethered for periods of not more than 1 hour at the time of feeding milk or milk substitute.

- Floors shall be smooth but not slippery so as to prevent injury to the calves. Floors shall be suitable for the size and weight of the calves and form a rigid, even and stable surface. The lying area shall be comfortable, clean and adequately drained and shall not adversely affect the calves. Appropriate bedding shall be provided for all calves less than 2 weeks old.
- All calves shall be provided with an appropriate diet adapted to their age, weight and behavioural and physiological needs, to promote good health and welfare. To this end, their food shall contain sufficient iron to ensure an average blood haemoglobin level of at least 4.5 mmol/L and a minimum daily ration of fibrous food shall be provided for each calf over 2 weeks old, the quantity being raised from 50 g to 250 g per day for calves from 8 to 20 weeks old. Calves shall not be muzzled.
- All calves shall be fed at least twice a day. Where calves are housed in groups and not fed *ad libitum* or by automatic feeding system, each calf shall have access to the food at the same time as the others in the group.
- All calves over 2 weeks of age shall have access to a sufficient quantity of fresh water or be able to satisfy their fluid intake needs by drinking other liquids. However, in hot weather conditions or for calves which are ill, fresh drinking water shall be available at all times.

Source: European Communities (Welfare of Calves) Regulation 1995 and 1998 amendments.

4.9.1 Birth to weaning

Unless the cow is to calve outdoors, she should be confined in a spotlessly clean and disinfected calving box and well bedded down with fresh straw to minimize the risk of infection to cow or calf at the time of parturition. Assuming a normal delivery, the first tasks for the stockperson are to ensure that the calf can breathe properly, and then disinfect the navel with iodine or with an antibiotic spray. The next essential is to ensure that the calf drinks an adequate amount of the cow's first milk (colostrum) in the first 12 hours. Colostrum provides not only food but also maternal antibodies to protect the young calf against the common infections that it is likely to encounter in early life (see Section 4.12).

The teats of mature Holstein/Friesian cows may hang far below the abdominal wall and may be difficult for the young calf to locate. If the calf is left with its mother, the stockperson should ensure that it is feeding satisfactorily. Many good stock-people like to remove the calf from its mother as soon as possible, before the maternal bond has developed, so as to minimize distress for both cow and calf. If so, the cow should be milked out and the calf offered three to four feeds of colostrum during the first day of life. For calves born to Holstein/Friesian cows, each of these first feeds should be of 1.5 litres.

Having started the calf, it is a matter of choice whether to rear it up to weaning in an individual pen on restricted amounts of milk replacer fed from a bucket twice (or, later once) daily or to rear it in a group with free or controlled access to milk replacer sucked through a teat. The feeding options are given in Box 4.3.

Box 4.3   Systems for feeding artificially reared calves to weaning

Bucket feeding: twice daily

Week 1: 2×1.5 litres/day at 125 g powder/litre = 375 g powder/day fed at blood heat (40 °C). During week 2: increase intake to 2.0–2.5 litres/feed at 125 g powder/litre = 500–625 g powder/day.

Introduce a dry calf starter ration (based on cereals, etc.) and roughage in the form of hay or barley straw. Wean when intake of calf starter = 1 kg/day which occurs at approximately 5 weeks of age. By this time each calf will have consumed approximately 20 kg of milk powder.

Bucket feeding: once daily

Weeks 1 and 2: feed twice daily as above. Week 3: feed 2.0–2.5 litres/day in a single feed containing 450–500 g powder; offer starter feed and hay as before. It is essential to provide water for these calves. Intake of milk replacer prior to weaning will be approximately 16 kg.

Teat feeding

- Calves may simply be fed once or twice daily from buckets with teats attached. This is natural and healthy.
- Dispensers that deliver freshly mixed milk replacer at blood heat:
  1. *Ad libitum* dispensers. Most calves thrive on this system but intakes of milk powder to 5 weeks of age are likely to exceed 30 kg per calf, which substantially increases feed costs relative to bucket feeding. Moreover, calves that have had *ad libitum* access to milk powder may be eating much less than 1 kg/day of calf starter ration at this time. One strategy to encourage intake of dry feed is to restrict time of access to the teat for the last week before weaning or make it more difficult for the calves to drink by progressively constricting the milk supply line.
  2. Computerized dispensers which recognize individual calves, wearing transponders, dispense controlled rations (e.g. 400 g/day of milk powder) and provide records of any calf which fails to drink its full ration.
  3. Dispensers that deliver acidified milk replacer at room temperature. Acidification helps both to preserve the feed in the dispenser and to reduce the risk of diarrhoea by maintaining a low pH in the abomasum.

4.9.2 The bought-in calf

The artificial rearing of calves on their farm of birth can usually be accomplished without mishap. Unfortunately, the majority of beef calves from the dairy herd are moved off their farm of origin at about 1 to 2 weeks of age into specialist rearing units. This may involve trips through two or more markets, and transport, sometimes for the full length of the country. Such animals are deprived of normal food, water and physical comfort, and are confused, exhausted and exposed to a wide range of infectious organisms, of which the most important are the *Salmonella* bacteria. By the time they reach their rearing unit, they are likely to be infected, dehydrated and stressed, and need special care if they are to survive.

On arrival, bought-in calves should be rested in comfort in deep straw. In very cold weather, they may benefit from a little supplementary heating for the first 2 to 3 days. Water should be available, but they should be offered no milk replacer for at least 2 h after arrival. If they arrive in the evening, they can be left until the following morning. Some people feed 1.5 litres of milk powder at 125 g powder/litre for the first feed. It is probably wiser to give two 1.5-litre feeds of a proprietary glucose/electrolyte solution (or one tablespoonful of glucose and one teaspoonful of common salt in 1.5 litres of water) to rehydrate the calves and provide a minimal supply of energy but keep the gut empty of nutrients until the calves have been able to eliminate most of the enteric bacteria acquired in transit. Thereafter, feeding can be as described above. An injection of fat-soluble vitamins A, D and E is also advisable, especially for calves purchased in the late winter. A preferable alternative to this remedial action is for specialist calf rearers to negotiate contracts with dealers who can guarantee to supply calves from their farm of origin to the rearing unit on the same day and with the minimum of disturbance and mixing.

4.9.3 Feeding after weaning

After weaning, calves are fed a concentrate ration plus hay, straw or silage *ad libitum*. The amount of concentrate fed and its protein concentration are governed by how fast the calf is expected to grow. If it is to be turned out to grass in the spring and reared for slaughter at 18 to 24 months, it should get no more than 3 kg/day of concentrate with a protein concentration of 180 g/kg plus hay or silage *ad libitum*. Calves in contract-rearing units, which need to achieve as much weight gain as possible by 12 weeks, and barley beef calves, will probably be given unrestricted access to concentrates and consume more than 4 kg/day. In this case the protein concentration in the post-weaning concentrate diet should be no more than 160 g/kg, and it may pay to feed roughage in the form of straw rather than hay or silage. Since calves are likely to eat less barley straw than hay or silage it follows that they will tend to eat more concentrates when straw is the only source of roughage. If the calves are to be reared intensively on a high concentrate ration and slaughtered at 12 to 16 months of age, it pays to adapt them to a high concentrate ration as quickly as possible. If the mainstay of their subsequent diet is to be grass or maize silage then, equally, it makes sense to introduce these feeds as soon as possible.

4.9.4 Housing young calves

The basic requirements of calf housing are:

- construction which can provide clean, dry, draught-free accommodation without risk of injury to the health of animals and workers;
- design which allows feeding, cleaning, disinfection and general hygiene;
- design which allows a thorough inspection of calves and easy stock management;
- adequate air space and ventilation;
- accommodation for the isolation of sick calves.

Calves may be kept in single pens, in groups, or in a combination of both. When group penned, the minimum permissible pen floor space per calf of less than 150 kg is 1.5 m^2 but 1.7 m^2 is recommended. For calves between 150 kg and 220 kg, the minimum space is 1.7 m^2 per calf; and for calves over 220 kg, 1.8 m^2. However, as a general guide a total floor area of 2.3 m^2 per calf with a cubic air capacity of about 7 m^3 per calf should be provided. For larger herds a double range of pens with a central feeding passage is suitable. The passage shall not be less than 1.2 m wide. Movable pen divisions may be used to facilitate different space requirements and cleaning systems. Individual pens shall be a minimum of 1.0 m wide by 1.5 m in length, but 1.7 m length is recommended, especially for isolation pens.

4.9.4.1 Pens

European Union Regulations state that individual pens for calves except those for isolating sick calves should not have solid walls but shall have perforated walls which allow the calves to have direct visual and tactile contact. Calves more than 8 weeks old may not be kept in individual pens unless a registered veterinary surgeon certifies that its health or behaviour requires it to be isolated in order to receive treatment.

The greatest threats to the health and welfare of the young calf are infections which may cause septicaemia, enteritis (leading to diarrhoea or scours) and pneumonia (see Section 4.12). The organisms responsible for these conditions are widespread and young calves, especially those which are moved through markets, are practically certain to be exposed to some degree of infection. The prime specification for a calf house is, therefore, that it should be as hygienic as possible, not only on the surfaces of the walls, floor and feeding utensils, but also in the air itself. It should be power-washed with hot water or steam and disinfected before the first calves of the season arrive, and this process should be repeated between successive batches. Whenever possible, the rearer of bought-in calves should practise an 'all in, all out' policy and avoid introducing new baby calves into an already infected building. Hygiene and humidity are also controlled by ensuring effective and appropriate drainage under the individual group pens.

Air hygiene is determined mainly by air space per calf and, to a much lesser extent, by ventilation. This is because the animals are the prime source of pathogenic organisms, but ventilation only removes a small proportion of these organisms from the air in the building; most die *in situ* (for further explanation, see Webster, 1985). Unweaned calves require 6 m^3 air space per calf to ensure reasonable air hygiene, and post-weaning calves 10 m^3. In temperate climates, effective air movement (a minimum of four air changes per hour) can be achieved by natural ventilation through strategically placed inlets and outlets. Whether reared in groups or individual pens prior to weaning, calves are normally grouped after weaning and reared in follow-on pens. The simultaneous stresses of mixing and weaning can increase the risk of disease at this time, especially pneumonia. One advantage of rearing batches of calves in groups and feeding them from a teat is that they can be kept in the same group and in the same accommodation from the time of arrival until turnout. Calves are initially restrained in the back of the pen by straw bales, which are taken down at weaning and used as bedding. The small increase in feed costs prior to weaning may be more than offset by reductions in the cost of housing and of disease.

4.9.5 Rearing calves for veal

The intensive production of veal in Europe and North America in the latter part of the twentieth century involved the confinement of calves for life in individual wooden crates and the feeding of a liquid milk replacer diet, deficient in iron, to ensure white meat. The European Communities (Welfare of Calves) Regulation (1995, 1998 see above) have now prohibited the worst welfare excesses of this system. Calves over 8 weeks of age must not be penned individually and the food for all calves shall contain sufficient iron and a minimum daily ration of fibrous food. Nevertheless the system continues to present many welfare problems. Group housing is typically on slatted floors, which can become very slippery, especially given the liquid, projectile nature of faeces from calves on liquid diets. This problem is exacerbated when entire bull calves, reared to heavier weights, approach sexual maturity and attempt to mount one another.

4.9.6 Alternative husbandry systems for veal calves

Several alternative husbandry systems for veal calves have been explored in an attempt to discover one that is more humane and also economically competitive with the intensive method. The aims of these systems are to ensure good welfare by keeping calves in groups with access to straw or other bedding and to provide sufficient fibrous feed to promote good health and normal behaviour in consequence of normal rumen development. Liquid milk replacer still forms the major part of the diet in order to promote rapid growth and produce quality 'pink' veal that attracts a high price. Veal is perceived as a luxury meat by those prepared to eat it, and shunned by others as unacceptable on welfare grounds. It should follow, therefore, that high welfare standards become a major selling point for those seeking to produce high-premium veal for the luxury market. A few honourable entrepreneurs have sought to exploit this market with approval from bodies such as RSPCA Freedom Foods. However, the economic returns to date are not encouraging.

4.10 Finishing Beef Cattle

This section describes the management of cattle reared for prime beef from weaning, in the case of suckled calves, or 6 months of age, for artificially reared calves, to the time of slaughter.

4.10.1 Winter feeding
Two classes of beef animals will require winter feeding in yards:

1. weanlings from the suckler herds and store animals from dairy/beef systems animals entering their first winter and at least a year from slaughter;
2. finishers – animals being finished for slaughter over the winter.

From a feeding viewpoint, the main difference between the two types is that weanlings have time after the winter to exhibit compensatory growth whereas the finishers do not. However, weanlings are still immature and relatively underdeveloped so a minimum rate of gain is necessary to ensure essential bone and muscle growth. For dairy calf-to-beef production systems this minimum has been set at about 0.5 kg/day.

Grass silage is an integral part of most beef production farming systems in northern and northwestern Europe. Besides silage being an important feedstuff for cattle, especially when they are housed indoors, silage production can be integrated into farming systems in a manner that makes an essential positive contribution to both effective grassland management and internal parasite control with grazing animals. Furthermore, nutrients collected from housed livestock can be best recycled by spreading the manures on the grassland used for producing silage.

Generally, the level of concentrates fed to weanlings and store cattle in winter is low. Reducing or eliminating concentrate feeding towards the end of winter is sometimes practised. Within the EU, beef production has been influenced by legislative requirements, such as age limits for the application of premiums and the ban on the sale of animals over 30 months of age (to control the threat of BSE). Such requirements have been gradually removed and animals are likely to be finished at an age that best suits market demands.

Most beef finishing systems use a confinement system based on conserved forages (e.g. grass or maize silage) and concentrates composed mainly of grains (e.g. barley), protein sources (e.g. soya bean meal) by-products (e.g. non-forage fibre sources), minerals and vitamins. Concentrates are a major cost element in feeding beef cattle in winter, particularly finishing cattle. The optimal feeding system is one that takes into account daily live-weight gain, feed efficiency, seasonal variations in market prices and regional variations in perception of beef quality. When forages are supplemented with concentrates, forage intake declines. This is known as substitution. The present economic level of concentrate supplementation for finishing steers offered silage *ad libitum* is in the range 4 to 7 kg per head daily depending on factors such as concentrate costs, type of animal being finished and anticipated carcass price. Concentrates are normally fed at a flat rate throughout the finishing period either as one or two discrete meals per day or as part of a mixed ration. In recent years, mainly because of the need to hold cattle until specific dates to collect premiums, the practice of varying the level of concentrates throughout the finishing period has developed. Feeding a lower level early on prevents animals being finished before their eligible premium dates, and then if they are not finished as the eligible premium date approaches, the level of concentrates is increased to permit rapid disposal after the retention date has passed. Manipulating growth rates in the finishing period can have an adverse effect on meat quality as there is evidence that a declining rate of gain before slaughter predisposes to poorer-quality meat. Furthermore, Mediterranean markets require carcasses with muscle which is light red in colour and fat which is white in colour. These colour traits are more likely when animals are fed a high level of concentrates towards the end of the finishing period.

4.10.2 Housing and welfare

Housing protects animals from adverse weather conditions and provides structured management (feeding, drinking, health check etc.) under controlled conditions. In many Irish beef production systems, animals are generally housed in a concrete slatted-floored facility for a 4- to 5-month winter period at $2.2\,m^2$ per head for 500 kg animals (Dodd, 1985) and fed *ad libitum* grass silage with concentrate supplementation. Provision of adequate space allowances during the housing period for cattle determines their welfare status. High stocking densities of less than $2.0\,m^2$ per head have been shown to adversely affect the frequency and duration of lying and levels of aggression within groups. Animal behavioural studies indicate that intensive stocking rates on slatted floors can present a significant challenge to the successful adaptation of cattle to confinement. Cattle are social animals and establish social bonds and hierarchy among themselves. In large groups (>100 animals) with minimum space allowances, individual animals appear to have difficulty in memorizing the social status of all peers, which increases the incidences of social aggressiveness and oral stereotypies in cattle. The abrupt breakage of the social bond or hierarchy through regrouping and relocating may lead to social stress and an animal may respond with abnormal behaviour and impaired performance.

4.10.3 Summer grazing and pasture management

The allocation of summer pasture for all animals should be sufficient to meet their feed requirements. A supply of clean fresh water should be available at all times and the pasture area should be free of hazards which may cause injury to the animals. An adequate supply of good-quality pasture for suckler cows in spring and early summer ensures rapid weight recovery, good milk production and good reproductive activity. Paddock grazing or the use of a buffer area allows better budgeting of the grass available, thereby matching the demand of the animals with grass supply. A flexible approach to grassland management is essential to control within- and between-year variation in grass growth.

Overstocking resulting in cows losing weight is not acceptable. It may be necessary to reduce stocking rate in autumn or during dry summers in order to maintain adequate feed supply. Overstocking in the autumn has an undesirable effect on calf and cow performance. The calf will be unable to meet its requirements for growth and the cow will not establish adequate body reserves at pasture to help sustain her in the winter period. Undue delays in weaning on scarce autumn pasture can also result in rapid loss of body condition in suckler cows.

The two most important species of parasitic roundworms affecting grazing cattle are *Ostertagia*, which causes gastritis, and *Dictyocaulus*, which causes pneumonia. Both species overwinter on pasture and, therefore, can affect calves shortly after turnout. If, as is likely, the pasture was grazed by cattle the previous year, it pays to delay turning out young calves until early May, by which time most of the over-wintered *Ostertagia* larvae will have died. If calves do become infested and excrete eggs on to the pasture, there is a second build-up of larvae on the pasture by the middle of July. Ostertagiasis in cattle can be controlled effectively by pasture management, but many beef farmers consider it necessary to dose young calves with anthelmintic drugs in their first summer at grass. Cows and yearling cattle that have previously been exposed to a low level of parasitic challenge develop an effective immunity.

The lungworm, *Dictyocaulus*, is a much more dangerous parasite which causes husk or hoose, a severe, incapacitating parasitic pneumonia. Affected animals have difficulty in breathing, develop a characteristic deep, husking cough and lose condition extremely fast. The most elegant way to control husk is to vaccinate the calves with two oral doses of irradiated (and thus attenuated) larvae before turnout. It is, however, often cheaper to control the condition with appropriate anthelmintics.

4.11 Routine Procedures

This section describes routine procedures in husbandry and preventive medicine common to most beef farms. The skills that enable the stockperson or veterinary surgeon to carry out painful procedures like castration and de-horning with speed, safety and humanity are not to be learnt solely from textbooks but by direct, practical instruction from trained operators.

4.11.1 Castration

Castration is performed on calves because it reduces management problems associated with aggressive and sexual behaviour. The production of beef from castrated male cattle is still preferred in Ireland, and in numerous other countries such as the UK, USA, Australia and New Zealand. Castration is a husbandry procedure, which can cause pain and discomfort and if done incorrectly may result in subsequent health problems.

The legal requirement for the use of anaesthesia for castration in cattle varies considerably between different countries depending on the method involved and the age of animals. In Ireland, use of anaesthesia is required for surgical/Burdizzo castration of cattle over 6 months of age. In contrast, castration of calves without use of anaesthesia must be done before they reach 2 months of age in the UK. In Ireland and the UK, rubber ring castration (or use of other devices for constricting the flow of blood to the scrotum) without use of anaesthesia can only be performed in calves less than 7 days of age. In New Zealand, cattle over 9 months of age must be castrated using an effective anaesthetic. In Germany, castration of cattle without use of anaesthesia is allowed only in animals less than 4 weeks of age. By contrast, there is no legal requirement for the use of anaesthesia for castration in the USA. In all of the countries mentioned above, where the administration of anaesthesia is required for castration, the procedure must be done either by a veterinarian or under veterinary supervision. This is a technicality based on the fact that anaesthesia constitutes an act of veterinary surgery. So far as the welfare of the calf is concerned, anaesthesia would bring relief from pain at any age.

4.11.1.1 Castration methods

Burdizzo castration is based on the principle that crushing destroys the spermatic cord carrying blood to the testicles, leaving the skin of the scrotum intact. A Burdizzo emasculatome (or clamp) is used to crush the spermatic cord, but blood supply to the scrotum is preserved. Each spermatic cord is crushed twice (second crush below the first) for 10 seconds each along the neck of the scrotum with the Burdizzo clamp to ensure completeness of the castration procedure. With this technique, the testicle is left to atrophy in the scrotum, and because of the lack of an open wound the potential for haemorrhage or infection is minimized.

Banding castration involves use of a specially designed elastic band with the aid of an applicator around the neck of the scrotum, proximal to the testicles. This will cause ischaemic necrosis of the testicles, eventually leading to testicular atrophy and sloughing of the scrotum.

Surgical castration techniques for male cattle involve opening the scrotum with a scalpel or sharp castration knife, to expose the testicles. Traction is then applied manually to the exposed testes and spermatic vasculature to allow complete removal of the testicles. Manual traction usually provides adequate haemostasis for small calves. However, the use of an emasculator in place for 30 seconds that crushes and cuts the spermatic vessels is recommended for all ages to improve haemostasis. Proper surgical hygiene must be observed during the castration procedure to avoid any unnecessary cross-contamination, infections or sepsis. Concurrent clostridial immunization is recommended.

Everybody who rears male calves for beef should ask himself the question 'Is castration necessary?' If the cattle can reach slaughter weight in 18 months or less, the answer is almost certainly no. Entire male cattle grow lean tissue faster than steers or heifers, and the population advantages of bulls have increased in importance since the ban on the use of anabolic steroids as growth promoters for beef cattle.

4.11.2 Disbudding

The most common method of disbudding is to remove the horn bud under local anaesthetic using a hot iron when the calf is at least 3 weeks old and the horn tip can be clearly felt. An alternative approach is to destroy the horn tip with hot air. Both techniques should only be attempted after personal instruction from a competent operator.

Disbudding of calves should be carried out within 3 weeks of birth. Animals should be administered a local anaesthetic in order to minimize pain and stress responses.

4.11.3 Emergency slaughter

The most humane procedure for slaughtering casualty cattle is for either a veterinary surgeon or a licensed slaughterperson to kill the animal on the spot using an approved procedure such as shooting it with a captive bolt and then cutting the throat. If, however, the animal can be transported to an abattoir, it is more likely to be killed and butchered in such a way as to render the meat fit for human consumption. Within the EU the welfare of the animal is now largely covered by the EU Council Regulation (EC) No. 1 of 2005. On 5 January 2007 new EU rule (Council Regulation (EC) 1 of 2005 on the protection of animals during transport and related operations) on the protection of animals during transport came into operation. The Council Regulation has been given legal effect in Ireland by the European Communities (Animal Transport and Control Post) Regulations 2006 (S.I. No. 675 of 2006). (For UK legislation see DEFRA, 2009b.) The general rule is that unfit animals may only be transported if the intended journey is not likely to cause them unnecessary additional suffering.

Sick or injured animals may be considered fit for transport if they are:

- slightly injured or ill, and transport would not cause additional suffering; in cases of doubt, veterinary advice shall be sought;
- transported under veterinary supervision for or following veterinary treatment or diagnosis. However, such transport shall be permitted only where no unnecessary suffering or ill treatment is caused to the animals concerned.

(For a complete list see Annex 1, Chapter 1 of Council Regulation (EC) No 1/2005.)

Transport of weak, sick or injured cattle to a slaughterhouse will clearly cause unnecessary suffering if the animal is in severe pain which is exacerbated by movement; a broken leg is an obvious example. A calf that is too weak to move could reasonably be transported to a slaughterhouse if it is carefully carried on to (and off) the lorry. The larger animal, such as the downer cow that collapses and develops paralysis post-calving, presents a more difficult problem. She may be reasonably comfortable where she lies and equally so if on deep bedding in a lorry. Any procedure that involved dragging the live recumbent cow over the ground to enter and exit the lorry would constitute unnecessary suffering and the owner should arrange for the animal to be killed on the spot. The whole issue of the moving of casualty animals is complex. For advice see the *Fitness to travel: guidance note* (DEFRA, 2009b) and EU Council Regulation (EC) No. 1 of 2005. The method of disposal of carcasses should be in accordance with the requirements for the disposal of waste as laid down in Council Regulation 2002/1774/EC (as applicable) (see Annex 1, chapter 21, Disposal of carcasses).

4.12 Calf Health and Welfare

The objective of a well-designed herd health programme is to address multiple areas of management in order to reduce the likelihood of disease outbreaks occurring in calves and adult animals and is a necessary step if economic returns are to be realized. The aim of successful calf rearing is to produce a healthy calf which is capable of optimum performance throughout its life from birth through to finishing. A suitable calf-rearing system has the following characteristics:

- good animal performance with minimal disease and morbidity and optimal growth rates;
- low cost input;
- low labour input.

The survival of the calf involves all of those factors, plus a suitable post-birth environment, management and nutrition.

4.12.1 Colostrum

The first and most important feed given a newborn dairy calf is colostrum. Maternal colostrum provides the main source of immunoglobulins for the newborn calf. Immunoglobulins help to maintain the animal's health and reduce mortality rates by helping to eliminate foreign agents in the body such as bacteria and viruses. In the bovine species, immunoglobulins do not cross the placenta in utero, and the newborn calf is, therefore, dependent on antibodies obtained through ingestion of colostrum. The two main classes of immunoglobulin are IgG class (approximately 80%) and IgA (8–10%). IgG protective antibodies operate within the general circulation; IgA provides protection at mucosal surfaces, especially the gut wall. It is of vital importance that all calves are fed two litres of colostrum within one hour of birth and receive a second 2 litre feed 4 to 6 hours later to ensure that sufficient IgG is absorbed across the gut wall.

Colostrum feeding should continue as long as possible after birth. While immunoglobulins are not absorbed after 24 hours they continue to provide local protection in the intestinal tract. The timing of colostrum feeding is important due to the loss of absorptive sites in the intestine over the first 24 hours and competition from bacteria in the intestine. Calves that receive inadequate colostrum are more susceptible to neonatal infections. This problem can be particularly severe in calves that that have been moved off their farm of origin and through markets. In these circumstances, there is greater risk of exposure to infection. Circulating IgG levels may be lower due to inadequate colostrum feeding on the farm of origin and less effective when challenged by pathogens from a different source.

4.12.2 Calf mortality

Calf mortality can best be subdivided into four main categories:

- abortions (foetal loss at less than or equal to 270 days' gestation);
- perinatal mortality (foetal loss at greater than 270 days' gestation and mortality during the first 24 hours of life);
- neonatal mortality (death between 24 hours and 28 days);
- older calf mortality (death between 29 and 84 days).

Morbidity and mortality of the young calf represent a major cause of economic concern for beef producers. Septicaemia and enteric disorders caused by strains of *E. coli*, Rotavirus, *Neospora*, Coronavirus, *Cryptosporidium* or by *Salmonella* species are the main cause of neonatal mortality. Older calf mortality is mainly dominated by respiratory infections and salmonellosis.

Disease is not a simple matter of exposure of a susceptible animal to an infectious agent such as a bacterium, virus or fungus. Calves are exposed to infectious organisms from the moment of birth, and natural defence mechanisms usually prevent the establishment of disease. Animals develop disease because of a complex relationship between the host (animal), the infectious agent and the environment. Control of the agent is largely based on prevention of exposure, immunity and chemotherapeutic agents (drugs). Diagnosis and correction of health problems usually involves clinical, immunological, haematological and therapeutic approaches.

In recent years there has been major emphasis on reducing the reliance on antibiotics in animal production, which demands nutritional management procedures aimed at elevating passive immunity in calves.

4.12.3 Calf diarrhoea

Outbreaks of diarrhoea in calves are associated with the interaction of potentially pathogenic enteric micro-organisms with the calf's immunity, nutritional state and environment. An outbreak may be triggered by a single infectious agent but is mainly due to mixed infections. The most common organisms involved are *E. coli*, *Salmonella* species, Rotavirus, Coronavirus and *Cryptosporidium*. Dehydration, acidosis, impaired growth rate or death are the major consequences. A number of preventive measures have been adopted to control calf diarrhoea. Control of *E. coli* infection may be achieved by hyperimmunization of the dam with an *E. coli* antigen, thereby providing passive immunity to the calf (via ingested colostrum) during the first 2 to 3 weeks of life, before it can produce its own antibodies.

4.12.3.1 Salmonellosis

Salmonellosis in calves is mainly caused by the organisms *Salmonella dublin* or *S. typhimurium*. *S. typhimurium* DT104 is highly pathogenic to calves, resulting in a high incidence of mortality. Furthermore, it has a wide range of antibiotic resistance and is capable of rapidly developing new resistance patterns. It is also an important cause of human food poisoning. In acute cases of calf salmonellosis, a septicaemia may occur, accompanied by blood-stained diarrhoea. Calves that are affected more severely have an elevated body temperature (greater than 40°C), are debilitated and have reduced feed intake. The calf may become infected as early as the second day of life, with highest incidences occurring at 1 to 5 weeks of age. Outbreaks of *S. typhimurium* are usually associated with purchased calves. Salmonellosis superimposed on calves with pre-existing pneumonia leads to an exacerbation of clinical signs and pulmonary damage. Thus, purchased calves should be carefully examined on arrival so that any infection may be quickly diagnosed. Prevention is again highly dependent on ensuring that the calf receives adequate colostrum after birth.

4.12.4 Respiratory disease

The underlying cause of bovine respiratory disease (BRD) is extremely complex, with the involvement of viruses, bacteria and *Mycoplasma*. The incidence of infection (morbidity) is usually high, but the mortality rate is variable. Viruses that have been predominantly isolated from outbreaks of calf pneumonia are infective bovine rhinotracheitis (IBR), respiratory syncytial virus (RSV), parainfluenza-3 virus (PI-3 virus) and bovine virus diarrhoea–mucosal disease (BVD-MD virus). Predisposing factors are those that affect the magnitude of the infectious challenge (e.g. over-stocking, poor hygiene, inadequate ventilation) and those which affect immuno-competence (ability to fight infection). These include stress, draughts and fluctuating temperatures, poor nutrition and/or concurrent disease. In most cases it would appear that the primary infective agent is viral, producing respiratory tract damage that is subsequently extended by *Mycoplasma* and secondary bacterial infections. Viruses are unaffected by antibiotics; however, antibiotic treatment is usually administered to treat secondary bacterial infections. *Mycoplasma* species are resistant to antibiotics which act on the cell wall, and an antibiotic specific to the cell nucleus is required to inactivate it. In order to direct the appropriate treatment strategy, nasal swabs should be submitted to the appropriate regional veterinary laboratory for accurate identification of the pathogen(s) involved. In addition, *Mycoplasma* species are known to suppress the calf's immunity to disease. Of these, *M. bovis* is the most pathogenic and can act in unison with *Pasteurella* species to produce a very severe form of pneumonia. Following suppression of immunity the animal's ability to withstand an attack from *Pasteurella* and other organisms is reduced. *P. haemolytica* is an important secondary agent in respiratory disease. Pathological changes occur in the lung tissue, leading to consolidation and respiratory distress. Negative consequences for the welfare of animals that survive a respiratory disease attack are that they may end up as 'respiratory cripples' with permanent lung damage.

Bovine respiratory disease, which can terminate fatally, affects both the dairy and beef industry and is the most important disease affecting calves in terms of animal welfare and agricultural economics. In an Irish survey in a slatted unit containing 6,399 beef cattle, over a 6-month period respiratory disease was the most frequently recorded cause of morbidity and mortality and this observation is in agreement with reports from large feedlots in the USA.

Outbreaks of respiratory disease occur throughout the year but are particularly common in late autumn and early winter when young animals are brought indoors. Disease occurrence is most common in herds of 2–6-month-old animals; in severe outbreaks the majority of calves in a herd are affected. Environmental factors and adverse animal management practices can also predispose animals to disease. Environmental factors include draughts, inadequate ventilation and poor air hygiene which facilitate the spread of infectious agents within the herd. The importance of sound animal management cannot be overlooked and factors such as adequate colostrum intake in early life, prevention of co-mingling of different age groups and avoidance of stressful procedures (e.g. weaning, castration, de-horning) during high-risk periods for disease cannot be overemphasized.

Numerous vaccines provide a range of combinations of live and/or killed antigens, active against IBR, RSV and PI-3 virus, *Pasteurella* spp. and *Haemophilus somnus*. Intramuscular modified-live virus vaccines quickly induce long-lasting immunity. Intranasal modified-live virus vaccines induce immunity at the mucosal surface. However, response to these vaccines is only evident in calves over 1 month of age when their own immune system is active. It is difficult to successfully vaccinate young calves against these diseases because protective colostral antibodies block the vaccine, resulting in maternal antibody interference with vaccination. Development of vaccines effective against the *Pasteurella* organisms and other bacteria that cause pneumonia has been difficult, and success cannot be guaranteed.

4.12.4.1 Prevention of pneumonia in calves
The following are important factors in prevention of pneumonia.

- Many vaccines provide a variety of combinations of live and/or killed antigens. However, experience indicates that responses to these vaccines were only evident in calves >2 months of age, when their own immune system was active.
- Good housing, good nutrition (including mineral and vitamin supplements) and good management, while not preventing an outbreak of respiratory disease

in calves, undoubtedly minimize the long-term negative effect of the disease. They allow a more rapid recovery, thereby preventing the development of chronic cases.

- Rear calves in groups of similar age in well-ventilated draught-free buildings.
- Work in close association with the veterinary surgeon. Collection of nasal mucus samples or swabs for laboratory diagnosis will direct the administration of the appropriate antibiotic treatment.
- Regular temperature checking is useful to guide both diagnosis and observation of treatment effect.
- Minimize exposure of the calf to the infectious agent. This may be achieved through the use of closed herds, screened replacements and positive herd immunity.
- Oral rehydration is particularly beneficial under practical conditions, as loss of body fluid is often associated with pneumonia.
- Vaccination may help to attain optimum livestock productivity through disease prevention. However, vaccination is effective only against specific organisms.
- Note the overall role of pre- and postnatal nutrition, including trace elements and vitamin supply.
- In those herds that are known to have trace element deficiencies, or to have a high tetany risk, young calves may need supplementary magnesium and trace elements for optimal health and immune status.

4.13 Handling, Transport and Slaughter

4.13.1 Handling
Although cattle are a domesticated species, the handling of cattle by humans can result in increased stress, agitated behaviour and even injury or death, especially if the animals are not used to being handled, or are handled in an inappropriate manner. The following recommendations are designed to ensure good welfare during the handling and movement of cattle.

- Animals should be treated and handled in a manner which avoids injury and stress. Goads or electric prodders should not be used.
- The movement of animals from one paddock to another, or to penning facilities, should be done without recourse to excessive force. Beating the animals, or the presence of an untrained aggressive dog which causes the animals to panic, is not acceptable.
- At the time of movement, check for any abnormal behaviour, lameness, reluctance to move or isolation from the remainder of herd.
- Cattle need to see where they are expected to move to, i.e. if going indoors or into a truck make sure that lights are on and corridors are clear.

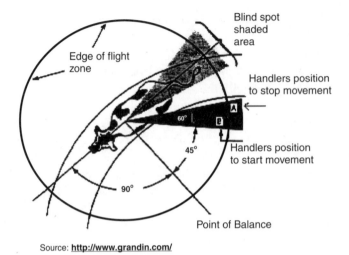

Source: http://www.grandin.com/

Figure 4.5 The flight zone. Source: Grandin, 2007. Reproduced with permission from Professor Temple Grandin.

Grandin (2007) has pioneered the design and management of high-welfare handling systems for cattle. One essential feature of these is proper attention to the principle of the flight zone (Figure 4.5). The flight zone is described as the area around an animal, which if penetrated by the handler, will be re-established by the animal by moving away. Flight zones can vary widely depending on whether an animal has been raised in extensive or confined conditions and its level of tameness or wildness. To avoid undue agitation of the animal, the handler should work at the edge of the flight zone. If the handler penetrates the flight zone too deeply, the animal may try to run back past the handler, or if it is in a race, rear up and attempt to escape (Grandin, 1992).

4.13.2 Transport

The transport of livestock can have major implications for their welfare, and there is strong public interest and scientific endeavour aimed at ensuring that the welfare of transported animals is optimal. Physical factors such as noise or vibrations; psychological/emotional factors, such as unfamiliar environment or social regrouping; and climatic factors, such as temperature and humidity, are also involved in the transport process. Alterations in immune function resulting from transport stress are particularly relevant to younger animals, and illness in young cattle following road haulage is not uncommon. The handling and marketing of animals prior to the journey to the abattoir must not involve extended periods of feed withdrawal as, in addition to the welfare consequences, this will result in bodyweight loss and reduction in meat quality. Feed withdrawal will also increase the impact on animal welfare, through hunger and metabolic stress.

While it is well established that transportation of cattle is a stressor that causes a quantifiable response measured, for example, by a significant increase in blood cortisol, stress during transport resulting in physiological or pathological changes can be reduced with good management practices.

The age of the cattle transported can have a great effect as instances of morbidity and mortality are greater in transported calves younger than 3 weeks of age, which may be compounded by the stress incurred by simultaneous weaning.

One of the most prevalent examples of transport stress is 'shipping fever' in transported cattle. The disease may have first appeared as early as the late 1800s to early 1900s when cattle were first transported by railroad. The aetiology of shipping fever is complex. However, the simple definition, 'the occurrence of pulmonary infections during or after transit,' is accurate enough.

4.13.3 Stunning and slaughter

The purpose of stunning an animal before slaughter is to render it unconscious and hence insensible to pain, before death occurs due to exsanguination. Conventionally, cattle have been stunned mechanically, such as by captive bolt, although there is some commercial use of electrical stunning, e.g. in New Zealand and the UK.

The captive bolt, when used correctly, has been shown to be an extremely effective method of stunning. Halal (Islamic) or Shechita (Jewish) ritual slaughter often involves the throat-cutting of cattle which have not been stunned. Since 1995 animal welfare legislation around slaughter has been covered by Council Directive 93/119/EEC covering a wide range of animals and slaughter circumstances. The European Commission has revised the legislation to reflect new knowledge and advanced scientific evidence and the new Regulation (Council Regulation 1099/2009) was published in 2010. Information on humane killing and slaughter methods, together with the relevant legislation, is provided by the Humane Slaughter Association (www.hsa.org.uk).

Methods of restraint causing avoidable suffering must not be used in conscious animals because they cause severe pain and stress:

- Suspending or hoisting animals (other than poultry) by the feet or legs;
- Indiscriminate and inappropriate use of stunning equipment;
- Mechanical clamping of the legs or feet of the animals (other than shackles used in poultry and ostriches) as the sole method of restraint;
- Breaking legs, cutting leg tendons, or blinding an animal to immobilize them; severing the spinal cord;
- The dragging of disabled animals and other animals unable to move while conscious is prohibited; stunned animals may, however, be dragged.
- Conscious animals should not be dragged, dropped or thrown (OIE, 2008, Animal welfare code http://www.oie.int).

References and Further Reading

Allen, D. (1990) *Planned Beef Production and Marketing.* Blackwell Scientific Publications, Oxford.

DAFF (2004) *Expenditure review of beef carcase classification scheme.* Department of Agriculture, Fisheries and Food, Dublin, Ireland.

DEFRA (2003) *Codes of Recommendations for the Welfare of Livestock: Cattle.* Department for Environment, Food and Rural Affairs, London. Available at: http://www.defra.gov.uk

DEFRA (2009a) *On farm animal welfare legislation.* Department for Environment, Food and Rural Affairs, London. Available at: http://www.defra.gov.uk

DEFRA (2009b) *Fitness to travel: guidance note.* Department for Environment, Food and Rural Affairs, London. Available at: http://www.defra.gov.uk

Dodd, V.A. (1985) Housing for a beef unit. *Veterinary Update,* April, 6–13.

Drennan, M.J.and McGee, M. (2004) Effect of suckler cow genotype and nutrition level during the winter on voluntary intake and performance and on the growth and slaughter characteristics of their progeny. Irish Journal of Agricultural and Food Research **43**, 185–99.

Drennan, M.J. and McGee, M. (2009) *Producing high quality carcasses from grass-based suckler beef systems.* Occasional report, Teagasc.

Earley, B., McGee, M. and Fallon, R.J. (2000) Serum immunoglobulin concentrations in suckled calves and dairy-herd calves. Irish Journal of Agriculture and Food Research **39** (3), 401–7.

Farm Animal Welfare Council (1986) *Report on the Welfare of Livestock at Markets.* RB 265. HMSO, London.

Grandin, T. (1980) Observations of cattle behavior applied to the design of cattle handling facilities. Applied Animal Ethology 6, 19.

Grandin, T. (1992) Handling and transport of agricultural animals used in research. In *The Well-being of Agricultural Animals in Biomedical and Agricultural Research*, Mench, J.A., Mayer, S.J. and Krulisch, L. (Eds.), p. 74. Scientists Center for Animal Welfare, Greenbelt, MD.

Grandin, T. (ed.) (2007) *Livestock Handling and Transport*, 3rd edn. CABI Publishing, Wallingford.

Humane Slaughter Association (2000) *Electrical stunning of red met animals.* Available at: http://www.hsa.org.uk

Humane Slaughter Association (2001) *Captive bolt stunning of livestock.* Available at: http://www.hsa.org.uk

Humane Slaughter Association (2004) *Emergency killing* (video). Available at: http://www.hsa.org.uk

Keane, M.G. (1999) Comparison of carcass grades of steers in the Republic of Ireland, Northern Ireland and Great Britain. Farm and Food 9, 6–9.

Keane, M.G., O'Riordan, E.G. and O'Kiely, P. (2009) Dairy calf-to-beef production systems, Teagasc, Report.

Ministry of Agriculture, Fisheries and Food (1983) *Codes of Recommendations for the Welfare of Livestock: Cattle.* MAFF Publications, London.

Ministry of Agriculture, Fisheries and Food (1984a) *Energy Allowances and Feeding Systems for Ruminants*, RB 433. HMSO, London.

Ministry of Agriculture, Fisheries and Food (1984b) *Cattle Handling*, B 2495. HMSO, London.

Ministry of Agriculture, Fisheries and Food (1986) *Annual Reviews of Agriculture*. HMSO, London.

Ministry of Agriculture, Fisheries and Food (1995a) *Agriculture in the United Kingdom 1994*. HMSO, London.

Ministry of Agriculture, Fisheries and Food (1995b) *Summary of the Law Relating to Farm Animal Welfare* (reprinted 1998) PB 2531. MAFF Publications, London.

Meat and Livestock Commission (1994) *Beef Yearbook*. MLC, Milton Keynes, UK.

Molony, A.P. (1999) *R & H Hall Technical Bulletin* Issue No. 4.

Montano-Bermudez, M., Nielsen, M.K. and Deutscher, G.H. (1990) Energy requirements for maintenance of crossbred cattle with different genetic potential for milk. *Journal of Animal Science* 68, 2279–88.

More O'Ferrall, G.J. (ed.) (1982) *Beef Production from Different Dairy Breeds and Dairy Crosses*. Martinus Nijhoff, The Hague.

Murphy, B.M., Drennan, M.J., O'Mara, F.P. and McGee, M. (2008) Performance and feed intake of five beef suckler cow genotypes and pre-weaning growth of their progeny. Irish Journal of Agricultural and Food Research 47, 13–25.

Petit, M. and Lienard, G. (1988) Performance characteristics and efficiencies of various types of beef cows in French production systems. *Proceedings of 3rd World Congress on Sheep and Beef Cattle Breeding*, 19–25 June 1988, INRA, Paris, 2, 25–51.

Sarzeaud, P., Becherel, F. and Perot, C. (2008) A classification of European beef farming systems, EAAP Technical series No. 9. in EU beef farming systems and CAP regulations 2008, pp. 23–31.

SCAHAW (2001) The welfare of cattle kept for beef production. Publication of the European Commission, Health and Consumer Protection Directorate-General by the Scientific Committee on Animal Health and Animal Welfare (SCAHAW) SANCO.C.2/AH/R22/2000. Adopted 25 April 2001. Available at: http://europa.eu.int/comm/food/fs/sc/scah/out54_en.pdf (accessed 20 December 2003).

Webster, A.J.F. (1985) *Calf Husbandry, Health and Welfare*, 2nd edn. Collins, London.

Webster, A.J.F. (1995) *Animal Welfare: a Cool Eye Towards Eden*. Blackwell Scientific Publications, Oxford.

Webster, A.J.F., Saville, C. and Welchman, D.B. (1986) *Alternative Husbandry Systems for Veal Calves*. University of Bristol Press, Bristol.

Williamson, M (1998) Straw in Europe. Chalcombe Publications, ISBN 0 Q48617411.

Sheep

5

PETE GODDARD

Key Concepts

Management and Welfare of Farm Animals: The UFAW Farm Handbook, 5th edition. John Webster
© 2011 by Universities Federation for Animal Welfare (UFAW)

5.1 Introduction

Since the previous edition of this book was published there has been a significant shift in the public view of how we treat farmed livestock and assess their welfare. With much more emphasis being placed on quality of life aspects there is a pressing need and responsibility to critically examine how diligent livestock management can deliver the greatest welfare benefit to sheep. By using a framework provided by the five freedoms and the increased use of proactive farm health plans and risk avoidance strategies, there is the opportunity to consider management actions (or inactions) from the individual sheep's perspective. Production requirements or environmental constraints create welfare challenges which the stockperson must work hard to address. Welfare challenges include lameness, perinatal lamb loss, undernutrition, internal and external parasitism (and the development of anthelmintic resistance) and the impact of management practices – castration, tail docking, transport and slaughter. The impact of these can be minimized or eliminated through knowledge-able shepherding and veterinary advice. This chapter builds on that in previous editions, for which I am greatly indebted to the work of Huw Williams, my teacher and later colleague at the Royal Veterinary College. The chapter provides informa-tion about many common sheep management systems and practices, and emphasizes those human actions which have the greatest potential to affect sheep welfare and how the success of these actions can be evaluated.

Methods to assess welfare and to evaluate how well a producer is achieving welfare goals are poorly developed in the sheep sector. The fact that the public already believes sheep systems to have an inherently high level of welfare (due primarily to the high degree of naturalness and lack of intensification) may have resulted in less focus on this sector. Consequently there is less consumer pressure to encourage sheep producers to adopt higher standards through the sale of welfare-premium products, for example through commitments to tackle issues such as lameness.

5.2 The Sheep Industry Worldwide

5.2.1 Development and structure of the industry

There are probably well over a billion sheep worldwide, living in widely different environments and managed in diverse ways, from nomadic subsistence systems to the intensive lowland production of fat lambs. In a number of countries, sheep (and other livestock) represent a family's financial reserve or bank, being sold in times of need but otherwise representing the family's status. This can lead to the number of head being more important than their condition. In many subsistence systems, knowing when to sell or slaughter livestock in the face of feed or water shortage is key to sustainability or even survival. In some harsh environments sheep are well suited to exploit the conditions. While Australia and New Zealand are dominant in many aspects of sheep production, the number of sheep in New Zealand is currently declining and China has the largest sheep population (almost 150 million in 2003). In many countries, sheep play an important part in the rural economy – particularly Iran, India, Sudan and the UK. A number of other African and Asian countries also have significant sheep populations and some South American countries (e.g. Brazil) are becoming more involved in sheep production. Ruminant numbers are increasing to provide protein for the world's rapidly growing human population, though within this general picture, the trend in sheep numbers is variable and in some countries the number is declining in favour of cattle. As a result of increasing ruminant numbers, there are concerns about rangeland degradation; many rangelands are already under severe pressure, a critical concern in countries where livestock production is paramount. A vicious cycle can ensue if carrying capacity is exceeded and overall animal production declines. In such areas, innovative management systems can provide solutions; greater use of crop residues/green by-products (e.g. rice straw) and mixed ruminant animal/plantation enterprises has been shown to be very effective at a local level. Climate change impacts will also play a part in the suitability or otherwise of areas for ruminant production; drought conditions have been a factor in the recent decline in sheep numbers in New Zealand, for example. Changes to government subsidy in a number of countries and, at a European level, the ongoing review of the Common Agricultural Policy (CAP) all have the potential to impact on the profitability of sheep production.

Sheep are amongst the earliest domesticated ruminants, probably arising from the mouflon around 11,000 years ago in the region around Iran and Iraq. Sheep produce a range of commodities useful to humans including meat, milk, fleece and hides, and can act as a bank or reserve to be realized through sale or slaughter. The relative importance of these features varies with the breed and system of management (Table 5.1). There are around 800 breeds (about 70 of these are found in the UK), each generally well-fitted to their environment and management conditions. These management conditions range from those which can deliver individual animal care, to large extensively managed or ranched flocks. Under these latter conditions, sheep may simply be gathered periodically to allow selection of animals for slaughter or release back for breeding. It is essential that sheep are well fitted to their environment and possess suitable fitness traits. However, within such systems there is considerable opportunity for poor welfare to arise; as animals are inspected only infrequently,

Table 5.1 Examples of sheep breeds and their main uses.

Type of sheep	Primary use	Example types
Hill/upland	Producing store lambs for finishing, replacements and draft ewes	Scottish Blackface, Swaledale, Welsh Mountain
Fat-tailed breeds (found mostly in arid regions)	Milk (pelts from Karakul lambs used for traditional fur coats)	Awassi, Karakul
Fine-wool	Wool	Merino types, Rambouillet
Mutton	Meat	Suffolk, Down breeds, Border Leicester
Dual purpose	Meat & wool	Polworth, Corriedale
Milking	Milk production	British Milksheep, East Friesian, Lacaune
Hair sheep	Meat	Soay, Persian, Peliquey

injury and disease will go undetected. Key management decisions in these systems relate to selection of the correct breed and breeding of individuals with desirable characteristics: good mothering abilities, resistance to parasitic disease and lameness, and a low incidence of lambing difficulty.

While there is a worldwide trade in sheep products, the movement of live animals for slaughter has declined over recent years as a result of good chilling and freezing technologies which preserve meat in excellent condition, and through public concern over live exports of stock for slaughter. Biosecurity requirements now often restrict the movement of genetic material to semen and embryos rather than live animals.

5.2.2 The situation in the United Kingdom

Sheep production in the UK, while embracing many recent technical advances, is still largely governed by the geographical conditions where production takes place. Sheep can be found in areas ranging from lowland pastoral and arable areas which can be readily cultivated, and where different enterprises can outcompete sheep, to upland and hill areas where conditions are potentially much more severe, with a predominately unimproved rough grazing. In these latter areas, which account for around one-third of the available agricultural land in the UK, there are few other options for converting the available biomass into food owing to the severity of the climate, difficulty of terrain and low soil fertility. Over the course of centuries, a number of sheep breeds have been developed to maximize the potential of the environment and nutritional resources available. (For an excellent brief description and picture of UK breeds, visit the National Sheep Association (NSA) website.) This is coupled with the development of integrated management systems to allow movement of sheep when natural resources become scarce. In addition to producers of meat and wool, sheep are agents for managing the countryside in hill and upland areas. Support payments have undergone a significant change from a headage-based system to one which provides incentive to maintain good environmental conditions.

There are around 18 million breeding ewes in the UK but numbers fluctuate depending on market forces. This number more than doubles in the summer if lambs are included. Flock sizes vary widely from small hobby farmers with tens of ewes to large commercial flocks with over 1,000 ewes. Recent changes to the agricultural subsidy arrangements and other pressures have resulted in a considerable reduction in the hill sheep flock in the UK.

The principal output of the UK sheep industry is prime lamb – the top-quality finished meat product – and also mutton from older animals. Prime lamb is produced from the offspring of terminal sires and pure-bred or crossbred ewes. Lamb meat production rose as the national flock increased in the 1980s but today the UK produces around 85% of its sheep meat requirements – approximately 300,000 tonnes. Other than in a small number of specialist flocks, wool accounts for virtually no income for the sheep farm; shearing costs are often not covered and wool removal is considered primarily as a welfare action. A small number of sheep are involved in milk production, something which is much more commonly seen in continental Europe and Asia, and a number of hides are processed.

In the UK, sheep production falls into two main categories: hill and upland systems, and lowland systems. These are dependent on each other but the distinction capitalizes on different environmental resources and the capabilities of different breeds and their crosses (Figure 5.1). This results in a stratified breeding and production system across the UK.

5.2.2.1 Hill and upland production

About half the national flock is found in hill and upland areas where ewes represent the main reservoir of the breeding stock. A primary output of this system is the crossbred ewe which goes on to form around 80% of the lowland breeding stock. Other animals sold include older pure-bred ewes which are unable to sustain further lamb production in the harsh upland environment (usually after three crops of lambs), ewe lambs (to be retained for breeding in the hill and upland system) and male lambs (usually castrated – called wether lambs) as store animals for fattening (finishing) with preferential feeding. The process of movement down the hill of these older ewes is referred to as 'drafting'. Hill ewes require characteristics of hardiness and good mothering ability and are generally more 'self sufficient' than lowland breeds. Lambing rates can be as low as 80%, i.e. 80 lambs born per 100 ewes. 'Easy care' breeds of sheep are being developed which combine these characteristics with health traits (e.g. resistance to foot rot and parasitism) and, possibly, a fleece which naturally sheds in the summer. In these systems we may find as few as one sheep per hectare overall, yet often there will be some improved grazing, usually close to the farm buildings ('in-bye') where stock can benefit from preferential nutrition at key times of the production cycle, e.g. at lambing; the extent of this may determine the carrying capacity of the enterprise. These areas may also allow conservation crops such as silage or hay to be made. Some upland farms, which have a more favourable environment for sheep, take the draft ewes from hill farms and cross them with a longwool breed. The resultant female lambs move to lowground farms to cross with terminal sires, and some males may go directly for slaughter from the farm. Lambing rates of upland farms may reach 125%. These farms also make better use of a two-pasture system whereby there is a relatively small area of improved pasture and a relatively large area of unimproved hill integrated into a complete management approach. The improved pasture can be utilized primarily during lactation and lamb growth. If a rest period can occur from mid-August (when grass can regrow) the area can be used again to provide a flush of improved nutrition during the pre-mating and mating periods.

5.2.2.2 Lowland production

The crossbred ewes from the above system move to lower ground and are bred to terminal sires of meat breeds to produce lambs with excellent carcass characteristics

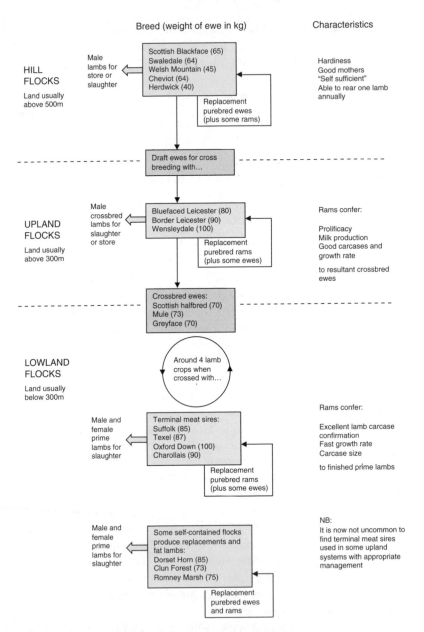

Figure 5.1 The stratified arrangement of the UK sheep industry.

for the prime lamb market. Compared to hill breeds, crossbred ewes have traits of increased body and litter size and the ability to produce sufficient milk for twin lambs – lambing at typically upwards of 160%. The potential for the crossing of a large number of breeds allows the industry to respond rapidly to changes in market demand. Stocking densities are much greater (around 12 ewes per hectare) and there is considerable scope for active pasture management.

5.3 Selection and Improvement

Traditional sheep markets and agricultural shows are places where breeders of livestock proudly displayed their best animals, yet superficial phenotypic characteristics are not necessarily correlated with important market or health requirements, e.g. for ewes to experience trouble-free parturition. Even the experienced stockperson's eye, while able to ensure animals remain of a particular type, is less able to evaluate the genetic potential of breeding stock. However, standardized classification methods, for example for overall fatness and conformation of crossbred animals, can have a place in pure-bred selection programmes. Much sheep breeding in the world has no coordinated improvement strategy but in a number of countries genetic improvement programmes identify animals with advantageous characteristics and disseminate this genetic superiority. As yet the use of genetic improvement in the sheep sector has not been fully exploited. The earliest examples related primarily to production traits and the recent focus has included health issues such as parasite tolerance/resistance and resistance to foot rot. With a move to more easy-care systems of sheep production, maternal traits and lamb survival are also key selection criteria. Some traits can be evaluated in contemporary comparison trials (either within- or between-flock comparisons) as part of a sire reference scheme which requires recording of a range of criteria to indicate the genetic merit/ superiority or breeding value of stock. In systems where feeding and disease are managed to a high standard, improved breeds can exploit these conditions. Recently, molecular techniques for the identification of specific proteins, genome sequencing or quantitative trait loci (QTL) are available to identify animals of high genetic merit. There are also known gene-specific characteristics (e.g. Boorroola sheep with increased fecundity, and greater muscle mass in Texel sheep). Accurate measurement of certain carcass characteristics *in vivo* has been achieved using ultrasound scanning of muscle and fat depth at key sites. The use of computed tomography (CT) carcass analysis has allowed an even greater precision and the resultant identification of the most superior meat sires and so more rapid genetic progress can be made. Video image analysis systems are being developed to objectively evaluate carcasses. Computer programmes are able to integrate a range of relevant material to generate multitrait selection indices for superior sires, related to the emphasis placed on the component traits – such as carcass weight, growth rate and maternal traits. Often, best linear unbiased prediction (BLUP) software is used to separate genetic and environmental effects on performance to generate estimated breeding values (EBVs) within sire reference schemes and maximize the speed of genetic progress. For example, the Signet Sheepbreeder service in the UK generates benchmark data for terminal sires. Such schemes have the potential to focus increasingly on health and welfare criteria but these aspects have yet to be fully exploited.

5.4 Natural History and Behaviour

The general characteristics of sheep are similar to those of other ruminant animals. In horned breeds, the horns of the males are much larger and often more elaborate than those of the female. An adult male of the most common breeds can weigh from 45 to around 150 kg. Litter size is generally from one to three, with lamb birth weight varying according to maternal size. Sheep can live for between 15 and 20 years. Wild sheep are still found, for example, the Rocky Mountain bighorn sheep (*Ovis canadensis*) and the mouflon (*Ovis orientalis*).

Factors that encouraged the early domestication of sheep included their gregarious, flocking nature, and their size, which made for easy control and individual handling. Sheep were not aggressive towards humans and, as ruminants, did not compete directly for the same food resources. Over the intervening years, animals with desirable behavioural and production traits have been selected (directly or indirectly) to fit animals to particular systems and environments. Early selection will have reflected the developing relationship between the shepherd and the flock in migratory systems, still evidenced in some modern-day practices. Although found in virtually all areas of the world, sheep tend to perform less well under moist, tropical conditions.

5.4.1 Social organization

Sheep in extensive or range systems have the ability to display innate patterns of behaviour. For example, they can develop a special knowledge of a particular hill and become linked or 'hefted' to this home range (or areas within this), with young learning about this from their mothers. This facilitates shepherding and sheep can better cope with adverse weather conditions if they are aware of favourable aspects of the terrain. Basic behavioural traits include strong flight reactions, a following pattern, a very strong bond between a ewe and her lamb(s) and a flocking behaviour, especially in the face of a perceived threat. If isolated, sheep become very agitated and show marked vocalization. Sheep-friendly handling systems should minimize isolation and encourage sheep to move of their own volition. While grazing, sheep will disperse across a given area, with different individuals displaying varying degrees of sociability. From a management perspective, advantageous flock behaviour tends to be lost in very small groups. Under more natural conditions (e.g. as seen in flocks of feral Soay sheep or rangeland flocks of Merino sheep in Australia) mixed groups of animals are found, though adult males tend to associate with the female flock only at breeding time; in managed populations, single sex/age groups predominate.

5.4.2 Inter-sheep behaviour

Sheep flocks display a complex social structure. Sheep have the capacity to recognize and remember a number of other individuals (and humans). Marked instances of aggression are shown between males during the breeding season, when significant injuries can occur. Competition for feed resources can occur in both sexes when limited supplementary feed is available or when sheep are housed, seen as butting or barging behaviour. Mixing groups of sheep does not generally cause difficulty. The strong mother–young bond is the most marked inter-animal behaviour displayed, yet early weaning does not appear to lead to prolonged behavioural effects in lambs. An early and effective ewe–lamb bond is critical in terms of lamb survival, and management practices must not impede its establishment. Moves to establish easy-care sheep flocks rely on the selection of individual ewes which demonstrate (among other qualities) a particularly strong maternal instinct.

Inter-sheep behaviour is determined by a range of sensory cues. Grazing sheep will frequently stop grazing and look around. If isolated, they vocalize to regain neighbour contact. Vocalization patterns between the ewe and her newborn lamb are a significant and specialized aspect of the ewe–lamb bond, with a preponderance of low-pitched bleats.

Sheep alert their immediate neighbours to perceived danger by standing alert and upright or moving off with a stiff-legged gait. If roused in this way, sheep will sometimes congregate at a vantage point which gives them a panoramic view of their surroundings, and turn to face the disturbance. Sheep show little mutually supportive behaviour such as grooming.

5.4.3 Reproductive behaviour

Ewes, in the absence of a ram, show little overt behavioural change when in oestrus. In the presence of a ram, ewes in oestrus sometimes seek out the ram and may show a tail waggling or fanning behaviour before standing to be mounted, though it is usually the ram that does most of the seeking. If the ewe is receptive she may urinate but this cannot be used as a definitive marker. Immediately prior to this, the ram will explore the perineal area of the ewe and display one or more of a number of specific behaviours: often he will raise his head, extend his neck in an exaggerated forward movement, curl his lip and expose his teeth in an extended sniffing action called 'flehmen'. He may also vocalize at this point and paw the ground. Some of these actions may be seen a short distance from the ewe. This pre-mating phase in the ram is generally short. The ram will then mount the ewe from behind and perform one or sometimes a small number of ejaculatory thrusts before dismounting. After dismounting the ram will often stand alongside the ewe with head lowered. After a few minutes the ram will go off to seek another oestrous ewe. If several rams are kept together in the pre-mating period, an increasing level of competitive encounters is seen, with rams challenging each other in head-to-head combat. This can result in serious injury. If several rams are used together, competitive encounters can occur if there are too few ewes relative to the number of rams, which may reduce the overall mating efficiency.

5.4.3.1 Behaviour at parturition

Lambing is a critical period in the shepherding calendar. If sheep are to lamb outdoors, the first sign of parturition is likely to be the ewe isolating herself from the remainder of the flock and seeking a desirable location to give birth. Thereafter, in both housed and outdoor situations, the ewe will become increasingly restless, often alternating short periods of standing and lying, possibly scraping the ground and turning around. The first stage of labour is indicated by evidence of abdominal straining and may last up to 6 hours, during which the cervix dilates and uterine contractions begin. Disturbance at this point may interrupt the process. The start of second-stage labour is often marked by a rush of foetal fluid as the allanto-chorionic sac (the first 'water bag') ruptures and the amniotic sac appears intact at the vulva in around 50% of births. Part of the foetus becomes visible within the amniotic membranes. During this period, the ewe may alternate standing and lying but she usually lies down as the lamb's head passes through the vulva. Further abdominal contractions are seen and the foetus is expelled, connected by the umbilical cord. Many lambs are born within the amniotic sac. The amniotic membranes are usually broken by either vigorous movements of the lamb or when the ewe turns around to lick her lamb. Failure to clear these membranes from around the lamb's nose will prevent respiration. Generally lambs are born head first (anterior presentation). Most ewes complete this second stage of labour in around an hour (range 0.5–2 hours). Third-stage labour involves expulsion of the placenta (afterbirth); the ewe will generally eat the foetal membranes and lick up fluid discharges. Most ewes pass the remaining foetal membranes within 2–3 hours (range 0.5–8 hours).

The lamb will thereafter attempt to stand (and usually be up within 5 minutes) and is stimulated to do this by the ewe's movement. The neonatal lamb will become attached to any moving object; this can be exploited in fostering proce-dures. Once standing, the lamb will attempt to locate the ewe's teats and begin to suck (usually within 20 minutes of birth and certainly within the first hour). Sucking by the lambs causes the release of the hormone oxytocin which promotes uterine contraction as well as milk letdown. Successful sucking is evidenced by the vigorous waggling of the lamb's tail and the bleats of the ewe and may be accompanied by the lamb butting the udder, though this is usually more apparent in older lambs. These actions may be hindered by the delivery of a further lamb, the overzealous actions of the ewe or the inappropriate actions of a maiden ewe. Many ewes attempt to position themselves to aid sucking by the lamb, or push the lamb towards the udder. As the lamb sucks, the ewe often vigorously licks the lamb's perineal area. This period is crucial in terms of lamb survival: development of an effective ewe–lamb bond, based principally on both sound and olfaction, is highly correlated with survival success. Disturbance during lambing can lead to rejection or desertion of the lamb by the ewe or subsequent mismothering. This bond facilitates letdown of milk by the ewe, sucking by the lamb and recognition of the individual mother so that an effective association and following pattern can develop. Characteristic low-pitched bleats from the ewe (compared to the high-pitched bleats such as made by distressed sheep) are made exclusively to the lamb and are considered care-giving. They aid establishment of the ewe–lamb bond. The lamb will feed initially from the ewe about 3 or 4 times per hour. Lambs which are quick to stand and suck after birth are likely to develop a better bond with the ewe. As the lamb matures, the frequency of feeding will decline, though intake increases over the early weeks of lactation. Ewes of some breeds are notoriously poor mothers, while ewes of a number of hill breeds and easy-care varieties are very self-sufficient. In any breed, abnormal behaviour during the lambing period (which may be due to fatigue after a long lambing or a long period between multiple births, disturbance, overcrowding in the lambing shed, or inexperience) can result in rejection or desertion of the lamb, or mismothering. Undernourished ewes may show poor maternal behaviour.

5.4.4 Daily activity pattern

On a daily basis, the main activities of sheep are alternating bouts of grazing (20–90 minutes) and resting (45–90 minutes). Depending on the quality of grazing (or supplementary dietary components) sheep will feed for around 8 hours per day. While resting, sheep ruminate for much of the time. They will also sleep for short periods.

5.4.5 Abnormal behaviour patterns

Abnormal behaviour patterns, sometimes suggesting environmental deficit in other species, are not commonly seen in sheep. Most behaviours of this nature are shown by sheep in individual pens (e.g. short-term – vocalization; long-term – pulling and eating their own fleece) and no true stereotypies are recognized. Maiden ewes may show poor behaviour towards their lambs which can result in a lack of imprinting or colostral deprivation which have serious consequences for the lamb. Occasionally, early rearing conditions can affect subsequent male mating behaviour.

5.4.6 Human–animal interactions: the stockperson

Different management systems inevitably result in different amounts of human contact. The quality of any interactions between the stockperson and their sheep is crucial in maximizing the value of positive experiences (supplementary feeding, for example) and minimizing potential negative impacts of handling. Since isolation from the flock is known to be distressing for sheep, attempts should be made to limit this. Good stockmanship brings benefit to the sheep and facilitates the stockperson's work. Handling systems which are fit for purpose, designed with knowledge of sheep behaviour in mind, facilitate the work of the stockperson and enhance sheep welfare. The Farm Animal Welfare Council (FAWC) suggested that for one stockperson, an upper limit of 1,000 sheep (with additional help at times such as lambing) was reasonable.

In some traditional transhumance[1] systems which have been practised for centuries, the continual presence of the carer results in the sheep becoming habit-uated to him or her. In contrast, the recent advent of large, extensively managed flocks where the individual contact between the stockperson and sheep is limited brings a new set of challenges. With infrequent handling, more procedures are likely to be applied to individual animals and it is likely that the sheep will find this aversive. There is limited scope for any positive human–animal interaction to reduce this negative impact. When large mobs of sheep are handled it is very difficult to deliver individual care. It is known that well-handled sheep show less avoidance of humans but in some extensive systems such opportunities to provide 'gentling' experiences do not exist. It is not known whether providing a positive experience (e.g. supplemen-tary feed) in relation to aversive procedures may attenuate the negative effects. Selection of sheep for traits suiting them to particular systems – beyond production, health and survival traits – does not appear to be a consideration in most breeding programmes. Stockperson behaviour is therefore likely to be particularly important at these times; this can be enhanced through training. Sheep should be cared for by sufficient personnel with adequate knowledge of sheep and the particular husbandry system adopted, and stockpersons should be able to recognize problems at an early stage. The stockperson should be able to recognize any shortcomings of the system and attempt to compensate for these. However, some aspects of stockperson behaviour are likely to be related to inherent personal characteristics – for a thorough exploration of this important area readers should consult Hemsworth and Coleman (1998). Unfortunately, changing demographics in the UK at least show that fewer young people are likely to seek appropriate vocational training to work with sheep, and continuing professional updating of skills is sometimes difficult to achieve.

5.4.7 Sheep–dog interactions

Dogs are perceived as predators by sheep and, while dogs are used to move or gather sheep over extensive terrain, close proximity to dogs is considered aversive to sheep and should be avoided. The natural behaviour of sheep towards herding dogs is flight or distancing, often to the edge of the sheep's flight zone. If dogs chase sheep in an uncontrolled way, sheep may injure themselves; on sheep farms adjacent to urban areas, dog worry is becoming an increasing concern. Disturbance of sheep prior to lambing is a particular issue following reports of subsequent abortion. Sheep dogs used for herding are generally not used in closely confined handling areas where sheep cannot display distancing behaviour. Dogs should be trained not to bite or grip sheep. While herding dogs need appropriate training, some breeds and lines within

---

[1] Seasonal movement of people with their livestock, typically to higher pastures in summer and to lower valleys in winter.

breeds have been selected to maximize innate herding traits. Breeds include the Border collie and the Australian kelpie. At lambing time, ewes may become aggressive towards dogs and this reaction is sometimes used by stockpersons to encourage the ewe–lamb bond in reluctant ewes by heightening their maternal instinct.

In contrast, dogs of certain breeds can be used for sheep protection, mostly in high altitude areas, where large predators such as wolves can be a problem, accounting for a significant number of losses. These dogs are very passive around stock and sheep appear to bond with the guarding animals from a young age. Breeds include the Maremma and the Anatolian shepherd. The use of guarding dogs appears to be increasing on a world scale.

5.5 Reproductive Biology

Basic reproductive data for sheep breeds in UK conditions are summarized in Table 5.2. All British breeds of sheep, except the Dorset horn, are seasonally polyoestrous (and even Dorset horn sheep may show an anoestrous period), and short day breeders, commencing cyclic activity as daylength decreases in late summer. In ewe lambs, puberty is reached at around 8 months of age if nutrition has been adequate and they have reached 50% of adult weight; a reasonable lamb crop cannot be expected if lambs are under 65% of their mature weight. Thus well-grown lambs could be ready to breed at the end of their first summer. While photoperiod and diet are influential in promoting the organized release of sex hormones, the introduction of the ram may trigger the onset of reproductive activity in suitable prepubertal lambs. In these lambs, ovulation occurs at least once before the first behavioural oestrus. Ram lambs may also reach puberty and be fertile in their first autumn, often at a lower percentage of mature weight than ewe lambs, but maximum fertility is not reached until around 2 years of age. The potential for such lambs to breed can pose a significant management challenge, for which castration is the often-adopted solution unless male lambs can be fattened for sale at an early stage.

In temperate latitudes, the onset of seasonal breeding activity is dependent on decreasing daylength; nearer the equator the breeding season may be extended over the whole year, though temperature and nutrition exert some control. The hormone melatonin, produced by the pineal gland during the hours of darkness, has a pivotal role in relaying photoperiodic information to the hypothalamus; a shorter period of secretion increases the sensitivity of the hypothalamus to oestradiol and reproductive activity is suppressed. As daylength shortens, a longer period of melatonin secretion reduces the sensitivity of the hypothalamus and seasonal reproductive changes are seen. (Administration of melatonin produces a similar effect and can be used to advance the breeding season.) Ewes in very poor body condition may not display oestrus. Rams are also influenced by similar

Table 5.2 Sheep reproductive data.

	Adult ewes	Ewe lambs	Comment
Seasonality			
Onset of oestrus (mean dates)	Dorset Down (14 August) Halfbreds (20 September) Blackface (9 October) (Dorset Horn aseasonal)	By 7–9 months old if achieving 50% of adult weight	Inter- and intra-breed variation, affected by early introduction of ram
Oestrous cycle events	Oestrus 24–40 hours Ovulation 24–27 hours after the onset of oestrus Inter-oestrus interval 16–17 days		First seasonal ovulation not accompanied by behavioural signs
Fecundity			
Puberty		7–9 months	Depends on reaching 50% mature weight
Live lambs per ewe lambed	Welsh Mountain: 1.2 Blackface: 0.8–1.4 Clun: 1.5 Mule: 1.8 Cambridge: 3.0	1.0–1.25	Affected by body condition, grazing quality and stage of breeding season
Lambing interval	Annual (restricted by breeding seasonality)		Dorset Horn and Poll Dorset can breed 'out-of-season' but rarely done
Breeding life	Up to 15 years but most culled by 6 years old		
Fertility			
Ewes per ram	Hill: 40–50 Lowland: 50–60 Synchronized: 10–15	20–30	
Percentage ewes lambing	Lowground target 95% Hill target 92%	50–67% (can reach 85% if lambs over 60% mature weight)	Investigate if lowground <93%, hill <90%
Pregnancy length	142–150 days		Breed and litter size effects

seasonal effects, again mediated by melatonin (though in many breeds, mating is possible all year round). As a result, in practice fewer ewes are allocated to each ram at either extreme end of the breeding season. Testis size, semen quantity and quality and sexual activity are all affected by seasonal influences and the libido of rams peaks with short daylength.

The introduction of males into a group of females at the start of the breeding season has the effect of causing the majority to ovulate within a week, providing there has been no male exposure prior to this. This 'ram effect' is primarily pheromonal. Since the first oestrus of the season is 'silent' (not accompanied by behavioural signs), it will be 18 to 20 days before overt oestrus is displayed in the majority of animals. Ovulation rate, which is highest in the early part of the season, controls litter size. Ovulation rates vary between breeds (Table 5.2) and exogenous melatonin has been shown to increase the ovulation rate. The natural ovulation rate is maximal by the third lambing. After the first oestrus, ewes generally come into heat every 16 to 17 days until pregnancy or anoestrus intervene. Following mating, spermatozoa must reach the site of fertilization (the midpoint of the uterine (Fallopian) tube) within 12 to 24 hours of ovulation (24 to 30 hours after the onset of sexual receptivity – i.e. around the end of oestrus). In hill flocks around 40 to 50 ewes are run per ram, around 50 to 60 in lowland flocks. Maternal recognition of the embryo commences at around day 12 and embryo invasion into the uterine mucosa occurs at around 16 to 18 days, with attachment to the maternal endometrium completed by around day 30. Twin foetuses are generally found in opposite uterine horns.

Sheep develop a cotyledonary placenta with specialized attachment zones. Gestation length is around 147 days (range 142–150 days depending on breed and litter size). The number of lambs born per ewe lambed varies with breed from a maximum of around 1.2 in hill breeds to over 2 in some specialist lowland breeds; these figures are affected significantly by nutrition and environment. The prime means of controlling litter size is breed selection. Ewes with a large litter size may need additional support at lambing time and, in hill flocks, ewes producing twins are often at a significant nutritional disadvantage. The main causes of foetal loss once implantation has occurred are serious feeding mismanagement and infection. While ewes can have a breeding life of up to 15 years, most are culled from the breeding flock by the age of 6.

5.5.1 Manipulation of reproduction

In order to achieve a higher lambing percentage, to encourage early lambing (or out-of-season lambing) or to facilitate a compact lambing period, a number of techniques are undertaken. If mating is condensed, ram power must be increased, with rams as well as ewes in appropriate condition. Lambing percentage should be set to best match the farm's resources. Early lambing or the assisted increase in litter size also dictates that, to ensure lamb survival and welfare, facilities, labour and feeding management must be appropriate. For example, early lambing may require the provision of enhanced shelter. No manipulative methods should be seen as a substitute for poor management and indeed they will work best where overall flock management is of high quality; in some flocks simply improving ewe condition at mating can have the biggest positive effect. The main methods employed commercially include the use of intravaginal progesterone-impregnated sponges or controlled internal drug release devices (CIDRs) which suppress the release of pituitary hormones and hence normal oestrous activity. On removal, 12 to 14 days after insertion, oestrus commences from around 24 hours later (a little sooner with CIDRs). Sponges are not generally recommended for maiden animals. Pregnant mares' serum gonadotrophin (PMSG) can be used in conjunction with progesterone treatment to control ovulation and initiate oestrus in anoestrous ewes. PMSG has also been used in superovulation regimes. Synchronization of oestrus is essential in flocks in which artificial insemination (AI) is practised. Where synchronization has been used, one ram is needed per 10 to 15 ewes.

Exposure to vasectomized males can advance the breeding season in certain breeds. In some flocks, melatonin implants are used to simulate short daylength and thus advance the breeding season in order to produce early lambs. Opinions vary as to whether melatonin should also be given to rams in these flocks.

Artificial insemination and embryo transfer (ET) are established techniques to accelerate genetic improvement in a flock (primarily through higher selection intensity) or to introduce a new genotype. AI also can be used in situations where biosecurity requirements prevent the movement of rams and thus can be particularly important in an international context, though some diseases (such as foot and mouth disease) can still be transmitted. Either laparoscopic, transcervical or intracervical AI can be undertaken with fresh or frozen semen around 12 to 18 hours after a synchronized oestrus as detected by teasers or (more usually for laparoscopic AI) 56 hours after progesterone sponge withdrawal and hormone injection (10–20 hours earlier if CIDRs are used). Using traditional mating systems an individual male could achieve around 50 pregnancies per year but with intrauterine AI this figure could approach 8,000. Semen collected using electro-ejaculation (EE) (Section 5.6.2.1) is usually inferior to that collected from trained rams using an artificial vagina, is more often contaminated and less suitable for freezing. The use of EE has been questioned on welfare grounds and, as a result, its use may be restricted to diagnostic applications by a veterinary surgeon in some countries. Similarly, performance of laparoscopic AI and ET is restricted to veterinary teams. Ovariectomized ewes serve as teasers at collection stations. Compared to AI, ET allows more selection pressure to be exerted on the female and requires multiple ovulations to be produced in donor ewes in a multiple ovulation and embryo transfer (MOET) programme. Embryos are collected 5 or 6 days after the onset of oestrus. However, variability in the superovulatory response remains a limiting factor. As with AI, although biosecurity is usually enhanced using ET, certain viral agents in particular can penetrate the zona pellucida and thus there is still a risk of disease transmission from infected donors. Laparoscopic embryo recovery and transfer (compared to surgical methods) has the potential to improve the welfare of the donor ewe but the repeated use of donor animals has raised concerns and the Farm Animal Welfare Council has urged caution when any new breeding technologies are introduced. An EU-wide code of practice for animal breeding techniques exists and includes consideration of individual animal integrity. With accelerated breeding practices, there is the inherent risk of the production of a large number of animals which are ill fitted to their environment. For more information on reproductive techniques see Williams (1995).

The production of transgenic animals (those with additional, extraspecific DNA incorporated into their genome) or cloned animals, while the subject of some public welfare concerns, is not a common practice and consideration is beyond the scope of this chapter.

5.6 Management

5.6.1 The range of management systems

In general terms, the way a flock is managed depends on the target end-product. This could be anything from prime lamb or a top-quality breeding ram to a supply of milk. The aim is to deliver this, based on the natural resources and facilities available through excellent stockmanship and appropriate breed selection. The timing of key activities in the shepherding year is predicated by the seasonal ability of a ewe to lamb and successfully rear her lamb(s) when grass growth sustains maximal lactation. (Note: there is a small number of flocks which lamb in the autumn.) Economic production requires the best available grass, supplemented by conserved forage and cereal crops. Given the annual production cycle and the fact that young females will not usually be recruited into the breeding flock until 1 or 2 years of age, it is not possible to make rapid changes to systems, and in the more challenging environments where sheep are kept there is minimal scope for alternative systems to develop. In these harsher, wetter areas of the UK, systems are primarily dependent on grass, with sheep gaining body condition over the summer and relying on body reserves (in the form of fat deposits) over the winter.

In the stratified system of sheep production in the UK (Figure 5.1), ageing ewes move from hill flocks to more equitable lowland conditions, allowing one or possibly two more crops of lambs. Store lambs also move down the hill and some hill sheep are moved to less harsh conditions each autumn. Central to the decision of when to move ewes is the capability of the ewe to sustain herself through natural grazing, as determined principally by incisor tooth presence and condition; once prehension is compromised the ewe's ability to survive on a grass-based diet declines. Sheep with missing permanent incisors are defined as 'broken mouthed'. While incisor teeth provide a benchmark for decision-making, the condition of cheek teeth (premolars and molars) is also important as they can be in poor condition, yet these are not easily (and so are rarely) examined. An indication of the eruption profile for sheep teeth is given in Table 5.3.

Table 5.3 Average eruption pattern for permanent sheep teeth. The dental formula is I:0/4 C:0/0 PM:3/3 M:3/3.

Teeth		Permanent teeth[1]	Common descriptor[2]
Incisors	I 1	1 year 3 months	Two tooth
	I 2	1 year 9 months	Four tooth
	I 3	2 years 3 months	Six tooth
	I 4[3]	2 years 9 months	Full mouth
Premolars (cheek teeth 1–3)	PM 1	1 year 9 months	
	PM 2	1 year 9 months	
	PM 3	2 years	
Molars (cheek teeth 4–6)	M 1	3 months	
	M 2	9 months	
	M 3	1 year 6 months	

[1] Temporary incisors erupt from around birth or up to 2–3 weeks.
[2] In the UK there are numerous regional terms to describe sheep of different ages.
[3] Sometimes not present, displaced or vestigial.
In the UK, lambs with evidence of one or more permanent incisor erupted are considered over one year of age for the purposes of the Specified Risk Material (SRM) controls in relation to TSE diseases.

5.6.2 Management of rams

5.6.2.1 Examination of rams

Rams should be examined about 10 weeks prior to use, in order that corrective actions can be effective before the breeding season; rams need to be in a fit and active condition, able to seek out ewes and mate successfully. The inspection should include body condition, teeth condition and lameness. Routine vaccinations must be conducted in advance of breeding (usually 4–6 weeks) in order that any associated handling stress or transient temperature rise occurs sufficiently in advance of sperm production: spermatogenesis takes around 50–60 days and once released from the matrix of the testis, spermatozoa spend from 2 to 5 weeks in the epididymis during which maturation for maximum fertility occurs. Anything with the potential to cause a rise in temperature (including environmental effects) can have an impact on semen quality. All young rams should be closely examined to exclude the possibility of transmitting hereditary problems to their offspring (e.g. entropion). Rams should also be inspected for evidence of superficial abscesses and, if found, the presence of caseous lymphadenitis (CLA; caused by *Corynebacterium pseudotuberculosis*) must be excluded. (Aspects of these physical examinations should also be undertaken periodically once the rams are in use.)

Palpation of the testes and accessory organs will reveal any obvious abnormalities or injuries, in which case veterinary advice should be sought. The testes should be equal in size, freely moveable within the scrotum and, prior to the breeding season, firm to palpate with no obvious irregularities. The tail of the epididymis can usually be palpated as a soft swelling at the base of the testis and the spermatic cord can be felt running into the inguinal ring. Ultrasonography is used increasingly in the examination of ram genitalia. In young rams intended for first use, extrusion of the penis should show that development is complete with no residual adhesion between the penis and prepuce. This will also reveal any abnormalities in older rams. In many flocks a number of rams are used in large groups of ewes, so underperformance by a single ram may go undetected, or a small overall reduction in flock fertility may be seen. When only one or two rams are used in a smaller group, the effect of underperforming individuals can be much more dramatic. Estimates of infertility and subfertility range from 3% to 10% in the UK.

To ensure that the ram can produce adequate good-quality semen, samples are sometimes collected using either an artificial vagina (AV) or electro-ejaculation (EE), which involves electrical stimulation of the nerve plexus near the pelvic genitalia with a lubricated rectal probe. In the UK, this latter technique is restricted to veterinary clinical use, on welfare grounds, as it is a potentially stressful and painful procedure. Semen is analysed for volume (0.7–2.0 mL), sperm count (around $2–5 \times 10^9$ sperm per mL), progressive motility, morphology and the absence of cells indicative of infection. Semen with more than 20% abnormalities should not be used for AI. The only true reflection of a ram's ability is in the subsequent pregnancy rate, a combination of libido (keenness to mate ewes) and fertility.

5.6.2.2 Feeding of rams

Rams are, for most of the year, usually maintained outdoors in bachelor groups on a grass diet. While it is important to maintain their condition, rams should not get too fat. Body condition score (BCS) should be monitored and should be around 2.5–3 during this maintenance period (see Table 5.4). Rams should not be overlooked in vaccination programmes or parasite control measures. Prior to the breeding season, rams should be placed on a rising plane of nutrition (starting at around 200 g/day of concentrates, rising to 500–700 g/d) to achieve, on lowground flocks, a BCS of around 3.5–4 on introduction to the ewes. Accustoming the rams to supplementary feeding facilitates continued feeding during the mating period, as at this time their natural grazing inclinations are significantly reduced and failure to maintain sufficient condition will reduce their reproductive success; rams can lose up to 15% bodyweight during a 6-week tupping period. Individual feeding also leads to rams being easier to catch for the purpose of undertaking routing tasks. When tupping has ended, rams are removed, inspected and placed on a maintenance diet. Underperforming rams should be examined closely (for details see Williams, 1995).

5.6.2.3 Introduction of rams to the breeding flock

Depending on the mating strategy, entry of the rams may be preceded by the use of a teaser (vasectomized) ram, up to a month before the rams are joined, to encourage the ewes to commence cyclic behaviour or to synchronize their oestrous cycles (when introduced to already cyclic females). (Note: teasers should be of the same health

Table 5.4 Sheep body condition scoring (BCS). Source: Meat and Livestock Commission (1988).

Score	Descriptor
0	Extremely emaciated and on the point of death. It is not possible to detect any muscular or fatty tissue between the skin and bone.
1	The spinous processes are felt to be prominent and sharp. The transverse processes are also sharp, the fingers pass easily under the ends and it is possible to feel between each process. The eye muscle areas are shallow with no fat cover.
2	The spinous processes still feel prominent, but smooth, and individual processes can only be felt as fine corrugations. The transverse processes are smooth and rounded, and it is possible to pass the fingers under the ends with a little pressure. The eye muscle areas are of moderate depth, but have little fat cover.
3	The spinous processes are detected only as small elevations; they are smooth and rounded, and individual bones can be felt only with pressure. The transverse processes are smooth and well covered, and firm pressure is required to feel over the ends. The eye muscle areas are full, and have a moderate degree of fat cover.
4	The spinous processes can just be detected, with pressure, as a hard line between the fat-covered eye muscle area. The ends of the transverse processes cannot be felt. The eye muscle areas are full, and have a thick covering of fat.
5	The spinous processes cannot be detected even with firm pressure, and there is a depression between the layers of fat in the position where the spinous processes would normally be felt. The transverse processes cannot be detected. The eye muscle areas are very full with very thick fat cover. There may be large deposits of fat over the rump and tail.

The technique is designed to produce a highly reproducible system and is based on the assessment of the prominence of the spinous and transverse processes of the lumbar vertebrae, the degree of fat cover of the latter and the presence of muscle and fat below the transverse processes. The fullness of the eye muscle (longissimus) is also assessed.

status as other sheep in the flock). If any form of synchronization has been used, the ratio of ewes to rams will need to be reduced. Young rams may be presented with fewer ewes or not used on the gimmers – females entering the flock for the first time. (Note: the regional use of traditional sheep terms can cause confusion!) Young rams are usually exposed to groups of experienced ewes and are generally not worked alongside older rams who would otherwise dominate them and inhibit their mating activity. It is common to use a colour marker (raddle), applied directly to the brisket of the ram or via a keel harness, to colour the rump of the ewe, indicating that mounting has occurred. The colour is usually changed after 14 days to allow successive oestrous cycles (or the work of individual rams) to be monitored. A lack of evidence of mounting or a succession of colour marks indicates a problem with either ram or ewe, such as infertility or embryo loss, and prompt veterinary advice should be sought, especially if more than 15% of ewes return to first service. Recording of colour marks is the main route by which some flocks predict lambing if ultrasonography is not employed. It is important that the area used for mating affords the sheep sound footing and is, for example, not unduly hilly or rocky. Often in-bye fields are selected to facilitate observation of the rams at work. When rams are used in teams, it is important to closely observe the rams for signs of excessive competition. This is a particular problem if rams are used in pairs. Vasectomized rams, turned into the flock 3 to 4 weeks after mating, can be used to identify non-pregnant ewes which continue to cycle.

5.6.3 Management of breeding females

Ewes must enter the breeding period in optimum condition. This may be difficult to achieve, given that most will have been lactating the previous summer. Particularly in hill flocks, the ewe will also need to be assessed for her ability to survive over the coming winter and allow her *in utero* lamb(s) to develop at the same time. The two months before tupping is a vital period if annual flock performance is to be maximized.

5.6.3.1 Examination of ewes

Legs and feet must be in good order, and, for hill sheep, the presence of a full set of incisor teeth is vital. Hill ewes whose tooth condition means that they are unlikely to be able to graze effectively should be drafted to lowground flocks where conditions are more favourable. Palpation of the udder in ewes which have reared a lamb will indicate whether subsequent lactation might be affected – e.g. if there are swellings, lumps or evidence of abscessation. These can indicate previous mastitis and a possible compromise to subsequent lactation and consequent lamb growth. These considerations should be applied to stock animals, home-bred replacements and bought-in animals, for which biosecurity considerations also apply (Section 5.13.2). Culling criteria thus include poor teeth, unresolved lameness, mastitis, previous reproductive problems which may prejudice normal fertility and easy birth, and failure to achieve, on lowground flocks, a BCS of 3 by one month after weaning. If required, ewes should receive vaccinations against diseases such as enzootic abortion and toxoplasmosis in advance of the breeding season. Certain vaccines should not be given concurrently and so adequate time must be allowed. This is a good point in the year to review the flock's health plan with the unit's veterinarian, who may examine a selection of animals.

5.6.3.2 Feeding of ewes before mating

For those ewes that reared a lamb the previous summer, correct nutrition during lactation should prevent excessive weight loss. However, for hill sheep in particular, although generally only rearing a single lamb, this may be difficult to achieve. As for rams, breeding females must be in appropriate condition at mating to encourage optimum fertility. Ewes are often placed on an increasing plane of nutrition prior to mating (a process known as 'flushing') to enhance ovulation rates and so produce more lambs. However, this does not compensate for ewes being in an underlying poor body condition. It is important to begin a planned build-up to mating as soon as weaning has occurred, with the aim to have, on lowground flocks, ewes with BCS 2.5–3, 3 to 6 weeks before the rams are joined. This gives the opportunity to concentrate efforts on poorer individuals and sheep which are still growing (ewe lambs (6–8 months old) and gimmers (18–20 months) and ensure that all animals gain about 0.5 BCS point by mating to be at BCS 3.5 in flocks where high lambing percentages are the target (about half a point less for hill ewes). As an indication, this would need an 80 kg ewe to gain about 2 kg bodyweight per week. For hill flocks, achieving a high proportion of twins may be a disadvantage. If ewe lambs are to breed in their first autumn they need to reach 60% of their mature bodyweight; two-tooth ewes (gimmers) can be expected to be at 80% of their mature weight (Williams, 1995). It is particularly important that ewes are in good condition as early as possible in the breeding season since there are market advantages to be realized from the production of early-season lambs. In later-breeding flocks, pasture resources alone may be unable to provide an adequate level of nutrition at this time. More detailed information can be found in the publication by the Meat and Livestock Commission (1988), *Feeding the ewe*.

5.6.3.3 Joining with the rams
Depending on the system, groups of ewes are joined with the rams to achieve lambing at particular times in the spring. For hill and upland flocks ewes and rams are joined in October–November; for grassland flocks at a lower altitude this happens around a month earlier. Ewes are often split into mating groups to facilitate management. Maiden females, which may be reluctant to seek the ram, are often not included in the main flock but mated in small groups to experienced rams, after the main flock.

5.6.4 Pregnancy
Once the rams are removed, ewes should be maintained on a good plane of nutrition with no abrupt changes, to support embryo implantation. While most embryo loss is thought to occur at this time, in hill flocks it may be difficult to avoid some weight loss, unless sufficient quality in-bye grazing remains available. It has been suggested that certain forage crops such as kale or rape, eaten immediately before mating, might lower fertility so it is prudent to allow simultaneous access to pasture. Younger animals (ewe lambs but also two-tooth ewes) which have just entered the breeding pool should continue to receive a high-quality diet to allow their own growth to continue. In many systems it is recognized that adult ewes, in adequate condition at the start of pregnancy, can tolerate a reduction in body condition and a loss of weight of up to 5%. Target live weights for lowland breeding ewes are given in Table 5.5.

From around 40 days post-mating it is possible to examine ewes using B-mode ultrasonography to determine pregnancy and foetal numbers. However, the most accurate diagnosis is made at around day 80. To allow for an average spread of matings, flocks are generally scanned between 11 and 15 weeks after ram introduction. In the UK this has become the principal method used, though sometimes

Table 5.5 Target liveweights (kg) of lowland ewes at various ages and in different reproductive states; values represent percentage of mature weight at conception.

Type of sheep	Stage of pregnancy		Lambing			Lactation
	Conception	Day 90	Day 120	Pre-	Post-	week 8
Ewe lamb (bearing a single lamb)	60	65	70	75	64	62
Two-tooth ewe (bearing twin lambs)	80	85	90	97	80	77
Mature ewe (bearing twin lambs)	100	96	100	112	90	83

stockpersons simply rely on the presence of the keel mark (though embryonic death and the presence of oestrus in up to 20–30% of pregnant ewes can reduce the accuracy). Beyond 100 days of gestation, palpation of the foetus through the abdominal wall may be attempted. Ultrasonography, performed at an early stage, will show if there have been any foetal losses in early or mid-pregnancy; this information may prove useful in diagnosing nutritional or disease problems in the flock. The main value in scanning ewes is to allow nutrition in the last third of pregnancy to be tailored to maternal needs, based on foetal load. For most flocks, nutrition in mid-pregnancy (months 2–3) should aim to avoid excessive weight loss; only individual sheep may need supplementary feeding. Ewe lambs and two-tooth ewes will need particular attention and access to the best available grazing. For early-lambing flocks, abundant natural vegetation may still be available and lead to some sheep becoming too fat. Over-fat ewes can have difficulties at parturition and during mid- and late pregnancy may suffer from the metabolic condition, pregnancy toxaemia, particularly if subjected to sudden food restriction. They may also produce small lambs. Undernourished ewes are at greater risk of diseases, which may prejudice their own and their offspring's survival.

From around 6 to 8 weeks prior to expected lambing, at a time when naturally available feed is at its nadir, around 70% of growth of the foetus occurs, with consequent demands on the mother. It is usual to place ewes on an increasing plane of nutrition and to provide food in a form which they can consume, given that the enlarging uterus reduces available space for the rumen. Voluntary food intake may also decline at this time. While the basis of the diet at this time may be good-quality conserved grass or root crops, there is also a need to feed concentrates to achieve an overall energy provision of 9–11 MJ/kg, particularly as lambing approaches. Adult sheep need to be monitored to ensure that their BCS does not decline significantly. For hill sheep bearing single lambs there is reliance on natural resources and body reserves to meet the doubling in feed requirement of even a single-bearing ewe. Ultrasound scanning allows the separation of ewes with multiple foetuses for increased feeding over this period. For sheep bred for the first time, their nutrition will need to allow for

Table 5.6 Feeding regime for ewes in late pregnancy.

Feedstuffs (kg/day)	Ewe weight and foetal load					
	50 kg			70 kg		
	Single	Twin	Triplets	Single	Twin	Triplets
Hay	0.83	0.83	0.83	1.00	1.00	1.00
OR Silage	2.60	2.60	2.60	3.50	3.50	3.50
6 weeks before lambing						
Hay or silage as above plus concentrates	0.18	0.30	0.34	0.24	0.37	0.44
4 weeks before lambing						
Hay or silage as above plus concentrates	0.28	0.45	0.51	0.36	0.56	0.66
2 weeks before lambing						
Hay or silage as above plus concentrates	0.37	0.59	0.68	0.48	0.75	0.86

their own development as well as that of their foetuses. Supplementary feeding can also accustom ewes to the type of feed which will be available if they are housed for lambing and, for hill ewes which remain outdoors, it accustoms them to emergency feeding as may be required in storm conditions (Table 5.6).

Better nutrition during pregnancy has significantly reduced ewe and lamb mortality over the last half-century. As well as avoiding metabolic problems around the time of parturition, correct nutrition promotes the birth of vigorous lambs of good birthweight with adequate nutrient reserves to allow them to stand and suck within a short period, crucially important in terms of survival in cold and wet conditions. In practice, feeding in the weeks immediately prior to parturition balances some degree of loss of body reserves with natural resources and supplementary feedstuffs. Conducting a BCS evaluation of a selection of sheep 3 to 6 weeks prior to lambing will allow final adjustments to be made. The condition of the poorest ewes should not be allowed to fall below BCS 2 at lambing.

During the last third of pregnancy, ewes may receive booster vaccinations to maintain their protection and increase the amount of colostral antibody available to their lambs. Potentially stressful procedures should be avoided immediately prior to expected lambing. For the same reason, if ewes are to be housed, they should be moved to sheds well in advance of lambing.

5.6.5 Lambing management

5.6.5.1 Preparation for lambing

The loss of lambs (and some ewes) in the perinatal period is a significant welfare challenge to sheep. Lambing also represents the culmination of the stockperson's reproductive management, the foundation for which was laid at tupping time through the selection of a genotype appropriate for the environment and correct nutritional provisioning from before mating until lactation. Preparation is crucial as stockpersons find this a potentially challenging period, often working long hours under arduous weather conditions. The first 24 to 48 hours after birth are the most critical in terms of lamb survival, and present a significant window of opportunity for stockpersons to provide support.

Preparations for lambing will depend on the system and must address the likely events which could lead to significant welfare problems. Where more close supervision is available, key issues relate to assisting (at the right time) during parturition, resuscitation, dealing with hypothermia, ensuring early sucking and the consumption of adequate colostrum, the adequacy of the ewe–lamb bond, and fostering or artificial rearing if required. For hill and upland sheep lambing outdoors, it is not possible to deliver the same quantity of care and thus it is critically important that self-sufficiency traits are present. In addition, ewes should be in the target body condition and be on familiar land, hefted to where they can find shelter if required or artificial shelter provided. In these systems, with possibly one stockperson for over 1,000 ewes, individual care will generally not be provided to the same extent as in lowground flocks. Knowing when to intervene is a key stockmanship skill.

Ultrasound scanning allows the segregation of ewes based on foetal load. In addition to allowing correct late-pregnancy nutrition, this facilitates preparations for cross-fostering of triplet lambs onto single-bearing ewes. A prerequisite to using scanning information is easily read identification and accurate individual records.

Particularly for indoor lambing and where mating was synchronized, arrangements must be made for adequate experienced surveillance. Everyone involved should know when to intervene in case of a protracted birth (sometimes becoming involved too early is counterproductive), which manual methods can be employed to resolve dystocia, and when to seek help. Stockpersons should know how to attempt resuscitation, how to ensure adequate colostrum has been taken by the lamb (and what to do if not) and the importance of hygiene measures such as navel dipping. There needs to be good access to pens (and ways to move sheep around easily), adequate lighting, facilities to care for sick ewes and those which abort, and arrangements for the collection of placental material, dead lambs and dirty bedding. A marking and recording system must be agreed by all involved before lambing starts (not least to ensure correct bonding when ewes and lambs join communal groups).

It is usual to prepare a lambing toolkit which contains in a single place a number of commonly required items (Box 5.1). During slack periods used items must be replenished.

5.6.5.2 Ewe behaviour at lambing

It is important to be able to recognize the signs of labour (Section 5.6.5.4) and know when to provide assistance to ensure the welfare of both the ewe and lamb(s). Hill sheep and other more self-sufficient or 'easy-care' breeds may not benefit from

Box 5.1   Contents of a good lambing toolkit

General

- Record book/pencils, marker sprays/crayons, torch and spare batteries
- Water, buckets, soap, disinfectant solution, hand towels
- Rubber rings and applicator
- Disinfectant for lambing pens

Assistance at lambing

- Obstetrical lubricant, disposable gloves
- Strong iodine solution for dipping navels (and suitable dip cup)
- Digital thermometer (works quickly and no chance of broken glass)
- Lambing ropes/tapes/aid for repositioning lamb's head
- Scissors

Support for lambs

- Towels for drying lambs, heat lamp/hairdryer
- Warming box for hypothermic lambs
- 20% glucose solution (10 mL/kg), 50 mL syringe/19 G 3 cm needles/antiseptic swabs
- Respiratory stimulant (e.g. Doxapram drops)
- Oral rehydration solution

Support for ewes

- Calcium borogluconate solution for injection (and means for administration)
- Magnesium sulfate solution for injection
- Propylene glycol for oral administration
- Prolapse retainer/harness
- Antibiotics (as prescribed by vet)
- Needles and syringes

Artificial feeding

- Stored (frozen) colostrum
- Stomach tubes, large syringes/feeding bottle
- Graduated plastic jugs
- Bottles, teats and disinfectant
- Ewe milk replacement powder
- Hypochlorite solution for disinfection

human intervention which may delay the lambing process and jeopardize lamb survival. Here stockpersons observing their sheep in order to spot ewes in difficulty are unlikely to be able to deliver major benefit to the majority of animals. For housed sheep or those with poorer maternal traits, individual attention will be more helpful. Care of the indoor lambing environment needs considerable effort if infectious disease is not to become a problem. If ewes have been housed for part of the preceding winter, some clipping of the fleece on housing facilitates supervision at lambing – it is easier to observe what is happening – and makes it easier for the lambs to locate the ewe's udder.

Once lambed, the housed ewe must be observed for signs of acceptance of her lambs and her willingness to let them suck. Other events which can lead to lamb morbidity include ewes failing to groom lambs or rejection of second lambs (sometimes seen if there has been an unduly long interval between the birth of siblings). Those sheep lambing for the first time will more frequently need encouragement to allow the lamb to suck and obtain a good supply of colostrum. Colostrum contains a high level of energy, minerals and vitamins and also provides immunoglobulins – antibodies against specific diseases, which must be ingested since no antibodies pass to the lamb across the placenta. This helps the lamb to resist diseases endemic in the lambing environment (e.g. watery mouth which is seen when lambs ingest environmental organisms such as *E. coli*). It also confers non-specific immunity and is a direct source of heat to a cold lamb. Colostrum also has laxative properties. It will generally not be possible or desirable to provide a high level of support to hill or easy-care breeds. Although a stronger ewe–lamb bond exists, human disturbance at the birth site may cause the ewe to abandon the new lamb. However, it is still possible to provide some pens for ewes and lambs and protection from the worst of the weather by building shelters from large straw bales.

Ewes housed for lambing are often kept with their lambs in individual pens for around 24 to 48 hours. Placental material (afterbirth) is collected for hygienic disposal and pens are cleared of contaminated bedding, disinfected and re-bedded prior to reuse. Alternatively, lambing ewes are housed to lamb in indoor groups. Depending on the weather conditions, they are then turned out in small groups to sheltered paddocks which allow ready observation in case of mismothering, poor maternal behaviour or ill health. If ewes with young lambs remain for too long in the relatively confined conditions of housing, they risk mismothering and infection rates increase.

5.6.5.3 Newborn lambs

To ensure its survival, the newborn lamb must rapidly become dry, stand, consume an adequate amount of colostrum and develop a bond with its mother. Lamb birthweight varies with breed and litter size: single Blackface lambs weigh between 3.5 and 4.5 kg; twins will each weigh around 0.5 kg less. During periods of poor weather, particularly when wet and windy conditions combine, the core body temperature of wet or even partially dry lambs can fall quickly, leading to hypothermia. It is estimated that in the UK between 2 and 3 million lambs die of hypothermia each year, as a result of exposure and/or starvation. Lamb survival is enhanced if they stand and suck quickly to replenish energy reserves; lambs slow to stand have greater difficulty in maintaining body temperature. Sucking in lambs is often accompanied by vigorous tail wagging. Ewes in poor condition predispose their lambs to the risk of hypothermia. Lambs may also be at risk if ewes are very old or if they demonstrate poor ewe–lamb bonding. Lambs from large litters or where there have been problems during birth are also at risk. Other causes of lamb death include stillbirth and infectious disease, with a small percentage due to congenital abnormalities. From a welfare perspective it is important to recognize that a large proportion of these losses is avoidable.

It is imperative that lambs receive adequate colostrum as soon as possible (ideally within 2 hours) and certainly within 6 hours of birth before 'closure' of the gut wall to immunoglobulin passage. Ingestion of colostrum (and later milk) into the abomasum (the true, glandular stomach) can be assumed in lambs whose abdomens have a full appearance on palpation behind the last ribs. Some stockpersons collect colostrum from ewes with multiple lambs in order that this can be fed artificially to later-born littermates. Colostrum can be stored and fed to orphaned or weak lambs and be deep frozen in advance of the next year's need. Colostrum has laxative properties which help the lamb to pass contents from the foetal gut (meconium). Moving ewes to new locations to give birth can mean that there is an absence of colostral antibody to 'local' disease organisms. The colostrum from suitably immunized cows or goats can also be used but bovine colostrum can lead to anaemia in lambs.

5.6.5.4 Assisting during parturition

Manual delivery of the lamb(s) must be undertaken with care and rigorous attention to hygiene. This is to prevent inter-animal transmission of disease and to protect the stockpersons. A number of organisms prevalent at this time can cause serious disease in humans (i.e. they are zoonotic) and, even if all appears normal, their absence cannot be assumed. *Chlamydophila abortus* is among the organisms of particular concern to pregnant women, leading to the recommendation that pregnant women should not work with sheep (since these may abort if infected) and particularly lambing ewes, the products of lambing (or abortion) and lambs needing artificial rearing. Flocks with specific disease problems or those buying in young females or receiving pregnant ewes should seek veterinary advice about the risks and control measures which can be adopted. For more details see Eales *et al.* (2004).

Stockpersons must be able to recognize the stages of parturition, act appropriately when a ewe needs assistance and be able to correct malpresentation of lambs. If a ewe has been straining hard for 15 minutes or more and there is no sign of progress she should be examined to determine the cause: principal reasons include inadequate dilation of the cervix, abnormal presentation or dystocia due to the disproportionate size of the foetus. There is not the opportunity to develop this area adequately here but inexperienced attempts at foetal repositioning can seriously harm the ewe and lamb. Birth injuries sustained during a difficult or prolonged birth (either natural or with overzealous human assistance) can result in stillbirth, failure to thrive or morbidity. This may be as a result of physical injury or anoxia in lambs deprived of oxygen from placental exchange before respiration commences. Dystocia is responsible for many ewe deaths and is a significant welfare concern.

Good hygiene is absolutely crucial at lambing time, given the number of infectious agents which can be spread. It is common practice to dip the navels of housed lambs (Figure 5.2a) – a strong iodine solution is usually used at birth and ideally 4 to 6 hours later as part of the disease control strategy. It is important that the solution covers the navel right up to the abdomen. Iodine speeds desiccation of the remaining umbilical cord (Figure 5.2b) and reduces the chance of infectious organisms causing navel ill or subsequent joint ill.

5.6.5.5 Resuscitation

Some newborn lambs need encouragement to start breathing, especially if the birth process has been long or difficult. For lambs with a heartbeat (which can be easily felt at the front of the chest just behind the forelimb) but no obvious respiration, a number of simple actions are often sufficient. The nose and mouth must be cleared of foetal membranes and the lamb should be vigorously stimulated, for example by rubbing with clean straw. The nose can be tickled with straw, which often stimulates sneezing followed by breathing. Gently swinging the lamb by the hind legs is often found to prompt respiration and facilitates drainage of foetal fluids from the chest and airways. Respiratory stimulants can be applied to the underside of the tongue. While artificial respiration could be attempted using a purpose-made device, direct 'mouth-to-mouth' methods should not be practised due to the zoonotic disease risk.

5.6.5.6 Dealing with hypothermia

Hypothermia is the cause of the majority of perinatal lamb death in the UK. Because hypothermia can dull cognitive experience and consciousness, it is possible that noxious experiences of hypothermic lambs are reduced and so it is difficult to assess the overall welfare impact of this state. Even if lambs are healthy and in a good nutritional state, weather conditions at lambing time, particularly in hill and upland areas, may be such that they are unable to rapidly dry, stand and suck and the ewe may have failed to select a sufficiently sheltered birth site. The body temperature of lambs that have not dried or stood up within a short period can fall rapidly. Any lamb showing signs such as lethargy or failing to follow or suck from its mother should be assessed by taking its temperature: the normal temperature of a lamb is 39–40 °C and lambs at risk can have temperatures of 37–39 °C. In individual cases, drying the lamb

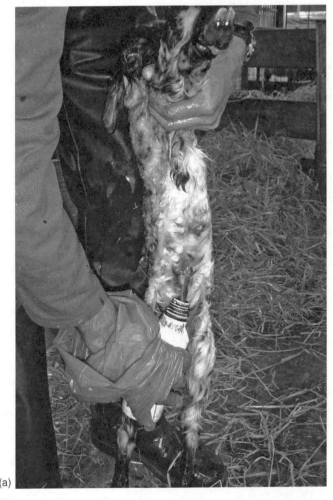

(a)

Figure 5.2 Use of iodine for navel dipping: (a) applying strong iodine solution soon after birth; (b) a dry navel and withered umbilical cord. Photographs by permission of Kay Aitchison.

and either stomach tubing (see Section 5.6.5.7) with warm colostrum or intraperitoneal injection of a warm glucose solution may be effective. Lambs with temperatures below 37 °C require urgent attention if they are to survive. For lambs more than 5 hours old, which will have exhausted their built-in fat reserves, the sequence of events should be to dry, then provide energy (by intraperitoneal glucose injection if it is weak and unable to support its own head), then warm the lamb. If a hypothermic lamb is warmed abruptly in the absence of an energy supply it can die from shock. A further aid to reduce the incidence of hypothermia is the temporary use of jackets for newborn lambs.

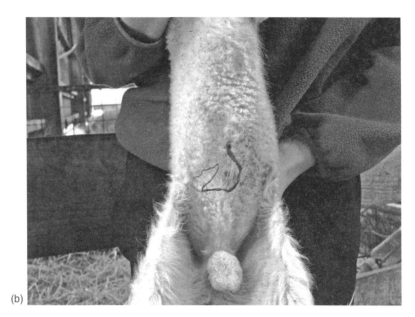

(b)

Figure 5.2 (Continued).

5.6.5.7 Stomach tubing

The procedure is to use a rubber catheter of around 4.5 mm diameter, 30 cm long. This should have a smooth, rounded end with an offset opening. With the lamb sat across the stockperson's lap, the lamb's head is raised and the lubricated tube gently introduced over the back of the tongue. The tube can be easily advanced as the lamb swallows and force is not required. Its advancement down the oesophagus (gullet) can then be observed externally as it passes down the left side of the lower neck in the jugular groove. It is crucial that the tube is not located in the trachea. This is unusual, but fluids introduced into the lungs of a debilitated lamb will likely lead to death. As this may occur in weak or unconscious lambs, stomach tubing is not recommended for them. If the tube is in the trachea its advancement down the neck will not be seen and in some cases – but not all – the lamb may cough and exhibit signs of discomfort. The tube is advanced until around 20–25 cm is in the lamb, when the tip should be in the stomach. A graduated feed bottle or syringe is attached to the external end of the tube and warm (body temperature) colostrum or milk, as appropriate, is delivered under gravity or gentle positive pressure. The tube is then gently withdrawn with the bottle still attached. The equipment should then be cleaned for subsequent use (e.g. using hypochlorite solution) and a record made of the time and amount given to the lamb.

5.6.5.8 Early sucking: provision of colostrum

It is important that stockpersons can recognize hungry lambs (Figure 5.3) and take appropriate action. Hungry lambs have an arched back and it will not be possible to

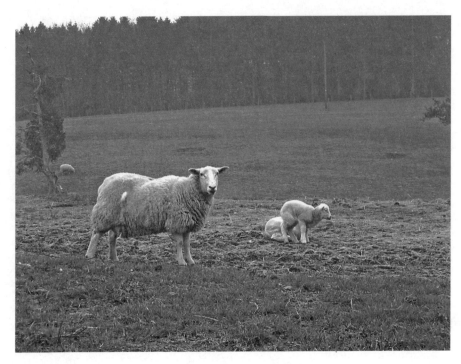

Figure 5.3 A hungry lamb showing a characteristic stance. The lamb should be fed and the ewe checked for mastitis. Younger lambs adopting this stance may also be hypothermic. Photograph by permission of Paul Roger.

palpate a full stomach. Using a rule of thumb of 50 mL/kg, a 5 kg lamb will require 250 mL colostrum (and later milk when the special properties of colostrum have waned) per feed, four times a day. Weak lambs may need initial feeding by stomach tube.

5.6.5.9 Artificial feeding, fostering and adoption

Intervention will be required if ewes die or fail to lactate sufficiently well. Lambs which exhibit a strong suck reflex, even those which have yet to take colostrum, can be fed via a bottle. As with tube feeding, it is important to ensure that feeding implements are scrupulously clean and milk substitutes correctly formulated. While lambs may need individual attention to teach them to suck, they can very easily be moved to automatic systems (lamb bar) which, from the stockperson's perspective, is vital if a large number of orphans are expected. More simple systems such as buckets with teats attached are also effective. From about 3 weeks a palatable creep feed in pelleted form and high-quality hay are introduced. It is then possible to consider weaning lambs at around 6 to 8 weeks of age if solid feed intake is adequate. Artificial rearing does not maximize the use of ewes which have either lost lambs or have the capacity to accept an additional lamb.

Vigorous lambs can be fostered on to ewes using a number of methods, some of which involve coating the lamb with birth fluids from the recipient ewe or using the skin of a ewe's dead lamb to mask its own individual smell. It is helpful if the weight of the lamb to be fostered matches that of the ewe's own lamb. Sometimes cross-fostering can be done before the ewe has established a bond with its own offspring, and this method is used to move one lamb from triplet-bearing ewes to a ewe with a singleton. If there has been a delay in the fostering process the acceptance rate can be improved by manually mimicking the cervical sensation of the lamb passing through the birth canal. Alternatively ewes are retained in a yoke system where they have no choice but to accept the foster lamb. This latter method may take up to 3 days but in any case the sooner the process is initiated following the birth of her own lamb(s) the easier the new bond is to establish. Often the welfare of the ewe is overlooked in these systems: there must be ready access to feed and water, with a minimum period of restraint. Some stockpersons utilize the protective response ewes demonstrate towards their lambs on exposure to a dog to strengthen the ewe–lamb bond, but this technique has the potential to cause unacceptable distress to the ewe. Some ewes will never take foster lambs.

5.6.6 Lactation

The udder of the ewe should have been checked prior to tupping, but if lambs fail to thrive the ewe must be examined again for evidence of adequate milk production. In the first 6 weeks, the lamb's growth is dependent primarily on the ewe. Thereafter, milk remains a crucial component of the lamb's diet as it begins to eat herbage and until this can adequately compensate for the nutrients supplied by milk. In order for the ewe to produce sufficient milk, the diet must be adequate and she must remain healthy. The ewe's nutritional needs are greatest in early lactation and in most systems this is planned to coincide with available spring grass; for early-lambing flocks, considerable supplementary feeding will be needed. For ewes with a high lactation potential (up to around 2.5 L per day), voluntary food intake may not be sufficient to meet demands and further weight may be lost (up to 5% of bodyweight) as fat reserves are utilized. This is not usually a problem if ewes are in the target condition at lambing time and if there is sufficient protein in the diet. There may be an advantage in the separate feeding of ewes rearing multiple lambs (which produce up to 40% more milk) in order to provide them with a higher plane of nutrition (or providing supplementary 'creep' feed to lambs). It is common to continue the pre-lambing feeding regime of a diet with high digestibility. The periparturient increase in shedding of roundworm eggs by the ewe (resulting from perinatal immunosuppression) may affect maternal condition and thus milk production. Maximum milk yield is seen around the third lactation and vigorous lambs have a positive effect on milk production.

5.6.7 Weaning

Weaning is usually undertaken when lambs reach 14 to 16 weeks of age but the timing is dependent on the system. Weaning is done abruptly across the whole group. By this time, though still sucking, lambs are not primarily reliant on ewes. Early weaning of lambs in milk breeds or frequent lambing systems requires the young lambs to be provided with appropriate concentrate diets. If lambs are weaned onto grass too early, they will fail to thrive or reach their growth potential. However, early weaning may be part of a farm strategy to control intestinal parasites by moving lambs, following anthelmintic treatment, to pasture with a predicted low level of infectivity (e.g. previously ungrazed by sheep that year or used for conservation crops).

5.6.8 Autumn lambing

A small number of flocks based on the Dorset Horn or Poll Dorset breeds, with their less pronounced reproductive seasonality, can be managed for autumn lambing in order to target Easter markets which are otherwise short of fresh lamb. The system can also capitalize on an otherwise slack period in the conventional shepherding calendar. However, this system requires a high standard of management and the availability of freely draining land if the ewe flock is to be outwintered during the lactation period. Alternatively, ewes and lambs are kept indoors with early weaning of lambs at around 6 to 8 weeks with the move to high-quality creep feed available *ad libitum* and the provision of good-quality hay. Lambs can reach a market weight of 40 kg by 16 weeks of age. In some southern counties of the UK it is common to fold (move across) ewes and lambs on winter roots and brassicae, e.g. direct-drilled kale, rape and turnips.

5.7 Management of Hill Sheep

Within the stratified system of UK sheep production (Figure 5.1) hill sheep represent the starting point for many enterprises. Reliance is primarily on nutrition from uncultivated natural hill vegetation with its inherently low nutrient value, but this does not mean that supplementary feeding is not required. Sheep can tolerate low environmental temperatures providing they are of adequate nutritional state, in good fleece and this remains dry. Sheep have been selected to tolerate the conditions experienced, primarily through their ability to efficiently utilize body reserves over the winter (i.e. during pregnancy and early lactation), ease of lambing and the development of local knowledge (hefting) allowing them to take advantage of protective natural landscape features. On some farms, shelter belts of trees are established for the same purpose. Pure-bred sheep are generally found in these systems. The market requirement for leaner sheep has the potential to be at the expense of desirable traits required by sheep in extensive environments such as reserves and insulation provided by fat.

Key management activities are usually focused on late pregnancy and early lactation when body reserves can become depleted and ewe deaths due to inanition (exhaustion) (particularly if ewes entered the winter in too low a body condition) are a real possibility. Actions at this time include provision of supplementary feed through conserved forage, root vegetables or feed blocks. The main triggers of the start of feeding are BCS and the advent of bad weather, rather than the time of year *per se*. Alternatively, some ewes are routinely moved to areas of improved or more sheltered grazing such as in-bye land or areas of improved hill grazing. This also facilitates supplementary feeding of concentrates and minerals if required. Additional planning actions in these systems include consideration of supplying emergency rations in case of storm or heavy snowfall or moving sheep to relative shelter if adverse weather is forecast.

The current poor economic climate for extensive hill and upland systems in the UK is resulting in a significant reduction in the number of hill sheep. This, coupled with what are often considered poor working conditions and the low recruitment rate of young stockpersons, leads to the conclusion that such systems will likely decline further. This has a knock-on effect on sheep systems requiring crossbred ewes.

5.8 Management of Lowland Flocks

The main advantages for lowland flocks compared to hill systems are the more favourable weather conditions, the longer grass-growing season and the provision of housing. These combine to allow a more flexible management programme to be developed.

Shelter or more permanent housing are provided primarily to protect ewes and lambs at lambing time or more generally over the late winter and early spring when weather conditions, combined with an increased nutritional demand on pregnant ewes, are most challenging. Simple shelters (either adjacent to the farm buildings or on protected pastures) can be erected for use by lambing ewes for periods of 24 to 48 hours. A variety of readily available materials can be employed; most frequently shelters are made from straw bales with a simple form of covering, and a hurdle at the front, with the closed side towards the prevailing wind. An additional advantage of these temporary shelters is the avoidance of a long-term build-up of infectious disease agents. Corrals of large straw bales can also be used at pasture to provide additional shelter to groups of ewes and lambs once turned out to grass.

Alternatively, permanent housing is used for lambing ewes, either in the form of traditional barns or, where weather conditions allow, polythene tunnels. While the latter have a more limited lifespan they offer a cost-effective solution and can be erected in areas where a more substantial structure would not be possible.

Individual indoor pens for lambing ewes are generally constructed against the inner sides of buildings using wooden or metal hurdles (Figure 5.4), with provision for temporary feed and water supply. Pens need to be of suitable size – around 1.5 m

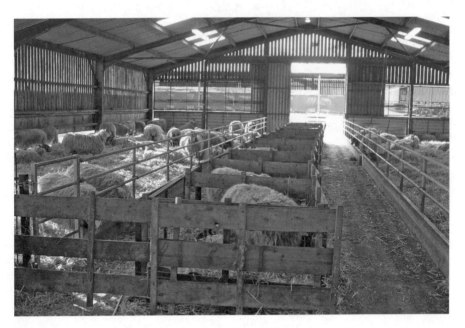

Figure 5.4 A well-ventilated lambing shed with individual pens for ewes and lambs. Photograph by permission of Kay Aitchison.

by 1.5 m is ideal. There should be at least one pen per eight ewes but more pens may be needed for synchronized flocks. Either ewes are moved to these pens in anticipation of lambing or are moved from a communal pen, with their lambs, soon after birth to facilitate bonding and individual care. Pens should be constructed so that it is easy for the stockperson to remove bedding and clean and disinfect them between lambing ewes, since preventing disease spread at lambing time is a key challenge. Slatted-floor pens are not appropriate for lambing sheep. There needs to be provision for fostering lambs and for orphan lambs. Orphan and sick individuals need additional heat, usually provided by a suspended infrared lamp. Arrangements must be made for the hygienic disposal of bedding, foetal membranes and stillborn lambs.

5.8.1 Winter housing

Housing sheep for all or part of the winter is common practice in some areas, typically on mixed enterprise farms, where unoccupied buildings are available. There is no need to provide supplementary heat, but it is important that the effect of the wind and draughts at sheep height is reduced, for example using space boarding or suitable netting. Adequate air movement is needed to avoid hot and humid conditions which predispose sheep to respiratory disease. Conditions underfoot must remain dry and sheep need to lie on a dry bed. While slatted floors are sometimes found, and do ensure a dry surface, more generally solid floors covered with straw are seen. These require more regular maintenance to avoid dampness and resultant foot problems such as foot rot; it is important that sheep are introduced to the house having been subjected to an adequate foot care programme. Slatted floors should not be used for lambing ewes or ewes with lambs at foot. Poor quality or incorrectly spaced slats result in foot and leg injury and have high maintenance costs.

Winter housing provides compensation for energy needed to maintain growth and production when weather is poor and allows the adoption of early-lambing systems. There is a relative ease of management of sheep with the ability to stock at a high density (especially if sheep are shorn on introduction to the house, which reduces the required floor space by 20–25%), at the same time resting available pasture. Recommended floor space is given in Table 5.7. Disadvantages include the potential higher prevalence of infection, particularly respiratory disease and neonatal infection, and the need for greater attention to foot care. The provision of adequate care will be aided by good working conditions for the stockpersons, including adequate lighting and the ability to isolate individuals or small groups to receive special attention. It is generally unhelpful to house sheep in excessively large groups (more than 30); larger groups do not allow stable social structures and make it more difficult for stockpersons to deliver individual care.

Feed and watering arrangements must reflect group size. Ideally feeding is facilitated by providing gangways between pens (Figure 5.5). There should be sufficient trough space to allow all sheep access to concentrate feed at the same time: for example, large ewes will need around 50 cm of trough space and 22.5 cm of hay rack access. Housed lambs following autumn or winter lambing will require access to a creep area for preferential feeding. Feeding of silage leads to a high output of urine, which can increase the bedding needs.

Table 5.7 Recommended space allowances (m²) for housed, unshorn sheep*.

Type of sheep	On slats	On straw
Large ewe in lamb (70–90 g)	0.95–1.1	1.2–1.4
Large ewe with lambs	1.2–1.7	1.4–1.85
Small ewe in lamb (45–70 kg)	0.75–0.95	1.0–1.3
Small ewe with lambs	1.0–1.4	1.3–1.75
Large hoggs (32 kg)	0.55–0.75	0.75–0.95
Small hoggs (23 kg)	0.45–0.55	0.65–0.95
Lambs up to 12 weeks old	Not recommended	0.5–0.6
Lambs and sheep 12 weeks to 12 months old	0.55–0.8	0.75–0.9
Lamb creep area	Not recommended	0.15–0.4

*Shorn sheep will require around 20% less space.

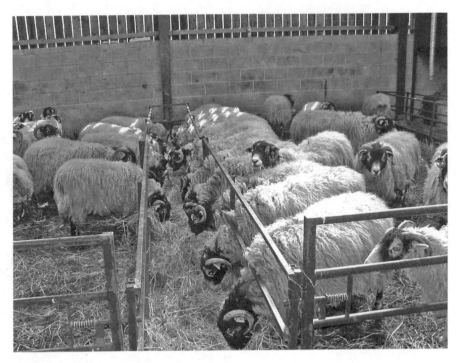

Figure 5.5   Housed sheep being fed from a gangway between pens, facilitating the stockperson's work. Photograph by permission of Paul Roger.

5.9 Management of Fatstock

The end product of prime lamb production is the fat lamb (see Figure 5.1). With the majority of lambs born in the spring, there is a market advantage to early lamb production, either through advancing the birth date or ensuring maximal growth rates through optimizing nutrition and parasite control. The choice of breed (particularly through the terminal sire, which has the ability to confer desirable carcass characteristics) is of great importance. Carcass classification or grading incorporates measures of fatness, muscling, carcass conformation and the type of animal – from new-season lamb to mature sheep. Weight is also important. Lambs are generally sold at around 50% of their mature weight with a killing out percentage of up to 50%. Stockpersons will select batches of lambs for sale when they reach an adequate weight and condition to maximize their market potential. Assessing fatness is an important acquired skill, principally based on assessing the fat cover at the tail root and loin area. From the market side, the regular provision of lamb of even quality is important. In particular, consumers require carcasses which have a low fat content. The move towards leaner carcasses has resulted in lambs being marketed at slightly lower slaughter weights.

Lambs can be sold off the ewe (i.e. while still taking milk) and if the ewe has been well fed lambs can be sold from 10 weeks of age when they weigh around 20 kg. Beyond this age, provision of high-quality pasture and control of intestinal parasites are important if lambs are to be marketed early and feeding costs controlled. Most lambs are sold at some point after weaning (at around 16 weeks of age) with weaning generally dictated by the need to allow ewes to recover condition prior to the next breeding season. These lambs will generally be finished on late summer grass and sold as dictated by the prevailing market conditions.

A number of European markets exist for lambs of a particular weight at certain traditional times of the year. In the UK, lambs which are not sold off grass at the end of the summer are usually sold on for fattening for sale in the autumn or winter (store lambs). As grass growth declines, additional foodstuffs are substituted to maintain growth rates, including root crops, grass or arable by-products. Concentrates may also be used if there is a need to target a particular market window of opportunity. If sheep are closely confined outdoors on poorly draining ground in wet winter weather, poaching can be a serious problem, resulting in foot problems and disease, especially if there is no dry lying area, though this should be provided. Any problems can be exacerbated if root crops are fed since these increase urine production and the moisture content of faeces.

5.10 Organic Sheep Production

The number of sheep in organic systems in the UK increased rapidly during the first decade of the present century but remains small compared to 'conventional' production. Organic farming continues to receive strong support for philosophical, ethical and economic reasons. Organic principles require a whole-system approach which precludes the use of synthetic inorganic fertilizers, pesticides, growth regulators, livestock feed additives and genetically modified foodstuffs. Livestock must be fed on organically produced foods: on sheep farms, this implies a reduction in forage production when inorganic nitrogen inputs are removed. While organic farmers have an explicit motivation to care for the land, most other farmers do likewise. From a sheep farming perspective, organic systems rely primarily on efficient grassland management, crop rotations (where the land allows cultivation) and animal manure to maintain soil fertility, with minimal inputs from outside the system; this too is in line with the practice in many conventional systems. For hill sheep systems this does not have a major impact and so, for some producers, conversion, in relation to feed inputs, is relatively straightforward. Organic cereal rations need to be provided for supplementation of prolific ewes in late pregnancy and early lactation and for finishing young stock. Gross margins per animal are 15 to 20% above that of conventionally produced livestock. Organic regulations place restrictions on husbandry procedures such as tail docking, which can only be allowed with the use of an anaesthetic and, for example, from 2010 not allowing the housing of sheep in the final fattening stages.

There is a compulsory requirement to develop a plan to promote health and introduce disease control measures that lead to progressively less dependence on conventional medicines. Thus organic systems focus on health and welfare promotion, in tune with flock health planning (Section 5.13.1). If veterinary treatments are required, complementary or homeopathic products are chosen above conventional medicines. Animals treated with the latter may be subject to extended withdrawal periods or possibly exclusion from organic sale. The requirement for the preferential use of homeopathic remedies above allopathic, proven products (except in some cases of known disease risk), needs justification since the comparative advantage of organic farming in terms of disease control has yet to be clearly demonstrated. Requirements of organic standards restrict the use of anthelmintics on a routine basis, favouring pasture management to avoid exposure of susceptible stock (principally lambs in their first grazing season) to infection. This may not always be entirely satisfactory. For example, significant gut damage can be caused by some worms (e.g. *Nematodirus* species) before there is evidence of parasite eggs through faecal counts. Even with exemplary management some use of anthelmintics is almost always essential to ensure effective control of internal parasites. The restricted use of some preventive medicine strategies (including the restriction on the use of organophosphorus dips to control sheep scab) is, to some, less acceptable from an animal welfare perspective than providing a comprehensive disease reduction and prevention programme incorporating conventional medicines. Some of the reported reductions in health problems on organic farms may be the result of reduced stocking density.

5.11 Hobby Sheep-Keeping

For many of the same reasons that sheep were among the first domesticted animals, sheep are increasingly kept in very small flocks, sometimes aiming to produce a niche product or satisfy local demand. Sheep in small numbers are also found increasingly as pets – often accompanying a range of other species. Hobby sheep-keepers, while sometimes extremely knowledgeable, may equally be ignorant about the welfare needs of their sheep and the legal requirements in relation to livestock – for example, the need to register their holding to facilitate national disease control measures. In hobby situations, overweight sheep and sheep with ill-kept feet are frequently encountered. Ideally, sheep should not be kept singly.

5.12 General Nutrition and Feed Management

The key to economic sheep production is to maximize the contribution of home-produced resources, primarily grazed grassland (including silage aftermaths) during the summer months and conserved fodder over the winter months. This usually allows the feeding of concentrates to be reserved for ewes in the last few weeks of pregnancy (Table 5.6) or in early lactation if sufficient spring grass growth has not yet occurred (especially in early-lambing flocks). Concentrates may be fed to fattening lambs to supplement grass. Other feedstuffs are used for overwinter feeding of store sheep and ewes in upland areas: these include a range of arable by-products and root crops such as fodder beet. There are a number of excellent publications providing sound advice about all aspects of sheep nutrition, for example, Meat and Livestock Commission (1988), and regional advisory services provide contemporary advice on economic feeding practices.

5.12.1 The importance of good pasture management and conservation

Since grass supplies around 90 to 95% of the overall energy requirement – either through grazing or conservation – it is of vital importance that good grassland management is practised. Elevation and climatic conditions influence grass growth. Thus different systems are encountered as production moves north and 'up the hill'. On lowland farms grass use is concentrated on the summer growing season and maximized through high stocking densities. Depending on the stage of grass growth and the deviation of grass height from an optimal 4 cm in the active growing season, the pasture will support a variable number of sheep over the summer. Early in the season, about 15 ewes (and their lambs) per hectare could be supported. However, the increasing cost of nitrogen fertilizer to support grass growth and the increase in organic rearing systems means that high sheep densities are not easily sustained. In addition, high sheep densities encourage the build-up of gastrointestinal parasites. Thus densities of ewes are more commonly around eight ewes per hectare on managed grassland. In contrast, sheep on extensive or upland/hill farms may rely solely on poor quality natural (rough) grazing. These sheep will usually need supplementary feeding, particularly towards the end of pregnancy, often through the provision of hay or feed blocks.

Once grass growth declines or ceases, sheep in lowland systems rely on conserved feeds – primarily hay or silage. Silage must be of adequate quality which is maximized at a low moisture content (dry matter above 25%) where an adequate level of acidity has been achieved through efficient manufacture and storage. (Silage feeding of sheep is not suitable for very small numbers as, once the anaerobic conditions of bales or clamps have been breached, spoilage can rapidly occur.) The making of field-cured hay is very sensitive to the weather and in the UK the balance in production has shifted to a major extent to silage. Commercial assessment of both hay and silage is available. Correct storage is also important if the nutritional value is to be preserved.

5.12.2 Root and forage crops

Once natural grass growth declines towards the end of the summer, particularly on lowland farms, there will be a need to provide supplementary food to bridge the feeding gap and allow the sheep to continue to be held at reasonably high stocking rates while continuing to extract the maximum value from the grass at a time when lamb growth is accelerating. This is often achieved through feeding a range of green fodder crops such as kale or rape, root crops such as turnips, or a number of arable by-products, though these alone may not provide sufficient nutrients for rapidly growing fatstock. Store lambs can be moved to graze arable areas where surpluses exist. These crops can subsequently form an important part of the early winter diet, often fed in combination with conserved grass (usually hay) to avoid digestive problems. Root crops can also be harvested to be fed later in the winter and around lambing time. If free access is required through the autumn and winter, the land must be suitable to carry the sheep if conditions become very wet; poaching of the ground and inadequate dry lying areas can lead to significant health and welfare concerns and incomplete use of the available crop. Some of these crops have a low dry matter content (e.g. DM of swedes is 12% compared to grass silage 25% and hay 85%). Access is usually through strip grazing controlled by electric fencing; however, electric net fencing should not be used if horned sheep are present. Broken-mouthed sheep or those with erupting incisors ('four tooth' – in their second winter) may be unable to eat root crops sufficiently and can lose condition rapidly.

A regional supply of crop by-products, undersown cereal crops and aftermaths can be utilized in the autumn, providing adequate note is taken of their nutritional contribution. In many lowland areas, good supplies of sugarbeet tops can be obtained. (It is necessary to allow adequate wilting of sugarbeet tops to avoid oxalate toxicity and digestive problems.) This feed is highly attractive to ewes, which can become over-fat during pregnancy, and if fed as a high proportion of the diet will need supplementing from 8 weeks before lambing.

5.12.3 Concentrate and compound feeds

Concentrates are cereal-based and rapid ingestion can lead to ruminal acidosis; though generally mild, this can result in reduced appetite. For this reason, concentrates are usually introduced gradually, with amounts built up over a few days. This may be more difficult to regulate in large groups of sheep where some consume more than others. Generally cereals are fed in an unprocessed form ('straights'), even if a little is observed undigested in the faeces. Compound feeds are usually pelleted or cubed feedstuffs made to a specific protein, energy, mineral and vitamin composition. Suitable feed mixtures can also be home produced through the use of grains or, for example, brewing by-products, with appropriate additions of protein-rich components (such as soya bean meal), minerals and vitamins. Compound feeds are generally expensive and reserved for feeding to match the nutritional needs of ewes in the last 6 to 8 weeks of pregnancy and early lactation. Store lambs may benefit from additional feed input in the last stages of fattening depending on the cost benefit. Such compound diets alone do not provide sufficient fibrous roughage to ruminants; therefore good-quality straw may also be provided *ad libitum*. A further method is the feeding of a complete diet to housed sheep, generally based on pelleted dried grass with vitamin and mineral additions. Sheep that are unaccustomed to supplementary feedstuffs may not take them in an emergency.

There is increasing use of feed blocks, which weigh 25 to 30 kg, as a dietary supplement especially for sheep wintered outdoors. These have a high energy density and can contain urea (as a non-protein nitrogen source) and balancing minerals – the exact composition varies. Adequate quantities of roughage should be available when blocks are fed. Blocks can also contain anthelmintics but this route may not provide a therapeutic dose to all animals, in which case anthelmintic resistance could develop. Blocks are particularly useful in areas where access is difficult. They resist weathering and last a considerable time but can be expensive and not all sheep will use them to the same extent.

5.12.4 Minerals and vitamins

Two main factors affect the adequate supply of minerals and vitamins in the diet: the local soil type and the content of any supplementary feedstuffs. A number of areas of the UK are recognized as being deficient in key minerals or trace elements, principally copper, cobalt and selenium. Livestock advisers can assess the likely availability of these essential dietary constituents at farm level. In addition, some trace elements (e.g. molybdenum) act in a competitive way, so reducing availability. Subclinical effects of deficiency can affect productivity through reduced growth rates or suboptimal reproductive performance. Provision of mineralized feed blocks or appropriately supplemented concentrate feed are ways to compensate for deficiencies, though not all sheep choose to use feed blocks. Supplements can be given on an individual basis, often through oral dosing of slow-release boluses, which lodge in the rumen, or depot injections. Copper supplementation, though often necessary, should be used judiciously as it is relatively easy to provide a toxic overdose. Magnesium supplementation may be needed in spring as rapidly growing grass has a low concentration. When required, vitamins are usually provided in compound feedstuffs. Fat-soluble vitamins have a limited shelf life so it is important to observe 'use before' indications and to store feed correctly. In emergency cases, a number of vitamins and trace elements can be given by injection.

5.12.5 Water

A supply of clean water should be available at all times, even though non-lactating sheep eating high moisture-content grass may not drink regularly. In extensive conditions, water is often provided from reliable natural sources. Where water is provided artificially, the supply must be checked and cleaned regularly. Indoor watering arrangements must minimize the chance of faecal or food contamination. If sheep are gathered around a water trough this suggests that either the supply has failed or the source has become contaminated. Sheep unfamiliar with automatic watering devices such as might be encountered at markets or slaughterhouse lairages may be reluctant to drink. Transported sheep often choose to eat rather than drink following unloading from a vehicle.

5.12.6 Nutritional disorders

5.12.6.1 Pregnancy toxaemia/'twin lamb' disease

Occurring in late pregnancy and around parturition, this condition is due to an imbalance of energy supply and utilization with low maternal glucose availability due to foetal demand, coupled with a reduction in rumen volume. Twin-bearing ewes are most at risk. Over-rapid mobilization of body fat reserves results in the appearance of ketones in the blood – the sheep's breath may smell sweet. A toxic condition ensues which, if not rapidly corrected, leads to coma and death. Following early signs of depression and apparent unawareness of their surroundings, ewes may become recumbent, and anorexia exacerbates the situation. If signs appear shortly before parturition, the birth of lambs can be hastened, for example by steroid injection or a caesarean operation. In some cases, ewes may spontaneously abort. Feeding of high-quality hay and concentrates and administering oral glucose or propylene glycol over a number of days can also be effective, if diagnosis has been prompt. In many cases treatment is futile and euthanasia of the ewe may be necessary. The condition is best avoided through correct ewe nutrition based on foetal load. Blood sampling a selection of ewes 4 weeks before lambing can indicate diet adequacy by measuring betahydroxybutyrate.

5.12.6.2 Urolithiasis

Urolithiasis is a disease seen primarily in castrated (wether) lambs receiving a highly concentrated diet. There is a blockage of the urethra, usually as it curves sharply over the ischium, by mineral sediments and proteins which precipitate in the urine. Clinical signs are primarily abdominal discomfort, straining, sometimes kicking at the abdomen, possibly accompanied by urine dribbling. A number of surgical approaches can be attempted but usually the long-term prognosis is poor and efforts should be made to correct the nutrition of at-risk stock.

5.12.6.3 Copper deficiency and toxicity

Many soils of the UK, and consequently the grass growing in these areas, are unable to provide sufficient dietary copper for sheep. The availability of copper is reduced in the presence of competitive elements, principally molybdenum but also sulfur. Copper gained during the grazing season is stored in the liver. Concentrate feeds for sheep usually contain adequate amounts of copper. Copper is an essential trace element needed, for example, for red blood cell formation. A true assessment of the copper status can only be achieved through liver analysis, though blood samples are often taken to provide a general guide. The classical sign of copper deficiency (hypocuprosis) is congenital swayback in newborn lambs where a defect in the nervous system (demyelination) leads to lambs being unable to coordinate their hindlimbs or even stand. In these cases, it is difficult to effect a cure and euthanasia must be considered for welfare reasons. In growing lambs which appear normal at birth, signs of swayback (enzootic ataxia) include failure to thrive and the fleece may develop a characteristic appearance of dullness, dryness and lack of crimp in the wool. Adult ewes experiencing copper deficiency may show ill thrift. An adequate copper status in the ewe may not necessarily prevent symptoms occurring in her lambs. The margin for copper excess over adequacy is relatively small and there is a real danger of overdosing sheep; copper toxicity is the most commonly diagnosed cause of poisoning in sheep. Providing copper supplements by way of intra-ruminal slow-release boluses should not be undertaken in sheep receiving a diet which is supplemented with even a small amount of copper (e.g. compound feeds, mineral blocks or mineral powders with added copper). Copper poisoning results in hae-molysis, jaundice and kidney failure and is usually the acute result of chronic copper accumulation. It is occasionally seen in sheep gaining access to cattle feed which has a greater copper content.

5.12.6.4 Cobalt deficiency

As with copper, many areas are deficient in cobalt which is a constituent of vitamin B12 (cobalamin). Thus sheep which rely mostly on grazing are more likely to suffer and rapidly growing animals are more at risk and can even die. The onset of cobalt deficiency is usually insidious, with sheep failing to thrive, a condition referred to as 'pine'. Signs include poor appetite, loss of weight, anaemia and a poor coat. Diagnosis is through blood sampling. Remedial action on an individual basis may involve a vitamin B12 injection (this may need to be repeated) or the use of an intra-ruminal slow-release bolus if sheep are of an adequate size to accept the bolus. Treating ewes will facilitate the passage of increased amounts of vitamin B12 in their milk. For long-term control, pasture dressing with cobalt may be considered but this is very expensive. Toxicity through overdosing is unlikely.

5.12.6.5 Selenium deficiency

Nutritional muscular dystrophy, known colloquially as white muscle disease or stiff-lamb disease, is due to either selenium or vitamin E deficiency. Young lambs (often under 4 weeks old) appear stiff or unable to stand. Emergency treatment requires individual supplementation (usually via injection) of affected lambs. Both selenium and vitamin E can be included in diets for ewes in late pregnancy or in lamb creep feed if problems are expected in a particular locality. Excessive selenium can lead to toxicity.

5.12.6.6 Hypomagnesaemia (grass tetany/staggers)

Though not common, this problem is sometimes encountered in early lactation, during periods of rapid grass growth. The low concentration of magnesium (Mg) available in rapidly growing spring grass, often in relation to high levels of fertilizer application (and sometimes at the end of the growing season) and the coincidence with maximum milk production, places a large demand on body magnesium reserves. In acute cases, ewes may be found dead. Affected ewes appear nervous, excited or apprehensive with muscle trembling, particularly around the face.

Clinical signs may be precipitated by strenuous events (e.g. gathering or transport). This is an emergency condition and treatment involves intravenous administration of a suitable electrolyte and mineral solution (which may contain calcium since hypocalcaemia often occurs concurrently). Recovery can be very rapid. Flock management should ensure a sufficient quantity of magnesium in the complete diet or the provision of a suitable mineral mix or feed block where concentrates are not fed at pasture.

5.12.6.7 Hypocalcaemia

This condition usually occurs around the time of lambing, though can occasionally occur prior to lambing if feed intake is interrupted (e.g. by snowfall). It occurs as a result of disturbed calcium metabolism and the inability of the ewe to maintain circulating calcium concentrations. Over-provision of calcium in the diet prior to lambing may precipitate the condition as the ewe will not develop an efficient calcium regulation mechanism geared to responding to peak demand. Clinical signs include muscle tremors, incoordination, rapid breathing and recumbency. Untreated ewes become paralysed and coma follows quickly; if ewes receive intravenous calcium borogluconate (usually followed by a subcutaneous 'depot' injection to prevent a relapse), recovery is rapid.

5.12.6.8 Listeriosis

Listeriosis is primarily seen as a rapidly deteriorating encephalitis in adult sheep which initially appear disorientated and may collapse on their front legs. They may also circle and drool saliva, with food impacted in their mouths. Organisms may gain entry to the body through mouth lesions associated with erupting teeth. It is associated with feeding silage (usually big bale silage) which has been contaminated with large numbers of *Listeria monocytogenes*. While this organism is relatively common in the soil and herbage, in silage which has become spoiled through not achieving sufficient acidity, bacteria present can multiply and pose a threat to sheep. If individual cases are seen, a thorough investigation of the feed source should be made to restrict the number of further cases.

5.13 Health and Disease

5.13.1 Risk-based health planning and preventive strategies

Flock health planning (see Box 5.2) is fundamental to all sheep enterprises and a requirement of farm assurance schemes. It provides a structured way to evaluate the disease and welfare risks to the flock, based on previous experience and local knowledge, and to develop a strategy to minimize or eliminate these risks. Reactive, 'fire brigade' measures to deal with day-to-day problems are inefficient for the farmer and are likely to have a negative impact on the sheep (e.g. the need to gather sheep more frequently to apply treatments). Health planning is also a way to incorporate

---

Box 5.2   Important general areas for flock health plans

Relevance
Adaptability
Ease of use
Cover all stock
Calendar to schedule routine treatments and activities, e.g.

- Condition scoring
- Vaccination
- Worm egg counts/oral dosing
- Ectoparasite control
- Lameness control

Address specific conditions on the unit
Focus on biosecurity and likely new diseases

Record key production data, disease incidence and medicine use
Set intervention levels for key problem areas, e.g. lameness
Describe carcass disposal policy
Integrate with (not duplicate) farm assurance scheme requirements
Ensure compliance with standards
Allow review/reflection/updating

---

best practice in disease control (e.g. the strategic use of vaccination) and welfare standards through advice from the farm's veterinary adviser. Depending on the sophistication of data recording it also provides the opportunity for benchmarking health and production against previous performance and/or that of similar local enterprises. There is opportunity to incorporate a range of targets which can range from essential or aspirational (e.g. reducing lamb losses or the reliance on anthelmintics). Being a risk-based activity, it provides an opportunity to focus on diseases which have the greatest effect on the health and welfare of the sheep. Veterinary advice will allow the selection of cost-effective strategies and computer-based sheep health planning packages are available.

For any health and welfare programme to succeed, stockpersons must be able to identify signs of illness, yet these initial signs can be subtle and often non-specific. Generally, behavioural signs appear first; e.g. a sheep may spend more time lying down, be slow to rise when approached or hang back behind the rest of the flock. Sheep may be listless and adopt abnormal postures. Of more diagnostic help are symptoms such as coughing or rubbing up against solid objects. The state of the fleece can be a useful guide to general condition, especially when compared to the remainder of the flock. A good stockperson will always be vigilant to signs such as these, and any sheep giving cause for concern must be subject to more detailed examination.

5.13.1.1 Routine treatments to enhance health and welfare

While a number of treatments relate to specific diseases (Section 5.13.4), a calendar can be developed to capture important elements of the flock health plan. An example of a simple calendar of preventive actions is given in Table 5.8. Drawing up and amending a calendar in the light of actual or possible disease threats is a key part of the health planning review.

Particularly for lambs in their first grazing season, enteric parasites are a problem, with control attempted largely by pasture rotation and strategic or responsive anthelmintic dosing. Adult stock may require dosing to reduce pasture burdens and, in wetter areas, where the intermediate snail host is present, the control of liver fluke is important. When dosing groups of animals it is important to batch animals according to weight and set the dose for the heaviest animal in the group; under-dosing results in reduced efficacy and encourages resistance to develop. A liver fluke forecast may be available to help with strategic actions; the effects of climate change mean that with warmer, wetter conditions in the UK, fascioliasis can now be seen at almost any time of the year. Sheep dogs should be wormed regularly to control tapeworm. Prophylactic foot care (including regular foot bathing) also needs to be programmed into the cycle and also undertaken when levels of lameness exceed action thresholds. The timing of treatments against ectoparasites is the most variable and dependent upon seasonal conditions.

5.13.2 Flock biosecurity

In general terms, biosecurity concerns the prevention of introduction of new diseases to the farm and the spread of disease on the farm. This can be achieved principally through regulation of the arrival of replacement stock or contact with neighbouring sheep through fences, but also through the movement of humans (e.g. stockpersons attending gatherings where sheep are present). For flocks sharing common grazing or where animal contact commonly occurs, it is sensible for adjoining properties to have broadly similar policies for mutual benefit. Disease can also arrive via a number of other routes – for example, wind-born spread of foot-and-mouth disease virus. Biosecurity may be practised within the farm with different groups of sheep of different disease status or at increased risk of disease. Biosecurity also concerns the export of disease agents from the farm to neighbouring properties and the control of diseases transmissible to humans. The safe disposal of dead animals and the products of lambing must be considered and appropriate arrangements put in place.

The fewer new sheep introductions the better. It is vital that new arrivals undergo a quarantine period to allow surveillance for diseases in incubation, performance of

Table 5.8 An example of indicative timing for some basic preventive actions in a northern hemisphere, spring-lambing flock.

Month and key events	Preventive action
October – mating	
November	Bluetongue vaccination within the vector-free period
December	Check for fluke eggs
January	Booster vaccination for pregnant sheep: costridial disease/pasteurellosis
February	Worming of ewes before move to clean pasture
March – lambing	Check for fluke eggs
April	Dip or spray ewes
May – shearing	Regular dosing of lambs for gut parasites if indicated – begin worm egg counts, depending on grazing
June	Ectoparasite control
July – weaning	Spraying/dipping/pour on against ectoparasites. Active foot care for all stock. Vaccination against abortion agents.
August	Pre-breeding inspections begin: feet, teeth, udders
September	Start replacement stock on clostridial/pneumonia vaccination programme. Booster vaccination for rams 4–6 weeks before mating

In tick areas, additional control measures will be needed. Liver fluke treatment to be added depending on risk factors and forecast. Strategic sampling will be required depending on specific disease risks e.g. internal parasites. Trace element monitoring may be indicated.

any screening checks and application of treatments such as vaccination, foot treatment or parasite control to bring new arrivals up to the same health status as resident animals. It is particularly important that anthelmintic-resistant worms and drug-resistant liver fluke are not introduced, through correct treatment during the quarantine period. Quarantine should be for at least 3 weeks, preferably 4. If possible, bought-in pregnant ewes should lamb separately from the main flock. The disease risk imposed by the arrival of new stock can be reduced through purchasing replacements from flocks of known disease status and which may be assured or monitored through a number of national schemes (e.g. enzootic abortion; Maedi-Visna; caseous lymphadenitis). However, for some diseases such as Johne's disease, it is impossible to be sure that incoming sheep are clear. Veterinary advice should be sought to maximize the value of the quarantine period. If quarantine arrangements are to be truly effective, stockpersons must adopt a high standard of cleanliness between handling incoming and resident animals, the latter usually being handled first in the working day.

For many 'closed' flocks it is often only rams that are brought in so the effort of applying a quarantine period is quantitatively reduced.

5.13.2.1 General hygiene

A high standard of general hygiene will minimize the opportunity for newly introduced diseases to spread around the farm. Simple cleaning methods and the use of an approved disinfectant should not be overlooked. It is particularly important to adopt a high standard of hygiene at lambing time when abortion agents are spread by foetuses and discharges from infected ewes, yet busy working conditions and long hours can militate against this. It is important to ensure cleaning and disinfection of lambing pens between occupants and the hygienic disposal of soiled bedding and the products of lambing. Fostering and rearing pens should also be kept in a hygienic condition. Thorough cleaning and disinfection are also required after de-stocking of buildings. This must include fixtures and fittings. Pressure washers make the work much less physically challenging and are very effective. Specific cleaning and disinfection regimes are required in cases of notifiable disease.

Hygienic practices should extend to keeping equipment clean, disinfected or sterilized and in good condition both during and after use – e.g. dosing guns and foot trimming shears. This also applies to the stockperson's protective clothing; wearing potentially contaminated work clothes and footwear in a domestic environment can put family members at risk. Vaccination equipment must be kept as clean as possible and needles changed at the recommended frequency as they can act as a route for disease spread and lead to abscess formation. Blunt needles are likely to damage the sheep and will cause unnecessary pain.

5.13.3 Vaccination

Vaccination to provide protection against a range of serious diseases should be considered as part of each flock's health plan. On organic units, specific approval for prophylactic vaccination will be required unless control is required as part of a statutory programme (e.g. bluetongue). The timing of primary and repeat vaccination needs to precede the peak risk periods and, for lambing ewes, booster vaccinations are given 2 to 4 weeks before lambing to maximize the antibody content of colostrum. It is important that ewes are handled calmly to avoid stress at this time. It is considered inadvisable to vaccinate rams in the 4–6-week period prior to tupping. Some vaccines should not be given concurrently, and advice should always be obtained as part of the flock health planning process.

5.13.4 Diseases with a significant impact on sheep welfare

While the presence of any disease will reduce the welfare status of an individual sheep, a number of specific disease entities are of major importance in the UK and around the world.

5.13.4.1 Lameness and foot care

Lameness in sheep can be due to a range of infectious and physical causes, though scald, classic foot rot and, recently, contagious ovine digital dermatitis (CODD) are most often responsible. Non-infectious causes include injuries, foreign bodies, laminitis, interdigital fibromas and congenital abnormalities (e.g. corkscrew-shaped claws). Sometimes, poor general body conformation may place abnormal load on the limbs. Exposure to a very high plane of nutrition such as a particularly lush pasture can result in laminitis, a painful inflammation of the sensitive laminae of the foot; affected animals can be lame in all four feet and rendered immobile due to the pain associated with this condition. Laminitis usually resolves once the plane of nutrition is lowered. Post-dipping lameness has sometimes been observed due to the build-up of *Erysipelothrix rhusiopathiae* organisms in the dipping solution.

Along with perinatal mortality, lameness probably represents the most important welfare problem for sheep both in terms of the impact on individual sheep and the sometimes high proportion of affected sheep in a flock. Lameness results in pain and suffering. It is a problem obvious to the public and one which attracts considerable concern. From an economic perspective, rams which are lame will not work efficiently and other individuals will exhibit suboptimum productivity so there is a financial penalty in addition to the welfare disbenefit. In the UK, most flocks struggle to keep lameness under control, sometimes despite a determined approach, and it is unrealistic to think that all lameness can be eliminated. Control rather than eradication is usually the goal. For effective control, an accurate veterinary diagnosis is first needed.

Some conditions such as interdigital granulomas ('strawberries') will require specific veterinary treatment but generally there is reliance on regular inspection with action as necessary. This often involves trimming (paring) the feet to approach what is deemed to be a normal conformation through the removal of overgrown or infected hoof horn. Correct trimming of a sheep's feet is a skilled action and is made much easier if the animal is held in a purpose-built turnover crate (Figure 5.6), enabling the stockperson to concentrate on trimming, not restraining. Overzealous

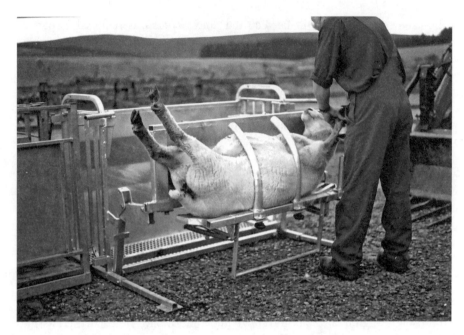

Figure 5.6 Stockperson attending to a sheep's feet using a turnover crate. Photograph by permission of Bob Ritchie.

foot trimming can be harmful and may lead to increased lameness in the flock. If bleeding occurs this indicates that the sensitive structures of the foot have been damaged. Sheep will be lame as a result of the pain and a route for infection has been created. Interdigital toe granulomas may form where the foot has been damaged. It is not necessary to draw blood to demonstrate that trimming has been sufficient. All those responsible for trimming a sheep's feet must be suitably trained to protect sheep welfare. To aid trimming, the feet should be clean, which can be achieved by the sheep first walking through a suitable footbath which can incorporate brushes. Foot shears or knives must be disinfected between animals as the organisms causing foot rot can be spread easily (it is also best to leave the most infected sheep until last). There are different views about the necessity for and value of routinely trimming feet in the absence of a specific need.

Sheep should pass regularly through a footbath containing formalin or, more commonly, zinc sulfate solution. (Formalin is usually supplied as a 40% solution of formaldehyde in water and requires further dilution before use on-farm.) Formalin solution, even as a 3% solution for routine use, can cause pain to the sheep, particularly if sensitive tissues are exposed by paring, and sheep may rush through baths with a leg held up, thus minimizing contact with the solution. (Formalin is potentially harmful to humans too and so the concentrate in particular must be handled with care.) Zinc sulfate (10% solution) is less painful but, to be effective, sheep with foot disease need to stand in the solution for up to 15–30 minutes to ensure adequate penetration of the hoof horn (surfactants to improve penetration may be added). Both solutions need to be kept clean and of adequate concentration. The efficacy of formalin is affected by the presence of organic matter. Manufacturers' recommendations for concentration of baths, and the safe use and disposal of chemicals, must be followed. In many systems, sheep are regularly put through footbaths and it is helpful to have an arrangement which cleans the feet of mud first before the bath is entered. This allows maximum exposure of the hoof to the solution. After bathing, sheep should have access to a dry standing area.

Sheep with evidence of infection in the foot should be identified for rigorous action (which may include effective antibiotic treatment), isolation from other stock and early culling if treatment is ineffective. Occasionally a high proportion of the flock will appear lame, sometimes after exposure to abrasive stubble or similar, with abrasion to the interdigital skin which is moist and painful. This condition of scald, ovine interdigital dermatitis (OID), one of the commonest forms of lameness, is caused by *Fusobacterium necrophorum* and is seen in warm, wet conditions, especially if the grass is long. Treatment can be frustrating and often involves weekly footbaths.

Foot rot is another widespread disease causing lameness in sheep. A large number of flocks in the UK experience lameness due to foot rot. It often starts as scald, with the subsequent invasion of a second bacterium, *Dichelobacter nodosus*. Delay in diagnosis and treatment can lead to prolonged pain, slow recovery and possibly irreparable damage to the foot and increases the level of disease in the environment. Chronic foot rot, through alterations in neurological mechanisms involved with pain, can result in sheep becoming hyperalgesic, responding to a noxious stimulus in an exaggerated way. Studies have shown that use of non-steroidal anti-inflammatory drugs (NSAIDs) may be useful in reducing this effect. Sheep with chronic lameness should be culled on welfare grounds. The flock health plan should identify management actions (including the use of a vaccine) to control the incidence and severity of foot rot. Since the organisms responsible are easily spread, adequate consideration must be given to how raceways or handling areas may act as a reservoir of infection. The flock can be split into groups of different foot rot prevalence so less affected animals can be handled first and chronically affected sheep can be identified for culling. On the other hand, sheep showing sound feet and natural resistance to foot rot should be retained for selective breeding.

Recently, a severe form of lameness, CODD, has been identified as a condition distinct from foot rot, with infection first apparent at the coronary band, then spreading down the hoof. Veterinary advice should be sought to ensure an accurate diagnosis is made and correct treatment applied.

5.13.4.2 Internal parasites

Strategies to control parasites in the intestinal tract and liver should be one of the major components of flock health planning. There is not space here to explore fully the various factors which should form part of a control programme. The most important elements are: sound pasture management in relation to nematode parasite epidemiology; the use of faecal egg counts (to assess worm burdens) which can be conducted on-farm using proprietary kits; selection for breeding of animals with greatest genetic resistance; and, lastly, the strategic use of anthelmintic treatments. The use of rams with resistance to worms can be achieved through estimated breeding values for faecal egg counts. While oral dosing of sheep (Figure 5.7) with liquid anthelmintics is a straightforward task, it does need to be done carefully to avoid damaging the pharyngeal area of the mouth.

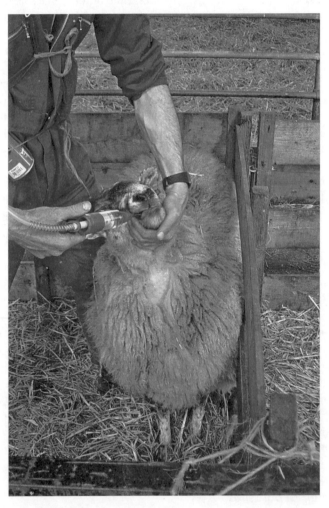

Figure 5.7 Administration of an anthelmintic drench to a ewe using a properly calibrated dosing gun. Photograph by permission of Kay Aitchison.

Lambs in their first grazing season are at greatest risk of nematode infection. Not only will disease lead to health and welfare concerns but lambs with a high worm burden will not thrive. Strategic worming of ewes is also needed as they show a periparturient rise in worm egg output which can lead to the contamination of early grazing. Maximizing the use of clean grazing (land not used for sheep since the last season, or used previously for hay or silage crops) or rotational grazing with cattle is possible on some lowland farms. However, some parasites can remain a threat from year to year, particularly *Nematodirus* species which are a threat to 6–10-week-old lambs eating increasing amounts of grass. Changing climatic patterns have resulted in a northerly extension in the range of parasites such as *Haemonchus contortus*. Tapeworms are generally controlled by adherence to regimes for nematodes and regularly worming farm dogs. The protozoon parasites, *Coccidia* spp, can cause particular problems in lambs of 4 to 6 weeks of age where there is a rapid increase in infectious organisms from older to younger lambs, particularly if the lambing period is extended, before natural immunity develops. *Cryptosporidium parvum* affects younger lambs and is a zoonosis.

Primarily as a result of worm-induced diarrhoea, sheep with soiled perineal areas are more prone to blowfly attack and fly strike (cutaneous myiasis). The necessity for tail-docking of lambs may be reduced if worm control strategies led to reduced faecal soiling. Given the seriousness of poorly controlled parasitic disease, a number of initiatives have been developed to provide targeted advice on control strategies. For example, the Sustainable Control of Parasites in Sheep (SCOPS) programme aims to provide an overall control strategy with less reliance on anthelmintics. This is particularly important as there is widespread resistance to many of the currently available wormers. Resistance is more likely to develop if sheep receive a suboptimal dose: when treating a group of sheep, always adjust the dosing gun in relation to the weight of the heaviest sheep in the group and ensure that the dosing gun itself has been calibrated accurately. Anthelmintics can be grouped into three main families based on their active principles. On veterinary advice, products from these families can be used together or on an annual rotation but on some properties multiple resistance means that none of these is entirely effective.

5.13.4.3 Ectoparasites

One of the major ectoparasitic diseases affecting sheep welfare is sheep scab, caused by the mite, *Psoroptes ovis*. The mite's abrasive mouthparts inflict an intensely irritating bite to the sheep's skin, causing the sheep to rub, leading to self-inflicted injury. Thus one of the first signs of scab is patchy fleece loss and rubbing against fixed objects. The disease is most prevalent in the autumn and winter and can be easily diagnosed by looking at a skin scraping taken from an active border of the lesion. While the sheep is the permanent host to the mite, suggesting that control might be straightforward, the ability of the mite to remain viable in the environment and the sometimes less-than-complete efficacy of treatment results in persistence and spread of infection. In the UK, a national control policy had reduced the incidence through a coordinated treatment across all flocks. Since scab ceased to be a notifiable disease a large rise in disease incidence has occurred which is now being brought in check through a number of local initiatives which aim to ensure coordinated treatment. The SCOPS programme is also targeting widespread eradication programmes. Some injectable agents are available to treat or protect sheep against mites but many flocks rely on immersion dipping with organophosphorus (OP) compounds. The use of OPs has been questioned on human heath grounds (and health and welfare impacts on the sheep too) and strict measures are needed to reduce human exposure, with stringent requirements for the safe disposal of spent dip. Synthetic pyrethroid compounds are also effective but since the beginning of 2010 cypermethrin sheep dip products are no longer available in the UK.

A range of other ectoparasites affect sheep and cause stress, have a considerable nuisance value and can transmit important diseases (e.g. the sheep tick (*Ixodes ricinus*) which transmits louping ill virus, lice, keds and mange mites). Of particular note are the greenbottle (*Lucilia sericata*) and bluebottle (*Calliphora* spp.) which are the major cause of fly strike/cutaneous myiasis, the most commonly reported ectoparasite problem in many flocks. Regular inspection of sheep around periods of fly activity is crucial in order to identify affected sheep for immediate treatment. Blowfly eggs are laid on moist, faecally contaminated wool, usually around the tail area. When these eggs hatch the larvae (maggots) burrow into the sheep leading to large ulcerated areas, subject to secondary infection. Fly strike is more common in warm, wet areas and when sheep are more tightly stocked. It is a life-threatening condition and can lead to significant losses. To control a range of ectoparasitic conditions, strategic dipping, spraying or topical, 'spot-on' or pour-on treatments are used to coincide with local risk periods. Showers and spraying races have not yet been shown to be as efficacious as plunge dipping for complete control but are used in many countries. If lambs at foot are dipped along with their dams, it is important to handle them carefully and ensure proper mothering after dipping, when olfactory cues will be disrupted. Dipping to control ectoparasites is stressful and should not take place if sheep are hot, thirsty, wet, tired or fully fed. Sheep should not be dipped during the hottest period of the day.

5.13.4.4 Mastitis

Mastitis (inflammation of the mammary gland) in sheep often goes undiagnosed until a pre-breeding inspection. Since mastitis occurs mainly in the first month of lactation, it should be suspected if lambs fail to thrive as milk production will be affected. It is more commonly seen in lowland flocks. Ewes with clinical mastitis can become systemically ill and require prompt treatment to reduce inflammation and restore lactation. On inspection, the udder will be swollen, hardened, hot and inflamed, often with superficial purple discolouration, and only watery fluid may be drawn from the teat. This is a severe condition and even some treated ewes may die or ultimately lose, through sloughing, the affected part of the udder. Milk production will be lost for the current season and the udder may be permanently damaged. Unfortunately affected sheep may often go undetected and so untreated. Subclinical mastitis is also responsible for significant problems for sheep, again including poor lamb growth. Since the organisms responsible may be spread in the environment, for housed ewes in particular, a high standard of hygiene must be employed and ewes with mastitis should be segregated from other sheep. Selection of ewes based on mastitis resistance is rarely practised.

5.13.4.5 Zoonoses

Zoonotic diseases are those capable of being transmitted from animals to humans. Sheep can carry a number of zoonotic infections, many of which are prevalent at around lambing time. As with any diseases of this nature, immunocompromised individuals are more at risk but, in particular, pregnant women represent a high-risk group in terms of the potential impact of diseases causing abortion in sheep. A number of diseases may be acquired following contact with sheep and sheep tissues including tissue fluids, or through ingestion of infected meat or milk, offal or meat products. For untreated wool coming from some countries, anthrax may be a risk. Any sheep with enteritis could be carrying *Salmonella* spp. or other zoonotic organisms such as *Campylobacter* spp. and *Cryptosporidium parvum*.

The highest-risk materials are the products of abortion or infected lambings – foetal fluids, afterbirths and the lambs themselves (even if lambs are viable). Since abortion due to *Chlamydophila abortus* can occur from some weeks before lambing and ewes with infection (and the products of abortion) may remain infectious for some time after, it is recommended that pregnant women (and those attempting to become pregnant) should not work with sheep. Disease organisms can be carried on protective clothing and so stockpersons with pregnant women in their household must be very careful. Disease symptoms in humans can range from flu-like signs through to life-threatening placentitis, foetal abortion, metritis and possibly disseminated intravascular coagulation (DIC).

Enzootic abortion of ewes (EAE), caused by *Chlamydophila abortus*, is the most commonly diagnosed type of abortion in sheep (stockpersons should aim for <2% abortion in the flock and instigate investigations if this is exceeded). It is spread from infected and susceptible sheep at lambing time through the products of an infected birth. Aborting sheep become immune thereafter. Sheep infected for the first time will abort at the next lambing. Abortion 'storms' can occur when infection is introduced and spread in a naïve flock. Thereafter around a third of ewes could abort annually. If sheep abort sufficiently far in advance of lambing it is possible for sheep infected at that time to abort during that pregnancy – a risk which can be reduced by the use of prophylactic antibiotic on a whole-flock basis. While a tentative diagnosis can be made by eye (since infected afterbirths show a characteristic, 'leathery' thickening between the cotyledons) it is important that, especially for early abortions or where a number of ewes abort in a season, a definitive diagnosis is made if possible since more than one abortion agent may be present. All afterbirths, dead lambs and contaminated bedding should be carefully disposed of as indicated in the farm's biosecurity plan. Maintaining a closed flock or purchasing replacement females from certified EAE-free sources is one way to avoid abortion through this cause. Alternatively a highly effective live vaccine is available in the UK which is administered to susceptible animals (primarily gimmers entering the breeding flock) prior to mating. The vaccine can also cause illness in humans and should not be administered by pregnant women.

Toxoplasmosis, caused by *Toxoplasma gondii*, a protozoan parasite, is another common cause of abortion in sheep. Toxoplasma has a complex life cycle involving a final host – usually the cat – and an intermediate host – the sheep. Young cats usually have a high shedding rate. There is not thought to be inter-sheep transmission. A vaccine, administered prior to mating, is available for use in flocks where toxoplasmosis is a problem. While humans may contract disease at lambing time, it is more likely due to the exposure of pregnant women to infected raw meat (through either handling or consumption) or the organisms present in cat faeces. A relatively high proportion of the UK population shows serological evidence of exposure.

Salmonella spp., *Campylobacter* spp. and a number of other organisms can cause abortion or enteritis in sheep and result in zoonotic disease.

Orf (contagious pustular dermatitis) is a viral disease causing skin lesions, and lesions at junctions of the skin and mucous membranes, for example, around the mouth of lambs. This results in transmission to the ewe's teats and udder. Orf can also affect the lower limbs and genitalia and can lead to ill thrift. In cases of severe infection, a live vaccine should be considered. Humans can experience, sometimes, quite severe lesions following exposure to both field cases and the vaccine and so should be careful to wear protective gloves when handling affected sheep or administering vaccine. The virus can remain viable in the environment for a considerable period.

In some areas of the world, *Brucella melitensis* causes human disease, mostly through the consumption of unpasteurized milk and milk products.

5.13.4.6 Notifiable diseases

A number of diseases of ruminants are defined as 'notifiable', requiring notification of suspicion to the competent authorities who will instigate an investigation. Prior to reaching a definitive diagnosis, the farm holding will be placed in quarantine, recent animal and human movements may be traced and surrounding premises may also be subject to movement restrictions, the extent of which depends on the disease. If disease is confirmed, a range of actions may ensue including slaughter of stock and thorough cleaning and disinfection. After a rest period, re-stocking is usually permitted. Notifiable diseases of relevance to sheep in the UK are foot and mouth disease, bluetongue, anthrax and scrapie.

5.14 Routine Husbandry Procedures

5.14.1 The balance of welfare benefit

Some 'routine' husbandry procedures are applied to all animals in a flock in order to prevent a number of animals (but possibly not all of them) from experiencing a particular problem. The potential welfare benefit (to some) and the likely disbenefit (to all) need to be weighed. While the 'cost' is always to the individual sheep, the 'benefit' may not be so easy to assign. It can be argued that when the benefit of any management action is focused on the individual sheep (e.g. treatment of injury or disease) the welfare cost can be more easily justified. When the benefit is primarily to the enterprise (e.g. transport or slaughter) the welfare cost imposed on the individual sheep, arguably, should be less than in situations where sheep might receive some benefit. Describing some procedure as 'routine' does not absolve the stockperson from the need to critically evaluate whether there is a need for the procedure to be undertaken, especially when a common generic description for some such activities is 'mutilation'. For example, it may be possible to stop castrating male lambs which, through correct nutrition, could reach market weight before reproductive precocity was a problem, or reduce the incidence of fly myiasis through proper control of gut parasites rather than relying on tail docking to partially mitigate the effects.

5.14.2 General handling

The interaction between the stockperson and individual sheep in a flock is key to ensuring a high standard of health and welfare. Handling should only be undertaken by those with sufficient knowledge and skill to understand and work with the normal behavioural characteristics of sheep, in order to reduce the stress inevitably associated with handling procedures. Handling facilities designed from the sheep's perspective will make working with sheep much easier, so enhancing both sheep welfare and stockperson job ease and satisfaction. Stockpersons must have a working knowledge of the relevant guidelines which explain the legal and recommended requirements to be followed (e.g. *Codes of Recommendations for the Welfare of Livestock*). Stockpersons must also be conversant with the additional health and welfare requirements of local marketing or farm assurance schemes.

Depending on their temperament and familiarity with the stockperson, individual sheep can be caught, either in the field or in a large pen, with the aid of a crook to hook the sheep above the hock. If sheep are too flighty to approach they will need to be herded into a small handling pen, which can be of a temporary nature in the corner of a field or gateway. Sheep can then be held by placing, for example, the open left hand under the lower jaw, raising the head slightly and, having manoeuvred the sheep to a convenient position, using the right leg to hold the sheep against a solid object. While the horns can be employed to steady an adult sheep of a horned breed, this should not be done with younger animals since the horns can be seriously damaged. Sheep must not be caught and manhandled by their fleece as this will cause pain and bruising; if this is done immediately prior to slaughter the carcass may be downgraded.

For some activities it is necessary to cast a sheep – tipping it over to rest with its hindquarters on the ground and its back against the stockperson. In this position, most sheep tend not to struggle and procedures such as foot trimming and removing soiled wool from around the breech (dagging) can be accomplished single-handed. However, if a large number of sheep are to be examined on a regular basis, it is preferable to invest in a turning crate. This is probably less stressful for the sheep (which is securely restrained) and allows the stockperson to concentrate attention and energy on the task itself. Sheep which are to be sheared still require to be handled manually. There are a number of methods of casting in which a skilful manipulation of the sheep should be substituted for large amounts of energy! Light sheep are usually cast by a lifting method whereby the handler (on the left side of the sheep) standing against the sheep and with the left hand controlling the head, leans across, and holding the sheep by a fold of skin and wool in the area in front of the right stifle, lifts the hind leg off the ground. At the same time, pressure from the handler's knees against the left hind leg prevents the sheep from bracing itself and the sheep can easily be turned to rest between the handler's knees. For heavier sheep, the process starts in the same way but with the right hand under the tail. By bringing the head and hindquarters together the sheep eventually falls onto its left side and can then be rolled up on to its rump in the same way. It is not advisable to restrain late pregnant ewes in this position for long periods.

5.14.2.1 Gathering and moving sheep

One common underpinning need in any sheep system is to move animals between grazing areas or to collect them together for selection or other husbandry treat-ments. For hill flocks, gathering is a major exercise sometime involving the collaborative efforts of a number of local farms whose sheep share the same open hill. The use of well-trained herding dogs is essential – a poorly trained dog has the potential to completely disrupt the activity and lead to panic amongst the sheep. The advent of four-wheel-drive motorbikes has facilitated the task of gathering but, since there is the potential to increase the speed of the gather, it is all the more important to be aware of fatigue in the flock if gathering is over a long distance or of a long duration (often many hours). In the same way, gathers on hot days are often avoided but, if necessary, must be conducted in such a way that sheep do not become fatigued and dehydrated. Similarly, dogs should not be allowed to harass straggling individuals or those at the back of a large mob whose forward movement is restricted by stationary sheep. Sheep should be given the opportunity to dem-onstrate their innate following ability, which is thwarted if they are rushed too much. Thus gathering by stockpersons, whether on foot or using a vehicle, can be a difficult task if sheep welfare is not to be compromised. Because of the labour element required and the potential loss of production or injury to sheep that occurs on each occasion, in large, extensive flocks, gathering is limited to only a few occasions each year – with the corollary that more may be done to individual sheep on each occasion. If ewes with lambs at foot are to be gathered, additional time must be allowed; if the lamb cannot keep up with the ewe she will usually turn back and make the overall process more difficult. In some situations, supplementary feed may be on offer and ewes and lambs will be attracted by the sight and sound of a rustled feed sack or rattled bucket.

Because of the natural following behaviour of sheep, young ewes introduced to the main flock will follow the behaviour of older animals. This following trait has been used to facilitate the movement of animals through an abattoir raceway system by the use of trained 'Judas' sheep which have learnt the route. In some countries there is a restriction on keeping resident sheep at the abattoir on animal health grounds.

5.14.2.2 Handling facility design

The design of and construction materials used for handling facilities are varied, depending on need. Most sheep farms need at least one purpose-built handling system (Figure 5.8). This must be designed with a sound knowledge of sheep behaviour in mind and must also take into account the need to work, sometimes, in bad weather conditions and the need to allow adequate cleaning and disinfection as part of the farm's biosecurity arrangements. Thus these areas benefit from a solid surface which allows the sheep to stand on a clean substrate and with pens built of materials which are easily cleaned and do not tend to harbour disease organisms. Since sheep find

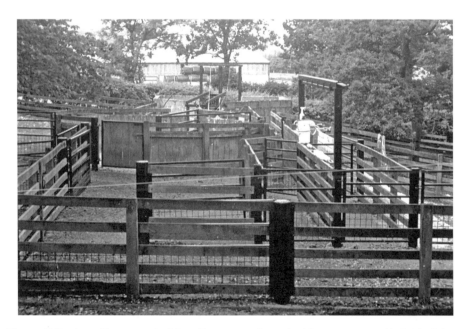

Figure 5.8 A small, purpose-built handling system. Pens, shedding raceway and individual sheep handling area are to the right. It is difficult to thoroughly disinfect wood. Photograph by permission of Kate Phillips.

isolation aversive, the pens should allow as much visual contact as possible and the working methods should minimize the times when sheep are isolated. In yards and buildings, sheep are easily disturbed by shadows and loud noises. Individual handling is also stressful to the sheep and most common practices such as dosing, vaccination or condition scoring do not require individual isolation and can be conducted in small pens or raceways with the stockperson working alongside.

It is desirable that as much of the area as possible be covered to allow work to be conducted in the dry and to prevent sheep becoming overheated in the summer under the direct sun. At the very least, the handling area needs to be sheltered.

Handling systems should include a gathering pen, of sufficient size to accommodate the largest mob, a way of easily encouraging sheep into smaller pens (such as some form of crowding gate), a raceway system by which sheep can be moved from these smaller pens and a working area where, for example, husbandry treatments are applied. Arrangements which funnel sheep towards passageways where they can see the sheep ahead facilitate a smooth flow. Conversely, sharp corners (which can cause bruising injuries) or apparent dead ends impede natural movement patterns. Handling systems usually incorporate a footbath, the size of which will depend on whether a walk-through or a stand-in protocol is adopted. There is often an immersion dip and draining area, though requirements imposed by environmental authorities for the safe disposal of spent dip have resulted in an increase in the number of self-contained contractor services. Finally, there need to be shedding arrangements and release pens. Some handling systems incorporate a loading area and ramp. For more information on the subject of handling and facility design, readers are referred to Grandin (2007).

5.14.3 Identification

A number of temporary or permanent identification and marking methods are used for sheep. These include, tattooing, horn branding, electronic identification (EID), ear tags (metal or plastic) of a variety of designs, ear notching, aerosol marker sprays and colour marking (e.g. raddle). The use of these is dictated by national, breed society and individual flock owner requirements. In order to help trace where animals have come from and to aid in control of the spread of animal diseases in the UK, it is necessary for sheep-keepers to register with their local animal health office. Animals that are not properly identified may not be allowed into the food chain. In the UK requirements include that sheep born after January 2008 need two identifiers if they are not intended for slaughter before 12 months of age or will be exported. (One identifier can be a tattoo for animals not for export.) Currently, a single UK tag can be applied if an animal is intended for slaughter in the UK before 12 months of age (usually the left ear is tagged).

Commonly, metal or plastic tags of a number of designs are placed in the lower ear margin, avoiding major blood vessels or cartilaginous ridges. When using closed loop tags in young animals, allowance must be made for the growth of the ear. The plastic 'flap' type tag is often preferred. When fitting two-piece plastic tags, the male part of the tag is fitted from the back of the ear as centrally as possible. There is a variation in the retention rate and the damage to the ear on insertion, and so tags should be chosen carefully and those inserting tags should be suitably trained. Equipment must be kept in good working order and regularly cleaned to ensure that infection is not transmitted between animals. It is best practice to apply tags in cooler weather to avoid fly nuisance or possible fly strike and infection; hygienic measures might include the application of insecticide.

In the UK a phased introduction of the EU requirement for individual sheep recording is planned. Coupled with this is the introduction of electronic identification (EID) which has recently become available using a special ear tags. Subcutaneous implants, usually placed at the base of the ear or, much less commonly, intra-ruminal boluses are also available. One disadvantage of implanted or intra-ruminal EID is that there is no visual element. Providing unique identification, these electronic tags require the use of a hand-held reader or a device which can be incorporated into the weighing crate of a handling system. This allows information to be collected automatically for downloading to a farm's management database.

5.14.4 Transport

Sheep are transported regularly for management and trade purposes. It is generally accepted that transport, even under optimal conditions, is stressful to the sheep and thus should be minimized. The containers used are as varied as are the distances involved – from one or more ewes and lambs in a trailer towed around the farm by a four-wheel-drive motorbike to large numbers of market-weight sheep transported in pens in the holds of ships between Australia and the Middle East. It is important that, when assessing the welfare impact of the overall transport process, all elements be considered – from the initial collection, possible movement through a market during a journey break, and novelty following arrival at the final destination, often an abattoir lairage.

It is a widely supported view that the long-distance transport of slaughter sheep should cease in favour of moving frozen or chilled products. Within Europe, there are considerable movements of live sheep to satisfy particular seasonal demands – for example, from Poland to meet the Easter demand for sheep in Italy. Long-distance transport can cause many problems for sheep and potentially compromises all of the five freedoms; it is unequivocally to the detriment of sheep welfare. Much of the long-distance trade by sea of around 4 million sheep annually is to satisfy religious requirements for Halal slaughter, yet this could be undertaken in the country of origin – and some arrangements of this nature have been made to provide Halal-certified meat. Sometimes large numbers of live sheep are required for religious festivals and this requirement can only be reduced through negotiation. For sheep which are not killed immediately on arrival, the environmental conditions may also be aversive to them. Welfare considerations should include a number of pre-shipment practices – gathering, shearing and collection in feedlots to accustom them to transport conditions, including feeding from troughs. These alone can introduce a range of environmental and psychological stressors. During the sea journey, mortality can be high, though has declined over recent years following the introduction of veterinary standards. The main problems leading to mortality are failure to eat, salmonellosis and heat stress. (Heat stress occurs when poorly adapted sheep fail to cope with a high heat load, despite panting and other short-term heat-reducing physiological changes.)

Inter-country or inter-region transport of any livestock has the potential to introduce exotic disease (the rate of shedding of organisms by infected animals increases too) and to make individual transported animals more susceptible to disease through the negative effect of stress on the immune system. In addition, the increased contact between unfamiliar animals increases the opportunity for disease to spread. For this reason and because of the general welfare disbenefit, the European Food Safety Authority notes that transport should be avoided wherever possible and journeys should be as short as possible. In many countries, there has been considerable public pressure to end live animal export and to slaughter animals as close to the point of production as possible.

Within the EU, there are comprehensive rules relating to distances, journey duration and transport conditions, but enforcing the legislation is demanding on resources. There are requirements for vehicle design in relation to materials (e.g. non-slip flooring), and operation (e.g. ventilation systems and hygiene measures). In many cases (depending on journey distance) a route plan is required which should allow for contingencies such as delays or injury to any of the animals. In the UK, implementation of the EU transport regulations means that in 'basic' standard vehicles, the maximum journey time is 8 hours. In vehicles of higher specification, the maximum journey time for adult sheep is 14 hours' travel, at least 1 hour of rest (and the provision of water – and feed if deemed necessary) and then a further 14 hours' travel. In particular circumstances the journey can extend a further 2 hours if close to the destination at the end of the prescribed time. Otherwise a 24-hour rest period must follow before further transport is possible. The regulations, currently under review, should be consulted for more specific information. Rules also include an assessment of driver competence; it has been shown that one of the main impacts on the welfare of transported sheep is the care with which a vehicle is driven, e.g. avoiding rapid acceleration and sharp cornering in order that sheep may more easily retain their balance. This reduces energy demand (and possible fatigue) and the chance of injury. The road quality is also important and drivers should avoid minor or unmade roads with many corners. Drivers should receive bonuses related to the condition of sheep on arrival, not for minimizing journey duration. Driver liability for slaughter losses (e.g. bruising injury sustained during shipment will reduce carcass value) could also be an effective mechanism to improve welfare.

In addition to driving quality, the care taken on loading and unloading will have a major impact on sheep welfare. Sheep should be allowed to load at their own pace and this is encouraged by the provision of suitable handling pens and loading bays. Where sheep are regularly loaded, it is worth constructing a simple ramp to allow the sheep to walk on a level surface into a livestock vehicle. When it is necessary to manhandle individual sheep they must not be pulled or dragged by their fleece, and if on the rare occasion they need to be lifted, this can be done (providing the sheep is not too heavy for the handler) by holding the sheep by the flank area with one hand and the other under the jaw and pulling back towards the handler's body, taking the weight of the sheep.

Fitness to travel for the whole journey also needs to be assured prior to departure. This is a particular issue for many cast-age ewes, some of which should be euthanized on-farm. All sheep should be afforded the same care during transport. In many areas, the closure of local abattoirs has a negative welfare consequence as even cull animals have to undergo increasingly long journeys. Closure also thwarts the public desire to establish transparent local production chains. Major meat buyers have the power to encourage more local production and abattoir facilities (reversing this closure trend) and the enforcement and enhancement of standards.

5.14.5 Markets

Livestock markets present sheep with a range of novel experiences, many of which may be stressful. There are often many humans in close proximity to pens and raceways, the market can be very noisy and feed and water may be unavailable. Standards for droving – moving animals around the market – must ensure that animals are given the opportunity to move at their own pace. Drovers must be properly trained and be experienced in responding to sheep behaviour and not use excessive force. There must be adequate provision for the care of sick or injured sheep and all facilities must be well-designed and maintained to prevent injury and the build-up of disease organisms. Certain classes of sheep are marketed separately to preserve their disease-free status. A range of agencies have representatives at markets to ensure animal welfare but it is not always entirely clear who is explicitly responsible. Because of the high visibility of market activities, it is in everyone's interest to ensure that standards of animal welfare are maintained at a high level.

While markets may be required to set a price for classes of livestock and to batch up small numbers of animals, it is preferable if animals for slaughter go directly from farm to abattoir. For breeding stock, Internet sales have a useful place. This mechanism also reduces the opportunity for disease transmission. Internet marketing is more attractive as purchasers place greater weight on performance records rather than phenotypic appearance.

5.14.6 Shearing

Shearing presents a cluster of aversive elements, from gathering, penning, possible food and water deprivation, individual handling and the immediate shearing process. Individual animal care is difficult to deliver when large mobs of sheep are handled in a situation which is stressful for the handlers too. While wool in some countries is a valuable commodity, in others the value is sometimes too low to offset the shearing cost. In these situations, shearing is undertaken primarily to protect sheep welfare and as a result there is increasing interest in using breeds of sheep with a natural propensity to shed their fleece in the summer. Failure to shear sheep on an annual basis due to economic pressures can lead to welfare problems (e.g. greater risk of ectoparasitic disease or the inability to regain their footing if they become cast with a heavy, wet fleece).

An average yield for a wool breed of sheep (e.g. Merino) is around 8 kg but for a hill breed could be as little as 2 kg. There is a gradation in price premium: as wool becomes finer a price premium is generally paid. Fine-wool breeds grow wool of less than 24 μm in diameter. Wool is the main output from the Australian sheep industry. The power of international animal activist groups to influence the market has led to concerns that sheep numbers in Australia could decline dramatically if designers refuse to buy wool from sheep subject to conventional mulesing (see Section 5.14.8).

The whole process from gathering to wool removal has to be designed to be as 'sheep-friendly' as possible. Wool removal itself appears to be the most stressful component overall. Shearing must be conducted skilfully to minimize injuries to sheep (primarily cuts from the shears). Some stockpersons house sheep the night before shearing to ensure that fleeces are dry. Shearing should not be undertaken on days when adverse weather is forecast, particularly if undertaken early in the season when shorn sheep can become severely chilled and may even die. Thought should be given to the need to provide short-term shelter for such sheep. Winter shearing of sheep prior to housing allows animals to be kept at a lower space allowance (especially at the feeding face) and facilitates supervision at lambing but must not be undertaken in the absence of housing. An appropriate comb leaving a covering of wool on the sheep should be used. Winter-shorn sheep should not be turned out until at least 15–20 mm of fleece has regrown. Housing alone can be stressful to sheep and 'wool slip', a partial baldness, may occur as a result of the combined stressors of shearing and housing.

5.14.7 Castration

Castration, one of the major mutilations and a painful husbandry procedure of male lambs, has been the subject of considerable public concern and research effort. Before considering which method to employ, the need for castration must be questioned seriously since many systems have the capacity to produce market-weight lambs before sexual development and behaviour become problematic. However, the presence of sexually active young males could lead to major welfare problems through indiscriminate breeding and the resultant uncoordinated lambing and the birth of lambs with poor survival chances. Unplanned mating of immature females may adversely affect their welfare. Groups of uncastrated male lambs with insufficient space may fight and injure each other. Castrated adult males are easier to handle than entires, and with the increase in conservation grazing there is a demand for such wether sheep. In some situations meat from older, castrated males is desired by the market. Entire young animals grow faster but may be harder to finish (fatten). Almost half of the male lambs in New Zealand are left entire – probably because of the extensive production system, also found increasingly in many other countries.

Since castration is a management action primarily for the benefit to the enterprise, it should only be conducted when absolutely necessary and then with the least possible welfare disbenefit to the lamb.

Castration should be performed by a trained stockperson using the least aversive method. Some methods cause more suffering than others: surgical castration (removal of the testes) without the use of pain relief is considered worst by the Farm Animal Welfare Council. Methods are prescribed in legislation and are often time-limited. For example, in the UK the use of rubber elastrator rings applied around the scrotal neck is not permitted after 7 days of age – yet there is no evidence to support the implication that pain perception is less during the first week of life than at a later age. The restriction to the first 7 days presents problems in extensive hill flocks. In the UK, for lambs older than 3 months, an anaesthetic must be used and castration under-taken by a veterinary surgeon. Castration results in handling stress and acute and chronic pain. The extent of these varies with method and competence of the stock-person. While local anaesthetic could be used in some situations, it is not often applied and will not provide analgesia extending beyond the duration of the acute pain: in the case of rings this lasts for around 2 hours but will be followed by further pain and inflammation which can last until the affected tissues drop off. The availability of anti-inflammatory drugs and analgesics for sheep is generally poor and their use is not widespread; they are rarely, if ever, used following castration. A simple, efficacious analgesic protocol which stockpersons are willing to apply is urgently needed.

Although castration is sometimes delayed to allow the selection of breeding rams, the techniques are more usually applied to young lambs. Commonly, a rubber (elastrator) ring is applied around the neck of the scrotum to restrict the blood supply to the scrotum and its contents, which die and eventually drop off distal to the ring. This method results in acute and chronic pain. Rings can be applied by a single operator with the lamb sitting between the stockperson's knees. It is important not to catch excess skin or rudimentary teats in the ring. If only one testis is present, the lamb should not be castrated at this time. Short scrotum castration is also undertaken whereby the ring is applied distal to the testes to force them into the lamb's body, where increased temperature restricts sperm production. Rubber rings should not be used in the first 24 hours due to the risk that the resultant acute pain interferes with establishment of the ewe–lamb bond and reduces sucking. Another common approach is surgical, opening the scrotum with a sharp knife and removing the testes by traction. Every effort must be made to ensure a high standard of hygiene to prevent infection entering the open wound. This technique is best performed by two people, one responsible for holding the lamb, the other performing the technique in as clean a way as possible. Less commonly, the spermatic cords are crushed using a bloodless castration device (Burdizzo).

5.14.8 Tail docking

This procedure, another mutilation, involving removal of the distal part of the tail, is performed to reduce the risk of fly strike. It is again useful to attempt a cost–benefit analysis. A welfare disbenefit accrues to all sheep which are docked, yet the potential benefit is unpredictable as some sheep would never have suffered fly strike. However, strike is a serious, debilitating, sometimes life-threatening condition and represents an unacceptable welfare problem. Predisposing factors include soiled breech areas often as a result of heavy burdens of gut parasites. Thus good parasite control (e.g. through selection of sheep with genetic resistance to nematode parasites) is an effective way of reducing the chance of strike. Equally, effective prophylaxis against blowfly attack is important. Some breeds of sheep have reduced fleece in the breech area or shorter tails and selective breeding could be better employed to increase the penetration of these desirable traits. Tail docking is not practised in hill flocks, where the chance of myiasis is less and the tail provides additional protection against the cold.

Methods include the use of elastrator rings within the first week of life, cauterization using a hot docking iron, or the combination of Burdizzo and elastrator rings. Many lambs are docked surgically using a sharp knife. The pain and distress caused by tail docking is considered to be less than following castration. Enough tail must be left to cover the vulva in females and the anus in males.

For some Merino and Merino-type sheep bred with deep skin folds to increase skin surface area and thus yield of wool, the technique of mulesing has been adopted whereby some of the folded skin around the breech and tail regions is surgically removed. The contraction of resultant wool-free scar tissue reduces the chance of subsequent faecal soiling. The welfare cost to individuals of this procedure, usually undertaken without anaesthetic, is likely to be considerable (the existence of post-mulesing aversion to humans supports this) and mulesing has engendered considerable public opposition. Selective breeding of sheep with reduced fleece or less skin folding in this area is a solution to be exploited, together with selection of strains of sheep more resistant to internal parasites, as noted above. However, these measures may be insufficient, particularly during long spells of warm, wet weather. The current practice of surgical mulesing is planned to be phased out in Australia by the end of 2010 and alternative ways to prevent fly strike, such as injections to induce skin necrosis or plastic skin clips, are being investigated.

Dagging of sheep using clippers is undertaken to remove excess wool around the breech area, tail and down the inside of the hind limbs to discourage faecal soiling. It is often undertaken prior to shearing to ensure that a clean fleece can be produced for sale, but also on a more individual needs basis if excessive soiling is evident at any time. Dagging of ewes can be undertaken prior to mating and before lambing.

5.14.9 Slaughter

Methods of commercial slaughter and killing are prescribed by legislation in many countries. In every case the purpose is to spare sheep any avoidable excitement, pain or suffering during slaughter/killing and related operations inside and outside the slaughterhouse. This includes the period of lairage (holding in pens following arrival at the slaughterhouse); legislation prescribes provision of feed, water and bedding. The slaughter process itself should render the sheep insensible as rapidly as possible and ensure that death through exsanguination occurs before consciousness returns. Methods of slaughter include captive bolt, concussion and electro-narcosis. That slaughter and killing occur efficiently and consistently is dependent on the training and skill of all those handling sheep *ante-mortem*. In the UK, closure of local abattoirs can make it difficult to slaughter sheep close to the point of production.

5.14.9.1 Emergency slaughter

There may be situations in which a sheep that has sustained an injury or a disease has progressed to the point when slaughter is the most humane option. Although the presentation to an abattoir of some animals described as 'casualties' could be an option, very few sheep can go via this route in the UK – the unit's veterinary adviser should be consulted. For many animals suffering a traumatic injury, transport is not appropriate as it is likely to exacerbate pain and suffering.

The flock health and welfare plan should consider, in advance, the inevitable need to destroy sheep on-farm. Whatever method is selected needs to be quick and humane; to achieve this, stockpersons need to be trained, competent and confident. In most cases, the method of choice is to use a shotgun to shoot sheep at close range. It helps if the sheep is still at the time, which may be achieved by offering some feed. With adequate safety precautions to remove bystanders, the sheep should be shot from in front of the head, just above the eyes, with the gun's muzzle 15–30 cm in front of the head, pointing down the length of the neck. The muzzle must not be placed any closer to or in contact with the sheep, as serious personal injury could result. A rifle could be also used from around 5 cm from the sheep's head. For those with a slaughterman's licence, a captive bolt pistol could be used. The animal should then be promptly bled out to ensure rapid death. The carcass should be subject to hygienic disposal, e.g. via the national fallen stock scheme. (Note: in most of the UK, on-farm burial is no longer permitted.) The farm should have a suitable vermin- and leak-proof container for storage prior to collection. Planning emergency slaughter options should also be done by those transporting sheep.

For young lambs (up to 5 kg), stunning and bleeding out could be considered. Stunning is best achieved by swinging the lamb by its back legs and hitting its head as hard as possible on a solid object. It is important that the stockperson is not diffident about this and achieves an effective blow. Alternatively give a powerful blow to the back of the head. With evidence of unconsciousness, the lamb is bled by cutting across the neck behind the lower jaw, and deeply to the vertebrae in the neck to ensure that both pairs of jugular veins and carotid arteries are severed to result in rapid death through blood loss.

Emergency slaughter may be required in disease epidemic control operations. There is evidence that foetuses of killed ewes, even right before term, will not reach a conscious state unless they are able to breathe and increase significantly their cerebral oxygen tension; thus their welfare is not compromised during this process, even though foetal sense organs operate and reflex movement can be detected. Safeguards should be put in place to ensure that the foetuses of ewes slaughtered in late pregnancy do not have the opportunity to breathe.

5.14.9.2 Religious/ritual slaughter

Killing/slaughter as part of the production process is regulated by national legislation in most countries, to minimize distress to the individual sheep. There is concern that certain religious slaughter practices, without pre-stunning to render the sheep insensible, compromise welfare since sheep are likely to experience very significant pain and distress, a view supported by the Farm Animal Welfare Council. As yet the UK government has chosen not to withdraw the exemption for religious slaughter without pre-stunning, although some religious authorities have voluntarily adopted this approach.

5.15 Welfare Assessment in Sheep

5.15.1 Using available indicators

The move to focus on outcome-based indicators of animal wellbeing across the range of farm animal and companion species has gathered pace recently, yet in the sheep sector this approach is poorly developed. Although it is recognized that welfare relates to the individual, sheep stockpersons frequently refer to flock welfare. Table 5.9 gives some suggestions for the type of welfare outcome indicators which could currently be applied to sheep. Many indices rely on data already available for flock management purposes, including BCS, evaluated at key times in the production cycle. For example, any flock with a significant number of individuals at BCS of less than 2 (for lowland sheep) and 1.5 (for hill sheep) must be regarded as demonstrating inadequate care and welfare – this needs the qualification of time in the production cycle as a score of 1.5 during pregnancy would be disastrous; lowest scores are usually seen at the end of lactation. Setting of intervention levels in relation to a range of parameters should be part of flock health planning and may form part of a farm assurance scheme. Success requires those recording the data to 'buy in' to the system and understand the value of the extra work involved and the need for accuracy. Benchmarking against other flocks is helpful, especially if common data collection systems are used. In the same way as monitoring animal-based indicators, medicine use can give a good indication of recurrent health problems. Observations made at the abattoir can give feedback and useful information to the producer – such as the incidence of particular diseases. This can inform on-farm preventive medicine programmes.

5.15.2 Welfare assurance schemes

While the general minimum standards for the protection of sheep have been set out in EU Directive 98/58/EC and deliberate acts of cruelty or neglect are covered by

Table 5.9 Some possible welfare outcome indicators for sheep.

Welfare indicator related to:	Example of good welfare	Example of poor welfare	Possible units
Behaviour	Demonstration of typical sheep behaviour including inter-animal interactions	Lameness; isolation from flock; slow to come to feed; lagging behind when driven	Number of lame sheep against target in health plan; increased vocalization; reaction towards the stockperson
Physiology	Measures may require blood sampling; carcass-related measures from abattoir; high levels of fertility	Increased concentrations of plasma cortisol etc; poor response to vaccination; altered reproductive patterns; presence of acute phase proteins	Incidence of poor protective immunity in vaccinated sheep; blood parameter units
Health/disease	Few animals with signs of ectoparasites; low faecal egg counts; fleece in good condition	Presence of chronic, treatable conditions; presence of skin disease (e.g. scab); patchy fleece loss; animals with faecal soiling; poor teeth; injuries	Number of cases of specific disease (compared to benchmarks); BCS at key times; mortality rate; use of medicines
Production	High weaning rates; marketing sheep at an early date; good feed conversion	Failing to make market weight on time; dirty fleeces; nutrition-related disorders	Production records; farm profitability; premium products

Note: Measures relevant to chronic welfare problems are poorly developed.

specific legislation, including the recently introduced Animal Welfare Act, requirements of retailers, producer groups and national schemes can encourage a higher standard. Often this is a seen as a required minimum for the producer to participate in a marketing chain. It can also be a mechanism to encourage a price premium for a product. As noted earlier, since the public already appear to consider that sheep benefit from a high standard of welfare (not least because of the 'naturalness' aspects of sheep production), there seems little scope for producers to further enhance their systems in the public's eye – at least in welfare terms. However, initiatives which address, specifically, important welfare compromises for sheep – perinatal mortality, lameness, avoidance of castration and tail docking – may be able to generate this added value. Even without specific welfare schemes, producers who strive for a high level of welfare in their sheep should benefit from a better price for high-welfare products, more job satisfaction, fewer losses from injury or disease and overall time saving. Sheep welfare elements appear in most major farm assurance schemes and, while in the UK only the RSPCA's Freedom Food initiative would claim to specifically focus on animal welfare, some organic certification schemes address this through a whole-system approach. The message the purchasing public takes from any scheme is often unclear and the profusion of own-brand schemes makes it difficult to establish the necessary clarity in this area.

References and Further Reading

Aitken, I.D. (ed.) (2007) *Diseases of Sheep*, 4th edn. Blackwell Publishing, Oxford.

Appleby, M.C., Cussen, V., Garces, L., Lambert, J.A. and Turner, J. (eds) (2008) *Long Distance Transport and Welfare of Farm Animals*. CABI Publishing, Wallingford.

DEFRA *Codes of Recommendations for the Welfare of Livestock: Sheep*. Available at: http: www.defra.gov.uk/animalh/welfare

DEFRA (2003) *Lameness in sheep*. Defra guidance booklet. Available at: http:www.defra. gov.uk/animalh/welfare

DEFRA (2004) *Improving lamb survival*. Defra guidance booklet. Available at: http:www. defra.gov.uk/animalh/welfare

Dwyer, C. (ed.) (2008) *The Welfare of Sheep*. Springer, New York.

Eales, A., Small, J. and Macaldowie, C. (2004) *Practical Lambing and Lamb Care: a veterinary guide*, 3rd edn. Blackwell Publishing, Oxford.

Farm Animal Welfare Council (1994) *Report on the welfare of sheep*. FAWC, London. Available at: http://www.fawc.org.uk

Grandin, T. (ed.) (2007) *Livestock Handling and Transport*, 3rd edn. CABI Publishing, Wallingford.

Hemsworth, P.H. and Coleman, G.J. (1998) *Human-Livestock Interactions: the Stockperson and the Productivity and Welfare of Intensively Farmed Animals*. CABI Publishing, Wallingford.

Henderson, D.C. (2002) *The Veterinary Book for Sheep Farmers*. Old Pond Publishing, Ipswich, UK.

Jensen, P. (ed.) (2009) *The Ethology of Domestic Animals*, 2nd edn. CABI Publishing, Wallingford.

Meat and Livestock Commission (1988) *Feeding the ewe*. MLC, Milton Keynes, UK.

National Sheep Association (www.nationalsheep.org.uk).

Ørskov, E.R. and Ryle, M. (1990) *Energy Nutrition in Ruminants*. Elsevier Applied Science, London, New York.

Russel, A. (1984) Body condition scoring of sheep. *In Practice* 6, 91–3.

Sargison, N. (2008) *Sheep Flock Health: A Planned Approach*. Blackwell Publishing, Oxford.

Scott, P.R. (2007) *Sheep Medicine*. Manson Publishing, London.

Williams, H.L. (1995) Sheep Breeding and infertility. In *Animal Breeding and Infertility*, Meredith, M.J. (ed.), pp. 354–434. Blackwell Science, Oxford.

Pigs

SANDRA EDWARDS

Management and Welfare of Farm Animals: The UFAW Farm Handbook, 5th edition. John Webster
© 2011 by Universities Federation for Animal Welfare (UFAW)

6.1 The Natural Biology of the Pig

Modern agricultural pigs have descended from the European wild boar (*Sus scrofa*). While their appearance and productive characteristics have been greatly changed by selective breeding, many of their basic behavioural instincts have been largely conserved despite many generations of domestication. Understanding the basic biology of their wild ancestors is therefore very important in designing good management and husbandry systems.

Wild boar are omnivores living in forest margins in small family groups of four to six related sows and their offspring of the last 1 to 2 years. Males live as solitary individuals or in bachelor groups, joining the sows only at the time of breeding. The wild pig is a seasonal breeder, coming into heat and mating in the autumn, and farrowing 4 months later in early spring. Sometimes a second farrowing may occur later in the year in August and September. This seasonality appears to be primarily determined by photoperiod, but food supply has also been shown to influence the timing of onset of ovarian activity in the autumn. Sows about to give birth isolate themselves from the main group and build a nest, where they give birth and initially nurse their young. After 1 to 2 weeks, they abandon the nest and lead their young back to rejoin the main group. The piglets show a gradually reducing frequency of suckling and increase in foraging for solid food, until they are finally weaned at an age of 3 to 4 months. Wild boar are not territorial, but have home ranges without a well-defined boundary. The family groups range over an area of 100 to 2,500 hectares, depending on season and food availability. These areas contain resting places and nests, watering places and wallows, rubbing and scratching places, regular rooting areas, and a network of regularly used interconnecting paths. The family disperses over a wide area while foraging, but comes back together for communal resting during the day and at night in simple nests made in areas of dense cover. Foraging activity occupies more than 50% of their active time, with a diurnal pattern of activity peaks at dawn and dusk, and comprises a mixture of grazing and rooting behaviours. The principal feeds are grasses, roots and tubers in the summer and mast crops, nuts and fruits in the autumn and winter, supplemented by invertebrates and carrion when these can be found.

Because of wild boars' forest habitat, their need to seek out food which is hidden or underground and to be aware of approaching predators, the senses of smell, touch and hearing are more important than vision. The snout is a highly developed organ for olfaction and rooting. Scent marks from glands on the face and neck, anogenital region, and feet are used to map their home range, and to identify members of the group. The pigs also have a complex repertoire of vocalizations, with grunts used in maintaining social contact, barks indicating alarm and squeals indicating distress.

Within the group, overt aggression is rare because of the existence of a dominance hierarchy based on age and size which gives priority of access to resources without conflict. This is maintained by use of signals based on threatening and submissive postures. Physical aggression occurs only if there is competition for some highly prized resource, such as when males compete for breeding opportunities, or when unfamiliar animals encounter each other.

These patterns of behaviour seen in the wild boar can all be observed in modern feral pigs, or when modern domestic pigs are placed in semi-natural environments. They can also be seen in some traditional extensive farming systems, such as those for indigenous Iberian pigs grazing in the oak forest 'dehesa' regions of Mediterranean countries. In more intensive farming conditions, expression of many of these patterns of natural behaviour is limited and this can give rise to some animal welfare problems, even where the physical needs of the animals are met by other means.

6.2 Domestication and Adaptability

Domestication of the pig was favoured by its social nature, adaptability and omnivorous habits. It occurred in Neolithic times, possibly by capture and habituation of wild pigs foraging on sown crops. Their ability to reproduce prolifically and deposit large stores of body fat favoured their value to humans. The development of distinct breeds of pig involved the promotion of these characteristics by the introduction of genes from smaller, early-maturing breeds (*Sus vittatus*), originating in Southeast Asia. In medieval times, village pigs were driven in groups to forage in woodlands and fatten in the autumn on mast, berries and roots. This system, known as pannage, gradually reduced in the Middle Ages as access to woodlands became more restricted and the role of the pig changed to utilize their ability to exploit human food wastes. Pigs were more often housed on a household basis and fed on kitchen wastes, while pigs kept in towns were often allowed to scavenge for food during the day. These keeping styles can still be seen around the world in subsistence living conditions. The intensification of pig production initially developed in conjunction with availability of specialized sources of by-product feeds such as dairy or brewery wastes. As the nineteenth and twentieth centuries progressed, the growing demand for pig meat and availability of cheaper cereals gave rise to the current systems of specialized farms with permanently housed animals fed predominantly on cereal-based diets.

Because of their adaptability, farmed pigs are found in almost all regions of the world, although their use for human food is restricted in some regions by religious taboos. Both Moslems and Jews believe their meat to be unsuitable for human consumption. Over the world as a whole, pigs constitute the most important source of meat, supplying about 40% of world meat supply. The global distribution of pig numbers is shown in Table 6.1.

Table 6.1 Pig population in the world (million head). Source: FAO statistics (http://faostat.fao.
org).

	1995	2000	2004
Africa	18	20	22
Asia	512	528	574
Europe	215	200	193
North America	93	95	99
South America	56	55	57
Oceania	5	5	5
Developed countries	304	289	285
Developing countries	595	614	667

6.3 The Basic Production Cycle

The basic production cycle of the pig under modern farmed conditions is shown in
Figure 6.1. Piglets are now born all year round to ensure a reliable source of meat in
all seasons. On most farms, production is organized so that a regular proportion of
the farrowings take place on a weekly basis, although on some smaller farms a
batched system will operate, with animals grouped to farrow in cohorts, typically
every 3 or 6 weeks. The breeding animals reach puberty at about 6 months of age. In
the female, the oestrous cycle lasts 21 days and animals will continue to cycle at all
times of the year until pregnant. Pregnancy lasts 115 days (3 months, 3 weeks, 3
days), after which the female gives birth to a litter of typically 8 to 16 piglets. These
piglets suckle for a period of 2 to 6 weeks, most typically 3 to 4 weeks, before being
artificially weaned and housed separately from their mother. The sow then comes
back into oestrus in 5 to 7 days and is bred again. The weaned piglets grow on for
meat production, reaching a typical slaughter weight of 90 to 120 kg by 5 to 6 months
of age.

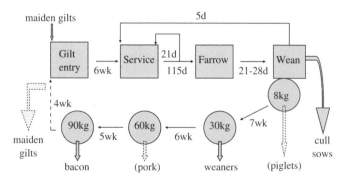

Figure 6.1 The typical production cycle of the pig.

Table 6.2 Pig performance standards for different countries in 2007. Source: BPEX (2008b).

	EU average	Denmark	USA	Brazil
Pigs born alive per litter	11.9	13.8	11.0	10.7
Pre-weaning mortality (%)	12.9	14.3	11.0	6.9
Litters/sow/year	2.25	2.23	2.39	2.01
Pigs weaned/sow/year	23.2	26.4	22.9	20.0
Post weaning mortality (%)	5.8	7.4	6.1	7.4
Finishing daily live-weight gain (g/day)	759	869	755	788
Finishing feed conversion ratio (kg feed/kg gain)	2.92	2.67	3.05	2.54
Average live-weight at slaughter (kg)	117	108	123	109
Carcass meat production/sow/year (kg)	1956	2003	1945	1470

The farm may buy in replacement breeding animals, or may breed its own in a specialized within-herd system. It will sell cull sows at the end of their reproductive life, and the progeny at a defined stage of growth. Many farms are 'farrow to finish', keeping the progeny until slaughter for meat production. While this is most typically at 100–120 kg live-weight, slaughter may take place at lighter weights in some specialist markets for fresh meat (the pork pig) or at heaver weights in markets for processed meat and ham (e.g. the Italian Parma ham pig may be 170 kg at slaughter). Some farms specialize only in piglet production and sell their progeny soon after weaning at 20 to 30 kg live-weight. These pigs are purchased by specialist finishing farms, who complete the rearing period until slaughter for meat. Occasionally farms sell newly weaned piglets directly from the sow, but this is less common because of the greater vulnerability of the animals at this time.

Typical levels of pig performance are shown in Table 6.2. These are based on national recording schemes in different European and American countries. They demonstrate that the production processes and outcomes are very similar in intensive systems around the world, with sows producing on average 20 to 23 weaned piglets each year. In Denmark, a combination of breeding for greater litter size and good management has now resulted in a national average of more than 26 weaned pigs per sow annually, a figure reached only by herds in the top 10% of achievement in other countries.

6.4 Housing Systems for Pigs

The housing systems for the pigs are typically, but not always, divided up by reproductive stage for breeding animals, and by age for growing and finishing animals. In intensive pig farming throughout the world, the systems used for production are relatively similar, although with some variations in housing design dependent on the regional climate. Less intensive systems also occur, ranging from traditional silvopastoral systems in Mediterranean countries, backyard pigs in developing countries or large-scale outdoor systems found in some parts of Europe and America.

In some countries, constraints on housing are set by legislation. This is generally the case in Europe, where the EU has agreed Directives to safeguard pig welfare. Directive 91/630 was the first of these which specifically addressed pig systems, and was subsequently supplemented by Directives 2001/88/EC and 2001/93/EC which increased legislative requirements. Additional constraints on systems of pig management arise from environmental legislation in Directives 1996/61/EC and 2003/87/EC. Some individual countries have yet more demanding national legislation, either for environmental or animal welfare reasons, as will be highlighted in individual sections of this chapter. Production systems may also be determined by the requirements of special labelling schemes. Some of these, such as organic production, have agreed international standards. For example, within the EU, the rules for organic pig production were first defined in Regulation 1804/1999. Other schemes are voluntary and may focus on different traits of interest to consumers. Examples of schemes which are designed to provide higher welfare for the animals by specifying more extensive housing systems and limiting certain contentious managements practices are the Freedom Food Scheme, run by the RSPCA in the UK, or similar initiatives such as the 'Certified Humane Raised and Handled' and 'American Humane Certified' programmes in North America. There are also larger-scale schemes run by industry bodies such as the Assured British Pigs scheme in the UK, the QSG scheme in Denmark, IKB scheme in the Netherlands and QS scheme in Germany. Such schemes typically require evidence of good practice within the current legislative framework, rather than setting additional constraints to building type or management system. They operate according to European requirements for quality assurance of products under the framework of EN 45011, combining a set of specific published standards with regular independent inspection of the farm to check compliance.

Housing systems adopted by pig-keepers can be divided into three major categories: outdoor systems, bedded indoor systems handling solid manure and slatted indoor systems handling liquid manure.

6.4.1 Outdoor systems

Large-scale outdoor production typically occurs in more temperate regions and comes in two distinctive forms – those supplying the commodity pig-meat market and those supplying specialist niche markets. In some European countries, particularly the UK but also to a lesser extent in France, and in some regions of North and South America, there are a significant number of outdoor herds contributing to conventional pig-meat supplies. These developed because of low establishment and overhead cost. Most commonly only the breeding animals are maintained outside, with the progeny transferred to more intensive housing at the time of weaning. These systems stock the sows relatively densely, at 12 to 15 sows per hectare, as part of an annual rotation with arable cropping. They only function well in areas with light, free-draining soils of sand or chalk and low annual rainfall of <750 mm. The pigs are kept in groups according to reproductive stage, in paddocks separated by electrified fencing and with simple wooden or metal shelters.

This conventional outdoor production contrasts with a smaller number of farms keeping pigs outdoor for production to supply local niche markets or according to organic standards. It is a requirement of the EU Directive on organic standards that breeding animals have access to pasture. Some national certification schemes also require that the progeny be kept at pasture, but this is not universal and in many countries the growing and finishing pigs are kept in housing with an outdoor run area which may be of concrete. It is not possible to have an organic pig enterprise in isolation, since they must be kept within an organic whole-farm system. In general, breeding sows and boars are kept in outdoor paddocks with simple shelters in the same way as conventional outdoor production. Weaned and growing pigs can be kept in similar paddock systems, in outdoor hut-and-run systems, or in more permanent housing with an outdoor exercise and dunging area.

A third major European outdoor system is the traditional Mediterranean silvo-pastoral system. This system, found most commonly in Spain, Portugal and Corsica, involves indigenous breeds that are extensively pastured in natural forests of oak or chestnut for the production of high-value dry-cured hams. Typically, all phases of production take place outdoors, with the finishing period taking place during the autumn when animals convert large quantities of acorns or chestnuts into fat deposits.

6.4.2 Indoor systems

Indoor housing is most commonly classified according to the method of manure management. The most common system throughout the world is to have pigs kept on fully or partly slatted flooring, so that the faeces and urine fall through the floor into a collection pit below, and are handled as a liquid slurry by pumping systems. In smaller, more traditional or high-welfare systems, the pigs are housed in pens with bedding and produce solid manure, or muck, which must be removed by hand in small herd systems or by machinery in larger enterprises. The most common bedding is straw, but in some countries other materials such as sawdust, wood shavings or rice hulls may be used. Bedded systems may take the form of deep litter pens, where the animals determine their own zones for resting and for dunging, and manure removal is done relatively infrequently, or minimally bedded pens in which the material is largely confined to a specific lying area while the dunging area is cleaned out on a more regular basis.

6.5 Breeds and Replacement Policy

While a wide variety of indigenous breeds exist in the different countries of the world, modern intensive production has focused almost completely on a few specialized breeds. The Landrace and Large White (or Yorkshire) breeds predominate in maternal lines, with breeds including the Duroc, Hampshire and Pietrain used extensively in sire lines for their carcass conformation and meat quality characteristics. The indigenous breeds survive in specialized production systems, such as the Iberian breeds in the extensive Mediterranean systems, and in smaller farms producing for niche markets. In particular, the use of traditional breeds is recommended in organic standards and a UK survey of organic farms found a wide range of such breeds still in use in the UK, including the British Saddleback, Tamworth, Gloucester Old Spot, Large Black, Welsh and Berkshire breeds. These traditional breeds are hardy and often have good maternal characteristics, but have largely disappeared from conventional production because of their early maturing characteristics and consequent tendency to become over-fat at a very young age. This usually means that they need to have their feed carefully restricted and to be slaughtered younger and at lighter weights, and are hence less profitable for conventional markets.

While pure-bred animals are still used in these niche systems, large-scale intensive systems typically use crossbred animals to exploit the benefits of hybrid vigour. Breeding females are most commonly first crosses between the Landrace and Large White breeds. However, in outdoor production systems the Duroc breed is often included to supply 25 or 50% of genes in a three-way cross with these breeds to give the greater robustness necessary to cope with the varying climate and greater social competition. Boars used in both intensive and extensive systems may be pure-bred Large White (Yorkshire), but are commonly synthetic lines blending a range of different breeds to give a 'terminal sire'. Although breeds are still described by their traditional names, in reality much of the selection and differentiation in recent decades has taken place within breed. Thus, a Large White line selected as a 'damline' for maternal characteristics of prolificacy and good lactation performance will vary markedly from a 'sireline' selected more heavily for traits of growth, feed efficiency and carcass conformation. The development of these specialist lines and synthetic breeds has been carried out very effectively by large international breeding companies, who can use sophisticated statistical methods to select animals for the most desirable combination of traits over large populations. By these means, rapid genetic progress can be made. For example, carcass backfat thickness in the UK slaughter pig was reduced in the late twentieth century by 0.4 mm per year, or 50% over 25 years, in response to consumer demand for leaner and healthier meat. More recently, litter size in Danish pigs has been increased by 15% in only 5 years.

To exploit this rate of progress, many farms purchase their replacement breeding animals from a specialized breeding company. The maintenance and development of the pure-bred 'grandparent' lines takes place in nucleus units owned by these companies. Animals from these units are transferred to multiplication units, also usually owned or managed on contract for the breeding companies, where the

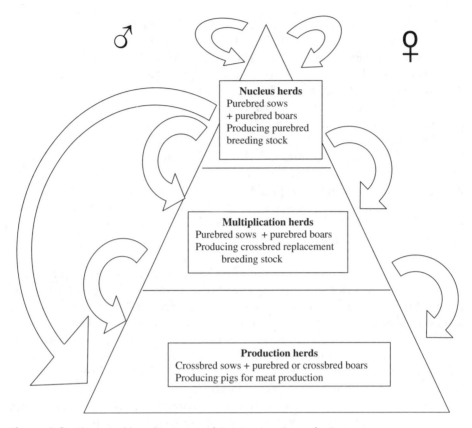

Figure 6.2 The typical breeding 'pyramid' in intensive pig production.

appropriate crosses are carried out to produce the crossbred production animals sold as breeding stock to meat-producing farms (Figure 6.2).

To minimize the risk of introduction of disease, some farms breed their own replacement females. In order to do this, they must either maintain a nucleus of pure-bred animals in the herd, to generate the most productive first-cross gilts, or adopt a reciprocal crossing policy between two breeds, known as 'criss-cross breeding'. In this system, boars of two different breeds (e.g. Landrace and Large White) are used in alternate generations so that a sow is always mated to the breed which was not her father. In this way, each generation has some hybrid vigour, having one-third of the genes from one breed and two-thirds from the other. This is an attractive option for a smaller unit, since no specialist pure-bred animals need to be maintained, but does require good animal identification and record-keeping to ensure the correct cross is always made, and gives a slight reduction in hybrid vigour which is equivalent to 0.5–1.0 fewer pigs produced per sow per year.

6.6 The Breeding Phase

Domestication has largely abolished the seasonal breeding characteristics of the wild boar, and females will now come into oestrus year round. However, some vestiges of their ancestral propensity to seasonality still exist, as shown by the occurrence of summer infertility which is especially pronounced in outdoor animals subject to natural photoperiod and in animals in hot climates. On any pig unit, the most important phase of production is the mating, since poor management here will result in poor conception or litter size and under-utilization of all the other buildings on the farm. A well-managed farm will have a calculated pig flow pattern, working out the building capacity at each production stage, and planning the number of weekly matings accordingly. To maintain this correct number of matings, new gilts must be introduced to the herd to replace older sows which are culled for poor production or age. While sows can continue to breed for many years, the modern sow is usually replaced after six litters, when her productivity starts to decline. The maintenance of a stable herd size typically requires the introduction of 40% of the herd size as new gilts each year.

Breeding gilts (nulliparous females) are typically delivered to the farm at about 6 months of age and 100 kg live-weight, and at the point of puberty. Since, when imminent, puberty can be triggered by mild stressors, the stimuli from the journey, handling and new housing often result in oestrus within a week of arrival. However, animals are seldom bred at this first oestrus, for several reasons. The first is that newly introduced animals are typically held in quarantine for a period of 6 weeks. This allows the new owner to be sure that they are not incubating any disease before they are introduced to the main herd, and also gives the animals the possibility to settle in their new location and be gradually adapted to the microbial challenges on that farm. For this purpose, cull sows or finishing pigs are sometimes introduced into the quarantine accommodation. Breeding gilts can also be purchased and introduced to the farm at a younger age, typically at 3 months of age and 30 kg. This gives them a longer period to adapt to the herd and has been associated with an increase in reproductive performance when bred. However, the extra housing demands make this option unattractive for many farms. The second reason for delaying breeding is that litter size increases with each successive oestrous cycle in these young animals, so that delaying until the second or third oestrus is usually cost-effective and also gives an animal which is older at farrowing and better able to meet the heavy demands of lactation.

Sows which are already in production enter the service house after weaning, and the cessation of the suckling stimulus normally induces a return to oestrus in 5 to 7 days. However, a number of management procedures will ensure that this process is not delayed, and will optimize the expression of oestrous behaviour and the ovulation rate. Group housing of sows, as opposed to individual housing in stalls, and daily physical contact with a boar both reduce the weaning to oestrus interval in an additive way, while isolation of weaned sows from boars can delay the onset of oestrus. Gilts tested for oestrus by a stockperson show a stronger behavioural response when adjacent to a boar than when tested in the home pen. However, young females housed permanently adjacent to boars appear to habituate to boar stimulation, showing shorter duration of oestrous behaviour and reduced response to a back pressure test during oestrus.

The oestrous and mating behaviours of the domestic pig show few changes from those exhibited by their wild counterparts. The oestrous cycle can be divided into four phases, each characterized by certain physical and behavioural symptoms. Dioestrus or anoestrus is the period when the ovary is least active and there are no external symptoms. Pro-oestrus is a period of increasing ovarian activity in which symptoms of approaching heat can be observed, such as reddening and swelling of the vulva. At this stage, behavioural changes are also seen as sows increase their level of activity, begin to nose and lever the flanks of other females and try to mount other sows. Where the possibility exists, oestrous sows will seek out and associate with a boar. Follicular ripening reaches its peak at oestrus and then ovulation takes place. At this time the behaviour of the female is characterized by willingness to adopt the standing reflex, necessary to allow mating by the boar.

The reflex is characterized by a flattening of the back and elevation of the perianal region, a posture also called lordosis, with a characteristic pricking of the ears in some breed types. This behaviour is shown most strongly in response to stimuli provided by the boar, but at the time of peak oestrus can also be induced by other sows or by a human who provides the appropriate tactile stimulus of pressure on the back. This period, often called 'standing oestrus', when the female accepts copulation, lasts on average 48 hours.

The most fertile period for the sow is towards the end of standing oestrus, when ovulation occurs. Detailed studies of ovulation by ultrasonography in the sow have shown that, irrespective of the total duration of standing oestrus, ovulation occurs after approximately two-thirds of the duration of oestrus. Where boars and sows are housed separately, it is normal to allow natural service or artificial insemination of sows once or twice daily throughout the period of standing oestrus so as to maximize the chances of hitting this fertile period (Figure 6.3).

Although sows may be bred by natural service or artificial insemination, some boars are always needed on the farm to ensure good oestrus stimulation. Where natural service is used, it is normal to keep one boar for every 20 sows in the herd. However, where group mating systems are used, such as in outdoor production, a higher ratio of one boar to 15 sows is required. The number of sperm and volume of an ejaculation increases from puberty until 18 months of age. This production level is maintained for about 5 years and then declines. Boars are normally culled after 2 to 3 years because of large size and the need for continuous genetic improvement. Indoor boars are normally housed singly and fed 2–3 kg of pregnant-sow diet. Present EU legislation specifies a minimum pen area allowance of $6\,m^2$ per animal and $10\,m^2$ if this pen is also used for service. It is possible to house familiar boars together in pairs or groups, but their management and handling is

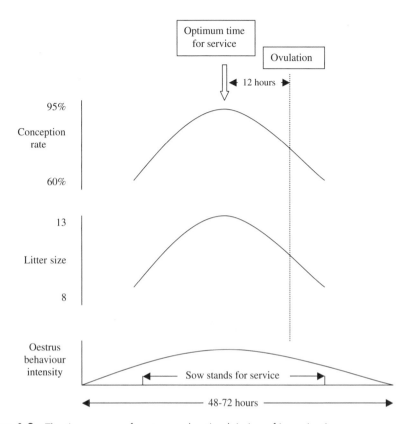

Figure 6.3 The time course of oestrus and optimal timing of insemination.

then more difficult. Mature boars will fight if unfamiliar animals are mixed and severe injury can result.

Domestic pigs show the same patterns of courtship behaviour as wild boar, with chanting (rhythmic grunting), sniffing and licking of the vulva, and pushing and nudging of the flanks preceding mounting, intromission and ejaculation. In commercial circumstances, where an oestrous sow is introduced to a boar in a limited area, boar courtship behaviour sometimes lasts less than 1 minute, but is very important as a higher level of courtship has been shown to increase conception and litter size. When the female shows the standing response, the male mounts and makes thrusting actions with the penis. Ejaculation occurs after 3 to 20 minutes (average 4.5 min). The use of a specially designed mating area of $10\,m^2$ with no obstructions, a non-slip floor and stimulation from other adjacent boars has been shown to give better breeding results than allowing mating to take place in the boar's home pen.

The use of group mating systems, in which a team of boars are placed with the weaned sows and mating takes place without significant supervision, is also adopted in some situations. While mating systems involving groups of boars housed together are still relatively uncommon in indoor production, this is historically the most common method used in outdoor production. However, a detailed study of this system highlighted its weaknesses, since the number of successful matings per sow varied from 0 to 7, while the number of matings performed by individual boars over the peak 4-day oestrous period varied from 0 to 13. Of the 45% of all mating attempts which failed to achieve copulation, half were due to intervention of a second boar. In a UK survey of breeding records from outdoor herds, it was found that 80 herds using outdoor group mating with three or more boars per group had an average farrowing percentage of 73%, 18 herds using outdoor mating with 1 or 2 boars achieved 75%, while herds adopting indoor mating achieved 79% success. For this reason, an increasing number of outdoor herds now house the sows temporarily during the breeding phase in nearby buildings or tents in the field where individual boars are kept and controlled mating or artificial insemination can be carried out.

The dynamic service system is another variant on group mating which has been developed as a means of overcoming some of the problems experienced in the existing outdoor group mating systems. Newly weaned sows are initially grouped in their weekly batch with *ad libitum* feeding. As they come on heat, they are transferred into one of a number of large dynamic groups according to body size. Each of these groups contains a resident team of boars (two to four boars depending on the scale of operation) and the number of sows added weekly is such that a 1:1 ratio of sows on heat to boars is maintained in each group. Service takes place within the group, and the sows remain until late pregnancy, when they are regrouped back into contemporary farrowing groups, and elevated late pregnancy feeding levels can be applied. Thus a 200-sow herd, weaning nine sows per week, might run three dynamic groups for small, medium and large sows respectively. Each group would comprise a team of three boars and 33–36 sows, with addition of three oestrous sows and removal of three late-pregnancy sows each week. While most uptake of the dynamic service system to date has been in outdoor herds, some pig units have adopted the system in large deep-litter buildings, either for sows or for breeding of synchronized groups of gilts in larger herds. The benefits of such a system are cheap housing and minimal labour demand. However there are many potential risks – aggression directed to the new sows, particularly at the critical times of service and implantation, could reduce conception rate and litter size because of the well-known detrimental effects of stress on reproductive physiology. Boar management is also still problematic, with the risk of uneven work rates, late detection of infertile boars and reduced service quality because of aggression between boars.

To allow exploitation of the best genetics, most mating in large conventional units is carried out by artificial insemination (AI). Since one ejaculate of semen can be used to inseminate 20 sows, AI offers the advantages of purchasing and keeping fewer boars, and the ability to invest in fewer but genetically superior boars. It also allows the semen to be checked for quality before use. While some larger farms will collect and process semen from their own boars, the majority will purchase the semen from a specialized stud. Semen from boars with the highest breeding values for desirable traits is made available by breeding companies, or in some countries by government-owned studs. In pigs, a large volume of semen is required for insemination relative to other species and, because the sperm do not survive well after freezing as a result of their higher lipid content than other species, most semen is delivered and used fresh. The development of special diluents with which the semen is mixed can prolong its effective lifetime for a period of 5 to 7 days, but this means that correct prediction of the time of oestrus in the sow and correct handling and storage of the temperature-sensitive semen is vital for good conception and litter size. Successful use of AI requires good operator skill for oestrus detection and insemination. The close proximity of a boar helps to elicit clear signs of oestrus, provide olfactory and auditory stimulation at the time of insemination and promote good conception.

6.7 The Gestation Phase

The two major objectives of management of the pregnant sow are to establish a large number of embryos in the uterus and to feed the sow in such a way that she is best prepared for the high demands of the subsequent lactation. It is important to avoid stress during the implantation period (10 to 18 days after service is a particularly sensitive time) as this can increase embryo mortality and reduce litter size. This can be helped by avoiding mixing or a change of environment during this period. If the sow does not return to oestrus at 21 days after service, she is likely to be pregnant, but this is generally checked by ultrasound pregnancy diagnosis at 4 weeks after service. The equipment most commonly used detects the increased blood flow in the uterine vessels using the Doppler effect. It is now possible to carry out pregnancy detection at 19 days after service using ultrasound scanning to observe changes in the appearance of the uterus, but this equipment is more expensive and the method requires more skill.

6.7.1 Pregnancy stalls

Gestation in the pig lasts for 115 days, with little variation about this average. This period of the sow's life has been the subject of much debate about welfare issues. Traditional systems, in which groups of pregnant sows were housed in outdoor paddocks or in covered straw yards, fell into disfavour as herd sizes increased and they became more difficult to manage. The 1960s saw the large-scale development and adoption of individual housing systems for sows, and these rapidly became the norm in many pig-producing countries. Such systems offered the attraction of low space requirement and ease of management. Sows could no longer fight and individual feeding could ensure that the nutritional needs of all animals were precisely met. With the small space allowances and enclosed buildings associated with individual housing, automated air temperature control was possible but provision of bedding and daily cleaning out presented a difficult and laborious manual task. In consequence, this was automated in many buildings by using fully or partly slatted floors, through which all excreta passed for storage away from the animals as a slurry. The slurry could then be mechanically removed from the building at any convenient time. To ensure that all urine and faeces were deposited over the slurry collection area, which was essential to avoid manual pen cleaning and keep the animals clean and dry, it was necessary to prevent sows from turning around in their pen. This was achieved either by enclosing them in a stall too narrow to permit this, or tethering them within their pen by means of a neck collar or girth strap. The resulting form of housing offered a relatively low-cost, simply managed system for large-scale pig production enterprises under all farming conditions. However, the very restrictive nature of such systems has given rise to serious public concern about sow welfare, and individually confined sows are often seen to develop stereotyped behaviours such as bar biting or vacuum chewing. As a result of these concerns, legislation to ban such housing systems has now been passed in many countries. In the UK, it has not been permitted to keep sows in individual stall or tether systems since 1999 and they are also banned in other countries such as Sweden and Switzerland. In the rest of the EU, tether systems have been banned and legislation will ban gestation stall systems after 2012, although the use of stalls for the period between weaning and the first 4 weeks after service will still be permitted. Elsewhere in the world, stalls are still the predominant housing system for gestation although their use is being reviewed in many countries and has been banned in some states in the USA.

6.7.2 Group housing for pregnant sows

There is a wide variety of alternative group housing systems in use during the gestation stage, made up from all combinations of their key components of group size, floor type, lying area design and feeding system. Group sizes vary depending on herd size, frequency of batch farrowing and whether small stable groups or large dynamic groups are adopted. Stable groups are formed at the time of weaning and remain together throughout pregnancy. This avoids any mixing and fighting to re-establish the dominance hierarchy. Dynamic groups have sows at all stages of pregnancy, with animals added, after service or pregnancy diagnosis, and removed, shortly prior to farrowing, on a regular (often weekly) basis. These large groups allow cheaper housing cost and provide more total space for exercise, escape from aggression and choice of location for the animals. However, because of the regular introduction of unfamiliar animals, they tend to have more aggression as the dominance relationships are repeatedly being re-established, and therefore need a higher standard of management.

As with all production stages, pens can be deep-bedded, shallow-bedded or without bedding, in the latter case usually having fully or partly slatted flooring. Slatted floors reduce labour and cost of bedding, but must be of good quality if lameness is to be avoided. In the EU, legislation now requires a minimum slat width of 80 mm and a maximum gap of 20 mm for concrete floors to reduce the risk of foot injury. Straw-based systems are often preferred because the straw provides not only additional thermal and physical comfort, but also a source of gut fill and occupation which is particularly important to reduce aggression in the pregnant sow.

Because of their restricted feeding level, the thermal comfort zone for a pregnant sow is relatively high (18–20 °C when individually housed without bedding). While this does not pose a problem in tropical countries, in more temperate regions ambient temperature often falls below this. To avoid the wasteful use of feed to maintain body temperature, sows in stalls or slatted systems are usually kept in insulated, controlled environment buildings, where the air temperature is regulated by changing ventilation rates of fans. However, systems in which animals are housed in larger groups on straw require access for machinery to enter the building to deliver straw and remove muck. These systems are therefore often found in large, uninsulated buildings where temperature is difficult to regulate. Covering the lying area with a false roof to form a kennel allows the sows to make a microclimate and conserve heat. This benefits both sow welfare and feed efficiency, but makes inspection and access to animals for routine tasks such as vaccination or pregnancy diagnosis more difficult.

6.7.3 Feeding systems for sows

Feeding of the non-lactating sow is an area of great importance. There are specific times when the level of feeding can directly impact on productivity, while at other times the objective is to minimize feed cost. Between weaning and breeding, a high plane of nutrition is important to stimulate a high ovulation rate. It is usual to continue feeding with the higher-quality lactation diet during this period and to feed *ad libitum* or at a generous allowance of 3–4 kg/day. For gilts coming up to their first service, this 'flushing' should be applied for 12 to 14 days before ovulation, since this can increase litter size by one or two piglets. However, once mating has occurred, continuation of this high feed level can adversely affect the hormonal balance and impair embryo implantation. It is therefore advised to reduce feed level to 2–2.5 kg from the day after mating until pregnancy diagnosis is positive. After this time, the objective is to feed the minimum amount necessary to achieve optimal body condition at farrowing of 3–3.5 on a 0–5 scale (see Figure 6.4). A sow which is thinner at farrowing will have lower birthweight piglets and fewer body reserves to support high milk output during lactation. Conversely, a sow which is too fat will have greater risk of prolonged parturition and increased stillbirths, and a lower appetite during lactation which will make her utilize body reserves to produce milk and adversely affect her subsequent breeding. To achieve the ideal body condition, sows are typically fed 2–3 kg of a gestation diet with 13 MJ/kg of digestible energy (9.2 MJ/kg of net energy) and 14% crude protein (4–5 g/kg of ileal digestible lysine). The exact amount of feed will depend on their size, body condition and housing, where the needs for exercise and keeping warm may differ. In the final stages of pregnancy, the foetal piglets show exponential growth rate. The birthweight of the piglets can be influenced by the feed level of the sow but the response is quite small (it takes ~100 kg of sow feed to increase individual piglet birthweight by 100 g). However, it is common practice to increase the feed level for the pregnant sow in the last 3 weeks before farrowing to 3–3.5 kg to reduce her mobilization of body reserves at this time of high demand. The food is typically reduced again to 2–2.5 kg

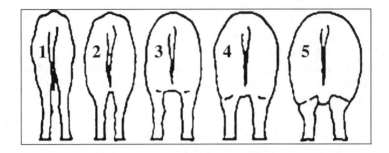

Score	Body condition	Prominence of backbone, ribs and pelvic bones
1	Emaciated	Bones visible
2	Thin	Bones felt by flat of hand without pressure
3	Optimal	Bones felt by flat of hand only with pressure
4	Fat	Bones felt only by pushing with finger tips
5	Obese	Bones cannot be felt

Figure 6.4   Body condition scoring in sows.

in the last 3 days before farrowing, since this can reduce the risk of health problems in the immediate postpartum period.

Outdoor sows have higher feed requirements because of greater activity and the lower temperatures experienced during winter. Their annual feed use in temperate regions is typically 15% higher than animals living indoors. Because the feed is usually scattered widely on the ground so that all sows in the group can obtain access, a special large pellet or 'cob' is manufactured to prevent wastage from blowing away in the wind, becoming lost in mud or carried off by small birds. The outdoor conditions give sows the advantage of a more natural environment, allowing them to forage for vegetation and invertebrates. However, for much of the year they obtain little additional nutrition from these activities and their vigorous rooting can rapidly destroy any vegetation cover on their paddock, leaving a bare surface which can become very muddy in wet weather. To prevent this, some farms insert nose rings in the sows to prevent them from rooting. Traditionally, two or three small rings were clipped through the upper rim of the nasal disc. While initially very effective in preventing rooting without impairing grazing, these rings are easily dislodged and may need to be replaced a number of times during the life of the sow. More recently, an alternative design has been favoured in which a larger 'bull ring' is fastened through the nasal septum and protrudes in front of the snout. The welfare implications of nose ringing are the subject of debate. The insertion of the rings is a painful procedure and the inability to express motivated rooting behaviour when hungry can be a source of frustration. These adverse effects for the animal must be offset against the better living conditions if a dry and grassy paddock can be preserved. The maintenance of vegetative cover also has important environmental benefits, since it allows plant capture of excreted nutrients throughout the growing season, and helps to maintain soil structure. This reduces the risk of leaching and run-off of nitrogen and phosphorus which can pollute waterways, and the undesirable emissions of gases such as ammonia and nitrous oxide into the atmosphere. At present there is no legislation against the use of nose rings and they are widely used in both intensive and more traditional outdoor systems according to environmental needs and the preferences of individual farms. Their use is even permitted in many organic schemes, where utilizing natural vegetation as a contribution to nutritional requirements is favoured.

The concentrate feed allowance for the pregnant sow is designed to meet all her nutrient requirements (typically about 1.3 times maintenance need) and is adequate for good health and performance, but does not satisfy her appetite and leaves her in a state of chronic hunger. This situation is now known to give rise to the stereotyped behaviours in sows in restrictive environments, where the food-seeking behaviours generated by this hunger have no appropriate outlet for expression. In group housing, it also causes aggression during competition for feed, and the abnormal injurious behaviour of vulva biting. To minimize these problems, it is recommended to feed the sow once daily, since one large meal is more satisfying both physically and physiologically than a number of smaller meals, and to provide additional roughage which can give greater gut fill and feelings of satiety. This can be in the form of supplementary hay or silage, or fresh straw bedding or by formulating the compound diet to have a higher fibre content.

Because the feed amount is so limited, it is important to ensure that each individual is able to eat her own appropriate share. This need has given rise to a variety of housing systems with different methods of feed provision designed to meet this challenge. More traditional systems often adopt simple group feeding options, placing the allowance for a number of sows in a long trough or spreading it widely over the ground. This approach can be mechanized using automated canisters, suspended over each pen and filled from a pipeline, to measure the group feed allowance and then dump it onto the floor at feeding time (dump feed systems) or with spinning discs which spread the food over a much wider area (spin feed systems). While this is a cheap housing option, it can cause significant welfare problems for the animals. Older and larger sows eat at least twice as fast as small ones, and can dominate areas of food resource. This can result in uneven sow condition, aggression as the hungry sows compete for the limited feed and the failure of young and timid sows to thrive. Housing systems with provision for individual rationing, while more costly in terms of space and equipment, prevent aggression over food and allow all sows to reach the time of farrowing in ideal body condition. Because of these advantages, many different systems of ensuring individual feed intake have been developed.

The most traditional method is to house sows in pens with individual feeding stalls in which the animals are enclosed only during the feeding period. Each animal can then be offered the appropriate amount of food, and remains protected while she consumes it. The communal area may be deep bedded, comprise a kennelled lying area and scraped dunging passage, or be unbedded with a slatted dunging area. While this is perhaps the ideal system from the perspective of sow welfare, it has a high labour requirement for confining and releasing sows each day and hand feeding the correct ration for each animal. It also has a high space requirement for provision of individual feeding stalls which are used for only a short period each day, and hence a high capital cost. Space allowance and cost can be greatly reduced by combining the feeding stall and lying area, as is done in systems with cubicles or free access stalls. Animals are free to leave the stalls during the day to spend time in a communal exercise and dunging area, but the space provided for this is very limited. If aggression occurs, it is difficult for the lower-ranking sow to escape and there is a danger that she becomes trapped in a stall by a following aggressor. This risk is lessened in systems where the length of the feeding stall is reduced, such that only partial barriers separating the head and shoulder are used. However, this increases the risk that faster-eating sows will finish their own ration and then bully their slower-eating group-mates away from their feeding place to steal additional food. To minimize this possibility, a more complex feed delivery system known as the Biofix or trickle-feed system has been developed. This uses a method of 'biological fixation', in which feed is dribbled out by an auger at the same controlled rate to each individual place. Since the sows cannot then eat at a differential speed, movement between feeding places gives no benefit and only short partitions along the trough are necessary to protect the feeding sows. Correct selection of the dispensing rate is essential to the success of the system, since too slow a rate will lead to restlessness in fast-eating sows, while too fast a rate will overwhelm the slow-eating animals. Experiments have shown that the number of aggressive interactions and changes of place during feeding increase as the dispensing feed drops below 100 g of pellets per minute. However with rates of more than 120 g per minute, more sows have food accumulating in the trough and the number of aggressive interactions when feed dispensing stops is increased. This system has the disadvantage that it is a flat-rate delivery and it is not possible to feed different amounts to individuals within the same group. It is therefore best used with small groups of sows where size and condition of animals within the group can be closely matched.

Because the nutritional requirements of individual sows can vary significantly, depending on such factors as live-weight, body condition and stage of pregnancy, the development of a system in which individual rationing could be automated was highly desirable. This was made possible by the development of electronic sow feeding, or transponder feeding, systems (Figure 6.5). In this system animals are identified electronically by a device carried on a collar, ear tag or implant, and feed sequentially at one or more feeding stations controlled by a central computer. The sow entering the feeder is automatically locked into a protective stall, recognized by her electronic tag and dispensed the appropriate amount of food according to her preset ration. On completion of her feeding period, the gates are unlocked and she is replaced by the next sow. Sows in stable groups using this system soon develop a relatively stable feeding order, with dominant sows feeding at the start of the cycle

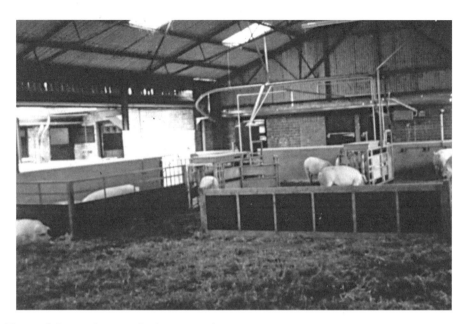

Figure 6.5 An electronic feeding system for gestating sows.

and low-ranking sows waiting until a quieter time of day. However, to maximize use of this expensive feeding technology, a large number of sows (typically 40 to 60) must share each station. This means that, except in very large herds, the system must operate with dynamic groups. Sows newly introduced to the group generally begin low in the feeding order, establishing themselves over time as longer-term group members are removed to farrow and other new sows are introduced. However, the constant introduction of new sows can disrupt the settled feeding order and cause more aggression and competition for feeder entry. There can also be problems when sows which have already consumed their daily ration return to the station in the hope of obtaining further food. These may try to circumvent protective devices to eject a feeding animal, or may occupy the feeder for long periods of time and prevent unfed sows from entering.

This problem can be avoided by operating a 'two yard' system, in which sows enter the station sequentially from one yard and, after feeding, exit via a side gate into a different yard. Sows which have not fed remain in the first yard to await attention if they have problems. Such systems may be operated either with individual electronic identification, or with a simple mechanical system and flat-rate feeding. Although simple in concept, some practical problems exist. Unless the size of the two pens is changed by moving of gates during the day, both pens must be large enough to house the majority of the group and total space requirement is high. Problems can also arise if sows pass through the feeder without stopping to eat and cannot then re-enter the feeder or be easily identified as not having fed.

Table 6.3 A comparison of dry sow housing systems.

System	Advantages	Disadvantages
Outdoor production	Low capital cost Large space and enriched environment	Group feeding on ground Exposure to climatic variation Higher feed wastage
Floor feeding (by hand, dump or spin feeding)	Simple and flexible Lowest capital cost	Group feeding only High aggression during feeding Higher feed wastage
Small groups with individual feeding stalls	Stable groups Individual rationing	High space requirement High capital cost
Cubicles	Individual rationing	Limited social space
Free access stalls	Lower space requirement	Visibility poor in covered cubicles
Trickle feed Biofix	Reduced space requirement with only partial feeding stalls Individual feeding	All sows in group receive same feed level Correct feed delivery rate critical
Electronic sow feeding	Individual rationing controlled by computer Low cost because feed station shared between many sows	Large groups often involve dynamic grouping Individual sows harder to check Equipment failure causes aggression
Wet feeding	Greater bulk gives quieter sows Cheap liquid by-products can reduce feed cost	Group feeding only High initial capital investment

In general, as summarized in Table 6.3, the different systems offer a trade-off between simplicity and the ability to provide for individual sow needs, and between mechanization, and hence capital cost, and labour input. However, it must be recognized that mechanization always carries a greater risk of malfunction and cannot fully replace the inputs of a skilled stockperson.

6.8 Farrowing and Lactation

The main objective for the farrowing and lactation period is to rear as large a number of piglets as possible, to achieve an even and adequate weaning weight and to leave the sow in good condition to commence the next breeding cycle. Because sows have become more prolific in recent years, these objectives now pose a greater challenge.

Sows are usually moved to special accommodation 5 to 7 days before their expected farrowing date to allow them time to settle before farrowing commences. In the wild, sows leave their group and walk long distances (10 to 30 km) in the days immediately prior to farrowing, before selecting a nest site and building a farrowing nest. In commercial conditions, the exact time of farrowing can be difficult to predict but the signs of imminent farrowing are restlessness, which typically occurs from about 24 hours before farrowing, and nest building which typically peaks at 6 to 12 hours before farrowing but can be very variable in time of onset. Shortly before farrowing, typically 6 to 8 hours but sometimes as early as 24 to 48 hours, it is possible to express milk from the teats of the sow and this is one of the more reliable signs that farrowing is imminent. Contractions can usually be seen from 3 hours prior to farrowing, but sometimes as early as 10 hours. Farrowing typically lasts 2 to 4 hours, being shorter in gilts than in older sows, with piglets delivered at varying intervals, averaging about 20 minutes.

The newborn piglet is born in a very vulnerable state. It is small, weighing typically 1 to 1.5 kg, and wet with birth fluid, and thus loses heat very rapidly. At the time of birth it has very low body fat reserves and therefore limited ability to maintain its core body temperature. Unless it suckles quickly it will become hypothermic, lethargic and likely to die. However, suckling is not a simple challenge. The newborn piglet must compete against its littermates for access to a limited number of teats, which can be difficult for small piglets born later in the birth order when older siblings are already well established. It also runs the risk of being crushed if its mother, weighing at least 200 times as much as the piglet, should move and trap it between her body and the floor. Occasionally, usually in gilts giving birth for the first time, the mother will be fearful and aggressive towards her piglets and may savage them. Given this scenario, it is not surprising that many piglets fail to survive the first few days of life. In the wild, the pig has evolved a strategy of producing a large number of young with low pregnancy investment. This allows the mother to rear a large litter in a good year, when food is plentiful, or to limit her efforts to fewer offspring if resources are scarce. For this strategy to work efficiently, surplus piglets should die quickly with least investment of resources, without compromising the survival of their littermates, and be those of poorest quality. The objectives of modern farming in keeping every piglet alive are therefore working against a long-term evolutionary strategy.

In modern farming, 18% of the piglets born do not survive until weaning and this mortality level has seen little improvement over recent years. More than half of these deaths happen during the farrowing period or within the first 48 hours. Stillbirths (piglets which die without ever breathing) account for 30–40% of all losses. Some of these piglets die during gestation as a result of infections, and are born in mummified form if this death happens a long time before farrowing. Others may die as a result of lack of adequate nutrients because of crowding in the uterus and lack of good placental supply. However, many die during the actual farrowing process as a result of asphyxia. This is a particular risk for those born later in the birth order, because the contractions of the uterus can disrupt their placental blood supply before they emerge and are able to breathe for themselves. Prolonged parturition as a result of sows being too old, too fat, too hot or experiencing too much disturbance during farrowing can exacerbate the problem. The level of stillbirth losses can be minimized by monitoring the progress of parturition and giving assistance if the inter-birth interval is too long (>1 hour). To facilitate supervision of farrowing, sows can be induced to farrow in more predictable, synchronous batches by injection of a prostaglandin, which will induce farrowing in 12 to 24 hours. However, sows should never be induced earlier than 2 days before their expected farrowing date, or piglet viability will be seriously impaired.

For the piglets which are born alive, most deaths are attributed to crushing by the sow. However, as described earlier, this is part of an interacting complex of risk factors (Figure 6.6) and is often only the final end-point of a path to mortality predisposed by other events. To prevent crushing, the majority of farms now house the farrowing sow in a crate, only slightly larger than her body size, designed to control her movements when lying down and prevent her from 'flopping' onto her piglets. The farrowing crate also offers other advantages when trying to improve piglet survival. Because the sow is fixed in one location, it is possible to predict exactly where the piglets will be born and to provide temporary extra heat at this place, thus reducing risk of hypothermia before suckling. A more permanent specialized resting area for the piglets, usually referred to as the 'creep area', can be provided close to the sow with supplementary heating by lamps or heat pads. This proximity of a warm area helps to encourage the piglets to lie away from the sow

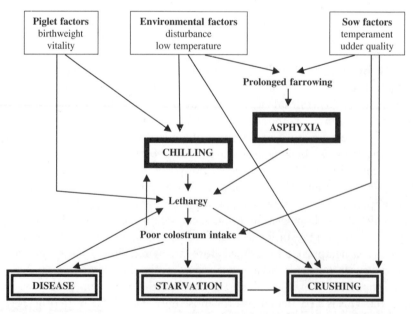

Figure 6.6 The interacting causes of piglet mortality.

between sucklings, at a location where they are at less risk of crushing. Confinement of the sow in a crate also means that small or weak piglets can be assisted by stockpeople in safety, without fear of maternal aggression.

6.8.1 Housing systems for lactating sows

When first introduced, the farrowing crate led to significant improvements in piglet survival and ease of management. However, it has also raised concerns about the welfare implications for the sow. The crate imposes severe restriction on movement during the period before farrowing when the sow is very active and motivated to build a nest. The nest-building behaviours are further thwarted if, as is commonly the case to facilitate management and hygiene, fully or partly slatted floors are used with little or no bedding provided to act as a substrate for the behaviour. It has been demonstrated that inability to express nest-building behaviour at this time causes expression of abnormal behaviours and a physiological stress response in the sow. Furthermore, as lactation progresses, the inability of the sow to escape from the attentions of her large litter can again induce stress. For these reasons, use of the farrowing crate has been banned in some countries, such as Switzerland, and its continued use is under debate in many others. However, finding an acceptable commercial alternative has not been simple.

Although it is the case that in the UK outdoor systems achieve comparable levels of piglet survival in very simple huts without any supplementary piglet protection or heating (Figure 6.7), this is probably due to a unique combination of circumstances. The genotypes used in outdoor production tend to produce a larger and more viable

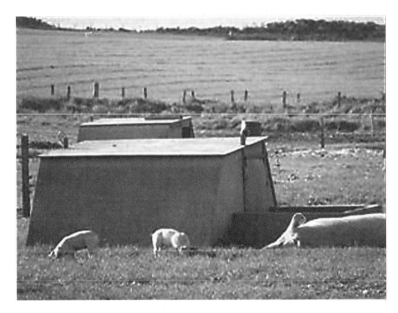

Figure 6.7 A typical farrowing system for outdoor production.

piglet, but the system itself also favours survival. The large space in the paddock means that the sow can farrow with minimal disturbance. The importance of this factor is shown by the increase in mortality which occurs in group, rather than individual, farrowing paddocks or when predators such as foxes are in the vicinity. Most importantly, the provision of a deep bed of clean dry straw allows the sow to fully express nest-building behaviour, which has been shown to lead to less rest-lessness during farrowing and better maternal behaviour. The sloping walls of a well-designed farrowing hut help to control the lying movements of the sow and provide escape routes for the piglets, while, if crushing does occur, the cushioning properties of the deep bedding can reduce the risk of injury.

Attempts to reproduce this non-crate approach in indoor conditions have so far met with only limited success. Where sows have been housed in groups, with free access to individual nests, there have been problems with animals which have given birth outside the nest in an inappropriate place, with disturbance of farrowing sows by others in the group, and with early desertion of the litter by some mothers. Where sows have been housed in individual pens without a crate, crushing of piglets has generally been higher and the workload and safety of stockpeople has been com-promised. Many different designs of non-crate system have been tried (Table 6.4). Sometimes these have given promising results during the development stage, but failed to be sufficiently robust under the more demanding conditions on large commercial farms. However, it is the case that countries which have banned or restricted use of the farrowing crate can achieve an acceptable level of survival, albeit usually on smaller family-run farms. New research and trialling of prototypes at the current time suggests that acceptable commercial alternatives will soon develop but these are likely to require higher capital cost and greater stockperson expertise in order to be successful.

Another approach used on some farms is to retain the farrowing crate for the period around parturition, but then to either give the sow more freedom of movement by opening up one of the crate sides so that the whole pen is available, or to move the sow and her litter to different accommodation where she is grouped with other animals at the same stage. This 'multisuckling' system allows both sows and piglets to co-mingle, typically from about 2 weeks after farrowing, so that no mixing and aggression occur at the time of weaning. However, there can be a major disruption of suckling at the time when grouping occurs which can increase risk of mortality for the piglets and induce a premature return to oestrus during lactation by the sows.

6.8.2 Management of the newborn piglet

The inputs of the skilled stockperson in the first days after farrowing are the key to good survival. The importance of rapid suckling after birth has been emphasized for nutrition and thermoregulation of the piglet, but it is also important for longer-term survival and health. Because of the nature of the porcine placenta, large molecules such as immunoglobulins cannot cross from the maternal blood supply. This means that the piglet is born without any protective immunity against infection. Until it starts

Table 6.4 A comparison of farrowing and lactation systems.

System	Advantages	Disadvantages
Farrowing crate	Control of sow lying Facilitates localized heating Protection for stockpeople Low space requirement Low labour requirement	Sow movement highly restricted Prevents sow nest building behaviour Sow cannot escape older litter
Modified crates (e.g. turn-around crate, Ottawa crate, ellipsoid crate)	Greater possibility for sow movement Control of sow lying Protection for stockpeople Low space requirement	Prevents sow nest building behaviour Sow cannot escape older litter
Swing-side crate (opened after farrowing period)	Benefits of crate during first days after farrowing Greater sow freedom in later lactation Feed intake and milk yield often improved	Prevents sow nest building behaviour Hygiene problematic unless slatted flooring
Open pens	Behavioural freedom for sow Simple, low cost housing	Little warmth or protection for newborn piglets High crushing levels common No protection for stockpeople Hygiene problematic unless slatted flooring Greater space requirement High capital cost
Designed pens (e.g. Schmid box, FAT pen, Werribee pen)	Behavioural freedom for sow Greater protection against piglet crushing Heated creep areas for piglets Zoned areas facilitate hygiene	
Indoor group farrowing (get-away pens, Free-dom farrowing, Thor-stensson system)	Large space for sow Individual nests for farrowing Social integration possible	Sows may farrow outside nest Farrowing may be disturbed Sows may desert litter Piglet mortality often high
Multi-suckling systems	Benefits of crate during first days after farrowing Behavioural freedom and social integration in later lactation Low cost lactation housing	Animals must be moved during lactation Suckling is disrupted when litters are grouped Lactational oestrus may occur
Outdoor farrowing (group or individual paddocks)	Plentiful space and enriched environment Isolation reduces disturbance Low capital cost	Exposure to climatic extremes Predators may take piglets Working conditions often challenging

to synthesize its own immunoglobulins in sufficient amounts at 4 to 6 weeks of age, it is dependent on the passive transfer of immunity via maternal colostrum. The colostrum produced by the mammary glands at the time of farrowing is a very concentrated source of immunoglobulin, providing both general protection and specific protection against the infectious diseases that the sow has experienced on that farm, or has been vaccinated against. For the first 24 hours after birth, the gut of the newborn piglet is permeable to these large molecules, allowing them to be taken up from the colostrum into the bloodstream of the piglet. This permeability gradually reduces with time, a process hastened by the ingestion of food, until closure is complete and no further transfer is possible. If the piglet fails to suckle, or suckles only poorly in the immediate postpartum period, it will be at much greater risk of succumbing to infectious disease during the lactation period, and may even be compromised throughout its lifetime. The skilled stockperson will therefore intervene if necessary to ensure that weak piglets, or small piglets in large litters, are able to obtain their adequate share of colostrum during the critical period. With very weak piglets, it is possible to feed them by hand after milking the sow, or to use colostrum which has previously been obtained and frozen for emergencies. However, a better solution for large litters of healthy pigs can be to adopt 'split suckling' where the bigger pigs in the litter which have already had a good feed are closed into a heated creep area for an hour to allow the less strong piglets the opportunity to suckle without competition.

This can be important because, from the minute of birth, each piglet tries to locate and defend the best teat on its mother. The sow typically has 14 functional teats, but not all are equally productive. Those at the rear of the udder are more likely to be low-yielding or damaged in older sows. Very early in life each litter forms a 'teat order' whereby each individual piglet always goes to the same teat to suckle and defends this teat vigorously against its siblings. The stronger piglets are able to appropriate the most productive teats, while the smaller and weaker piglets are relegated to the poorer-quality teats. In nature, this strategy is logical, giving the best chance to the fittest individuals, but in modern farming it is yet another challenge to the production of a large and even litter. To promote this teat fidelity, the pig has developed a complex suckling behaviour with a fixed sequence of interacting events. Milk is not available on demand, as is the case in many other species, except in the first few hours after birth. After this time, the availability of milk is restricted to a 20-second letdown period occurring during short suckling bouts taking place every 40 to 60 minutes. These bouts are initiated either by characteristic nursing grunts from the sow, or by the demands of many hungry piglets massaging the udder. As the whole litter assembles at the udder and starts vigorous massage, the nursing grunts increase in frequency until milk letdown occurs. After a period of quiet and intense suckling, the piglets again show active massaging of their teats once milk supply has ceased. The vigour of this massage has been shown to influence subsequent teat productivity and provides a mechanism whereby the larger and stronger piglets can stimulate better yield from their own teats. To defend its teat, the piglet uses its well-developed, and needle-sharp, canine teeth which can inflict serious facial wounds on its littermates. This can be problematic in large litters, where competition is higher, and is often prevented by the clipping off or grinding down of these teeth on the first day of life by the stockperson. Once again, the welfare implications of this procedure have been questioned; according to EU legislation it can only be carried out where the welfare risk of pain or gum damage during the procedure is outweighed by the reduction in injury to the faces of littermates and the udder of the sow if it is performed.

Where the number of piglets in the litter exceeds the number of functional teats, the surplus piglets have a high probability of mortality since supplementary feeding at this very young age is seldom adequate to sustain them. The best chance to reduce mortality in this situation is to foster some piglets to another sow that has spare capacity. Skilful cross-fostering allows litter sizes to be evened up and matched to the rearing capacity of each sow, and allows the size of piglets within each litter to be matched. This gives small piglets a better chance of survival if they are competing with piglets of similar size. Fostering should ideally be done soon after the end of the colostrum period, and before the teat order becomes well established. It is better to move the large, strong piglets when fostering, rather than disturbing the establish- ment of the smaller or weaker piglets, and to close the new litter together in the creep area for a period to give them a more uniform smell and make the process less apparent to the foster sow. As lactation progresses, some piglets may start to fall behind in size because of a poor-quality teat. While it is possible to foster piglets between older litters, this is best done only when absolutely essential. Because the teat order is strongly formed by this time, and any unused teats will have dried off within about 2 days, introducing a new piglet causes a major disruption of suckling and litter disturbance, which can increase crushing and starvation risk for both the newcomer and the resident piglets.

In addition to teeth clipping, other procedures may be carried out on young piglets according to the needs of the individual farm. Tail docking involves removal of the distal part of the piglet's tail using a scalpel, clippers or cauterizing iron. This is done to reduce the risk of tail biting later in life, which can be a major welfare issue on some units. It is believed that the shorter tail is either less attractive as a stimulus for this behaviour, or more sensitive to the initial nibbling which is not then allowed to progress to a damaging phase. Once again, EU legislation requires assessment of the welfare balance between the pain of carrying out the procedure and the known degree of risk of later tail-biting injury. Another surgical procedure carried out on the suckling animal in most countries is the castration of male piglets, which involves incision of the scrotum and removal of the testicles. This is done primarily to reduce the risk of 'boar taint' in the meat resulting from the presence of androstenone and skatole, induced by the hormonal state of the male after puberty. Only a few countries, including the UK, currently produce pig meat from entire male animals. In most countries, castration is performed in the first week of life without any anaesthesia or analgesia. However, this is the subject of great debate within the EU, and some counties such as Norway, Switzerland and the Netherlands have already put in place legislation or industry codes requiring that some form of general or local anaesthesia be used. A new alternative of immunological castration has also recently become available. This involves two injections in later life of an antibody which inactivates the production of male reproductive hormones, effectively castrating the animal only for a few weeks between the second injection and slaughter, without any surgical intervention.

The final procedure usually carried out on young piglets is the administration of iron. Iron is needed as one of the essential constituents of haemoglobin (the oxygen-carrying molecule in the blood) in the rapidly growing young pig. Sow's milk contains a very low level of iron, supplying only 1 mg/day against a requirement of 7 mg/day. Because of limited body reserves at birth, the piglet therefore begins to become anaemic after about 7 days. In the wild, piglets get iron from rooting in the soil, as do piglets in outdoor herds unless on very sandy ground. In indoor herds, it is normal practice to supply iron to the suckling piglet at 3 to 6 days of age by intramuscular injection, although oral dosing is also possible. This is necessary because piglets will eat very little solid food before about 3 weeks of age, although they will drink substantial amounts of water, electrolyte solution or milk substitute if this is offered, especially if the sow is lactating poorly. By 3 weeks after farrowing, the milk yield of the sow reaches a plateau and then begins to decrease, and no longer supplies the needs of the growing piglets. It is therefore normal to supply a palatable, high-quality creep feed, starting from 10 to 14 days of age, to supplement the milk supply and make piglets familiar with solid food before weaning.

The best determinant of good piglet weaning weights is a good milk yield from the sow. This is achieved by ensuring that the sow farrows in the correct body condition, neither too thin nor too fat, and achieves a high intake of a good-quality diet during lactation. If the sow is nursing a large litter, it is common for her to mobilize some body reserves in early lactation to support milk production. However, if this mobilization is excessive or prolonged, she will be weaned in poor body condition and her next reproductive cycle will be compromised. Either she will fail to come back into oestrus after the expected period of 5 or 6 days, or she will fail to conceive to the first mating, or she will produce a small litter at her next farrowing. To avoid these risks, everything possible should be done to encourage a high feed intake. The sow should be given fresh feed twice daily, building up the amount offered as her appetite increases over the week after farrowing until *ad libitum* intake is achieved. By the middle of the second week she should be eating 6 to 8 kg/day of a high-quality diet containing 14 MJ/kg of digestible energy (9.9 MJ/kg of net energy) and 18% crude protein (8 g/kg of ileal digestible lysine). Intake can be promoted by ensuring good feed hygiene, removing any uneaten stale food, and by ready access to fresh water, adding water to the daily feed and ensuring that the drinker has an adequate flow rate of at least 1 litre/minute. It is also important to avoid excessive room temperature. While a room temperature of 20 °C is often maintained during the farrowing period to reduce chilling risk for the piglets, reducing this to 18 °C as soon as the piglets have learnt to use a heated creep area will benefit the sow because of her high metabolic heat production. In hot climates, feeding in the early morning and evening when air temperatures are cooler can also be beneficial.

6.9 The Weaning Phase

The age at which piglets are weaned is a compromise between the need to have a robust piglet, able to weather the nutritional and social changes inherent in the process, and the desire to minimize the time between successive farrowings of the sow to obtain maximum piglet production and profitability. In most commercial systems, this compromise is at 3 to 5 weeks after farrowing, depending on housing and nutritional circumstances. Under natural conditions, weaning is a gradual process in which the frequency of sucklings gradually reduces and the intake of solid food gradually increases until final completion at 12 to 16 weeks of age. During later lactation the sow comes back into oestrus and becomes pregnant again while still nursing. Oestrus is suppressed by suckling and, although it is possible to induce oestrus during lactation under commercial conditions by a high plane of nutrition, disruption of regular suckling and the stimulus of a boar, the timing of this event is not always predictable.

In commercial production, operating a well-controlled batch system is very important for health management and efficient utilization of buildings. This means that all sows in the batch should be served at a similar time so that stable groups can be maintained and entry and exit from farrowing rooms can be synchronous, allowing thorough cleaning and disinfection between batches to avoid carry-over of any infectious agents. A similar 'all in, all out' policy is very important for the newly weaned piglet, which is particularly vulnerable to health challenges because of its immature digestive and immune systems. The key to maintaining this planned batch schedule is the weaning time, since correctly managed sows weaned in the first month of lactation are unlikely to show lactational oestrus, and a synchronized oestrus will be stimulated to occur 5 to 6 days after weaning.

Theoretically, each extra week of lactation reduces the average sow output by about one piglet per year. However, research has demonstrated that weaning earlier than 3 weeks can be counterproductive because the recovery period after farrowing is too short, resulting in increased rebreeding interval and poorer conception rate. The optimal weaning time to maximize sow output is therefore between 3 and 4 weeks. However, the piglet is still quite immature at this stage, since it only starts to eat significant quantities of solid food at about 3 weeks of age and its digestive enzyme capacity to deal with non-milk diets is very limited. When weaned at less than 3 weeks, the piglet experiences a significant growth check while the transition to solid food takes place. During this period, the limited digestive capacity makes it very prone to enteric disease, while its poorly developed immune system means it is also at higher risk of other infectious challenges. By 4 or 5 weeks, the piglet is much more robust and the weaning process involves less growth check and health risk. For these reasons, current EU legislation specifies that piglets should not be weaned at less than 4 weeks of age, although a special clause allows litters to be weaned up to 7 days earlier to facilitate all-in all-out batch management. In organic systems, weaning is not allowed at less than 6 weeks of age and some national certification schemes recommend 8 weeks of age.

There are particular situations in which weaning before this time may be permitted and may give some benefits. Because the passive immunity of the piglet declines with time after colostrum ingestion, and because a number of endemic disease agent are passed from the sow to her piglets during the suckling period, it can sometimes be advantageous in breaking a disease cycle to wean the piglets at 10 to 14 days of age, while their immune protection is still high, and remove them from the vicinity of the sow to prevent cross-infection. This system, known as segregated early weaning (SEW) or 'isowean' has been widely adopted in large enterprises in some countries such as the USA, but poses particular challenges in both the rebreeding of the early weaned sow and the establishment of the immature piglet.

Abrupt weaning at any age younger than the natural weaning age imposes some degree of challenge for the piglet. As the change from milk to solid feed generally involves a break in the regular pattern of feeding and a reduction in total nutrient intake, the piglet generates less body heat and requires a higher environmental temperature to be comfortable and less susceptible to disease. It can take up to 2 weeks for nutrient intake to regain its previous level during suckling, during which period the piglet needs a temperature of 27–30 °C to achieve thermal neutrality. Its susceptibility to enteric disease at this time also means that a high standard of hygiene is essential. For these reasons, newly weaned piglets are often housed in heated, controlled-environment buildings on fully slatted floors called flat-decks. A cheaper alternative to heating up the whole airspace of a room is to create a lying area with a microclimate by providing a kennelled system. Such systems include 'bungalows' with an enclosed insulated lying area and an outdoor slatted dunging area, or the provision of a kennel within a strawed system inside a simple building shell. On larger units, it is possible to house large groups of weaners together in deep litter systems, with a temporary kennel made of straw bales which can be broken down for bedding as the pigs grow. The use of large group systems (100 or more pigs in a group) for newly weaned pigs has been quite widely adopted in larger herds because they offer the scope to cheapen housing and simplify management, as well as avoiding the need for regrouping of unfamiliar pigs in later growing stages when fighting is likely to result in lost performance. Although initially used in straw-based housing in large kennelled yards, such systems have also been developed for controlled-environment, fully slatted nurseries. Trial results have sometimes indicated reduced growth rate in controlled-environment large group nurseries compared with smaller groups, but this reduced growth can be compensated by better subsequent growth, resulting in no reduction in overall lifetime performance. The poorer initial growth in large groups seems to be related to the ease of accessing resources. The newly weaned piglets are less willing to move long distances to find food on a frequent basis, instead reducing their total daily intake. More recently, the popularity of large group systems has declined because of the emergence of a devastating new disease known as post-weaning multisystemic wasting syndrome (PMWS). This results in a high proportion of piglets which suddenly begin to lose body condition from about 2 weeks after weaning and fail to respond to any therapeutic intervention. At peak virulence, mortality rates can be as high as 20%. Until the recent development of vaccines against the putative disease-causing agent, porcine circovirus 2, the only method of control was to minimize all possible stressors and prevent transmission between animals. This led to an increase in systems with minimal mixing of piglets, where weaners were housed in their litter groups.

The housing of large groups of piglets in deep litter systems was most popular for the weaners from outdoor breeding herds, which already form large groups for exploratory activities in the field while still sucking. Mobile outdoor kennel-and-run systems are also used by such enterprises, and generally give performance as good as that seen in more intensive systems. Piglets weaned from outdoor systems are better able to manage the weaning transition, being faster to explore and ingest food and experiencing less growth check, despite the fact that practicalities dictate that they do not receive any special creep feed before this time. It may be that the greater experience of separation from the sow and exploration of a diverse environment are of benefit.

The most critical part of an early weaning system is correct nutrition. The sucking piglet has an enzyme system specialized for digesting the components of a milk diet, and the ability to digest starch and plant proteins is poorly developed. Only after it starts to eat significant quantities of solid food is the induction of these enzymes triggered. If given a poor-quality diet at the time of weaning this can only be partially digested, limiting the nutritional value and inducing diarrhoea. It is therefore necessary to formulate special diets for the weaned piglet containing milk or whey powder and readily digestible protein such as fish meal. The starch component can be made more digestible by cooking the cereals to break up their starch molecules, while a highly digestible fat source provides concentrated energy. Such ingredients are expensive, but are important for successful weaning at an early age. As the pig becomes older, the inclusion level of cheaper ingredients such as uncooked cereals and plant proteins can be gradually increased, and nutrient density reduced, until the pig can thrive on these components alone. When pigs are produced according to organic standards, the choice of dietary ingredients is more limited and many of the high-quality ingredients needed for successful early weaning, such as synthetic amino acids, are not permitted. Organic weaner diets consequently tend to be of simpler formulation and lower digestibility, but the greater weaning age of the piglets can offset these disadvantages.

6.10 The Growing and Finishing Phase

Once the weaned piglet is established, the main objective is to grow the pig to slaughter as rapidly and efficiently as possible. This requires attention to disease prevention, environmental quality and nutritional specification.

Table 6.5 Guideline temperatures and feed specifications for growing pigs.

Category of pig	Temperature range (°C)[†]	Diet specification[‡]	
		Energy (MJ/kg)	Protein (g/kg)
Newly weaned piglets	25–30	16.0 DE	220 CP
(weaned at 3–4 weeks of age)		*11.0 NE*	*13 idL*
Weaners (15–25 kg)	21–24	15.0 DE	210 CP
		10.5 NE	*12 idL*
Growing pigs (25–50 kg)	18–21	14.0 DE	200 CP
		9.8 NE	*10 idL*
Finishing pigs (50–100 kg)	15–18	13.0 DE	180 CP
		9.0 NE	*8 idL*

[†]Lower temperatures are required if pigs are housed on deep bedding.
[‡]Assuming entire males and females of improved genotype fed *ad libitum*. Traditional breeds have lower requirement.
  DE, digestible energy; NE, net energy; CP, crude protein; idL, ileal digestible lysine.

As with the other stages of pig production, housing for growing and finishing pigs varies widely. The most common form of housing across Europe is in controlled-environment buildings with fully or partly slatted flooring. This has the advantage that pigs can be maintained at the optimal temperature to maximize efficient use of feed (see Table 6.5) while labour for cleaning is minimized and the separation of the pig from its manure helps to maintain good health and reduce risk of zoonotic diseases such as salmonellosis. Temperature and air quality are regulated by use of thermostatic fan systems, or by automatically controlled natural ventilation (ACNV) in which ventilation flaps open or close according to internal temperature levels. In more tropical regions, building construction tends to be simpler, with open-sided buildings to maximize air flow or the use of curtains in colder seasons. Finishing pigs fed *ad libitum* can be particularly prone to heat stress, since they possess no sweat glands in the skin, and the provision of showers or wallows when ambient temperature is high can be beneficial to both welfare and performance. If they have no other possibility for cooling, they will seek to wallow in their own excreta, increasing risk of disease transmission.

Within the EU, legislation exists about the minimum space requirement at each production stage and design of slatted flooring to avoid injuries to pigs' feet (Table 6.6). Controlled-environment buildings can also be designed to incorporate solid flooring and use of some bedding material, when cleaned out regularly by tractor scraping of dunging passages or under-slat scrapers, or by use of sloping floors in 'straw flow' systems where the straw gradually moves down the sloped lying area into a scraped dunging channel at its base. More extensive forms of housing are provided by kennelled housing with tractor-scraped passages or deep litter systems in cheaper, naturally ventilated buildings. These incur additional costs in purchase of

Table 6.6 Space requirements and flooring specifications for pigs (to comply with EU Directive 91/630).

Category of pig	Space requirement (m²)	Specifications for slatted floors (mm)	
		Maximum void width	Minimum slat width
Breeding boar	6.0		
	(10.0 if service pen)		
Sow (group housed)	2.25	20	80
Growing pig:			
<10 kg	0.15	11	50
10–20 kg	0.20	14	50
20–30 kg	0.30	18	80
30–50 kg	0.40	18	80
50–86 kg	0.55	18	80
85–110 kg	0.65	18	80
>110 kg	1.00	18	80

bedding material and labour to provide straw and remove muck, but offer some benefits for pig welfare if managed in a hygienic way. Comparison of fully slatted and straw-bedding housing for growing and finishing pigs has shown that risk of enteric and respiratory disease is greater in the bedded housing, where the pig is in contact with its manure and dust levels can be higher, but the risk of lameness, gastric ulcers and tail biting is greater in slatted housing.

6.10.1 Tail biting

Tail biting is an injurious abnormal behaviour which occurs sporadically and unpredictably on many farms. It involves progressive chewing of the tail from a mildly scratched condition to one in which the whole tail is removed and the flesh of the victim may be eaten away up into the spine. Similar but less common abnormal behaviours causing lesions on other parts of the body include ear biting or flank biting. These behaviours are a major economic as well as a welfare issue, since they involve veterinary treatment of injury, mortality and condemnation of carcasses through infection. The widely used preventive measure of tail docking piglets soon after birth can reduce the risk of tail biting, but does not abolish it and a prevalence of about 5% is still recorded in most countries. The causes of tail biting, and its related injurious behaviours, appear to be multifactorial, with a genetic predisposition triggered by environmental or nutritional factors. It has been suggested that more than one type of causation may contribute to the expression of the behaviour. One form seems to be a result of redirected foraging behaviour in a barren environment. In this form, initial nibbling and chewing which might otherwise be directed to environmental substrates is directed towards the tails of penmates and gradually becomes more severe until blood is drawn. At this point, the attraction of other pigs to the blood results in a rapid escalation of the problem. Dietary deficiencies in protein and minerals, particularly salt, have been shown to increase tail-biting risk, possibly through enhanced attraction to blood. Another form of tail biting appears to erupt without a gradual build-up in chewing, and may be linked to frustration of animals unable to access resources such as food, water or preferred lying places. This sudden initial event is seldom directly observed but, again, once blood is drawn the behaviour spreads and escalates. It is often apparent that certain individual pigs, usually the smaller and unthrifty individuals, develop chronic tail-biting behaviour and move from tail to tail in an apparently obsessive way. Exactly what causes such pigs to develop is currently unknown, but their rapid identification and removal from the group is vital in controlling any outbreak. Other remedial measures involve removing all bitten pigs to eliminate traces of blood, painting the tails with unpalatable Stockholm tar, increasing the salt content of the diet to 0.4%, putting salt blocks into the pen and giving straw and playthings to distract the animals. Controlling an outbreak once under way is very difficult, and the objective should always be to prevent the onset of the problem by careful attention to housing and management.

The demonstrated role of barren environments in increasing tail-biting risk highlights the importance of environmental enrichment for the pig. Pigs are highly intelligent and exploratory animals and, although spending 70–80% of the day lying and resting when well fed, have a requirement for functional occupation during the remaining period if abnormal behaviours are to be avoided. When housed with straw bedding, the chewing and rooting of this material provides a good outlet for exploratory motivation. Even a relatively limited amount of chopped straw given daily appears to fulfil this function adequately. However, in slatted systems the provision of bedding may not be possible because it interferes with the management of the liquid manure if it falls through the slats and blocks up pipelines and pumps. Finding alternative forms of enrichment in these systems has proved to be a major challenge. Many items such as footballs and rubber tyres are initially stimulating but soon become ignored as lacking in novelty. In the same way hanging chains, widely used in the past, appear to generate only limited interest. The properties of enrichment which are able to attract and hold the attention of the animals have been shown to include deformability and destructibility, nutritional content, and lack of soiling. EU legislation suggests straw, hay, wood, sawdust, mushroom compost, peat or a mixture of these materials to be appropriate substrates for proper expression of investigation and manipulation activities. However, ropes, paper sacks and root vegetables have also been shown to be very effective.

Other forms of aggression within the group are usually uncommon provided that a stable group is maintained without introduction of unfamiliar animals, and access to resources is adequate. Where this is not the case, serious fighting can occur to establish and maintain social ranking and may even result in death in these larger and stronger animals. It has recently been shown that aggressive predisposition also has some genetic basis, and new breeding strategies may reduce the severity of aggression if mixing is unavoidable. However, with good planning and batch management this should not be necessary.

6.10.2 Feeding the finishing pig

The major nutritional objective of the finishing phase is to produce pigs at market weight which meet the specification for best carcass price. In most markets, this involves meeting a contract grading specification for both carcass weight and leanness, usually measured as subcutaneous fat thickness at one or more specified points on the back. Because they have been bred for leanness, it is possible for genetically superior pigs to be fed *ad libitum* through to slaughter and still give acceptable grading. This greatly simplifies the management of feeding since automated filling of feed reservoirs in each pen, which the pigs can access on a 24 hour basis, means that many pigs can share a limited feeding area provided from linear hoppers, circular pans or single space feeders. Such feeders vary widely in design and may supply dry meal or pelleted feed, liquid feed as a soup or incorporate integral watering devices in combination with dry food. Current recommendations in such systems are that up to 12 pigs can share a feeding place with dry food, and up to 20 with feeders which wet the food at point of delivery or provide liquid food. However, *ad libitum* feeding without development of excessive carcass fatness may not be possible with less improved genotypes, and particularly the castrated males, or when pigs are kept to much heavier weights before slaughter for some specialized markets such as Italian Parma ham. In these circumstances, feed restriction in the final stages of fattening may be necessary. When this is the case, adequate feed distribution is essential to ensure evenness of weight is maintained within the group and to minimize aggression at feeding time. The feed can be provided in long troughs or scattered widely on the floor. When troughs are used, the feeding space allowance per pig must be at least the width of an animal across the shoulders so that all can feed simultaneously. However, even when this space is provided, some individuals may dominate greater areas of the trough unless head or head and shoulder barriers are incorporated.

Feeds for the growing finishing pig are usually based on cereals and plant proteins, most commonly soyabean meal. However, feed costs can be reduced by the inclusion of industrial by-products from the human food and drink sector such as wheat feed, vegetable wastes and brewery and distillery products. Many of these products come in liquid form and can only be utilized with specialized feeding systems designed for this purpose. It used to be common practice to feed pigs on kitchen waste, particularly in smallholder systems. However, the disease risks associated with this procedure, where infected meat might be fed back into the food chain, have resulted in an EU ban on this practice. As the pig becomes older, its appetite increases and its need for protein relative to energy in the diet decreases. To maximize use of nutrients, it is therefore normal to feed a series of diets over the growing period which change in specification as the pig ages (Table 6.5).

6.10.3 Outdoor systems

While outdoor production systems for breeding sows are common in some countries, and outdoor systems for weaned pigs have increased, the outdoor finishing of pigs is still very uncommon. Constraints include land availability and soil damage, pollution potential, loss of performance and logistics of supplying the large daily requirement for feed and water in all weather conditions. A small number of herds have operated such systems for organic pig production, but information and experience outside this context is very limited. Outdoor finishing can be divided into two types. In the first, free-range pigs are provided with a large paddock and simple shelter, while in the second they are confined within an outdoor hut-and-run system. Paddock systems are the least common, requiring more land and being more difficult to manage.

In true paddock systems, pigs have the free run of a fenced paddock area. They are normally contained by a two-strand electric fence. The stocking rate suggested has been approximately 4,000 kg/ha, giving 40 to 50 finishing pigs per hectare, although this will depend on soil type and climatic conditions. In practice, even higher stocking densities have been used for limited periods in arable rotations (up to 500 pigs/ha), but have generally resulted in a high level of paddock damage. Housing for free-range pigs will depend on climate and group size. It must provide a warm, dry lying area in winter and, unless other provision is made, must also provide shade in summer. A minimum lying area of $0.5\,m^2$ for a 100 kg pig ($0.3\,m^2$ for a 50 kg pig) should be provided. Bedding should be provided in winter to provide floor insulation, and replenished frequently enough to maintain a clean, dry surface. Under UK conditions, a straw usage of 20–60 kg per growing-finishing pig per cycle has been reported. Housing is generally moveable, so that each new batch of pigs can begin in a clean paddock with a newly resited house. In UK conditions, housing comprising corrugated iron arcs or wooden sheds has generally been used, although tents have more recently been adopted on a few farms (see below). Feed is generally provided *ad libitum* via bulk hoppers, which can be filled mechanically (a group of 50 pigs requiring up to 1 tonne of feed per week). Water is generally provided from open troughs, allowing at least 12 mm of trough space per pig. These troughs need to have an adequate capacity and/or filling rate to provide at least 5 litres of water per pig per day, although this will vary with size of pig and environmental temperature.

An alternative system with tents and deep litter paddocks has been developed in Denmark, but not yet widely adopted. The objective has been to provide outdoor housing on a semi-permanent site while controlling pollution risk. The tents have roofs of 16-gauge double-skin transparent polyethylene film supported by a 10 m central pole and 16 shorter poles around the circumference. The walls are made of two layers of straw bales, protected by wire mesh. The inside area of $40\,m^2$ houses 100 pigs from weaning to slaughter. Smaller, $25\,m^2$ tents can be used to house 80 pigs from weaning to 30 kg. In summer, the high, conical shape gives good ventilation, while in cold weather, a canvas false-roof is installed at 1.6 m above floor level to maintain a higher house temperature. The outdoor area provides $1.8\,m^2$ per pig and is bounded by an electric fence. To prevent leaching of nitrate, the topsoil is removed from this area and banked around it. A 1 mm density polyethylene membrane is placed at the bottom, with 10 cm layers of sand on both sides. An 80 cm drainage layer of crushed shells is then covered by a top layer of 10 kg straw per m^2. Straw is replenished as necessary to maintain hygiene, giving an overall straw usage of about 600 g of straw per kg live-weight gain (9 tonnes per batch of 100 pigs from weaning to slaughter). After use, the straw and dung can be composted for manure, and the liquid manure in the shell layer used to fertilize crops.

The most common system of outdoor finishing in the UK involves a hut-and-run system, where pigs are provided with a hut and small outdoor run area bounded by solid fencing and bedded with straw to maintain hygiene. One common type features a wooden hut of 2.4 m by 6.1 m with an insulated steel roof, and an outdoor run of approximately 33 m^2 to house 25 pigs from 30 to 90 kg. The hut has an adjustable ventilator and contains and integral feed hopper with large capacity and water tank holding a one-day reserve supply. Between each batch of pigs, and even within-batch if the run becomes very soiled, the hut can be lifted and towed to a clean area of ground to reduce risk of infection. A further option for easier management and mechanization of feed and water supply is to place such units on a permanent concrete base. In this situation, the units are dismantled between batches, and reassembled after the base has been cleaned. Such systems start to resemble in approach the traditional brick pig houses with outdoor concrete runs which were used on small farms early in the twentieth century, or the systems used in many countries for organic pig production at the present time.

Information on performance levels of outdoor pigs is scarce, and controlled performance comparisons between indoor and outdoor finishing pig production are even less common. It would be expected that outdoor finishing systems would have poorer pig performance because of the additional energy losses associated with lower temperatures and greater amount of exercise, and limited trial data suggest a 5–10% poorer feed efficiency. Additionally, the genotypes of pigs commonly used in outdoor systems have been selected to better withstand adverse climatic conditions and, in consequence, have poorer lean tissue deposition potential and greater propensity to fatness than those used in intensive indoor systems. This results in poorer feed conversion ratios because of the higher energetic cost of fat deposition compared to lean deposition. However, respiratory health of the animals is generally better because of the plentiful supply of fresh air and lack of noxious gases which irritate lung tissue.

6.10.4 Handling and transport

The greatest challenges to the welfare of finishing pigs come during human interventions for procedures such as moving, weighing, transporting, catching and injecting. To facilitate ease of handling, and minimize the number of negative behaviours which the stockperson must carry out during the process, good housing design is critical. A thorough knowledge of pig behaviour can aid both the design of pig housing and the way in which animals are handled with least difficulty. The application of behaviourally based design criteria to pig movement facilities has been studied in some detail. Since pigs have poor depth perception, they are unwilling to cross shadows or high-contrast objects. Entering a strange dark space can take three times as long as entering a strange, brightly lit space. Therefore provision of even lighting and uniform flooring will facilitate movement. Since pigs have a wide-angled visual field, they can be easily distracted and hence solid-sided, gently curved races prevent movement being disturbed by outside events. Pigs raised in very confined and uniform environments have often proved more easily baulked and difficult to drive than those reared in more enriched environments. While pigs have less pronounced following behaviour than ruminants, they will follow a leader when it is an established member of their social group. Isolation from the group is very stressful and they will often panic if they become separated. Prevention of jamming at the entrance to a single-file race can be prevented by using an offset step at the race entrance, but use of a double race where two pigs can progress side by side is better. One of the greatest physical stressors is walking up a ramp, such as a loading bridge for transport. From their behaviour it seems that, to inexperienced pigs, a ramp with an angle of 30 degrees appears inaccessible to them.

The degree of stress during loading, transport, lairage and slaughter is important not only for the welfare of the animals but also for the quality of the meat. To assess the relative stressfulness of procedures carried out during transport, an artificial simulator has been used. Starting the motor which generated vibration and noise caused the greatest increase in heart rate, but this gradually declined as the test progressed, indicating some degree of adaptation. Similar results were obtained during real road journeys. By placing a switch panel inside the transport simulator, it was possible to study the motivation of pigs to avoid vibration and noise. Pigs quickly learnt to press the panel and temporarily switch off the simulator, indicating that they found it aversive. They pressed the panel more often if the level of noise and vibration was more intense, and continued to do so throughout the test period, indicating no degree of habituation. Pigs did not learn to press the panel to switch off noise alone, suggesting that it was the vibration which was important. When tested just after a large meal, they switched off the simulator more often, suggesting that transport was even more aversive at this time. Pigs appear to be particularly sensitive to travel sickness, and fasting them overnight before a journey is recommended.

6.11 Pig Diseases and Health Management

Pigs, especially when kept intensively, are susceptible to a number of infectious diseases which can spread rapidly within and between herds. Highly infectious exotic diseases, such as foot and mouth disease, classical swine fever and African swine fever, are controlled in many countries by national eradication programmes, in which all pigs in any herd where the disease is detected are slaughtered and their carcasses buried or burnt to prevent disease spread. Other, less serious diseases can exist endemically within herds where their effects on health and welfare can be minimized by good management. Many of these can be controlled by a vaccination programme within the herd. Use of vaccines against enzootic pneumonia (EP), porcine respiratory and reproductive syndrome (PRRS), erysipelas, *Escherichia coli* and PMWS is now widespread. However, for many respiratory and enteric diseases, maintaining a good level of hygiene and minimizing stressors for the animals, combined with rapid diagnosis and antibiotic treatment of clinical cases, prevents occurrence of serious herd losses. By maintaining a strictly controlled pig flow, with all-in all-out management of accommodation, thorough cleaning and disinfection between batches, and no mixing of cohorts of different ages, pen hygiene, air quality and hence infection pressure can be kept at a low level. The widespread adoption of these approaches has made it possible to reduce reliance on prophylactic use of antibiotics in feed or water, which has become unacceptable in many countries because of a possible association with the development of antibiotic-resistant strains of pathogen which might pose a threat to human health.

Because even well-managed endemic diseases result in slower growth and poorer feed efficiency, and hence significant economic losses, many herds seek to maintain a high health status. Provided that they are located far enough away from other infected herds, since some disease agents can easily be carried for distances of 3 to 4 km on the wind, good biosecurity precautions can prevent ingress of disease. The most important precautions relate to importation of diseased animals, or animal products. Therefore, high health herds will either run a closed breeding replacement system, or only take in animals and semen from herds of known and tested high health status. Any incoming animals must undergo a quarantine period, so that any incubating disease has time to be expressed. A perimeter fence around the unit, a good rodent control programme and bird-proofing of buildings prevent wildlife from bringing in disease. This fencing also allows control of visitors, with only those who have had no contact with other pigs in at least the last 48 hours being considered low risk. A requirement to shower at the entry point, and the provision of clean protective clothing and boots, further reduce the likelihood of importing disease agents. Similarly, all but essential vehicles are excluded, with feed deliveries and pig removal vehicles all operating from outside the perimeter. The use of disinfectant wheel dips and sprays at the unit entrance ensures that manure picked up on other farms is not brought in on vehicles, and foot dips outside each building prevent tracking around the unit. Where such precautions are rigorously enforced, high health status can be maintained with major benefits for both profitability and animal welfare.

6.12 Animal Welfare in Different Systems

The many welfare problems described with intensive indoor housing systems for pigs do not mean that welfare can only be good in an extensive situation; indeed, the opposite can sometimes be the case. The favourable consumer perception of outdoor systems results from the large area of free space, the environmental complexity and the choice of physical and social environment which is possible in these circumstances. There is evidence that outdoor systems may be better for health in some respects, since veterinary and medicine costs per pig are 10–20% lower in outdoor than in indoor herds. However, parasitism may be greater in the outdoor situation, where worm eggs can remain viable in the soil for extended periods and constitute a source of reinfection. This is a particular issue in organic herds, where routine use of anthelminthics is prohibited. Outdoor pigs face other welfare problems, particularly in relation to thermal stress and social competition. Low-ranking animals may be particularly disadvantaged in outdoor systems in comparison with the more controlled indoor situation, since they can receive only limited human assistance in attaining adequate access to resources such as shelter and food. Thus, when considered in the welfare framework of the 'five freedoms', the following conclusions about outdoor production systems can be drawn:

- freedom from hunger and thirst – no effect, or possible negative effect if reliant on natural foraging;
- freedom from thermal and physical discomfort – possible negative effect from climatic extremes;
- freedom from injury and disease – positive effect from reduced infection intensity, but possible negative effect from reduced biosecurity and increased parasitic burden;
- freedom from fear and stress – positive effect from greater space allowance and enriched behavioural development, but less human assistance for subordinate animals and possible negative effects at time of slaughter from unfamiliarity with confinement and handling;
- freedom to express normal behaviour – clear positive effects, although nose-ringing of breeding stock is an issue.

Organic production systems specify a number of conditions which are thought to improve the welfare of pigs. Permanent indoor housing of organic livestock is not permitted. Animals can be housed indoors for a maximum of 20% of their lifetime, but at other times must be kept either in fields or in housing where they have permanent access to an outdoor run. All housing must have a bedded lying area and slats, while permitted, must not exceed 50% of the total floor area (25% in some schemes). The space requirements for organic pigs are greater than those conventionally used. All pigs must be given access to roughage or fodder, and at present farmers use grazed grass/clover swards, conserved silage from such swards, from whole-crop cereals or from maize, and root crops such as fodder beet. However, a major current challenge for organic pig producers is to find enough organically produced feed of appropriate quality, especially for the newly weaned piglets. The objective of organic production is to maintain good health through the adoption of effective management practices. Organic production forbids the routine use of antibiotics, although it does not preclude their use for individual animals where there is a veterinary need. In such circumstances, longer withdrawal periods are specified (twice that required by law) before the animal can be slaughtered for meat. Animals which have received repeated antibiotic treatment cannot be sold for organic meat, presenting the risk that producers may withhold treatments to maintain their organic premium. Routine use of anthelminthics is not allowed, and the emphasis is on good pasture management and regular rotation to control parasite build-up. However, survey data suggest that parasitism can be a major problem in organic pig herds.

Build-up of parasites and other infectious agents can also pose greater challenges in bedded systems than in those where pigs are kept on slatted floors, and hence separated from their manure. However, such health benefits must be considered in opposition to many beneficial roles of bedding in provision of physical comfort, thermal comfort and environmental enrichment. As discussed throughout this chapter, each system has its own strengths and weaknesses which need to be addressed in the most appropriate way to ensure good pig welfare.

No matter which system is adopted, one of the most important determinants of pig welfare is the quality of the management and stockmanship that they receive. The importance of the relationship between the stockperson and their animals for productivity was first highlighted in a study carried out in the Netherlands. Twelve commercial units, each run by a single stockperson, were controlled by a large integrated company which dictated that all outside inputs (source of pigs, feed, management and veterinary advice) were similar. Despite this, the farms showed large differences in reproductive performance, with averages ranging from 17.9 to 22.5 pigs born per sow per year. To seek some explanation for this, the sows on each unit were subject to behavioural tests assessing their response to humans. It was found that sows on farms with poor reproductive performance showed more signs of fear of humans. When tested in their stalls, they had a greater withdrawal response to the approach of an experimenter's hand, and when confronted with a strange person in an open arena they showed less approach behaviour. This phenomenon was subsequently investigated in a series of controlled experiments, which demonstrated that pigs subjected to repeated negative or inconsistent handling developed a chronic stress response. This was reflected in poorer growth rate and reproductive performance. Subsequent studies have shown a relationship between the attitudinal and behavioural profiles of stockpersons and the level of fear of humans seen in their pigs. In Australia, implementing a training procedure which involved providing stockpeople with information on the sensitivity of pigs to negative handling and the practical benefits in ease of management and productivity when positive handling procedures are adopted, markedly reduced fear levels in the pigs and increased performance by five pigs per sow per year. Growing awareness of such benefits has led to the introduction of certified training programmes in many countries, and the highlighting of the importance of the human–animal interaction in both legislation and codes of good practice.

References and Further Reading

Assured British Pigs (2007) *AB Pigs Certification Standards*. Assured British Pigs, Cobham, UK.

BPEX (2008a) *Pig Yearbook*. BPEX Ltd, Milton Keynes, UK.

BPEX (2008b) *2007 Pig Cost of Production in Selected Countries*. BPEX Ltd, Milton Keynes, UK.

English, P.R., Fowler, V.R., Baxter, S. and Smith, B. (1988) *The Growing and Finishing Pig: Improving Efficiency*. Farming Press, Ipswich, UK.

English, P., Smith, W. and MacLean, A. (1982) *The Sow: Improving her Efficiency*. Farming Press, Ipswich, UK.

Faucitano, L. and Schaefer, A.L. (2008) *Welfare of Pigs from Birth to Slaughter*. Wageningen Academic Publishers, Wageningen, Netherlands.

RSPCA (2008) *Welfare Standards for Pigs*. RSPCA, Horsham, UK.

Straw, B.E., Zimmerman, J.J., D'Allaire, S. and Taylor, D.K. (eds) (2006) *Diseases of Swine*, 9th edn. Blackwall Publishing, Ames, IA.

Thornton, K. (1988) *Outdoor Pig Production*. Farming Press, Ipswich, UK.

Vaarst, M., Roderick, S., Lund, V. and Lockeretz, W. (2003) *Animal Health and Welfare in Organic Agriculture*. CABI Publishing, Wallingford.

Varley, M.A. and Wiseman, J. (eds) (2001) *The Weaner Pig: Nutrition and Management*. CABI Publishing, Wallingford, UK.

Whittemore, C. (1998) *The Science and Practice of Pig Production*, 2nd edn. Blackwell Science, Oxford.

Wiseman, J. (2000) *The Pig: a British History*. Duckworth, London.

Laying Hens

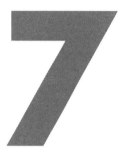

GRAHAM SCOTT

Management and Welfare of Farm Animals: The UFAW Farm Handbook, 5th edition. John Webster
© 2011 by Universities Federation for Animal Welfare (UFAW)

7.1 Introduction

When considering the welfare of laying hens it is essential to remember that birds are not egg-producing machines. They are living, sentient creatures and, human conscience might suggest, should be treated with respect. Chickens are capable of adapting to many environmental conditions. By adapting, they can become accustomed and cope with many types of change to their environment. Animal welfare is increasingly described in terms of animals being able to cope with such changes; if the animals cannot adapt and cope, then welfare is negatively affected. If humans can establish the limits of adaptability of laying hens we can provide a suitable environment that birds can adapt to easily and does not negatively affect the birds' welfare. Similarly humans can modify the production expectations (egg production per bird) so that welfare is not threatened. To do this we need an in-depth knowledge of the needs of the birds that we use.

In order to care properly for laying hens, it is important to understand the basic biology of the bird (in terms of anatomy and physiology). Chickens are complex organisms. Knowledge of the fundamental systems can assist in providing for the welfare requirements of the species. Since laying hens are producing eggs on a regular basis, the reproductive system of the female (hen) will be described in some detail, along with the skeletal and digestive systems. Behavioural needs of the hens may also relate to how birds perceive their environment and so sensory perception will be considered.

The keeping of hens for egg production will be put into context both in terms of the historical relationship between humans and hens for egg production, and the UK and global egg production industries. The permitted systems for the egg industry will be described and explained. This will include the rearing of pullets from day-old chicks to point of lay and then on to the production systems. The management requirements, biosecurity, disease control and common problems, including behavioural problems, and issues will be addressed. Bird welfare and larger welfare issues will be assessed. Egg quality systems, including provision for bird welfare, will be included before speculation on how egg production may evolve in the future brings the chapter to a close. While this chapter is addressed at an international audience, many of the descriptions of regulations and welfare organizations use the UK situation as an example.

7.2 Chicken Physiology

7.2.1 The reproductive system

Before discussing the way that chickens are kept, it is important to grasp the basic biology of the chicken to enable a better understanding of the birds. In birds (unlike mammals) it is the male that is homogametic, carrying two of the same sex chromosomes. So at the point of fertilization there are males (ZZ) and females (Z-). The female chick carries all of her undeveloped ova at hatch. However, only one of the female's ovaries (the left) is functional. At sexual maturity, under the control of hormones from the anterior pituitary gland, these Graafian follicles develop into mature ova, attached to part of the egg yolk. The yolk contains phospholipids (from the liver) which provide most of the nutrients required for a developing chick in the fertile egg. In the functioning ovary the follicles are different in size as they develop their attachment to the phospholipids. The larger yolks are the first to be shed from the ovary (Figure 7.1). The oviduct also changes at sexual maturity for it is here that the albumen (egg white), shell membranes, water and egg shells are attached. The pelvis of the bird widens to allow the passage of the egg and the cloaca (vent) changes to allow easy oviposition (egg-laying).

When the hen is in lay, this left oviduct will occupy most of the left side of the abdomen. Ovulation occurs daily and egg production (ovulation) is independent of mating. Hence there are no cockerels on most commercial egg production systems. It takes about 25 hours between ovulation and egg-laying (oviposition) so each egg is laid later each day. Most eggs are laid within 4 hours of dawn (or when the artificial lighting is turned on after the longest dark period for housed birds). Birds tend not to lay eggs in the dark period, retaining them to be laid early the following day. Thus we talk of birds laying 'clutches' of about nine eggs. Egg-laying behaviour is not related to the presence of an egg in the shell gland, but is connected to ovulation at least 24 hours earlier. Ovulation is controlled by luteinizing hormone from the pituitary gland. Once the egg is released from the ovary, it travels to the infundibulum where a thin layer of albumin surrounds the yolk. At the magnum, thick albumen, calcium, sodium and magnesium are introduced to the developing egg. Egg weight doubles until the two shell membranes are attached. In the uterus the egg spins and the calcium carbonate shell is added. This is usually done during the night as the bird is roosting. Finally the waxy cuticle is added in the vagina before the egg is ready to be laid. The non-functioning ovary remains dormant. However, in a small number of cases, it can become active. The outcome is that the hen will cease to lay eggs. The comb will grow and the hen will commence crowing like a cockerel.

Daily egg production puts a great burden on the hen. Her daily food intake will increase by about 35% from pre-lay to peak lay and the bird will need a great deal of calcium to provide for the egg shell formation. This is particularly important in later life as hens can mobilize the stored calcium from the skeleton, particularly from the long bones such as the tibia (Figure 7.2).

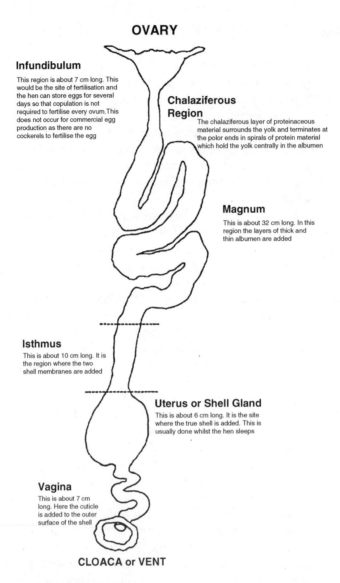

OVARY

Infundibulum
This region is about 7 cm long. This would be the site of fertilisation and the hen can store eggs for several days so that copulation is not required to fertilise every ovum. This does not occur for commercial egg production as there are no cockerels to fertilise the egg

Chalaziferous Region
The chalaziferous layer of proteinaceous material surrounds the yolk and terminates at the polor ends in spirals of protein material which hold the yolk centrally in the albumen

Magnum
This is about 32 cm long. In this region the layers of thick and thin albumen are added

Isthmus
This is about 10 cm long. It is the region where the two shell membranes are added

Uterus or Shell Gland
This is about 6 cm long. It is the site where the true shell is added. This is usually done whilst the hen sleeps

Vagina
This is about 7 cm long. Here the cuticle is added to the outer surface of the shell

CLOACA or VENT

Figure 7.1   The oviduct of a laying hen.

7.2.2 The skeleton

The skeleton of the chicken (like other flying birds) combines strength with lightness. The large sternum has a deep keel to accommodate the flight muscles. This keel can be vulnerable to damage when being handled, particularly during any rough handling when being extracted from the cage. It is important that birds are held properly and that the keel is supported (Figure 7.3).

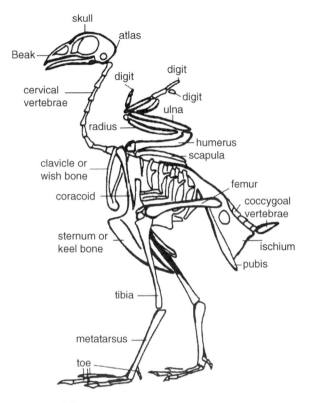

Figure 7.2 The skeleton of the laying hen.

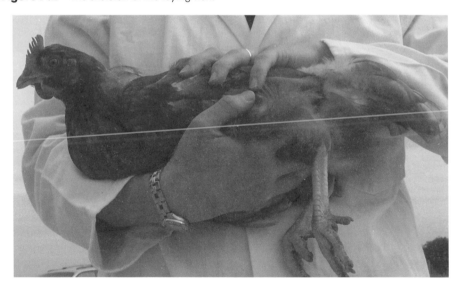

Figure 7.3 The correct way to hold a chicken, supporting the sternum and holding the legs with one hand with the other hand covering the wings.

On the ground, the whole weight of the bird is supported by the pelvic girdle and hips. The body weight is maintained close to the centre of gravity. Many of the bones are hollow (reducing weight). The long bones, such as the tibia, contain calcium which can be utilized by the hen for shell formation if there is insufficient other calcium available in the diet or other body reserves. Over a prolonged period this can lead to osteoporosis, or brittle bones, which has been termed 'caged layer fatigue'.

In general, during egg production in controlled-environment houses, feather growth is almost halted. In more traditional systems, during the 'winter months' when egg production stopped the birds would moult. Moulting involves new feathers pushing out old ones, calcium depletion in the long bones stops and calcium levels in these bones recover during the non-lay period. After about 3 months the birds come back in to lay, laying large numbers of eggs, larger than the corresponding eggs during the first period of egg production as point-of-lay pullets. Although laying hens can live up to 13 years, commercial laying hens are usually replaced after their first year of egg production (about 74 weeks of age).

7.2.3 The digestive system

Diet is particularly important to maintain output of good-quality eggs. Hens, like humans, are monogastric. They obtain nutrients directly by absorbing material from the food they eat, rather than relying on cellulose-digesting bacteria, like ruminants. The digestive system of the chicken is illustrated in Figure 7.4. The beak and tongue are used to investigate the environment and the taste of food. The beak tip is very sensitive with many nerves. Taste buds have been found on the base of the tongue and floor of the pharynx. The chicken's taste buds are morphologically similar to, but not

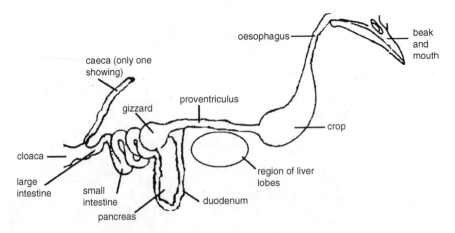

Figure 7.4 Pictorial representation of the digestive system of the laying hen. Note: the duodenal loop has been distended for clarity.

identical to, those of mammals. Chickens apparently avoid saccharine and sweet flavours, such as honey and strawberry, though they show a preference for sucrose and the butter-type flavours. Some producers use the appeal of ascorbic acid in water to get the birds to drink on arrival at the production system and to offset the effects of heat stress.

The crop is positioned in the neck region. It is an extension of the oesophagus with a thin, elastic membranous wall. Thus it is able to expand and act as a storage facility for food prior to digestion. This can be useful for flock-keepers since the neck can be palpated to determine if the birds are eating (a full crop). Occasionally birds can suffer a compacted crop, possibly from eating long grass. This can be treated by massaging after giving the bird a syringe of warm water, vegetable oil (or olive oil), melted butter or a yoghurt-type product. If this fails, veterinary assistance can be sought in order to make a small incision at the crop to remove the impacted material. Compacted crops can be fatal.

The proventriculus is at the anterior end of the stomach. This glandular section secretes hydrochloric acid and digestive enzymes into the food mix before the food moves down to the thick-walled muscular gizzard. Since birds do not have teeth and are unable to chew or mix their food prior to digestion, the gizzard performs a similar function. Birds deliberately swallow grit or stones and anything over 4 mm in diameter remains in the gizzard. The churning action of the muscular gizzard helps to break down the food particles by the mechanical, grinding action of these stones along with the digestive action of the material secreted from the proven-triculus. The controlled release of the resulting fluid into the duodenum enables the beginning of absorption. The bile and pancreatic ducts add further digestive enzymes or modify the pH in the gut to promote enzyme activity. The ileum (small intestine) is the major site of food absorption. Two blind-ended caeca occur at the junction between the small and large intestine. These caeca are involved in bacterial breakdown of cellulose, though the contribution to total food absorption by the bird is unlikely to be significant except in undeveloped village systems where the birds are expected to scavenge for most or all of their food. About every fortieth evacuation of faeces from the cloaca includes the watery contents of the caeca. It is wrong to believe that chickens urinate; though the kidneys do function as part of the waste removal system. They do not possess the essential metabolic pathways to produce urea. Nitrogenous waste from birds is in the form of solid uric acid (the white part of bird faeces). Some water reabsorption takes place in the large intestine along with storage of faecal material until evacuation takes place through the cloaca.

7.2.4 Sensory perception

The skin of a chicken possesses thermal and mechano-receptors (for pressure or 'touch') and receptors for vibration, particularly in the legs. This may allow rapid changes in body position when perched on a swaying branch, but could also be a warning mechanism if an unseen predator is approaching. Birds have a relatively large brain. They rely heavily on muscular coordination (for flight) and vision systems (eyes and visual acuity) for information about their environment. Hens have similar colour vision to humans, but their visual acuity covers a wide field, enabling large amounts of visual information, particularly movement, to be collected and assessed. Chickens perform rapid head movement to determine the location and distance of specific objects in their field of vision. The eye also appears to be capable of sharp focus, which is important during flight or moving between perches to avoid collision and injury.

Chickens possess olfactory receptors in the base of the upper jaw though smell does not seem to be an important stimulus compared to other types of stimuli for poultry. For example, birds can hear over a relatively narrow range of wavelengths but have very sensitive hearing (to pitch and volume) over that range. The ear system is similar to humans in that it is involved in hearing and balance. The outer ear has very little specialized structure. However, often producers use the colour of the feathers on the ear lobes as an indication of the colour of the egg shell. Chickens are capable of communication through body position and some vocalization. Vocal calls are produced at the syrinx, where the trachea forks into the bronchi.

7.3 The Poultry Industry

7.3.1 History of poultry in human society

The keeping of poultry dates back to classical societies such as Egyptian, Roman and ancient Chinese. Romans brought poultry to Britain when the Roman Empire expanded. It is possible that poultry remained in Britain through the centuries, but right up to the early 1900s poultry-keeping does not appear to have had the same cultural importance as, say, the keeping of swine, sheep or cattle. Even today, some influential agriculturalists appear to have a blind spot when considering poultry, compared to, say, dairy or other, more traditional, larger livestock. Yet, the poultry industry, of all livestock, is an expanding global industry with all of the sophistication of worldwide trading and supply chains, not seen in some of the more traditional livestock industries. The view that poultry is not important may result from outdated ideas of wealth and 'snobbery'. Presumably, being of lower individual value, there would not be the same prestige in owning a chicken compared to, perhaps, the ownership of a cow! Right up to the time of World War I, farmers' wives took care of chickens in the farmyard. Presumably, it was demeaning for the farmer (the man) to lower himself to do 'woman's work', looking after the farm chickens. Nevertheless, chickens seem to have a place deep in human culture.

From the days of Aesop, infants have been warned not to 'count the chickens before they hatch' or not to 'put all of our eggs in one basket'. We learned the importance of sharing from 'the Little Red Hen' and the foolishness of 'Chicken Licken' who thought the sky was falling. Male prowess has been likened to 'strutting roosters' and fussing mothers have been likened to mother hens. Eggs and chicks have become associated with Spring religious festivals and have come to symbolize new birth and fertility.

7.3.2 Poultry-Keeping in the UK

A cultural shift, to raise the profile of poultry production in Britain, occurred after World War I. The government realized the threat posed by submarine warfare, with the potential to disrupt food supply to the British Isles, and so looked favourably on any project that might improve self-sufficiency in food supply. At the same time, soldiers, sickened by their experiences in the trenches and the prospect of returning to a class-ridden society, expressed a desire to become (chicken) farmers. With government assistance several free-range units of about 500 dual-purpose birds were established. There was minimal environmental control for these flocks and pure strains such as Rhode Island Red and Light Sussex were common. The management of these relatively small flocks relied heavily on experience and intuition. The Egg Marketing Board ensured that all eggs were sold and prices were more-or-less guaranteed. This state of affairs continued through World War II. There was no real black market in eggs during the war since the Egg Marketing Board continued to purchase and distribute eggs.

Since the early 1900s some entrepreneurs in the UK had realized the potential gains to be had from properly organized poultry farming, following examples in the USA. Around this time poultry research was beginning to blossom, particularly in standardizing management techniques. Research was undertaken to increase production through breed selection, formulation of balanced diets and the development of improved, more intensive management techniques. Such research assisted in increasing production but a number of significant events occurred in the 1950s which laid the foundation for the modern egg production industry.

Perhaps the most important event of the decade was the derationing of wheat after World War II. The amount of feed wheat available effectively restricted the number of birds in a flock. Once this restriction was withdrawn, individuals could manage much larger flocks since it was this, and not labour, that was limiting at the time. A second, important event was the introduction of electricity on farms. This was probably of most significance in the later development of the egg production systems that relied on motorized automated delivery and egg collection apparatus. The third watershed occurred after a study group visited the USA and returned with a fast-growing strain of chicken 'designed' exclusively for the poultry meat trade. (One of the group smuggled hatching eggs in his luggage and these became the first broilers in Britain!) This effectively led to the parting of the ways for the poultry egg and the poultry meat industries. Instead of the dual-purpose birds, this enabled concentrated efforts in the development of birds selected either for egg output or for rapid muscle growth. These developments acting in unison with the research led to significant steps forward in terms of output.

The most significant consequences of research to improve egg numbers and quality have been the development of balanced, least-cost diets, notably incorporating the essential amino acids, lysine and methionine, and the establishment of management regimes in controlled-environment buildings. Perhaps the most significant was the determination of the importance of lighting on sexual maturity and egg production. Chickens possess a pineal gland which is associated with melatonin production. Since this hormone is produced during darkness, melatonin levels in the body are associated with daylength. Melatonin is involved in controlling other hormones and body systems. The detail will not be discussed here but can be found in any good chicken physiology text (e.g. Reece, 2009). There are critical levels of melatonin for the control of sexual maturity and sexual cycling (egg production). This is why such a discovery was critical for commercial egg production. Up to the 1950s or so, it was accepted that chickens generally stopped egg production during the autumn and winter months in Britain. Unfortunately, this clashed with one of the two main peaks in demand for eggs (i.e. Christmas, for cakes and puddings, and Easter, with egg-related festivities).

Putting the birds in sheds with electric lighting allowed for extended daylength with year-round egg production (with a significant economic advantage). The first indoor systems were simple 'deep litter' systems where the chickens were taken into a shed with an open-plan arrangement with a litter material on the floor (e.g. straw, sawdust or wood shavings), manually filled water and food dispensers, and nest boxes. This enabled housing of the birds for relatively little capital expense. However, the coprophagic birds suffered from disease and, in cases of panic, smothered each other in their attempts to escape. Also in large flocks, birds were aggressive and even cannibalistic. Such cannibalism was not found in cages and so caged birds were introduced into the controlled environment indoors. The more 'modern' egg-laying bird was relatively smaller than the previous dual-purpose birds and so producers put more than one bird in each cage. Since chickens are reasonably gregarious the birds were less frightened than birds kept individually, and output increased. Although simplified management and increased output with reduced marginal costs may have been the driving force, it could be argued that the caged system also improved the welfare of the birds by reduced aggression, reduced disease, lowered risks from predation and the provision of healthy food and a cleaner environment. The logical flow, however, was to increase the number of birds in cages and to put cages on top of each other to maximize the usage of the building. The increased use of electrical systems for environmental management and automated delivery of foodstuff and egg removal enabled increasing numbers of birds to be managed by a relatively small labour force. Eggs became more freely available at a lower cost and consumption grew.

As with any growing and developing industry, take-overs and mergers occurred. Relatively easy money was to be made and some of the businesses were bought by financial speculators. Strategic expansion within the industry led to vertically integrated companies, with more control over resources and quality control (Figure 7.5).

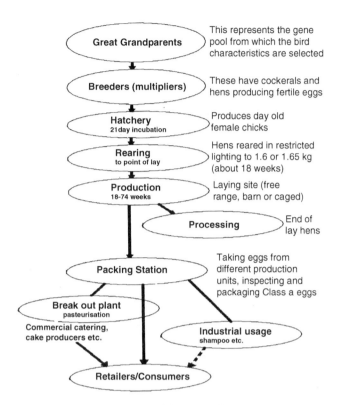

Figure 7.5 Diagrammatic representation of the vertically integrated laying hen egg industry. Note: breeders typically own all stages to the hatchery and producers from the rearing stage to the packing station.

A number of 'breeders' emerged on the international market, providing birds best suited to the requirements of egg production. These egg production companies expanded horizontally, purchasing other egg production units, and also purchased feed mills, rearing facilities, egg grading and supply chains to the newly developing supermarkets.

7.3.2.1 The structure of the egg production industry in the UK

The UK industry uses, almost exclusively, medium hybrid brown birds, supplied by well-established breeding companies. During the 1960s, a marketing decision assumed that consumers preferred a brown-shelled egg from brown-feathered birds (on the basis that they appear more 'natural' than the white-shelled variety). In the USA, the reverse is the case; white-shelled eggs are the standard (presumably on the basis that they appear more 'hygienic' than brown eggs). From the 1960s the birds were selected for several phenotypic characteristics such as egg output (in terms of numbers and quality), good food conversion (to eggs rather than muscle development and increased growth), hardiness (disease resistance) and docility (rather than aggressiveness). Once the breeding companies establish the bird type it is then the role of the multiplier farms to breed sufficient birds to meet the demands of the egg producers (Figure 7.5). These multiplier farms produce fertile eggs, having cockerels running with the hens (one cockerel for every 10 to 12 females). Sperm transfer is by natural copulation. Since the cockerels' testes are situated within the body cavity, there is little thermal shock at transfer into the females' bodies. Hence the sperm can survive in the females' bodies and go on to fertilize the successive eggs for several days without further copulation being required. These birds are maintained in these conditions from about 24 weeks to about 68 to 70 weeks. In this time the hens will lay over 200 fertile eggs. The eggs are taken to the hatchery and incubated for about 21 days. About 80% of the eggs placed in the incubators survive to hatch properly.

In modern commercial strains it is possible to identify the sex of day-old chicks from the down colour. Male chicks are removed and, since they do not lay eggs, are humanely killed by gassing at the hatchery. They are often sold as frozen chicks for food for captive birds of prey. The female day-old chicks are transported to rearing units.

7.3.3 World poultry keeping and egg production

Between 1970 and 2005 global egg production tripled. In the 1970s most of the world's eggs were produced from North America and Europe. This is no longer the case; most eggs in 2005 were produced in Asia (Table 7.1). In 1970 the USA was the leading producer of eggs (producing 4,053,000 tonnes) while China was fourth (producing 1,533,000 tonnes) and the UK was sixth (producing 892,000 tonnes). By 2005 China had overtaken the USA to be the major producer (24,348,000 tonnes), pushing the USA to second place (5,330,000 tonnes) and the UK was no longer included in the top ten producers.

The practices and problems of poultry-keeping are not the same between countries. Some of the main problems are often temperature dependent. For example, in tropical countries keeping the birds sufficiently cool can be a problem. Although the ancestor to the modern chicken was the Burmese jungle-fowl, it can be difficult for a large numbers of birds to regulate their thermal environment. In poorly ventilated sheds or in regions where air temperature and relative humidity are high (e.g. tropical countries) this is especially difficult. Some of the problems can be overcome to a degree by the breeding of birds adapted to these environments. Some keepers deliberately use, for example, naked-necked birds or birds with 'frizzle feathers';

Table 7.1 Trends in global egg production. Source: Windhorst (2007). Reproduced with permission from Reed Business.

Year	World output (000 tonnes)	Distribution (%)		
		North America	Europe	Asia
1970	19,538	25.3	30.9	23.7
2005	59,233	13.6	16.8	60.4

genetic strains producing relatively poorly feathered birds which may be less prone to heat stress. Some modifications to housing can also assist in maintaining the birds' environment. In some countries, curtain-sided buildings are used where netting material replaces solid walls so that air can circulate relatively freely. In other circumstances water or mist sprays are used as part of the control of the thermal environment. In some countries birds are kept on soil floors. Since it is difficult to disinfect these systems properly, they can often suffer relatively high levels of infection, parasitism and other health problems.

In many countries such as in Africa and Asia, where refrigeration units are not commonplace, chickens are kept in relatively small numbers in close proximity to the household. These birds are used to provide fresh eggs and meat and are not slaughtered until they are actually required for the table. These birds are often fed scraps or are allowed to forage for food items and insects. Birds are sold live at markets, coming into contact with many other birds. Biosecurity is difficult, if not non-existent.

Public concern as to the welfare of the laying hen seems to be most prevalent in northern European countries. This concern is directed mainly at the keeping of hens in the unenriched 'battery cage'. Some argue that this concern is the prerogative of more affluent, relatively well-fed societies whereas, in poorer countries, the need for food is more pressing. In other developed societies, such as the USA, the majority view, supported by legislation, continues to support the most intensive systems (although this view is strongly opposed by welfare groups within the same country). Where this approach prevails, extremely large numbers of laying hens are maintained to achieve the economies of scale that can arise from large intensive systems, producing large numbers of eggs. In the first quarter of 2008 there were on average 282 million laying hens in the US industry, producing 2.1 billion dozen eggs in that time (with an estimated 3.17 billion dozen eggs for the second half of 2008). Most of these eggs are produced in intensive systems. The significant increase in output from Asia is generally from intensive systems. In these countries welfare of poultry is of little concern, compared to food production. Welfare concerns may come with time or may be of importance if welfare becomes part of trade agreements with other countries.

7.4 Production Systems for Laying Hens

7.4.1 Pullet rearing

Flock rearers take the day-old female chicks and rear them to point of lay, usually around 18 weeks, though there are some variations, such as rearing to 16 weeks, before transferring to the production site. Generally, it is not the age of the bird that is important as much as the body mass. The target for hens for caged egg production is about 1.6 kg and, for free-range, 1.65 kg. If a bird is small when she lays her first egg, it is likely that she will lay smaller eggs (compared to her flock mates) for the rest of

Table 7.2 Lighting patterns for laying hens. Source: ISA, (2009–10).

Age (days)	Light period (hours)	Light intensity (lux)
1–2	22	20–40
3–4	20	15–30
5–6	18	15–30
7–14	16	10–20
15–21	15	10
22–28	14	10
29–35	13	10
36–42	12	10
43–49	11	10
50–105	10	10
From 133 days	Increase 0.5 h per week to 16 h	15–30

her life. Because there is such a strong link between daylength and sexual maturity in birds, these young birds are raised in lightproof sheds with restricted daylength (Table 7.2).

As the birds approach sexual maturity daylight hours are restricted to postpone the onset of sexual maturity. Because this involves artificial light restriction, some individuals have argued that it poses a welfare insult. However, 8 hours of light is similar to a winter day in the UK, thus not inherently unnatural. The argument that the birds never receive natural daylight depends on how important 'natural' light is to a species. Animals can adapt and so 'natural' light may be satisfactorily replaced with artificial light in terms of welfare 'needs'. However, hens are diurnal and are capable of utilizing sunlight for vitamin synthesis, suggesting that sunlight may be important to the birds. More research is required before 'natural' light is considered a welfare 'need' (rather than relying on an anthropomorphic 'natural is best' approach). Nevertheless, restricting birds to reduced light intensity may be another matter. Birds are often subjected to light intensities where they can see to eat and drink but to reduce 'vices' such as aggression and feather pecking or feather pulling. Keeping the birds under low light conditions has been a traditional management approach to minimize such problems. This may be more difficult to justify when reduced stocking, or some environmental enrichment, may be a more welfare-friendly strategy. Similarly, in production systems, interrupted lighting patterns have been used to reduce fuel and feed costs. In such situations light and dark periods throughout the day do not follow a 'natural' rhythm of one light and one dark period in 24 hours, but have shorter light periods with intermittent darkness. These can prevent birds from having extended dark, rest periods. This is of concern to welfare groups who campaign for at least 8 hours of uninterrupted darkness for the birds.

7.4.1.1 Vaccination

During the rearing period, mainstream commercial birds (but not organic birds) receive prophylactic vaccination. Some vaccines are administered at the hatchery either as a mist, allowing the birds to receive the vaccines by inhalation, through the conjunctiva or by ingestion from pecking at droplets on the down of their hatchery mates. Some may be given by injection (e.g. Marek's vaccine by injection at the back of the neck). Common vaccines in a typical vaccination programme for laying hens are listed in Table 7.3.

Such prophylactic vaccination programmes ensure that the hens are protected against disease outbreaks. It is not usual to routinely vaccinate hens once they are in lay (though some free-range flocks are vaccinated because of the greater risk of disease with the outdoor lifestyle). A major problem for free-range hens (or birds indoors on litter) is coccidiosis. This is only a risk where birds are liable to come into contact with poultry faeces or equipment (feeders and drinkers) contaminated with birds' faeces. The causative gut parasite produces fertile eggs as a contaminant of faeces from infected birds. Other 'clean' birds then ingest the eggs and become contaminated themselves (producing contaminated faeces). This disease, along with other gut parasites, can build up to the point where 'fowl sick land' is a problem (with a very high risk of contamination between birds and between successive flocks.

Some chick rearers use chick cages to rear the birds to point of lay (particularly for birds destined for the caged sector). These are relatively large cages for communities of chicks. As they grow, a proportion of the chicks are removed to adjacent cages to prevent overcrowding. Other chick rearers raise chicks on litter (such as white wood shavings) using systems which are similar to broiler rearing sheds. During rearing the birds may be subject to beak trimming.

Table 7.3 A typical vaccination schedule for laying hens. Source: Meunier and Latour (undated).

Week of vaccination	Type of vaccination
Day old	Marek's
15 days (1/2 dose)	Infectious bursal (iB)
20 days (1/2 dose)	Infectious bursal (IB)
25 days	Bronchitis, Newcastle disease, infectious bursal (typical brand name Combo Vec. 30)
30 days	Bronchitis, Newcastle disease, infectious bursal (typical brand name Combo Vec. 30)
49 days	Bronchitis, Newcastle disease, infectious bursal (typical brand name Combo Vec. 30)
10 weeks	Fowl pox and laryngotracheitis (commonly referred to as LT)
12 week	Combo Vac 30
13 week	Avian encephalomyelitis (commonly referred to as AE)
16 week	Newcastle disease

Once the birds are light stimulated (Brambell Report' 7.2), it takes about 10–14 days before they commence ovulation. This usually allows the birds to be transferred to the production site and settle in (finding the feeder and drinker systems, and so on) before the stress associated with laying an egg for the first time. The birds are often introduced at 18 weeks of age and come into lay in the following 2 weeks. Most birds are kept in controlled environments. The operating temperature in laying shed is around 23 °C. Of all the environmental controls it is, perhaps, lighting that has the most direct effect on egg production.

7.4.2 Production systems

The permitted egg production systems are:

- eggs from caged hens;
- barn eggs;
- free range;
- organic.

The requirements for these systems will be explained later. The initial eggs are quite small, though egg size can be manipulated, e.g. by increasing the oil components in the food. The birds will maintain egg output above 90% per day for up to 40 weeks. As the birds age, the egg numbers decrease but egg size increases. The birds remain in the shed until the egg numbers reduce to a level that the system becomes uneconomic (bearing in mind that the birds continue food consumption at around 110–120 g per bird per day) at about 72 to 74 weeks of age. Currently there are about 28 million laying hens in the UK, each bird producing between about 280 and 310 eggs. The systems will now be considered in detail.

7.4.2.1 Cage systems

According to classical scripts the Romans kept chickens in what we might recognize as a form of battery cage system. In the UK the first cages were introduced early in the twentieth century. Some of the first research cage systems were placed at the National Institute for Poultry Husbandry (NIPH). Chickens were put into cages to protect them from predators and to prevent coprophagy (muck eating) by the birds, which improved the welfare of the birds by reducing disease and mortality. The quality of the eggs was also improved since the contact of the eggs with the birds' faeces was reduced. The first cages were outdoors but these proved unsuccessful since it was difficult to maintain feeding for the birds, and the British climate meant that the birds ate more in the winter cold and less in the summer heat in order to maintain body temperature by adjusting metabolic heat production to meet the varying thermal changes of the environment.

In the early systems individuals were caged singly, enabling output to be monitored easily. If a bird ceased laying it was obvious and she could be replaced. However, when a second bird was added to the cage, productivity increased because the birds preferred the presence of conspecifics. To overcome the problems of the British weather, and to extend the laying period in an artificial lighting regime, birds were relatively quickly brought indoors (in cages) once electricity supplies became available on farms. The benefits of caged systems over deep litter systems quickly became apparent, in terms of bird health, egg quality and labour saving. Through the late 1950s and early 1960s the number of birds in individual cages and the number of cages in a shed grew quickly.

This escalation of large numbers of individual birds in large groups in a caged environment has obvious visual impact, and such intensive systems caused individuals and groups concerned with animal welfare to become increasingly alarmed. The need for legislative control to preserve the welfare of the laying hens was obvious and, as a result, the UK government set up a committee, which produced the 'Brambell, 1965 which considered the welfare of farmed animals. The Farm Animal Welfare Council was established, based on the recommendations of the report and successive governments have introduced legislation to improve the welfare of caged laying hens. In the mid-1990s floor space was increased to 450 cm^2 per bird. The 1999 EU Directive was incorporated into UK law in 2002 to create a major welfare improvement in 'enriched cages' in 2012. The major developments are listed in Table 7.4.

In the UK up to 2012 the majority of the national egg-laying flock will be housed in conventional cages, in groups of about five birds, in sheds of up to 120,000. The majority of the birds are on farms of between 100,000 and 2 million or so. The conventional cages will become obsolete in 2012, to be replaced by enriched cages.

Table 7.4 The differences in cages for laying hens *before* and *after* 2012.

Cage feature	Before 2012	New cages from 2003 and all cages from 2012
Stocking density (cm^2 per bird)	550	750 (600 usable area; at least 45 cm high)
Minimum total area (cm^2)	550 × no of birds	2000
Perch	x	✓ (15 cm per bird)
Dust-bathing/scratch area	x	✓
Nesting area	x	✓
Claw shortening device	From 2003	✓
Feeder space/bird (cm)	10	12
Drinker space/bird (cm)	10 (or access to 2 nipples)	Suitable for group size (or access to 2 nipples)
Minimum height (cm)	35 (at least 40 over 65% area)	20
Slope (rectangular mesh) (degrees)	8	Not specified
Slope (other floors) (degrees)	12	Not specified
Illegal after 2011	✓	x

7.4.2.2 Enriched cages

Enriched cages attempt to meet all of the behavioural and welfare needs of the hens. They were developed based on research from several countries. In the early 1990s, UK researchers such as Appleby in Edinburgh and Nicol in Bristol considered the inclusion of nesting devices in cages (Appleby et al., 2004). As part of the normal behavioural repertoire during egg-laying, hens need to find and investigate suitable nesting sites before the normal behaviour patterns continue. Where nesting sites are available the whole routine takes about 2 hours from the first signs of egg-laying behaviour and oviposition. In non-enriched cages the behaviours appear thwarted and the routine can continue for 4 hours until oviposition has to occur. Similarly, in barren cages dustbathing behaviour (usually associated with maintenance of feather condition) occurs in the absence of substrate as a vacuum behaviour, indicating that this is a behavioural need.

The Farm Animal Welfare Council produced their opinion on enriched cages in 2007. The Council was concerned that some designs of enriched cages continue to keep the hens continuously confined and do not allow expression of the full behavioural repertoire of the hens but, with adequate designs which pay attention to the needs of the hens, a more welfare-friendly system should result. The EU funded 'LayWel project, (2006) compared conventional cages; 'small', 'medium' and 'large' enriched cages and non-caged systems (Table 7.5). The main conclusions were that (apart from conventional cages which restrict behaviour to an unacceptable level) all systems had the potential to provide satisfactory welfare for laying hens (though the potential may not always be realized). Also, all cage systems tend to provide a more hygienic environment with low risks of parasitic disease.

Table 7.5 Welfare risks in different laying systems. Adapted from Laywel (2006).

		Cage type			Non-cage		Outdoors
	Conventional	Enriched			Single level	Multilevel	
		Small	Medium	Large			
Mortality (%)							
Mortality from feather pecking & cannibalism							
Red mite							
Bumble foot							
Feather loss							
Use of nest boxes							
Use of perches							
Foraging behaviour							
Dustbathing behaviour							
Air quality							
Water intake							
Welfare risk: code			low		medium		high

7.4.2.3 Barn systems

Until 2004 barn systems were also called perchery systems, but this is no longer included as a special marketing term (SMT) in the UK. Barn systems can trace their development from the deep litter systems that became common in the 1950s when electricity was introduced on farms. In order to improve management of the flocks, remove the effects of season and daylength on egg production, birds were brought indoors in an enclosed system. It was very simple and was similar to how modern broiler systems operate, apart from the provision of nest boxes and perches. The deep litter system required relatively low capital investment for a significant increase in production in a controlled environment. Birds were kept on a litter material (sawdust, wood shavings, etc.). The birds were stocked at seven birds per m^2. The system was very labour intensive, with manual egg collection and bird feeding systems. Nevertheless, the increased production and the levels of control made it a more attractive option. However, the high levels of labour requirements in the first systems (with manual feeding and egg collection), the relative high levels of floor-laid or dirty eggs and the disease risks to the birds in contact with their faeces meant that cage systems were preferred. More latterly, the legal requirement for no perches over litter made the pure deep litter system illegal.

Other non-cage systems developed with slatted areas (improving manure management). Some systems included perches and some had mesh-floored tiered systems or platforms to utilize the height of the building and increase stocking in the sheds. The permitted stocking density of such systems was set at about 25 birds per m^2. However, such high stocking often led to problems such as aggression, and in the early 1990s the author visited one site where over 30% of the birds were lost due to cannibalism. Many producers stocked at around 11–13 birds per m^2. This proved a bonus when in the 2002 legislation in the UK such producers were allowed to continue to stock at 12 birds per m^2 up to 2012, while anyone else had to stock at 9 birds per m^2. The feeder and drinking space per bird is strictly controlled. Nest boxes can be individual nests (1 per 7 hens) or communal (1 m^2 for up to 120 hens). The perch allocation (15 cm per hen) and location (at least 30 cm apart and at least 20 cm from a wall) ensures that slatted floors cannot be included in perch calculations and allows easier use by the birds. Since birds need to dust-bathe and scratch, 250 cm^2 per hen (at least one-third of the floor area) must provide a litter material. Any tiered system can have a maximum of four tiers (with 45 cm headroom between tiers) and faeces cannot fall on to birds on lower tiers.

In terms of market share, barn eggs do not appear to have caught the imagination of the UK purchaser, with a polarization between eggs from caged hens or eggs from free-range systems. The share for barn eggs remains between about 5% and 7% of egg sales. However, all free-range systems have to provide internal accommodation that meets the legal standard for barn eggs (the difference being that birds must have access to range).

7.4.2.4 Free range

For many consumers, free-range egg production conjures up ideas of traditional, non-intensive, low capital systems with relatively small flocks. The modern commercial systems may be very different, but are still strictly controlled in legislation. Birds must have daytime access to land mostly covered with vegetation. The popholes to the range must be at lest 35 cm high by 40 cm wide and along the entire length of the building, with 2 m opening per 1,000 birds. This was important because, in the past when the popholes were smaller, there was a tendency for the dominant birds to patrol the popholes and aggressively prevent subordinate birds accessing the range area. The maximum permitted stocking on the land was raised for 2004 from 1,000 birds to 2,500 birds per hectare (since at that time the term 'free range' was a merging of the existing 'free range' and 'semi-intensive' marketing terms). This caused some controversy at the time since welfare groups considered this a retrograde step in welfare terms. The RSPCA maintained the $10 \, \text{m}^2$ per bird stocking, though they are now considering a higher stocking rate for their Freedom Food farms.

Currently a number of UK retailers are stating that they will source all of their eggs from the non-cage sector. As a result of this, and the changes in legislation, the market share is increasing and currently accounts for about 25 to 30% of the UK market. There is some speculation that after the changes in 2012 the share in table eggs will increase to about 55 to 60% from the free-range sector. However, the current economic crisis may influence such changes as supermarkets that elect to sell cheaper eggs from enriched cages may increase their retail share.

7.4.2.5 Organic production

Over the past few decades consumers have become increasingly concerned by management practices in agricultural production. The supposed widespread use of growth promoters, medication and chemicals fuelled a backlash with some small-scale producers seeking an alternative. The United Kingdom Register of Organic Food Standards (UKROFS) (later superseded by Advisory Committee on Organic Standards (ACOS) in 2003, under the Department for Food, Environment and Rural Affairs; DEFRA) established standards for UK organic production. Current organic standards for laying hens state that no birds are kept in cages and there must be no more than 3,000 in the shed. There should be six birds per m^2, with 18 cm perch per bird. One individual nest is required per eight birds or $120 \, \text{cm}^2$ of communal nest per bird. There must be 4 m length of pophole per $100 \, \text{m}^2$ of the floor in the house. There should be $4 \, \text{m}^2$ per bird of range (with rotational land use). Permitted medicines rely heavily on homeopathic remedies. The use of disinfectants is strictly controlled, as are the permitted feedstuffs. Although the eggs are classed as organic, the birds, from non-organically produced parents, are not. Poultry must have access to an open-air area for at least one-third of their life. These areas for poultry must be mainly covered with vegetation and be provided with protective facilities and permit easy access to adequate numbers of drinking and feeding troughs. In the UK the Soil Association is an association of organic producers. The standards set are often in excess of those required in law. Members can use the Soil Association logo to demonstrate that the standards are met.

7.4.2.6 Backyard systems

In recent years poultry has become a popular gift in the UK (e.g. as a wedding gift, particularly in middle-class society) to be kept almost as pets. The birds are often pure breeds; the selling on of birds that have been 'rescued' at end of lay from caged systems is also a thriving (though small) business. DEFRA require that owners of 50 or more birds are registered. As of 16 June 2009, the GB Poultry Register holds details of 24,677 premises. A total of 262,937,612 birds have been registered. Small, backyard systems occur everywhere in the UK, mainly for showing purposes, pets or for production of fresh eggs for the kitchen. Bird pairs or trios are often kept in wooden arks or similar which are about 2 m long by 0.75 m wide with accommodation for the birds and a wire-framed cover over the garden area. Larger groups may be contained within an area (again using chicken wire mesh) with a small shed for accommodation. Alternatively the birds are allowed to range freely, returning at night to a secure shed for roosting. Paddocks may be fenced off to prevent entry by foxes and other predators. In such cases the mesh fence is often dug in to the ground with the fence curved outwards so that any digging fox cannot dig under the fence and gain access to the birds. There is very little legislative control over these small flocks (particularly flocks of less than 350 birds). However, most of these flocks are not kept purely for commercial egg production and the care focused on individual birds is usually higher than that which may occur in larger flocks. In many cases cockerels are kept with these groups (unlike in commercial flocks). Many systems rely on manual labour for food and water delivery, though some do have water and power supplies to the sheds. The food and equipment can be purchased in manageable amounts from agricultural or countryside-based stores and, in the UK, there is a thriving trade in supporting such small-scale groups or flocks. Thus such birds are generally fed balanced layer diets, supplemented with invertebrates and other scraps that the birds can forage.

In some countries, a few backyard chickens are kept as a source of both fresh eggs and meat for the family (rather than as a money-making enterprise). The birds live closely with their human keepers, often in their homes, and are generally free to roam and forage, feeding on scraps, etc. The level of direct care for the birds is relatively minimal as the birds tend to fend for themselves, but roost in close association with their keepers.

7.5 Management of the Laying Hen

7.5.1 Feeding and watering

It is important that the laying hens have *ad libitum* access to clean and safe food and water. Balanced diets have been researched and are readily available for laying hens. During the rearing period it is essential that the birds are fed sufficient calcium to ensure that, when they reach point of lay, the bone density is as high as possible to offset the problems associated with the calcium demand of sustained egg-laying. Traditional, manual feeding systems include simple hoppers, suspended through the barn, but these are not suitable for caged systems, which use a trough system in front of the cages. These are not used in large commercial systems as they are very labour intensive, but they offer an inexpensive system for smallholders and backyard flocks.

Mechanized feeders are available. These include chain feeders where a flat chain in the feeding trough operates to distribute food from a hopper. In barn and free-range systems this can be problematic in that birds can perch on the feeder and defecate in the food, or if they are in the trough when it begins to operate can be dragged through the trough (causing injury). Auger-filled pan feeders are often preferred since there is less risk of spoilage of the food. These systems are less labour intensive since they are capable of delivering food stored in bulk.

Similarly water delivery can be inexpensive with manually filled free-standing drinkers for barn, free-range and smaller-scale systems. These are very labour intensive and are not used on larger systems. Bell drinkers offer a relatively cheap automated delivery system. These are connected to a water supply and a simple spring valve opens when the weight of the water is reduced in the suspended trough. This occurs when the birds drink. When the weight of water increases the valve is shut off, which prevents overfilling. The problems of water spillage and potential (faecal) contamination of the water have encouraged a greater use of nipple drinkers. These are simple ball-stoppers in a tube connected to the water supply. As the birds peck at the ball, water is delivered directly to their beaks. To ensure adequate provision and to reduce the incidence of competitive aggression, DEFRA has recommended minimal feeder and drinker space allocation per bird (Table 7.6).

Standing water can become contaminated and so many commercial egg producers are turning to regulated mains water delivery. In situations where water is delivered from boreholes, regular water testing is important to ensure that the minerals and constituents are not hazardous and there are no bacterial or other biological contaminants. Monitoring of food and water consumption can be used as a systems or flock health check where deviations from the expected can be first indicators of potential problems.

Table 7.6 DEFRA Recommended water and food space per bird.

Feeders		Drinkers		
Linear	**Circular**	**Continuous**	**Circular**	**Nipple/cups**
10 cm	4 cm	2.5 cm	1 cm	1 per 10 hens OR (if plumbed in) at least 2

7.5.2 Lighting

Once the birds are in the laying accommodation, after a few days of continuous lighting the light duration is quickly reduced to match the lighting in the rearing accommodation. Once this is achieved the light duration is increased by between 20 and 30 minutes per week until about 15 hours of light per day is achieved. This is called a continuous lighting pattern. Birds produce eggs every 24.5 hours or so, so each bird lays her egg later in each consecutive day. Hens will generally lay eggs within the first 4 hours of 'dawn' so occasionally the bird does not lay but retains the egg to lay all the sooner the following day. Thus we talk about birds laying clutches of between six and nine eggs. There has been a lot of research on the effects of alternative lighting patterns, summarized in Table 7.7, where the egg size and number will be used as the standard, allowing other patterns to be compared. In general, in interrupted patterns, 'dawn' is the first light period after the longest dark period. Some welfare groups are concerned with the manipulation of lighting. Ahemeral (non 24-h) lighting strategies are not permitted in the UK, since they interfere with the diurnal rhythm of the birds. Some welfarists consider that birds should have at least 8 hours of darkness to enable them to rest. In terms of management, the dark period allows proper shell formation.

7.5.3 Egg collection

Manual egg collection is easy in small (e.g. backyard) flocks. In non-caged systems, eggs from places other than the nest boxes should be collected regularly to dissuade other birds from laying their eggs in the same location. If floor-laid eggs (in the litter) become a problem, agricultural electric fence wire can be used to stop the birds from laying eggs (particularly in corners or beside walls). Commercially only clean eggs laid in nest boxes can be sold as table eggs for 'in shell' consumption. In the UK it is illegal to wash or clean eggs from any contaminant if the eggs are to be in-shell table eggs. This is not the case in some EU countries and in the US, where a method has been developed to pasteurize eggs 'in shell'. Eggs should be stored 'pointed end' down, so that the air sac in the egg is at the upper end of the egg. In many larger commercial systems egg collection is carried out automatically. The birds stand on a sloping mesh floor so that the eggs roll to the front of the cage on to a conveyor belt. The conveyor operates at least once each day. It will operate more often during the period of peak lay (when the hens are between about 20 and 44 weeks old) to prevent a build-up of eggs on the belt and the risk of increased star cracks from collisions between eggs. In the UK, eggs are given their 'best before' date, which is ink-jet printed on to the shell (using food dye) at the time of sorting and grading, along with the code for the method of production (0 to 4, organic to eggs from caged hens) and a unique number associated with the farm or packing station from whence the eggs came. Legally the 'best before' date is 28 days from the day on which the eggs were laid and the sell-by date is 21 days from lay. Eggs sold commercially can only be packaged once and it is illegal to repackage them.

Table 7.7 Alternative lighting patterns and the influence on egg production.

Lighting pattern (light : dark (L : D)	Synchro-nized laying	Influence on egg size (egg mass)	Influence on egg number	Influence on shell	Main reason for use
15 : 9	Yes	Standard	Standard	Standard	Good number of medium-sized eggs
2 : 2 or 4 : 4 etc	No	Standard	Standard	Standard	Better food efficiency. Reduced energy costs
4 × (2L : 2D) 1 × (2L : 6D)	Yes	Possible increase (if birds eat more)	Standard	Can be reduced if the birds retain shells in the shell gland for less time	Better food efficiency. Reduced energy costs
14L : 14D (ahemeral)	Yes	Possible increase (if birds eat more)	Decrease	Can be increased if the birds retain shells in the shell gland for more time	Improve egg mass or shell quality/thickness

7.5.4 Disease control

There are many types of poultry diseases, from many causes. A number of important poultry diseases, and the major causes, are listed in Table 7.8. Although controls are listed, some diseases are difficult to control and in some cases mortality can be high (up to 100%). Note that in many cases the importance of good biosecurity is reinforced.

For those keeping small flocks it is important to take the greatest care not to introduce diseases to an established flock. If new birds are purchased or brought on to the site, a period of quarantine of up to 1 month is advised. If new birds are being introduced, it should be done carefully and strictly controlled, allowing birds to see each other, fenced off from each other. In an established flock there will be a hierarchy and new birds may cause an increase in aggression. This is not so pronounced if all the birds are at point of lay, as such social orders are generally created and quickly established around this time. In general it is the hobbyist's few birds and small pure-bred flocks that can pose a greater threat to the health of the nation's flocks: these tend to be the unvaccinated flocks and groups which are often transported around the country to shows and fairs.

Commercial flocks are managed to minimize disease risks. Breeding stock are valued highly and therefore are isolated; often such pedigree farms are situated in remote places or places where the sea borders the site to reduce the risk from airborne pathogens. In addition, access is strictly controlled and potential visitors may be subjected to a microbial test (e.g. from rectal swabs) in advance of a proposed visit. Parent stock are also regularly assessed for *Salmonella* spp., after the outbreak of *Salmonella enteriditis* phage type IV in the 1980s when a junior health minister (Edwina Curry) claimed that all eggs carried *Salmonella*. This strain was of particular importance in that it infected the ovaries of the hen so that when eggs were laid there was a potential threat of *Salmonella* being incorporated in the yolk as the egg was formed. By registering and screening the parents the risk of laying hens being infected is minimized. The laying flocks are also regularly checked for infection and receive vaccines for *Salmonella* at least twice during the rearing programme. Key vaccines are administered during the rearing period (see Section 7.4.1.1). Birds generally do not receive vaccines or treatments during egg production, in keeping with the statement on egg boxes saying that the eggs are from birds free of medication. Subclinical levels of disease in laying flocks will be tolerated. However, if there is an apparent problem, the first response would be to collect blood samples from a number of birds for laboratory analysis. Appropriate treatment is then administered, based on the results.

Hens are susceptible to many disease risks (Figure 7.6) and can carry several gut parasites such as tapeworms and nematodes as well as pathogenic bacteria. Recently attention has focused on *Brachyspira* spp., which is a type of bacteria found in birds' caeca. Some species can affect egg-laying performance. They can live for long periods in puddles and are thus capable of infecting the birds. Many gut parasites eject eggs;

Table 7.8 Important poultry diseases.

Disease	Cause	Control
Fatty liver syndrome	Imbalanced diet (sometimes seen with caged layer fatigue)	Correct diet at the correct point in bird's lifetime
Caged layer fatigue/ rickets	Calcium related deficiency or imbalance in diet	Calcium phosphate, vitamin D3 (some medication and mould toxins)
Infectious bronchitis	virus	vaccination
Avian encephalomyelitis	Virus (mainly vertical transmission)	No treatment. Prevent exposure. Vaccination against
Avian Influenza	Virus (mainly waterfowl carriers)	Vaccination against some. Prevent exposure. Can be 100% fatal
Chicken anaemia virus	Virus vertical transmission and horizontal (copraphagy of infected faeces)	Immunized parents. Prevention (biosecurity)
Infectious bursal disease (gumboro)	Virus	Vaccination against. Prevention (biosecurity)
Marek's disease	Virus	Vaccination against
Egg drop syndrome	Virus	Vaccination against. Prevention (biosecurity). EDS-free parents
Infectious laryngotracheitis	Virus	Vaccination
fowl pox	Virus	Vaccination. Prevention (biosecurity)
Lymphoid leukosis	virus	Virus-free parents. Biosecurity
Newcastle disease	virus	Slaughter. Vaccination. Biosecurity
Infectious coryza	Bacterial infection	Antibiotics. Vaccine. Biosecurity
Avian tuberculosis	Bacterial infection	Depopulation and biosecurity
Fowl cholera (pasteurellosis)	Bacterial infection	Sulphonamides and antibiotics. Vaccines. Biosecurity
Mycoplasmosis	Mycoplasmas	Mycoplasma-free parents. Antibiotics. Some vaccines. Biosecurity
Coccidiosis	Gut parasite	Anti-coccidial. Vaccines. Biosecurity. Natural immunity
Cryptosporidiosis	Gut parasite	Biosecurity
Histomoniasis (blackhead)	Gut parasite	Anthelminthics. Biosecurity
Toxoplasmosis (mainly backyard birds)	Protozoa in nervous, reproductive and musculoskeletal systems	Suppressing drugs. Biosecurity
Trichomoniasis	Protozoa in gut	Biosecurity
Round and flat worms	Gut	Medication. Biosecurity
Red mite	External	Topical treatments. Spray. Biosecurity
Lice	External	Topical treatments. Spray. Biosecurity

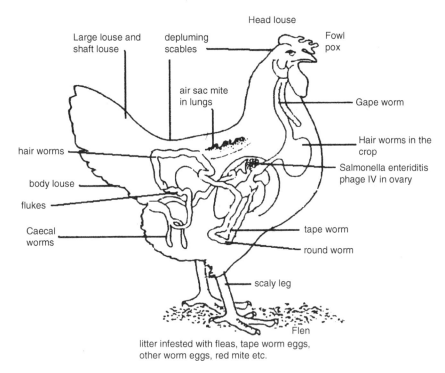

Figure 7.6 Pictorial representation of the potential threats to hens' health and welfare which can be spotted during bird (and environment) inspection. (Source: After ADAS, undated.)

some need to pass through other species as part of the life cycle, but the main problem is that eggs deposited in the range area can infect other birds. A sufficient build-up can lead to a high risk of bird infection. This 'fowl sick land' can cause many new birds or cleansed birds to quickly succumb to the parasites in the soil or on the grass. Because the risk of infection can be high for free-range birds it is usually free-range flocks that tend to receive vaccinations during their productive lifetime.

In the last decade attention has been focused on avian influenza H5N1, particularly following a number of deaths in Asia and Eastern Europe. The UK government has drawn up a strategy to deal with an outbreak of any zoonotic disease associated with poultry. Should there be an outbreak, flocks will be slaughtered, movement restrictions will be ordered and free-range flocks will not be allowed to range (preventing exposure to wild birds). Since commercial hens are kept together in large flocks, avoidance of disease risk is the major strategy for the industry. Therefore biosecurity is particularly important.

7.5.5 Biosecurity and hygiene
The benefits to be gained from economies of scale were quickly realized. Units of several hundred thousands of birds became the norm and units of up to 1.5 million or

so exist nowadays. However, such large flocks can also be problematic. One of the major risks is disease, which might influence the entire flock, or infect the eggs that they produce, with significant economic consequences. The poultry industry pays particular attention to biosecurity where potential risks of infection are identified and actions are taken to minimize the risk. Biosecurity activities are summarized in Table 7.9. The list is not exhaustive and some general hygiene has not been included.

7.5.6 Signs of health and disease

Good productivity and low mortality are obvious signs of good health. However they cannot be taken as the only signs of a healthy flock. Simple health checks, such as checking water and food consumption, can be first indicators of possible problems, if there is any deviation from the norm. However there are many potential causes (management of the thermal and physical environment and imbalanced diet, and so on) which can give the same results. A lot of information can be gleaned on entry to the flock. Listening to the birds can detect snicking (sneezing) or other unexpected sounds. A very quiet flock can also be suffering. By looking at the birds, information can also be obtained about the health of the flock. A stationary bird, stooped and with eyes closed, may be in pain. Birds with swollen heads or with liquid around the eyes can be suffering from diseases such as influenza or bronchitis. Bad smells in the shed can be caused by birds showing signs of diarrhoea, resulting from gut parasitic problems (e.g. coccidiosis) or one of many diseases. In brown-egg laying flocks, the appearance of white shells may be an indicator of mite infestation or subclinical disease. Soft-shelled or shell-less eggs or a drop in egg numbers could be signs of calcium problems or egg drop syndrome. Increased levels of aggression, feather pulling and cannibalism can arise from frustration, overcrowding, poor drinker and feeder management or poor environmental control.

7.5.7 Production disorders

7.5.7.1 Osteoporosis

Since the 1950s the physiological demands on the birds has increased remarkably. Expectations, in terms of egg numbers per bird, have almost doubled to the 300 eggs per bird expected from caged hens (or 280 or so from free range). The daily calcium requirements for egg shells is more than the diet can supply, or the bird can absorb, even though food is supplemented with granular calcium (traditionally as oyster shells). In times of calcium deficit, hens can mobilize skeletal calcium, particularly from the long bones (medullary bone) which become active as a calcium store around sexual maturity. Muscular paralysis and weak bones (osteoporosis) during peak egg production, caused by calcium deficiency, is known as caged layer fatigue. This can be offset by providing birds that have been light stimulated (i.e. about 2 weeks before the first egg, when medullary bone formation begins) with layer ration, rich in calcium. This allows birds to store calcium before the demands of egg-laying. A similar problem can occur towards the end of lay where sustained calcium demand

Table 7.9 Potential risks to birds or eggs and counter-measures (biosecurity).

Carrier	Threat	Biosecurity measure
Human	Flock	Prevent unwanted visitors Make feed lorries/bird deliverers disinfect before delivery and on entry (disinfectant wheel dips) Single entry with gate guard Visitors' book (signed by every visitor) Prevent access if visitor has been with other poultry in the last few days Prevent entry of individuals with illness Prevent staff keeping birds at home
Human	Flock/eggs	Minimize visitors to packing facility (apply biosecurity systems listed above) Provide overalls, boots and hair cover Make visitors remove 'outdoor' clothes and shower before access Remove jewellery Hand washing/sanitizers on entry Boot disinfectant at every entrance
Vermin (rats/mice)	Flock/eggs	Keep weed-free Have an open space (concrete) around and between sheds Do not allow scrap/unused equipment to languish on site (to become infested) Ensure doors close and fit properly Do not leave spilled food (clean up immediately) Do not store (new) litter on site Remove soiled litter at least 1 mile from shed Have a vermin extermination programme Maintain sheds properly (walls, etc) Clean between flocks (birds of the same age in each shed allows thorough cleaning of the shed)
Micro-organisms and pathogens	Flock/eggs	Disinfect thoroughly Prevent contamination Regular cleaning with deep cleansing as appropriate
Insect/flies	Flock/eggs	Electric 'Insecticutors' Fly-killing poisons where possible Prevent ingress Clean the environment to remove places where flies/fly eggs can survive
Wild birds	Flock/eggs	Ensure doors close and fit properly Do not leave spilled food (clean up immediately) Minimize exposure (bring free-range flocks indoors in times of risk (e.g. avian influenza outbreak)
Chickens	Flock/eggs	Remove dead/sick birds Dispose of dead birds quickly and efficiently (incineration) Test parents for *Salmonella* (if parents are free, offspring should be too) Regular cloacal swabs of laying flock to ensure free of *Salmonella* and other contamination

reduces the overall skeletal calcium. Eggshell thickness and quality is also compromised at this time if the shell glands are less efficient.

7.5.8 Behavioural problems

7.5.8.1 Feather pecking and cannibalism

Feather pecking is not a problem in itself. Feather pecking is misdirected investigative pecking as the birds investigate their surrounds. However, when feather *pecking* becomes feather *pulling*, this can lead to problems, particularly if the victim bleeds and the pecking bird starts to peck at the wound. This can quickly lead to damaging aggressive pecking and cannibalism. Cannibalism can occur from many causes such as sudden changes or a poor environment (high temperature, high light intensity, poor ventilation, overstocking, competition for insufficient numbers of feeders or drinkers, access to prolapsed or sick and dying birds,) poor diet (e.g. salt imbalance, lack of trace element or lack of sodium) or aggressive strains of birds.

In large groups of birds, such as free-range or barn flocks of several thousand birds, a stable social order cannot be established and general aggression can be extended in duration. This is recognized by Farm Animal Welfare Council, who have declared that system design should make escape routes available for bullied birds. Cannibalism is generally more frequent in barns and free-range units compared to battery cages. However, it can occur in battery cages. In such cases it has to be combated quickly since birds in neighbouring cages seem to develop cannibalistic tendencies and it can sweep through the system unless checked. Currently the main method of control is beak trimming, though this will no longer be possible after 2010.

7.5.9 Beak trimming

Chickens use their beaks for many different tasks. Apart from the obvious task of collecting food, it is used for aggression, investigation of the environment and as a gripping, breaking and ripping tool. The sharp beak has many nerve endings, suggesting that it also very sensitive. Because the beak is so sharp, poultry-keepers learned that the beak could be trimmed to remove the sharpness. This was found not only to reduce aggression (or at least reduce the potential damage birds did to each other) but it made the birds more careful when pecking for food. There was much less food wastage as the birds did not throw the food around as much. This is important to flock-keepers as food costs represent between 70% and 90% of production costs.

Trained beak trimmers can trim the beaks of young birds up to the age of 11 days. A maximum of one-third of the distance between the beak tip and the nostrils is permitted to be removed. This could be done for both the upper and lower beak at a cost of about 3p per bird. This was often done with a hot wire or blade that not only cut the beak, but cauterized the wound at the same time. It was important that during the procedure the bird's tongue was protected to avoid any further damage. Beak trimming also prevented cannibalism from spreading in flocks and so flock-keepers were allowed to beak-trim mature birds if cannibalism occurred. It would be wrong to understate the problem of cannibalism in some flocks of poultry. The causes are complex, ranging from dietary imbalance, stocking density, bird 'poise' and the level of arousal of the flock, to sudden environmental changes. Birds in large colonies are unable to establish cohesive social hierarchies and aggression, to establish status, is more prevalent in large flocks. Birds can recognize 15 to 20 individuals and have a 'general recognition' for about 100 birds in order to create and sustain a hierarchy, usually around sexual maturity. So birds can relatively quickly establish a hierarchy and then the levels of aggression associated with creating a hierarchy are reduced. This is not to say that levels of aggression are reduced in smaller flocks. There is a significant body of evidence demonstrating that aggression in flocks of about 100 birds can often be greater than in larger flocks. Nevertheless, in larger commercial barn and free-range flocks, there can be prolonged aggression if a stable social order cannot be established. In such cases, there tends to be a more polarized social arrangement, with an apparent extreme between the 'despot' birds and the 'omega' or 'pariah' birds. Where cannibalism occurs, it is often the individuals at the bottom of the order that become the early victims (unless another bird is injured). Once cannibalism becomes established in a flock it becomes difficult to eradicate and so prevention is the best approach.

Beak trimming is one method that has been chosen in the past to prevent aggressive pecking, feather pulling and cannibalism. Since it is impossible to identify individual aggressors in a free-range flock of several thousand, birds destined for barn or free-range systems are more routinely beak-trimmed as a preventive measure than in cage systems. Research has shown that some (but not all) forms of beak trimming can cause chronic pain associated with neuroma formation (Gentle *et al.*, 1990). Despite this there is a welfare argument to support beak trimming if it reduces the incidence of cannibalism. There is, however, no welfare argument to support beak trimming simply to prevent food wastage from birds flicking the food out of the feeders. Other techniques, including lasers and infra-red radiation, have been tested with varying degrees of success. Since June 2006, RSPCA Freedom Food has allowed commercial layer hatcheries to use an infrared beak-trimming device for chicks placed at Freedom Food laying farms and from December 2010 this is the only method permitted in the UK.

In 2007 the Farm Animal Welfare Council prepared a document advising the British government of the welfare implications of a ban on beak trimming (which was due to come into effect on 31 December 2010 but which has been postponed until 2016). The FAWC suggested that 'If injurious pecking could be eliminated by other means, for example through genetic selection, the use of controlled light for housed birds or other management practices, then the need for beak trimming would disappear and this mutilation would no longer be needed.' The current welfare codes for laying hens recommend that beak treatment should 'be restricted to beak tipping; that is the blunting of the beak to remove the sharp point which can be the cause of the most severe damage to other birds'. The FAWC view appears to be that beak trimming is a mutilation which goes against the 'five freedoms' of good animal welfare in that it causes pain and injury and possibly a deleterious change in behaviour. However, if this is not the case (particularly when it is done on young birds) then, if all other avenues of work (such as establishing a less aggressive strain of bird) are unsuccessful, beak tipping (of just the very end of the beak, and using the most humane techniques) should not be dismissed out of hand, if it prevents a worse welfare insult such as cannibalism.

7.5.10 Depopulation, transport and slaughter

Bird welfare during handling and transport is important. Birds should never be deprived of water before transport; however, feed may be withheld for up to 12 hours prior to slaughter (including catching, loading, transport, lairage and unloading times). This ensures that the birds do not have a full crop at slaughter. A full crop can burst and contaminate the carcass. The procedure should be coordinated to minimize the time that the birds are held in the handling crates or modules. Where possible any equipment (particularly equipment with sharp edges) should be removed if it may hinder the easy collection and transfer of the birds. The catching and handling of the birds must be done quietly, methodically and efficiently to prevent the birds from panicking, struggling or being injured. Reduced light intensity or blue lighting is often used to quieten the birds. The skilled catchers should be trained and demonstrate competence to ensure bird welfare throughout the procedure. If birds are in cages they should be taken out individually from the cage, being held by both legs in one hand and the breast supported in the other hand. Similarly birds in non-cage systems should be held by both legs. Any bird should be carried through the system by both legs and catchers must take care that the birds do not collide with anything in the system (particularly if the wings are flapping). Birds should never be carried by their wings, heads or necks and never more than three birds per hand. The distance birds are carried to the transport crates or modules must be minimized.

Although laying hens can survive longer than a decade, commercially most birds are removed from the laying site by about 75 weeks of age. Small, backyard flocks can be allowed to go through a moult, where egg production ceases and the birds refresh the plumage; the calcium in the bones is also replenished at this time. The birds return to almost peak egg production within a few weeks. This can occur several times and the birds can live a productive life for several years. Commercially, it is important that all of the birds in the same shed are removed at the same time to allow a thorough cleaning of the shed, for good biosecurity.

In the past, depopulation of laying hens from cages had significant welfare issues. End-of-lay hens have little economic value and the skill level of workers was low. Poor cage design meant that birds taken by the legs to be pulled from the cages risked significant damage to legs, wings and (in particular) keel bones. Studies showed that birds, already possibly suffering brittle bones (osteoporosis), risked bone breakage from poor handling when being taken from cages. Developments such as sliders over the food trough, better designed cage fronts and more careful handling have reduced the risks, but bird depopulation can still be a point where birds risk welfare insults. The depopulation of enriched cages may prove difficult in that the last few birds in the group have a relatively large space to avoid capture and in the ensuing struggle may be prone to injury. Also, once caught, the birds have to be carried to the doors and then stacked in modules. Collision injuries are possible and care has to be taken, even though catchers are compelled to complete the task as soon as possible.

The risk of injury is increased in barn and free-range systems where, as the population is reduced in the shed, the remaining birds can more easily avoid capture. Birds may be driven towards the catchers but seizing and restraining birds can be difficult and birds may be injured. Strategies, such as catching roosting birds in low light conditions, can be used so that the birds are less active.

Transport times are strictly controlled to avoid problems of hypo- or hyperthermia on board the lorries. As the number of slaughterhouses prepared to take end-of-lay hens has reduced in the UK over the last few years, distances and journey times have increased and the welfare of the hens during transport remains an important issue Commercially laying hens are slaughtered on lines usually used for broiler birds, though no broilers can be slaughtered on the line when it is used for laying hens. Smaller flocks can be slaughtered using hand-held stunners which render birds unconscious or dead by electrocution. Individuals may be killed by neck dislocation.

7.6 Welfare of the Laying Hen

There continue to be serious concerns for the welfare of animals used by humans for agricultural purposes. There are concerns for the welfare of the birds themselves, with continuing demands for increased productivity and efficiency (i.e. more eggs for less feed). A major historical problem with bird welfare and the poultry industry is one of profit. In the early development of the UK poultry egg industry, maximizing efficiency, producing more for least cost, was the driving force. Indeed, this was the aim of the UK government which provided minimal financial support for the developing industry but penalized the less efficient producers. When welfare issues were considered, from the 1960s onwards, any changes in production to improve bird welfare were seen as 'costs' to the industry, since it often meant that welfare requirements increased the costs of production, reduced stocking or negatively affected egg production per bird. Many producers argued that if the birds were alive and healthy then production itself demonstrated good welfare. The welfarists claimed that, while poor production was an indicator of poor welfare, high production levels were not indicators of good welfare *per se*. Another confounding problem for the industry has been that consumers may express a desire for higher welfare standards for laying hens (which would increase costs of production and therefore the price of eggs to the consumer) but actually elect to purchase cheaper eggs from caged hens. However, as stated earlier, the large increase in the sale of free-range eggs suggests that consumer demand is catching up with desire. Often proposed improvements for bird welfare have not been welcomed by an industry that perceives such moves as interference. Welfare improvements are often resented and the industry responds to minimize the effect of the proposals. For example, the response to the provision of 'litter' for dust-bathing in cages has been the use of Astroturf material, which is hardly a litter at all. Similarly a proposed increase in floor space per bird in cages was overcome not by reducing the number of birds per cage, but by the creation of an extension to the cage front.

Commercial free-range systems do not necessarily meet all of the welfare requirements of the laying hen. For example, large populations on inappropriate ground can cause birds to suffer disease risks, or smaller populations may exhibit high levels of aggression through frustration. The requirements of hens on range are not fully understood and there is a need to research birds' needs. The introduction of an enriched cage should be seen by the industry as an opportunity to create a system that not only meets the economic demands facing the industry but also best meets the welfare requirements of the birds. The compromise that often occurs between the scientific advice and the engineered systems means that the findings of academic research are not properly met and the expected welfare improvements are not guaranteed. This is apparently the case in some designs of enriched cages (e.g. where perches meet inappropriately and birds may be cramped) and some materials used may not provide the level of enrichment that might otherwise be provided (e.g. plastic matting instead of friable litter for dust-bathing). Despite such criticisms, it is important that producers are not seen as the villains. Ultimately they will produce eggs however society demands, *provided that society is willing to meet the extra costs of production*, which is not always the case.

An oft-used argument by UK producers is that the cost of implementing welfare legislation creates an 'unlevel playing field' in terms of costs of home-produced eggs versus cheaper imports. The EU has some newer member states with weak economies where preparations for the changes in 2012 may be difficult to afford. The EU has also stated an intention not to trade with nations outside the EU that do not have the same levels of welfare for the birds. The resolution of these issues will not be easy. Whatever happens, it is essential that the progression to higher welfare standards for laying hens continues, both in terms of the demands on the birds and the methods of production.

7.6.1 Welfare concerns for the hen

Agricultural production in the UK responded to the needs of the population and the drive from government after World War I, i.e. to become self-sufficient in cheap food production. This need was reinforced following World War II. The push for efficiency meant that other issues such as welfare were secondary. Much of the research on poultry has been on production, and funding to research diet, food efficiency and alternative food sources has been more abundant than for welfare. Breeding companies are still primarily driven to maximize output and make the birds more efficient. This assumes that the selection of laying hens has not yet reached their genetic limits. Thus, with some manipulation, breeders assume that they can unlock some new, previously unrealized level of production from the birds. However, reason would predict that this is not sustainable. Pushing the birds beyond an unknown limit represents a serious welfare problem. Already, commercial laying hens suffer osteoporosis, often associated with calcium depletion in the skeleton in response to the physiological loading of eggshell formation for the 300 or so eggs expected from the bird in 13 months of production. However, osteoporosis can result from dietary imbalance (e.g. calcium and phosphorus levels and ratio in the food). Also, birds can recover bone strength and bone density during a moulting process, though this is not permitted in Lion Code flocks.

Birds in traditional cages generally display more fear responses to novel stimuli presented at the cage front, than birds in non-cage systems. Whether this is the case in enriched cages is not yet known. It seems that birds regularly exposed to changing novel (non-threatening) stimuli are more receptive and less fearful when exposed to some novel stimulus, though not to the possibly more extreme novelty of handling and transport.

Some of the hybrids used in the past for commercial egg production were known to be aggressive. The popularity of such strains has dwindled in the past 20 years or so. DEFRA are looking to the breeders to produce a more docile strain of bird which is less prone to aggressive behaviour. Commercial flock size may also cause increased levels of aggression, but there can be many other causes. A few producers, with non-caged systems, are including cockerels in the flock in an attempt to reduce levels of aggression among the hens.

7.6.2 Welfare concerns in society

In the UK it is probably the welfare of laying hens in battery cages that was foremost in the minds of animal welfarists when concerns for farmed animal welfare were first voiced. In the early 1960s Ruth Harrison wrote a book about 'animal machines', stating concerns about (intensive) factory farming techniques. Pressure from lobby groups caused the UK government to set up the Brambell Committee in the 1960s to assess animal welfare. Some of the committee's recommendations to improve animal welfare were based on anthropomorphic evaluations (e.g. the recommended floor for laying hens was solid metal with circular perforations, which the birds disliked, preferring a mesh floor). On the positive side, the committee came up with the notion of 'five freedoms' for animal welfare.

In the early 1970s the FAWC was established, which continued this theme of 'five freedoms' which, although not the same as those of the Brambell Committee, can trace their ancestry back to it. The FAWC was established to undertake investigations of welfare issues concerning farmed animals and their management (taking advice from the farming industry and scientific evidence) and then reported to government as an informed body, allowing government to create advised welfare codes and recommendations for good practice and also to incorporate welfare in legislation through DEFRA. Although the *Codes and Recommendations for the Welfare of Livestock: Laying Hens* is not legislation itself, failure to comply with the codes can be used in court as evidence of cruelty, should a prosecution occur. Since its foundation, the FAWC has reported on a number of issues relating to the egg industry, such as:

- advice to the Agriculture Ministers of Great Britain on the need to control certain mutilations of farm animals (1981);
- report on the welfare of poultry at the time of slaughter (1982);
- an assessment of egg production systems (1986);
- report on the welfare of laying hens in colony systems (1991);
- report on the welfare of laying hens (1997).

In general, the FAWC report to the Government and then the Government, through DEFRA, responds, stating whether the current provisions are sufficient or how the recommendations are to be acted up on. There have been several pieces of legislation since the mid-1960s to improve the welfare of laying hens. These include:

- The Agriculture (Miscellaneous Provisions) Act 1968;
- The Welfare of Livestock (Prohibited Operations) Regulations 1982;
- The Welfare of Livestock Regulations 1994;
- The Welfare of Farmed Animals (England) Regulations 2000;
- Welfare of Farmed Animals (England) (Amendment) Regulations 2002;
- Animal Welfare Act 2006;
- Welfare of Farmed Animals (England) Regulations 2007.

The legal provisions have progressed from preventing offences such as: to cause or allow livestock on agricultural land (including intensive and 'back yard' poultry units) to suffer unnecessary pain or distress; prohibiting the devoicing of cockerels; the castration of a male bird by a method involving surgery, or any operation on a bird with the object or effect of impeding its flight, other than feather clipping. From 1994, legislation focused on cage construction (openings), dimensions and, in particular, space allocation per bird, currently standing at $550\,cm^2$ per bird but increasing in 2012 when enriched cages are introduced. General flock management (food and water provision), bird inspection and system checks are also included. In 2002 legislation encompassed the permitted stocking and management of non-caged systems, again focusing on 2012 as the target date for full compliance.

The more recent UK legislation for animal welfare (for farmed species *and* for animals in zoos) relies heavily on the provisions outlined in the FAWC's 'five freedoms' for good welfare. However, I feel that in poultry production and management, the 'five freedoms' have been misinterpreted as goals or aims. These 'freedoms' are often seen as a welfare 'ceiling' rather than a legal minimum welfare standard or 'floor'. Also, the concept of birds' 'freedoms' does not really reinforce the responsibility of the human keeper or carer of the animals. Freedoms (even in

Table 7.10 The 'minimum musts' for animal welfare (adapted from the Farm Animal Welfare Council's 'five freedoms').

1. The keeper/carer MUST prevent hunger and thirst. . .	. . .by providing ready access to fresh water and a diet to maintain full health and vigour
2. The keeper/carer MUST prevent discomfort. . .	. . .by providing an appropriate environment including shelter and a comfortable resting area
3. The keeper/carer MUST prevent pain, injury or disease. . .	. . .by prevention or rapid diagnosis and treatment
4. The keeper/carer MUST allow expression of socially acceptable behaviour patterns. . .	. . .by providing sufficient space, proper facilities and company of the animal's own kind
5. The keeper/carer MUST prevent fear and distress. . .	. . .by ensuring conditions and treatment which avoid mental suffering

human societies) are often abused and neglected. Increasingly, I am 'rebadging' the 'five freedoms' as the five 'minimum musts' (Table 7.10).

I appreciate that this is little more than a rewording of the five freedoms and I would not wish to be accused of criticising such an august body as the FAWC. However, these 'MUSTS' represent a change in emphasis and plant the responsibility for welfare of the animals firmly in the hands of the keeper or carer. A slight modification also changes the freedom to perform normal behaviours to 'socially acceptable' behaviour patterns, ruling out behaviours such as cannibalism in poultry. The means by which these 'musts' are provided remain the same as the FAWC recommendations, since they represent the most appropriate methods (Table 7.10).

7.6.3 Egg quality assurance and welfare enhancement

In the 1960s the Egg Marketing Board introduced a lion logo on eggs and slogans such as 'Go to work on an egg!' and 'Happiness is egg-shaped', using comedic actors of the day in advertisements on television. This was a particularly successful campaign. Following declining egg sales, resulting from the proposed potential health risk of heart disease associated with cholesterol levels in eggs and the impact of the 'Salmonella in eggs' scare in the 1980s, the industry relaunched the lion emblem to encourage egg sales. Unfortunately, the new generation did not readily embrace the image (its impact had been lost with time). The Lion Quality Code was launched and now represents a mark of quality control. The RSPCA have also launched a marketing tool (Freedom Foods) which is an assurance scheme that the flock management and systems used for egg production meet the required welfare standards. The Freedom Foods scheme cannot be applied to caged systems (since the RSPCA believes that cages are intrinsically cruel). This is not so for the Lion Scheme, introduced by the British Egg Industry Council.

7.6.3.1 The lion code

The Lion Code of Practice sets out procedures and inspections to maintain bird health and welfare and control egg handling and quality. The following is a short summary of some of the key points. Lion Quality eggs, carrying the little red lion on the shell, have a 'best before' date ink-jet printed (using food quality dye) on the shell and on the pack. For Lion eggs, the 'best before' date is up to 25 days from pack (or for inline operations up to 27 days from pack). Since the legally defined 'best before' date is 28 days from lay, eggs in the scheme must be sold sooner than the legal requirement. Most Lion Quality eggs are packed within 48 hours of lay.

The Lion Code was developed to establish quality standards for eggs fit for human consumption. The Codes of Practice address quality and bird welfare and apply to:

- breeding flocks and hatcheries;
- pullet rearing;
- laying birds;
- production practices (including health hygiene and welfare).

Along with bird management, the quality of the product is considered with reference to on-farm handling of eggs; distribution of eggs from farm; feed; hen disposal; packing centre procedures; advice to retailers, consumers and caterers; environmental policy and enforcement. All farms involved in breeding, rearing (to point of lay) and production, egg packing centres and feed mills in this scheme have to be approved by independent inspectors. All flocks have a passport certificate which contains the history and treatments associated with the flock. All egg movements require sufficient documentation to enable traceability. All hatcheries and breeding flock accommodation (and birds) are subject to regular microbiological monitoring, with the necessary slaughter of any *Salmonella*-positive flocks, and heat/acid treatment of feed.

As part of the scheme, all egg-producing flocks are vaccinated during rearing (as part of the standard vaccination programme) against *Salmonella enteritidis* using an approved vaccine. Pullet rearers are also required to undertake a hygiene monitoring programme before birds are taken onto the farm. These flocks are tested for *Salmonella*, with a disinfection programme for all bird transport systems. Records kept on the passport include:

- bird movements;
- testing for *Salmonella*;
- wild birds and rodent control measures.

For farms accommodating laying birds there are strict rules concerning:

- farm disinfection between flocks;

- prevention of cross-infection between birds on farms and between successive flocks;
- testing for *Salmonella*;
- wild bird and rodent control measures;
- record keeping.

The animal welfare requirements of the Lion Code exceed the legal requirements. These include:

- the banning of induced moulting;
- additional staff training procedures for the handling of end-of-lay hens;
- the Code mirrors the RSPCA's Freedom Food standards for free-range and barn egg production.

7.6.3.2 Freedom foods

The RSPCA has established a quality control system based almost entirely on bird welfare. Since the organization considers cages to be intrinsically cruel the society will only give accreditation to barn and free-range systems. The scheme is based around the FAWC's 'five freedoms' (reflected in the name of the scheme). Subscribers to the scheme pay a levy and are inspected by representatives of Freedom Foods Ltd. If proven satisfactory, the producer can use the Freedom Foods logo on the packaging. The main points of the scheme include the following.

Chickens must be fed a wholesome diet which:

- is appropriate to their species (meeting nutritional needs for good health);
- is available to them at all times (unless authorized by a veterinary surgeon);
- of known nutrient content with no mammal or bird protein;
- contains no antibiotic (except for therapeutic reasons);
- birds must be fed insoluble grit at least once per week;
- continuous access to an adequate supply of clean, fresh water (unless under the instruction of a veterinarian).

The environment in which birds are kept must:

- be designed to protect them from physical and thermal discomfort, fear and distress (coping with local weather conditions);
- a sign must be prominently displayed at or near the building entrance with the following information:
- total floor area available to the birds;
- total number of birds and stocking density;
- total number of drinkers and feeders;

- target air quality parameters;
- lighting levels and regimes;
- emergency procedures, i.e. actions in the case of fire, flood, etc.;
- nest box area per bird;
- lighting in the sheds should meet the welfare needs of the birds (including resting time) and be recorded.

It is not compulsory for laying hens in the Freedom Foods scheme to have free range. However, where it is provided there are requirements within the scheme, such as continuous access to the range during daylight hours. The RSPCA only allow 1,000 birds per hectare. This was the legal requirement up to 1 January 2004, but the 'special marketing terms' were simplified from the six or so possible production methods to only four (including organic production). The legally permitted number of birds on the range was increased to 2,500 (which previously had been the limit for 'semi intensive'). The RSPCA objected and maintained the reduced stocking level of 1,000 birds per hectare. For the RSPCA the maximum perimeter of range is 350 m from the house. Land use rotation must occur if there is a risk of accumulation of parasites (fowl sick land).

The scheme also includes the roles of managers and stock-keepers, bird inspection, health plans, and so on, along with requirements for transport and slaughter of the birds, but since these are not part of the bird environmental requirements, these will not be considered here.

7.6.3.3 Other schemes

Other marketing, quality and welfare assurance schemes exist within the UK. For example, for eggs to be sold as 'organically produced', the production methods must meet the legal requirements. The Soil Association is a sub-group within organic production. The Soil Association adds further requirements for organic production and its members can market the product under the Soil Association banner as a mark of distinction.

Supermarkets are also using eggs in advertising campaigns, attempting to use the perceived welfare concerns of society as marketing tools. For example, some major retail chain stores (claiming to take advice from the RSPCA) have committed to phase out sales of eggs from caged hens, and a well-known manufacturer of mayonnaise has recently stated that their product will only use eggs from the free-range egg sector.

7.6.4 Welfare monitoring protocols

In the past it was the responsibility of the State Veterinary Service to monitor egg production sites to ensure compliance with current, relevant UK legislation concerning general management, cage sizes, stocking densities, and so on. Inspectors could visit sites and make recommendations to the producer, or have the authority to close the unit if there was gross non-compliance. This caused some resentment among some producers who felt that, where EU legislation applied, other member states were not being as closely monitored, or the legislation as strictly upheld. In 2007 the State Veterinary Service merged with other groups, including the Egg Marketing Inspectorate. The Egg Marketing Inspectorate had the authority to inspect egg production sites and packing stations, etc., mainly to ensure compliance with legislation associated with hygiene, marketing standards, labelling and egg handling and storage sites, etc., rather than dealing with bird welfare *per se*. The Welfare of Farmed Animals (England) (Amendment) Regulations 2002 was one of the first pieces of legislation associated with egg production which made provision for inspection to be carried out by inspectors from other EU member states.

The RSPCA uses inspectors to assess the welfare of laying hens for farms included in the Freedom Foods scheme. These inspectors make farm visits and check bird welfare and ensure that all of the scheme's requirements are in place. This can be as simple as a tick-box check ensuring that requirements are in place, an examination of records and an assessment of the current flocks. Similarly assessors of the Lion scheme carry out farm assessments to ensure that all of the requirements of the scheme have been met.

There are other individuals and groups that are associated with the welfare of laying hens. Some research groups (e.g. the Roslin Institute in the past) and universities (e.g. Oxford, Cambridge and Bristol) have been particularly involved in research into animal welfare (including laying hens). Several welfare groups, such as Chickens' Lib and Compassion in World Farming, are also involved in promoting the welfare of laying hens. These have many publicity campaigns and lobby Parliament and the larger retailers to criticise cages and to promote higher welfare standards for farmed animals.

7.7 Conclusions: The Way Ahead

Eggs are a relatively cheap, highly nutritious food item or ingredient for other food products. As the human population continues to expand, the global demand for eggs will increase. It can be no surprise that the major egg producers of today are countries of high population (and rapidly developing economies). In fact history may be repeating itself, as it was in Britain that areas of rapid growth in the poultry industry coincided with rapidly growing population densities and industrial development (requiring cheap food for factory workers).

Optimistically, one would hope that consumers' concerns for the welfare of animals in society, and in particular farmed species, will continue to grow. Also, if this is a real concern, consumers may be more willing to pay the higher prices to meet the corresponding higher costs of production. Certainly, in the UK and in the EU, legislation increasingly seeks to safeguard the welfare of farm animals. The pressures from the UK's larger retailers on the nation's major egg producers may also bring about changes in the methods of production. The changes that are planned for 2012 could be significantly influenced if more retailers plan not to sell eggs from caged hens (from any cage type). Pressure from retailers and legislation appears more prevalent in European countries. These tend to be the more affluent economies.

In the current economic crisis it will be interesting to see if consumers' concerns for welfare are diminished in Europe. There has, in the UK, already been a reduced demand for organic produce. The dichotomy between consumers' concerns for bird welfare and purchasing patterns is well documented. As consumers in the UK change their purchasing habits, egg sales from the less prestigious retailers may increase. Such retailers are unlikely to stop selling the less expensive eggs from caged hens. If the more prestigious stores carry out their plans to not sell eggs from the caged sector, eggs from the UK enriched cage sector may be increasingly sold in these other stores, or eggs may be imported from other countries.

Welfare concerns may not be considered as important in developing economies. As the influence of Asian economies increases in global trading, the association between production and the welfare concerns for the animals may become secondary. The EU has stated that it will not trade with any third country that does not produce eggs with the same standards of welfare for the birds. Such threats may be interpreted as protectionist trading, possibly leading to some form of global trade war.

Notwithstanding these political issues, one might hope that concerns will continue to grow and develop for the needs of animals used in agriculture. It is also essential that this increased awareness and concern should lead to real improvements in farm animal welfare and protection. This will require continuing research to more fully understand the needs, and the limits, of the birds that are used for egg production. Humans have an important responsibility to look after the birds that are used for egg production. Let us hope that we take this responsibility seriously and provide the birds with a safe environment that protects their welfare.

References and Further Reading

ADAS (undated) *Poultry technical note*. Agricultural Development Advisory Service.

Appleby, M.C., Mench, J.A. and Hughes, B.O. (2004) *Poultry Behaviour and Welfare*. CABI Publishing, Wallingford.

Brambell, F.W.R. (1965) *Report of the Technical Committee to inquire into the Welfare of Animals kept under Intensive Livestock Husbandry Systems*. HMSO, London.

Council of the European Union (1999) *Laying down the minimum standard for the protection of laying hens*. Council Directive 1999/74/EC, 19 July 1999.

Department for Environment, Food and Rural Affairs. *Animal Welfare: Welfare of Laying Hens*. Available at: http://www.defra.gov.uk/animalh/welfare/farmed/layers (accessed 1 September 2009).

Department for Environment, Food and Rural Affairs (2002) *Laying hens: code of recommendations for the welfare of livestock*. DEFRA, London.

Department for Environment, Food and Rural Affairs (2006) *Compendium of UK Organic Standards*. DEFRA, London.

Department for Environment, Food and Rural Affairs (2007) *Guidance on legislation covering the marketing of eggs*. DEFRA, London.

European Food Safety, Authority (2005) Welfare aspects of various systems for keeping laying hens. Annex to *EFSA Journal* **197**, 1–23.

FAWC, (Farm Animal Welfare Council) (1982) *Report on the Welfare of Poultry at the Time of Slaughter*. Farm Animal Welfare Council, Surbiton, UK.

FAWC (1986) *An Assessment of Egg Production Systems*. Farm Animal Welfare Council, Surbiton, UK.

FAWC (1991) *Report on the Welfare of Laying Hens in Colony Systems: PB 0734*. Farm Animal Welfare Council, Surbiton, UK.

FAWC (1997) *Report on the Welfare of Laying Hens*. Available at: http://www.fawc.org.uk/reports.htm (accessed 1 September 2009).

FAWC (2009) *What is the Farm Animal Welfare Council?* Available at: http://www.fawc.org.uk (accessed 1 September 2009).

Gentle, M.J., Waddington, D., Hunter, L.N. and Jones, B. (1990) Behavioural evidence for persistent pain following partial beak amputation in chicken. Applied Animal Behaviour Science **27**, 149–57.

Harrison, R. (1964) *Animal Machines: the New Factory Farming Industry*. Vincent Stuart Ltd, London.

ISA (2009-10) General Management Guide: Commercials. Institut de Sélection Animale BV. Available at: http://www.isapoultry.com/

LayWel Project (2006) *Welfare Implications of Changes in Production Systems for Laying Hens*. Available at: http://www.laywel.eu (accessed 1 September 2009).

Meunier, R.A. and Latour, M.A.(undated) *Commercial Egg Production and Processing*. Available at: http://ag.ansc.purdue.edu/poultry/publication/commegg (accessed 1 September 2009).

Reece, W.O. (2009) *Functional Anatomy and Physiology of Domestic Animals*, 4th edn. Wiley-Blackwell, Ames, IA.

RSPCA, (Royal Society for the Protection of Animals) (2008) *RSPCA Welfare Standards for Laying Hens and Pullets*. RSPCA, Horsham, UK.

United Kingdom Register of Organic Food Standards (UKROFS) (2003) *UKROFS Standards for Organic Food Production*. Available at: http://www.defra.gov.uk/

Windhorst, H.W. (2007) Changes in the structure of global egg production. *World Poultry* **23** (6), 24–5.

Broiler Chickens

8

SUSAN HASLAM

8.1 The Industry

Broiler chickens provide humans with a relatively inexpensive source of high-quality protein which can be grown rapidly, with high food conversion efficiency and relatively low wastage through mortality. Husbandry systems have been developed over the last 50 years which produce high quantities of meat product per unit of land in production. Approximately 50,000 million broilers a year are produced globally. Broiler chicken meat is acceptable to all religious groups, other than those requiring members to be vegetarian or vegan, and is included in the diet of most countries worldwide. Broiler chickens may be readily produced on an industrial scale but are also equally suitable for small, low capital investment domestic production.

The international broiler industry consists, for the most part, of large integrated groups with the company supplying day-old chicks from a central hatchery, feed, medication and vaccination to company-owned or contracted farms. The company hires and often trains catching teams to depopulate houses and provides transport crates and transport vehicles to take birds to a central processing plant, or plants, for slaughter and often for further processing into convenience, higher-argin products for retail markets.

The typical, intensively produced broiler bird is slaughtered at between 36 and 54 days of age at a weight of between 1.7 kg and 3.5 kg. Most broiler chickens are kept in sheds on litter and fed *ad libitum*. Stocking density in conventional intensive units is likely to range from about 17 to 22 birds/m^2 (600–450 cm^2 per bird) as birds approach slaughter weight. Productivity is measured in terms of food conversion ratio (FCR, kg feed/kg live-weight gain) or food conversion efficiency (FCE, kg live-weight gain/kg feed, see Chapter 1), or as kg live-weight sold per square metre of floor space. By these measures, productivity has improved over the last 50 years by increasing the stocking density in sheds, and by genetic selection of birds for fast growth rate, improved FCE and higher breast yield. A modern intensive unit operating with a fast-growing strain of bird would have a target FCR below 1.8. In other words, it requires only about 4.4 kg of feed to rear a bird to a slaughter weight of 2.5 kg. However, this trend has had some effects on bird welfare.

Selection for rapid growth rate has created welfare problems, especially lameness and heart failure. High stocking densities have prevented birds from carrying out normal behaviour; poor litter management has led to problems such as contact dermatitis, where the skin is chemically burned by alkaline, wet litter. In developed, more affluent countries, there has been an increase in public concern relating to the welfare of broiler chickens and to the routine use of antibiotics to control infection in intensive units. This has led in recent years to an increase in alternative systems involving slower-growing strains of bird, lower stocking densities, and free-range, organic and other systems that claim higher welfare standards.

8.2 Production Systems

8.2.1 Chick production

Most broiler chickens in intensive units originate from two international breeding companies, Ross and Cobb, although each company produces several strains of bird with specific characteristics, which differ slightly in terms of breast yield, growth rate, FCE and other characteristics, to make them suitable for different husbandry systems or geographical regions. Strains of bird intended both for maximum growth rates and for less intensive systems tend to be hatched in the same large units. Eggs from breeder flocks are incubated on tiered racks in walk-in incubators. Bacterial load in incubators, which is high because of the sheer numbers of chicks hatched in close proximity, may be reduced by the use of chlorine gas. The welfare problems for chicks associated with the use of chlorine gas in incubators have not been studied, although this gas is known to be aversive to humans at relatively low concentrations, causing nose, throat and eye irritation. At higher levels, breathing chlorine gas may result in changes in breathing rate and coughing, and damage to the lungs in humans.

After hatching, chicks are vaccinated against various diseases, depending on local disease status. This usually involves release of an aerosol so that the chicks receive their vaccine through inhalation of droplets. Some vaccines (e.g. for Marek's disease) may be injected into the egg. Birds may then be individually sexed by trained operatives as, although the majority of flocks are mixed-sex, a minority of producers raise male and female birds separately. Traditionally this involved vent inspection, which required great skill and was rather stressful to the birds. Most modern strains can now be sexed according to feather appearance: day-old females have longer wing feathers than males. In high-throughput hatcheries, chicks are handled using mechanical systems, including high-speed conveyors, loaded into environmentally controlled vehicles and transported to growing houses.

8.2.2 Intensive rearing systems

Day-old chicks require house temperatures of approximately 32 °C at placement, which is gradually reduced throughout the flock cycle, according to a pre-planned programme, to about 21–23 °C when the birds are 5 weeks of age. House temperatures throughout the flock cycle are controlled by the use of in-house heaters and by changing ventilation rates, by altering the number of fans operating and inlets open. Management of house temperature and ventilation may be done manually or by computers, which are fed information on house temperature and ventilation from in-house sensors.

8.2.2.1 Brooding

Day-old chicks may be enclosed under brooders (gas-fired heaters) for the first few days of the flock cycle in order to prevent chilling; alternatively the entire house may be heated, known as whole-house brooding. Feed crumbs may be initially provided on paper to encourage pecking, as chicks are keen to peck small particles but do not initially distinguish between food and non-food items. Chicks may be further vaccinated during the flock cycle, delivered by aerosol or in the drinking water. Diseases controlled by vaccination include infectious bronchitis, infectious bursal disease, Newcastle disease and Marek's disease. Coccidiosis, a disease of the intestines caused by a ubiquitous single-celled organism, may be controlled by vaccination or the inclusion of drugs in the feed, such as the commonly used monensin and salinomycin.

8.2.2.2 Feeding

Feed may be provided via circular pan feeders or a continuous track feeder. Broiler rations are based on cereal, supplemented and precisely formulated to provide an optimal balance of metabolizable energy, amino acids, minerals and vitamins at all stages of growth. The starter ration containing 22–23% protein is usually fed as a crumb. After 3 weeks the feed will usually be pelleted and contain about 21% protein. Water may be provided in circular bell feeders or by rows of nipples which may be fitted with drip trays or 'cups', which reduce leakage and so tend to improve litter quality by reducing litter moisture. The ratio of bird drinkers or drinker space per bird and the overall length of track available per bird are critical to prevent competition for feed and water between birds. Feed and water are usually provided constantly, i.e. *ad libitum*, throughout the flock cycle. Water may be treated with peroxide or chlorine products to reduce bacterial contamination. Several successive diets, the composition of which are suited to the different stages of growth, are usually fed, with the final 'withdrawal diet' provided for the last 5 to 7 days containing no coccidiostat, in order to prevent residues of these medications entering the food chain.

8.2.2.3 Lighting

Lighting programmes are usually 24 hours of light during the first week of the cycle, to encourage young chicks to feed, and then again during the last week of the cycle to reduce 'flightiness' and so damage to birds when sheds are depopulated. However, light intensity is usually low (10–20 lux; see Table 8.1). A dark period of between 30

Table 8.1 Comparison between standards required for different systems for broiler chicken production. (For further explanation see text.)

	Max. stocking density		Age at slaughter minimum	Lighting minimum	Dark period minimum	Environment enrichment	Leg problems max permitted
	kg/m²	birds/m²					
UK Welfare Codes	34	15.5	Unspecified	10 lux	30 minutes	Not required	Unspecified
EU Standards (from 2010)	33	15	Unspecified	20 lux	6 hours*	Not required	Unspecified
Assured chickens (UK)	38	17	Unspecified	10–20 lux	4 hours	Not required	15%
EU Standards, Free Range	27.5 indoors	12.5	56 days	Uncontrolled	Uncontrolled	Outdoor access	Unspecified
	1,000 birds/ha outdoors						
Organic, Free Range							
fixed housing	21	12.5	81 days	Uncontrolled	Uncontrolled	Outdoor access	Unspecified
mobile housing	30	13.6					
RSPCA Freedom Foods	30	13.6	'49 days' wt. gain <46 g/d	100 lux	6 hours*	Straw, perches	4%

Except first 7 and last 3 days of life.

minutes and 8 hours in 24 hours may be provided during the remaining part of the flock cycle; this may reduce leg health problems and improve FCE. Dark periods are usually in a single block but may be split into several blocks over the 24-hour period. The EU Broiler Directive (2007), which came into force in 2010, requires a continuous dark period of at least 4 hours in every 24 hours. Birds given significant dark periods, of over approximately 4 hours, are metabolically different from birds kept under near-continuous light. They do not feed during dark periods but fill their crops ('crop up') immediately prior to the dark period and then again immediately after the lights come on. Lights may be controlled by a dimmer switch which allows a gradual reduction and increase in light levels at the beginning (dusk) and the end (dawn) of the dark period: this is known as dawn/dusk dimming.

8.2.2.4 Litter management

Broiler chickens are usually housed on deep litter, although litter may be shallow in some systems, including many houses in Sweden. Litter materials include long or chopped straw, wood shavings or chips, sawdust, straw/wood shaving combinations, paper products, hemp, rice husks, peat or earth. Litter may be replenished during the flock cycle if it becomes wet or greasy. In most European countries, it is routine to dispatch birds from all houses on the unit within a few days, remove all the litter and clean and disinfect and/or fumigate all houses, including feeder and drinker systems, before the next batch of chicks arrives. Swabs may be taken from house walls and equipment for bacteriology after cleaning and disinfection to check that these procedures have been effective, including sampling for *Salmonella*. In other countries, such as the USA, houses may not be completely cleared between flocks: new litter is placed onto that already in the house.

8.2.2.5 Stocking densities

For commercial purposes stocking densities are usually defined in terms of kg/m^2. In terms of bird welfare it is more useful to think in terms of the number of birds per square metre of house floor space, or the area available for each bird (cm^2/bird). The stocking rate at which the birds are placed in traditional, intensive commercial houses varies between different areas of the world. In the most intensive housing systems it may exceed 20 birds/m^2, (i.e. provide an area of less than 500 cm^2/bird). EU standards and UK Codes of Welfare recommend that stocking rates should not exceed 15 birds/m^2 (Table 8.1). Many companies have a policy of placing birds initially at higher stocking rates than 22 birds/m^2, then later taking part of the flock out during the flock cycle in order to make more efficient use of the floor area. This practice is known as 'thinning' and may be carried out several times during one flock cycle. Thinning is known to cause stress to both the birds removed and those remaining in the house. Many flocks tested negative for the food poisoning organism *Campylobacter* have been shown to become positive after thinning: thus thinning may represent a risk to human health as well as a compromise to bird welfare.

8.2.3 Less intensive indoor systems

Less intensive indoor systems typically stock at up to 30 or 34 kg/m^2 as birds approach slaughter weight (600 to 650 cm^2/bird) and may have other modifications aimed at improving bird welfare. Some use slower-growing bird genotypes and/or restrict feed in order to reduce growth rate. There may be various environmental enrichments, such as windows in the shed, toys, perches and straw bales. Misting systems, primarily introduced to prevent heat stress, may also be regarded as an environmental enrichment measure for indoor birds as these stimulate bathing behaviour. There may also be a policy of not thinning for some schemes. In Europe some large retailers incorporate these higher environmental standards as part of their ethical sourcing policy. The RSPCA farm assurance scheme, 'Freedom Foods', restricts daily growth rate of birds, prohibits thinning and requires environmental enrichment. These quality assurance schemes usually include regular audits to ensure that standards are being maintained (see Chapter 18). Birds from low-intensity, indoor systems cost more to produce than a traditional intensive bird but can sell at a premium price.

8.2.4 Free-range systems

Free-range birds also live in littered sheds but have daytime access to a ranging area, through popholes fitted at ground level in the walls of the shed. These systems have developed to meet demand from consumers who believe that free-range birds experience a higher level of welfare than intensively reared birds and that the meat quality and taste is better. Free-range birds sell at an even greater premium than low-intensity indoor birds. Slower growth rates and greater age at slaughter (56–81 days, Table 8.1) may contribute to improved meat quality and will certainly reduce the prevalence of leg problems (see section 8.3.2). There is potential for these birds to experience a 'richer' life, with opportunities and space to carry out most normal behaviour. However, problems can arise if the quality of husbandry is inadequate. Poor cover on range or inadequate perimeter fencing may increase the risk of predation or the fear of predation. Poor litter and fouled ground around popholes may increase the incidence of contact dermatitis on the feet, termed 'foot pad dermatitis', especially if stocking density in the shed is high. The provision of environmental enrichment, bird protection measures and contact dermatitis are discussed in more detail later in this chapter.

There is also a market for organically produced broiler chickens in some countries. The specific requirements of different certification bodies vary but all organic schemes require birds to be fed on organically produced food, have access to range, to be grown slowly, killed at a greater age than conventionally produced birds and to receive pharmacological products, such as antibiotics, only when they are essential to treat clinical disease. In the EU, the precise requirements for husbandry systems which label birds as 'free range' and 'traditional free range' are laid down in the Poultry Marketing Directive.

8.2.5 Comparison of production systems

Table 8.1 summarizes the main elements of broiler production standards set by EU legislation, the UK Code of Welfare for Broiler Chickens and some non-governmental quality assurance agencies. The UK Codes of Welfare (www.defra.gov.uk/animalwelfare) are not mandatory. EU legislation became mandatory in June 2010. Assured chicken production (ACP, UK) sets standards for and accredits about 95% of UK broilers. Both 'free range' and 'organic free range' are set out in EU law. Note that both ACP and Freedom Foods include an outcome-based measure of welfare, i.e. the prevalence of hock-burn.

8.2.6 Village chicken production

Chickens are a valuable source of high-quality protein in many rural areas in Africa and Asia. A comprehensive report on village chicken production system in rural Africa has been produced by he UN Food and Agriculture Organization (1998). Typical flock sizes vary from less than 10 up to around 100 birds, use indigenous, unimproved genotypes and birds are not segregated by age or gender. Smaller flocks are unhoused and receive little or no supplemental feeding; they are expected to scavenge for themselves. Birds are kept for eggs and meat. Approximately 20% of mature birds are likely to be in lay at any time. Birds eaten for meat are mature birds, including non-laying hens. The productivity of the birds is extremely low in comparison with large intensive units and characterized by low hatchability and high mortality due to disease and predation, especially of chicks.

The FAO report outlines a standardized methodology by which village chicken production systems may be improved, based on producer participation and aimed at increasing management skills, improving the way the final product is used and the use of marketing strategies (Figure 8.1). They recommend that the initial step in any programme aimed at improving bird productivity should be to identify and direct resources at the major problems occurring at village level. These are most commonly attributed to predators or infectious disease, especially Newcastle disease (ND). Locally run vaccination programmes for control of ND have allowed many families to expand their flocks without necessarily having to spend money on purchasing more feed. FAO also recommend the introduction of 'improved genotypes': birds with higher-yielding traits. The potential for this is obvious provided there is sufficient food for both humans and chickens. However, FAO (1998) cites several initiatives to increase productivity of village flocks that have not yet produced any sustainable improvement. The wisdom of some of these schemes is open to question. When chickens in family flocks are compelled to subsist for much of the year on what

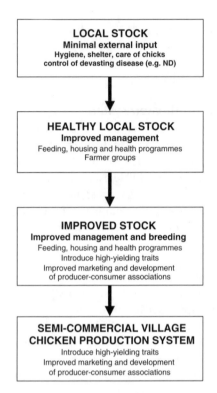

Figure 8.1   Step-wise improvement of village chicken production systems (FAO 1998).

they can scavenge for themselves, the introduction of 'improved' strains can become self-defeating.

8.3 Health and Welfare Problems in the Production Unit

8.3.1 Mortality

Mortality in broilers may be caused by infectious and non-infectious conditions, including heat stress, and pulmonary hypertension syndrome (PHS) or 'flip-over', which is right-sided heart failure.

8.3.1.1 Using mortality as a welfare assessment measure

Levels of mortality in groups of animals may be used as a welfare assessment measure. The EU Broiler Directive (2007) will require mortality levels to be recorded. At a typical slaughter age of 40 days, the maximum mortality permitted for stocking at over 39 kg per square metre will be 3.4% over the previous seven consecutive flock cycles. In a recent study of broiler chicken farms in the UK, the mean mortality level on farm was 4.1% (range 1.4% to 14.7%; Dawkins *et al.*, 2004). Mortality figures for broiler flocks should be interpreted with caution when used as a welfare assessment measure, since they will include birds which have been culled due to sickness or injury such as lameness. Where a farmer is rapidly and effectively identifying diseased or injured birds and humanely killing them, the overall welfare state of the birds on the farm may be good. Where culled birds are included in the mortality figure, a farmer with current bird mortality close to the legally imposed limits may be tempted not to cull lame or diseased birds, with the hope that they will live long enough to be loaded for transport to the slaughter plant. The suffering of these diseased birds will be prolonged and they are more likely to die due to stresses of handling and transportation, so increasing the number of birds found 'dead on arrival' at the slaughter plant.

8.3.1.2 Culling

Broiler chickens are customarily euthanized on farm by 'neck-pulling', which disarticulates the spinal column and breaks the spinal cord. However, disruption of the spinal cord without rupture of the carotid arteries in the neck, which supply blood to the brain, simply stops respiratory movement: there is evidence that birds killed by this method may be conscious for several minutes prior to brain death. A portable percussion stunner device is commercially available for bird euthanasia on-farm, which causes instant loss of consciousness: this device is more commonly used for turkeys but is effective for broiler chicken euthanasia. The use of this device, which is illustrated in Figure 8.2, is limited largely due to economic considerations, although more widespread use would greatly improve broiler chicken welfare.

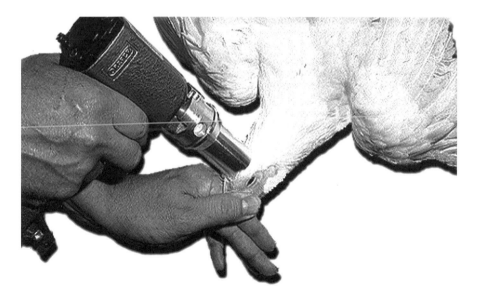

Figure 8.2 A percussion stunner for emergency slaughter of poultry (courtesy of Steve Wotton).

8.3.2 Lameness

Recent studies in the UK found that over a quarter of traditionally produced intensive birds are significantly lame in the week before they are slaughtered (Knowles *et al.*, 2008). The walking ability of a bird is usually described in terms of its 'gait score', which may be from 0, walking normally (e.g. a healthy free-range laying hen), to 5, completely unable to walk. Birds at gait score 3 are obviously lame, their movement is greatly restricted and this reduces their frequency of visits to feeders and drinkers. There is also clear evidence that these birds are in pain. Their overall activity is reduced, and they are reluctant to remain standing. There is even evidence that high gait-score birds will self-select feed which contains an analgesic drug (Danbury *et al.*, 1999). Many quality assurance schemes require birds with a gait score of 3 or above to be culled on humane grounds.

Most lameness in broiler chickens is due to developmental abnormalities of the leg bones and joints; lameness can also occur because of joint infections caused by bacteria such as *Staphylococcus aureus* and *Enterococcus caecorum*. These infections are, however, greatly exacerbated by the stresses associated with rapid growth. The main causal factor would appear to be damage to growth plates when the bones are very soft. The prevalence of lameness in broiler chickens may be reduced by using slower-growing genotypes or by restricted feeding during the first weeks of growth, e.g. by feeding in meals, rather than *ad libitum*, by providing feed which has a lower nutritional density or by increasing the duration of the dark period, during which birds do not eat (Knowles *et al.*, 2008).

8.3.3 Contact dermatitis

Higher stocking densities tend to cause increased litter moisture and ammonia, which may result in contact dermatitis, a condition where the skin is chemically burned, turning it black. Lesions of contact dermatitis are commonly found on the foot pads, termed foot pad dermatitis (FPD) (Figure 8.3), hock (hock-burn) and breast (breast-burn). Prevalence (mean and range) taken from a UK study (Haslam *et al.*, 2007) is shown in Table 8.2. Severe contact dermatitis lesions may penetrate the dermis, which is innervated, and are likely to be painful. A high incidence of contact dermatitis in a flock indicates that they have experienced poor litter and air quality during the flock cycle. Birds from houses with poor litter quality but with good leg health tend to have high prevalence of FPD, birds from houses with poor litter quality and poor leg health tend to have a higher prevalence of hock and breast burn, as they tend to spend longer periods of time with the hock and breast in contact with the litter.

The prevalence of contact dermatitis may be reduced by using wood shavings, by adding litter during the flock cycle, by using nipple and cup rather than bell drinkers, preventing drinker leaks, reducing water pressure to the drinkers, directing air intakes upwards and away from the litter, using less susceptible genotypes of birds, insulating pipes and water tanks, which may cause condensation, or relocating them to a position out of the area occupied by the birds. Litter may also be improved by

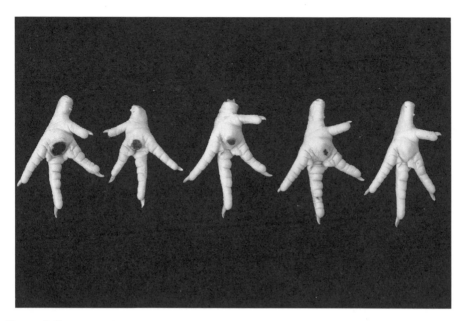

Figure 8.3 Foot pad dermatitis: examples of severity scored on a scale of 5–1.

increasing ventilation rates and, in cooler climates, through provision of under-floor heating.

8.3.4 Infectious disease

An outbreak of infectious disease on an intensive commercial unit containing many thousands of birds can be very costly for the producer. It also presents a severe cost to bird welfare. The effect on welfare of any disease may be described by the number of birds affected (morbidity), the number dying (mortality), and severity (pain and malaise) and duration of suffering. Most of the major infectious diseases can be controlled through vaccination. However, antimicrobial and anticoccidial drugs still play a major role in the control of infectious disease in poultry houses. Antimicrobial 'growth promoters', such as avoparcin, bacitracin, nitrovin and virginiamycin, have been routinely incorporated into the feed of broiler chickens worldwide for many decades. The overall effect of these antibiotics has been to improve FCE by destroying bacteria in the digestive tract. These include pathogenic strains of bacteria which

Table 8.2 Prevalence of contact dermatitis in UK broiler flocks. Source: Haslam *et al.* (2007).

	Mean %	Range %
Foot pad dermatitis	11	0–76
Hock-burn	1.3	0–33
Breast-burn	<0.01	0–0.12

may cause clinical disease, or reduce performance by causing subclinical disease, and non-pathogenic strains which can, however, compete with the host for nutrients.

The use of these antibiotics in chicken feed has been completely prohibited in the EU since 2006, after a gradual reduction in the number of permitted substances over the previous decade, due to the risk that their routine use might cause resistance to these, or similar antibiotics in bacteria which cause clinical disease in humans. However, since the use of antimicrobial 'growth promoters' has been prohibited, there is some evidence to suggest there has been an increase in the 'routine' use of therapeutic antibiotics used in human medicine. There is a real possibility that the ban on antibiotic growth promoters may increase rather than decrease the risk of transfer of resistance to antibiotics essential for the treatment of serious human diseases.

8.3.4.1 Biosecurity

Biosecurity is an essential element of disease control on intensive poultry units. Unnecessary visitors should be discouraged and essential visitors should either be required to leave vehicles outside the farm or use a wheel wash or even car wash installed at the farm entrance. They should be required to wear disposable, house-specific protective clothing and boots and use disinfectant footbaths and hand washes. Some farms use a barrier system at the entrance to the house, where people entering the house are required to put on house-specific clothing and boots which are kept on the house side of the barrier, leaving their own boots on the outside. In some countries, for example Thailand and Chile, for very large farms and for very high-value birds, extreme biosecurity measures are taken, which may include one or more showers and complete changes of clothes, disinfection of the interior of vehicles and fumigation of any equipment taken onto the farm. For large commercial farms worldwide, records of previous sites visited are usually kept in order to enable the source of any disease outbreaks to be traced.

8.3.5 Heat stress

High levels of mortality may occur in broilers due to heat stress caused by inadequate ventilation systems or system failure in bird houses, which prevent house temperatures being held down during hot and humid weather conditions. In large units with electric fans, large numbers of birds may die if the failure is not rectified within a very short time; potentially as short as 15 minutes. The sudden death of large numbers of birds due to heat stress may be prevented by the installation of high temperature alarms, which sound in the house and, usually automatically, call a pager or telephone a stockperson to alert him/her to the problem. Where ventilation systems are electrically powered, it is essential that a back-up generator, which can be started in the event of electrical failure, is immediately available. Where the ventilation system includes an auto-start generator, which starts automatically in case of mains electricity supply failure, it should incorporate an alarm which sounds if the auto-start fails.

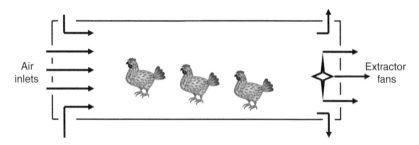

Figure 8.4 Tunnel ventilation for poultry houses and air flow patterns. (After Bucklin et al. 1998, Tunnel Ventilation of Broiler Houses.)

Houses in geographical locations where hot and humid weather is frequent may be fitted with 'tunnel ventilation', where very large fans fitted into the end wall on the short end of a house draw air along the length of the house, illustrated in Figure 8.4. The design of inlets and positioning of fans in relation to local prevailing winds, and in-house equipment, can lead to uneven air flow patterns and dead spots, where there is no air movement: such systems should always be installed by experienced experts.

When external air temperature exceeds 30 °C, it is impossible to prevent heat stress in poultry houses simply through control of ventilation. In these circumstances, the air may be cooled through the latent heat of evaporation of water. The house may be fitted with sprinkler systems, which operate sporadically to produce a very fine mist or fog, which evaporates before hitting the litter. Alternatively, evaporative cooling systems may be incorporated into the ventilation system. Misting systems and evaporative cooling systems need to be used with care to ensure that they do not create excessive humidity in the house. The relationship between safe temperature and safe humidity for broiler chickens is shown in Figure 8.5. This illustrates the combinations of air temperature and relative humidity (RH) at which birds are at risk. For example, a combination of an air temperature of 30 °C and a RH of 60% would just put birds into the danger zone. This chart can be applied worldwide to birds on farm, in transport and lairage. In all systems, including less intensive or hobby flocks, the effects of heat stress on birds may be reduced by reducing or withholding feed, which lowers metabolic rate and so reduces heat production by birds. If all else fails, it may be necessary to reduce bird numbers to reduce the amount of heat generated within the building. One broiler produces about 12 watts. Thus the heat load on a building containing 30,000 birds would be 36 kW!

8.3.5.1 Risks in naturally ventilated and free-range systems

Free-range and organic systems operating in temperate climates do not usually have electrically controlled ventilation with fitted alarm systems. However, birds in some large, more densely stocked, naturally ventilated houses, with no access to range, are at risk of death due to heat stress in hot weather. Such houses should

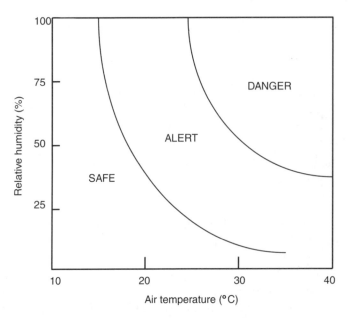

Figure 8.5 Temperature/humidity, thermal comfort and stress index. Reproduced from 'The Welfare of Poultry at Slaughter or Killing © Crown copyright 2007.

therefore be fitted with high temperature alarms and provision to increase air movement when necessary. Birds with access to range can escape the problem of heat stress in densely stocked buildings (provided they choose to go outside). It is important, however, to provide birds out of doors with cover from direct sunlight and from the fear of predation.

The range area should be designed and maintained so as to minimize both the real risk and the birds' perceived risk of predation. The farmer must then ensure that the perimeter fences surrounding the ranging area are constructed to exclude predators, either by height (for those that can jump), through the use of barbed wire or electrical fencing. In some areas it may be necessary to bury the fence below the ground to exclude burrowing predators. Perimeter fences must be regularly checked for integrity and maintained adequately. Electrical fences should be checked more frequently, kept free of vegetation which may cause failure of the fence, and consideration should be given to installing electrical failure alarms and having a back-up electrical supply to provide power in case of failure.

Provision of overhead cover on the range will encourage birds to use the range. It provides protection from direct sunlight and excessive air movement. It provides real protection from overhead predators and, more importantly in most circumstances, it provides birds with a sense of security since it reduces the perceived threat of predation. Cover may include shrubs, trees, long grass, biomass vegetation, netting, trailers or low plastic tables and should cover as much of the range area as possible.

Where separate shelters are provided, they should be sited close together to ensure that birds are not in the open for long periods when moving from one covered area to another.

8.3.6 Pulmonary hypertension syndrome

Pulmonary hypertension syndrome (PHS) may cause mortality or poor welfare due to right-sided heart failure. The prevalence is greater at low temperatures and at high altitudes, both of which increase the load on the cardiorespiratory system. It can also be precipitated by acute stress. The prevalence of PHS may be reduced by selection of less susceptible bird genotypes and careful control of house temperatures. It can also be reduced through the practice of dawn/dusk dimming, gradual rather than sudden switching between light and dark.

8.3.7 Bird behaviour and environmental enrichment

Bird welfare is thought to be improved by the provision of environmental enrichment, which is why some higher welfare accreditation schemes require such enrichments to be provided. Scientific evidence suggests that only enrichments that encourage natural exploration and foraging behaviours, such as the provision of straw bales, have a genuine effect in improving welfare. Access to range for chickens allows exploratory and ground-pecking behaviour, directed at different plant and small invertebrate species. Toys, compact discs or balls are sometimes provided to encourage exploration, although birds rapidly habituate to these so that, although initially attractive, they are soon ignored. Ground pecking on range is rewarding since it persists throughout the bird's life. Access to dry friable litter allows dust-bathing behaviour. Increased space allowance, in either indoor systems or those with range access, allows walking and running, dashing and sparring and wing flapping behaviour, which may not be possible in heavily stocked houses. Misting systems encourage bathing and preening behaviour and perches may allow normal perching and roosting behaviour. However, although younger birds tend to use perches, fast-growing strains of birds in intensive systems tend not to use perches. There are several probable reasons for this: pain caused by leg disorders, unfitness once birds become very heavy, and difficulty in maintaining balance in birds with abnormal development of the breast muscle.

Birds kept in environments with a significant dark period of over about 4 continuous hours in a 24-hour cycle are generally more active and more reactive to stimuli than birds with less than 4 hours or no dark period. They may also be more inclined to use perches, especially the slow-growing strains. Birds given significant dark periods throughout the flock cycle tend to have better leg health than those with short dark periods. However, there is evidence that birds which have had longer dark periods sustain more damage at depopulation than birds which have had shorter periods. This is presumably because more active birds are more difficult to catch. This problem can be reduced by shortening the dark period during the last 3 to 7 days of life.

8.4 Depopulation, Transport and Lairaging

In very small systems, chickens may be killed for human consumption by neck dislocation (or a percussion stunner, Figure 8.2) on the farm at the end of the flock cycle: this obviates the need for loading onto a transport vehicle, transportation and live shackling or gas stunning. Some very high-value birds may be killed on farm using a slaughter line on site but nearly all birds from nearly all systems are transported in crates on a transporter for slaughter at a central slaughtering plant.

8.4.1 Depopulation

The best technique for collecting birds for slaughter is to lift them individually, with both hands placed around the body to prevent wing flapping, so reducing bird stress and injury. Such best practice is followed in some Scandinavian countries that have well-enforced legislation to protect bird welfare, or where the value of birds is high, relative to labour costs, as in some South American countries. Houses may be depopulated at night to reduce the risk of heat stress and stress due to unaccustomed daylight in traditional, intensive birds, where light levels have been low throughout the flock cycle. Many large commercial broiler chicken producers run training courses in bird handling in order to reduce injury and stress to birds and reduce carcass damage due to handling: such courses may include a visit to the slaughter plant to view carcass damage to birds on the line. Routine monitoring of carcass damage, feedback of levels of carcass damage to catchers and their managers, and bonus payment schemes for low carcass damage all contribute to reducing stress and damage at depopulation.

There is nevertheless evidence that house depopulation procedures may often cause very poor bird welfare, especially where labour costs are high and broiler meat relatively inexpensive since this encourages very rapid loading and increases the occurrence of injury to birds. Up to five or six birds may be carried by the legs, five in each hand, exacerbating pain due to leg pathologies and causing new problems including hip dislocation (Gregory and Austin, 1992), out of the house and loaded into lorries with fixed, side-loading crates. Newer transport vehicles have metal-framed modules with drawers, which can be taken into the house, using a forklift truck, to limit the distance over which the birds have to be carried inverted.

Poor bird welfare and carcass damage at depopulation may also be reduced by the use of mechanical depopulation, using one of the various commercially available 'harvesting' machines. There is evidence that birds show little fear response to these machines, in comparison to human catchers, and may sustain less injury than with conventional methods of manual catching. However 'harvesting' machines are expensive and are only economically viable for large broiler production companies. They can only be used in large open-span houses, where there are no roof supports in the body of the house and, as yet, their reliability is open to question.

8.4.2 Transport

Levels of mortality due to heat stress may be high during transport of birds to the slaughter plant, or when held in the lairage, when ambient temperatures are high. Birds are at a greater risk of suffering from heat stress when there is a breakdown of transporter vehicles or delays at the slaughter plant due to line breakdown. Consequently, in countries with seasonal differences in ambient temperatures and relative humidity, the prevalence of birds found dead on arrival (DoAs) is usually considerably higher during summer, rather than winter months. Losses due to heat stress may be reduced by careful programming of catching and killing, to reduce waiting times in the lairage, reducing stocking levels in transport crate, separating crates in the lairage to improve air circulation between crates, providing covered lairages (to keep birds out of direct sunlight) and providing an adequate number of high-powered fans to cool birds by increasing air movement.

In countries where daytime temperatures are usually high, such as in southern Europe, birds are always collected and slaughtered at night and bird transporters are built with an air gap running longitudinally down the centre of the lorry trailer, between stacks of crates, to improve air flow around the birds. In hot climates, bird transporter vehicles may be placed under a shelter surrounded by 'curtains' of flowing water to keep temperatures low. The risk of heat stress in lorries and lairages may be monitored by routine recording of air temperature and humidity at bird level. However, heat stress can be assessed more reliably by observation of the birds themselves; especially the proportion of birds panting (mouth-breathing) with beak open. If over 50% of birds are panting, immediate action is required to reduce the risk of high mortality due to heat stress.

8.4.3 Stunning and slaughter

Birds may be stunned or killed using electrical stunning or in a controlled-atmosphere chamber and then slaughtered and bled by a neck cut that severs the carotid arteries. Both stunning and neck cutting are automated but there should always be a manual back-up neck cutter, who should be replaced every 20 to 30 minutes, to prevent fatigue.

8.4.3.1 Electrical stunning

For electrical stunning, birds are inverted onto a 'shackle line', a moving chain from which hang curved, metal shackles into which the legs of the birds are placed. Inversion of birds for shackling is stressful and birds with leg pathology experience pain when placed firmly into shackles, especially at high line speeds of up to 200 birds per minute in large plants, when the procedure must be performed very quickly. Bird stress at shackling may be reduced by providing a dark, noise-free environment, by ensuring that shackle size is appropriate for the size of bird being killed, and by training operators to shackle birds in a two-stage process: the first person places the bird loosely in the shackle, reducing pressure on the legs, the second then pulls each loosely hung bird firmly into the shackle. Bird stress at shackling points and in areas through which the live bird line passes may be reduced by providing blue lighting. 'Breast comforters', which consist of rubber strips placed in parallel with the bird line and along which the birds rub, also reduce bird stress and wing flapping. Live bird lines should be straight and birds should be suspended for just long enough to settle after hanging, approximately 10 to 12 seconds. The effectiveness of measures taken to reduce bird stress can be monitored by recording the number of birds flapping on the live bird line, which should be zero.

For electrical stunning, the head of the bird is immersed in a water bath and an electric current passed between the shackle line and the bird. Entrance ramps to electric stun baths should be constructed so as to provide a shallow incline to a sudden drop, thus ensuring that the head of the bird enters the bath suddenly. The adequacy of the entrance ramp to an electric stun bath may be monitored by recording the number of birds receiving a pre-stun shock in a given time period. Birds receiving an effective single stun display a single, immediate wing movement, to bring the wings sharply against the body. Birds receiving pre-stun shocks show multiple wing flaps and may attempt to 'fly the stunner', i.e. keep their heads out of the water bath by violent wing flapping.

The factors that determine the efficacy of electrical stunning are complex (see European Food Safety Authority, 2004). Many abattoirs use low-frequency stunning (50 Hz AC) and a current of over 105 milliamps per bird to ensure an adequate stun. Effectively stunned birds will not react to neck cutting, will show no rhythmic respiratory movement, no righting reflex (attempt to assume an upright position) or corneal reflex (i.e. they should not blink when the front of the eye is touched). The neck cut should be made as close as possible to the exit of the stunner. Effectiveness of stunning should be monitored by a manual operator standing immediately downline from the automated neck cutter. Birds may appear to be adequately stunned at the exit to the stunner, but may recover consciousness on the bleed rail if the cut is inadequate for the bird to bleed to death before it recovers from the stun. Birds that are conscious when they enter the feather plucker because they have not been cut or have been cut inadequately constitute a very serious welfare problem. Uncut birds are obvious as they appear as dark red carcasses on the line after the pluckers.

8.4.3.2 Stunning/Killing in controlled atmosphere chambers

Most controlled-atmosphere stunning chambers use high concentrations of carbon dioxide. However, inhalation of carbon dioxide causes some distress and, in the UK, may only be used under special licence from DEFRA. In some systems currently in use in Europe, a two-stage process is used. Birds are first exposed to a low-concentration 'stunning' exposure, followed by a high-concentration killing exposure. This may reduce the intensity of distress but prolongs the time to loss of consciousness. In recent years alternative methods using less aversive gases and gas mixtures have been developed and trialled for effectiveness in stunning/killing, effects on bird welfare

Table 8.3 Gas mixtures recommended for use in controlled-atmosphere stunning. Source: European Food Standards Agency (2004).

(a) A minimum of 1 minute's exposure to 40% carbon dioxide, 30% oxygen and 30% nitrogen, followed by a minimum of 2 minutes' exposure to 80% carbon dioxide in air; OR

(b) A minimum of 2 minutes' exposure to any mixture of argon, nitrogen or other inert gases with atmospheric air and carbon dioxide, provided that the carbon dioxide concentration does not exceed 30% by volume and the residual oxygen concentration does not exceed 2% by volume; OR

(c) A minimum of 2 minutes' exposure to argon, nitrogen, other inert gases or any mixture of these gases in atmospheric air with a maximum of 2% residual oxygen by volume
Compressed gases should be vaporized prior to administration into the chamber. In no circumstances should solid gases with freezing temperatures be used. Prior humidification of gases is recommended.

---

and carcass quality. Argon, for example, has been shown to be undetectable to birds thus much less stressful than carbon dioxide. It is, however, much more expensive than carbon dioxide and can give rise to skin haemorrhages and so impair carcass quality. Gas mixtures recommended for use in controlled atmosphere stunning by the European Food Safety Authority (2004), to protect bird welfare and carcass quality, are detailed in Table 8.3.

Stunning/killing in a controlled-atmosphere chamber avoids the need for shackling live birds, which is a positive step in terms of bird welfare. Ideally, birds are taken into the chamber while in their transport crates. In this system, birds which were dead on arrival at the plant can be distinguished from birds killed in the chamber by their bright red discolouration. Moreover, where birds are required to be killed, rather than just stunned in the gas chamber, the risk of recovery on the bleed rail is extremely low. It is, however, more common to tip live birds from crates onto a conveyor belt which takes them into the gas chamber.

8.5 Broiler Breeders: Parent, Grandparent and Great-Grandparent Flocks

Broiler chickens reared for meat production are sourced from flocks of parent birds, known as broiler breeders, which are in turn sourced from grandparent and great-grandparent flocks. Broiler breeders produce between 120 and 180 eggs in a laying cycle of approximately 47 weeks, depending on genotype. The birds are usually housed in climate-controlled, deep litter systems similar to meat birds but with rows of nest boxes, usually placed centrally along the longitudinal axis of the house on a raised, slatted area which constitutes approximately one-third of the house. Males and females are housed together throughout the flock cycle. Initially, the ratio of females to males is approximately 9:1. Broiler breeders are less heavily stocked than meat birds, at approximately 25 birds per square metre, including male and female birds.

8.5.1 Welfare problems for broiler breeders

8.5.1.1 Hunger

Broiler breeders are exposed to most of the same potential stresses as meat birds but also have additional, specific problems. The most significant of these, in terms of duration and severity, is hunger. Clearly, broilers have been selected for very fast growth rates; over 50 g per day for some strains. If fed *ad libitum* broiler breeders would become very heavy; some would die and most experience severe leg problems before reaching sexual maturity at between 16 and 21 weeks of age. Many of those that did survive would fail to mate. Growth rates are therefore controlled in juvenile broiler breeder birds by severe restriction of feed, in terms of both nutrient density and volume. Adult male broiler breeders must be more feed restricted than females, as females require additional resources for egg production. This is usually achieved by positioning of racks over some of the feeders, which are separated into individual feeding places. The dimensions of the feeding places are designed so that they are too narrow for the head of cockerels, while permitting access to hens. This food restriction creates severe hunger, especially in male birds, which manifests itself as increased drinking and feeder-directed stereotypical pecking behaviour. Competition between birds for food can lead to uneven growth in female flocks, which is very carefully managed by separating birds into groups by weight and moving individuals between the groups as they change between weight bands. Female juvenile broiler breeders should be weighed at least once weekly in order to control weight gain during growth (approximately 7% bodyweight gain per week) and weight control remains critical thereafter. Increase in drinking due to hunger can cause poorer litter quality and more severe contact dermatitis lesions.

8.5.1.2 Injuries and mutilations

Breeding hens may suffer from feather damage and skin wounds on the back due to mating. Damage to hens during mating is minimized by removing the spur bud on the back of the leg of day-old male chicks using a heated wire. The dew and pivot claws of male broiler breeders may also be removed at this time using scissors. Genetic selection for birds with short, blunt spurs has made this unnecessary in some genotypes. Damage to hens may also be reduced by progressively removing cockerels from the flock throughout the egg-laying cycle, to reduce the ratio of cockerels to hens. Cockerels which are less fertile are identified by pallor of the comb and/or wattles.

Broiler breeders, and especially male birds, may be beak-trimmed in order to prevent injury due to feather pecking and cannibalism. Beak trimming can cause severe, lasting pain. The welfare consequences of beak trimming are reduced if carried out in young chicks, prior to 10 days of age, and if only the tip of the beak, which is not innervated, is removed. Outbreaks of feather pecking and cannibalism are fairly common in broiler breeders. Feather pecking outbreaks are usually managed by reducing light intensity in the house, but could be further reduced by the use of appropriate environmental enrichment, as feather pecking is a form of foraging behaviour directed towards an inappropriate target.

The combs of birds may be removed at day-old stage using sharp scissors, a practice known as 'dubbing', ostensibly to prevent comb damage. This traditional practice is unnecessary in modern production systems. Removal of a specific toe at the first joint for the purpose of identification of pedigree birds, a practice which is distinct from de-clawing for protection of females during mating, is no longer considered as ethically justifiable. The welfare of broiler breeders has been examined in depth by the Farm Animal Welfare Council (1995).

8.5.2 Disease control

Broiler breeders are valuable birds and so receive additional protection in comparison to meat birds. Biosecurity measures in place at broiler breeder farms tend to be stricter than those in place at meat bird farms; birds tend to receive additional vaccinations, both at the hatchery and on farm and are likely to be vaccinated for protection against coccidiosis rather than have coccidiostats in feed. Birds may be treated for ascaris worms at transfer to the laying house at approximately 18 weeks of age. Additional precautions to ensure that water is bacteriologically clean may be taken, such as ultraviolet-light treatment of water supplied to the birds. Daily water consumption may be monitored routinely, as sudden changes in consumption acts as an early warning of a disease outbreak. Broiler breeders are at risk of red mite, a parasite which lives off the bird in the house and furnishings and which feeds off birds' blood, usually at night. Birds may become anaemic and may even die in cases of severe infestation. Thorough cleaning of housing and furnishing and the use of appropriate parasiticides are essential to control this external parasite.

8.5.3 Elite birds

The production of chicks for commercial rearing as meat birds is based on a breeding pyramid that usually involves four generations. At the top of the pyramid is the 'elite' flock genetically selected according to an index that gives most emphasis to the production traits of increased growth rate, breast yield and FCE. However, the selection index will also include traits relating to fitness such as leg and cardiovascular health, reproductive efficiency, disease resistance and good social behaviour. The health and welfare of specific strains of meat birds will be determined by the relative importance attached to fitness and production traits. The offspring of the elite flock are retained as the great-grandparent flock of broiler breeders. They produce the grandparent birds, which in turn produce the parent flocks, whose offspring become the chicks bred for delivery to the units producing birds for sale as poultry meat. This four-generation breeding scheme is designed to optimize the rate of multiplication of genetically superior birds.

In order to identify birds with the fastest growth and best FCE, it is necessary to feed birds in the elite flocks *ad libitum* up until normal meat bird slaughter weights, as are commercial birds. The birds selected for broiler breeder production, at the normal slaughter age of about 7 weeks, must then be very severely feed-restricted in order to prevent them becoming too heavy to walk, and thus mate, at sexual maturity, with all the consequences identified above for feed-restricted broiler breeders.

8.6 Broilers and Human Health

The principal risks to human health from broiler chickens are avian influenza, *Salmonella* and *Campylobacter*.

8.6.1 Avian influenza

Avian influenza is a zoonosis which primarily infects domestic poultry but can be passed to humans, causing severe flu-like symptoms. With some strains of avian influenza virus this can lead to death in approximately half of recognized cases. All strains of avian influenza are carried by wild birds, which rarely show clinical signs of disease. Human cases of avian influenza usually occur where there is very close contact between people and birds, such as small flocks in rural locations, where birds are still traded individually at markets. Not all strains of avian influenza are pathogenic to humans. The H5N1 strain is highly pathogenic for poultry, transmissible from poultry to humans and has been recorded as passing *between* humans in very isolated cases. Since strains of influenza virus have a tendency to mutate there is a risk that the ability of the virus to pass between people may be enhanced, resulting in a global pandemic. A vaccine has been developed to protect people against H5N1 vaccine in the USA and others are being developed elsewhere; however, two commonly used pharmaceuticals used to treat human flu have been found to be ineffective against H5N1 strains of virus. The use of routine hygiene precautions, including effective washing of hands and equipment, and adequate cooking of poultry products is recommended to reduce the risk of infection.

8.6.2 Salmonella

Salmonella bacteria are the most frequent causes of food poisoning in humans. There are many types and strains of *Salmonella*, some specific to poultry and some affecting many species. *Salmonella* infection in humans causes a mild to severe gastroenteritis, which may include fever, abdominal pain, diarrhoea, vomiting, dehydration and even death in immunocompromised individuals, the elderly or infants. Birds are rarely clinically ill as a result of carrying *Salmonella*, with the result that the risk to human health when handling birds is not as clear as, for example, avian influenza, where affected birds are obviously clinically ill. People usually become infected by eating undercooked poultry products which are contaminated with *Salmonella*, or with food which has come into contact with contaminated products. In the EU, there is a legal requirement for member states to have a surveillance system in place to identify poultry flocks infected by *Salmonella*. For flocks known to be infected, additional precautions can be taken during slaughter, such as killing last in the programme to minimize cross-contamination to uninfected carcasses.

Salmonella is transmitted via the egg from parent to chick and for this reason most control strategies aim to ensure that broiler breeder flocks are *Salmonella*-free, either by slaughtering infected flocks, or by vaccination. The risk of infection from outside is reduced by strict biosecurity precautions, discussed earlier. The prevalence of *Salmonella* infection of poultry meat have been reduced to below 5% of flocks in some countries where effective control strategies have been introduced, such as in the UK.

8.6.3 Campylobacter

Human infection with *Campylobacter* also causes fever, abdominal pain and diarrhoea, which is usually self-limiting. However, in about one out of 1,000 cases, the infection is followed 2 to 3 weeks later with Guillain-Barre syndrome, a debilitating inflammatory polyneuritis characterized by fever, pain and weakness that progresses to paralysis, which may be fatal unless intensive care facilities are immediately available. Many cases of *Campylobacter* infection are also caused by the consumption of undercooked poultry and/or the handling of raw poultry. *Campylobacter* does not cause clear signs of clinical disease in the live bird. It is not clear whether vertical transmission of *Campylobacter*, via the egg, is possible, but most infections in meat birds seem to occur while at the farm. *Campylobacter* is ubiquitous and birds are thought to be contaminated from the environment. All of the birds in a house tend to have the same *Campylobacter* status, i.e. they are either all negative or all positive, and there is clear evidence that common husbandry procedures, which cause stress to birds, increase the probability that a flock is positive and also increase the burden of infection, which will add to levels of potential contamination and cross-contamination at the slaughter plant. Most studies of the prevalence of infected flocks found that over 50% of flocks were positive for *Campylobacter*.

Control methods include the use of probiotics (competing microbial populations) in newly hatched chicks, chlorination or other treatment of drinking water, reduction of feed withdrawal periods prior to depopulation for slaughter, and reduction or elimination of the practice of thinning. None of these methods is entirely effective and *Campylobacter* contamination of poultry meat remains a common problem in most countries.

8.7 Assessing Broiler Chicken Welfare

Demands by consumers and retailers for evidence of ethical standards and satisfactory attention to animal welfare in food production has led to the development of farm assurance schemes and retailer assurance schemes, for which standards are set and farms regularly audited. At present these audits are based largely on assessments of resources necessary to ensure good husbandry. There is, however, an emerging trend to assess animal welfare using output measures, such as the percentage of lame birds, the prevalence and severity of foot pad dermatitis and the level of mortality for a flock, which are increasingly seen as more valid measures of welfare. A comprehensive discussion of resource and animal-based welfare assessment is presented in Weeks and Butterworth (2004). The development and implementation of methods for evaluating animal welfare on farm is discussed in more detail in Chapter 18.

8.8 Ethical Considerations, Summary and Conclusions

Since the food shortages in the West during and after the Second World War, the driver for agricultural production has been for more efficient production: more and cheaper food. More recently, there has been a greater consideration of the sustainability of systems, including food production systems, where 'development meets the needs of the present without compromising the ability of future generations to meet their own needs' (Brundtland Commission, 1987). This definition implicitly argues that the rights of future generations to have access to both raw materials and vital ecosystems should be taken into account in contemporary decision-making.

The broiler chicken industry has been conspicuously successful in achieving its primary aims, namely, a massive increase in supply of wholesome food (poultry meat) at a much lower cost to the consumer. The means to these ends have been genetic selection of birds for faster growth rate and more breast muscle, increased feed efficiency, intensification within housing systems, and control of disease through biosecurity and the development of vaccines and vaccination protocols. Intensification of production has allowed more food to be produced off less land and has made chicken meat affordable to a much wider population. However, a small, but significant, proportion of consumers in some developed countries are choosing to eat chickens produced in less intensive, free-range or organic systems. The reasons for this are complex; animal welfare is but one: However, the trend is significant and cannot be ignored by the poultry industry.

The principal problems arising from the intensification of broiler chicken production are poor bird welfare, the development of antibiotic resistance and the risk of contamination of poultry meat by food poisoning organisms. The main welfare problems occurring within intensive broiler chicken production systems are lameness, which is painful and affects the ability of birds to eat, drink and show most normal behaviour and is very likely to be painful, and contact dermatitis, attributable to poor litter and air quality in bird houses. Elite and broiler breeder birds suffer from severe hunger and pain due to feather pecking and mutilations in male birds. In addition fear, injury and distress are caused by: intensive methods of depopulation and transport; live shackling; ineffective electrical stunning, in some plants; and the use of aversive gases with long induction periods for stunning and killing, in the name of carcass quality. The use of such intensive systems, where each individual bird is worth so little in economic terms and is treated with total indifference, clearly breaks the covenant of respect for animals slaughtered for human consumption which is basic in all religions that allow the consumption of meat. This ethical concern has to be set against the undoubted success of the poultry industry in producing food that most of world wants to eat at a price most of the world can afford.

A widely accepted model of the relationship between animal welfare and productivity is the McInerney curve, and this is presented in Figure 8.6, as developed by Appleby (2005), who explains this model in the following way. The horizontal axis describes increasing animal productivity (thus benefit to humans); the vertical axis describes the quality of animal welfare. Point A defines the beginning of domestication and exploitation of farm animals by humans. Up to point B, animals and humans derive mutual benefit from their association so that point B marks maximum welfare for animals, with some benefits for humans. Maximum output of a commodity measured strictly in terms of human benefit occurs at point E, though this has incurred a cost measured in terms of bird welfare. Attempts to intensify further may become negative on both axes, e.g. through increased mortality and disease. Broiler chickens in the most intensive production systems are probably close to point D, optimal productivity but less than optimal welfare. Birds in village chicken systems that suffer from poor welfare due to disease, predation and poor nutrition might be said to be somewhere between points A and B. On ethical grounds it can be argued that the ideal compromise would occur somewhere between points C and D, or at a point where bird welfare was, at least, no worse than before the onset of domestication (point A).

While many communities in developing countries have a precarious food supply, and are regularly subject to food shortages and famine, the most serious health problems in the developed world are associated with the rapidly rising prevalence of obesity, including diabetes, stroke and cardiac disease. One of the main drivers of the

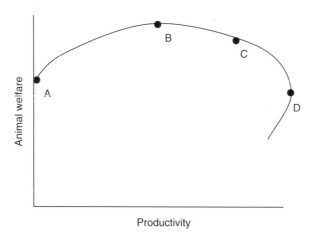

Figure 8.6 The 'McInerny Curve: a model of the relationship between animal welfare and productivity. (from Appleby 2005).

obesity epidemic is the fact that food has become cheap, and broiler production is one of the most conspicuous examples of this fact. In the affluent West, therefore, it is becoming increasingly difficult to justify the continuing emphasis on efficiency of production of broiler chicken meat, with the associated bird welfare, antibiotic resistance and food poisoning problems, in the face of the obesity epidemic. The challenge for the next 20 years is whether we can move broiler chicken production in developing countries to the right and in developed countries to the left to meet up close to point B on the McInerney curve. In this way we could both improve bird welfare globally while increasing food security in developing countries and sustainability in developed ones. When we make decisions with respect to which systems we ought to use in the production of broiler chicken, we need to consider the interests of *all* stakeholders: people in developed and developing countries, generations yet to come, and, of course, the chickens.

References and Further Reading

Appleby, M. (2005) The relationship between food prices and animal welfare. *Journal of Animal Science* 83, E9–E12.

Bruntland Commission (1987) United Nations 'Report of the World Commission on Environment and Development.' General Assembly Resolution 42/187. Available at: http://www.un.org/documents/.

Danbury, T.T., Weeks, C.A., Chambers, J.P., Waterman-Pearson, A.E. and Kestin, S.C. (1999) Self-selection of the analgesic drug carprofen by broiler chickens. *Veterinary Record* 145, 307–11.

Dawkins, M.S., Donnelly, C.A. and Jones, T.A. (2004) Chicken welfare is influenced more by housing conditions than by stocking density. *Nature* 427, 342–4.

European Food Safety Authority (2004) Welfare aspects of animal stunning and killing methods. AHAW/04-027. Available at: http://www.efsa.eu.int/EFSA/Scientific_Opinion

European Union (2007) European Union Broiler Directive (2007). Available at: http://eurlex.europa.eu/.

Farm Animal Welfare Council (1995) Report on the welfare of broiler breeders. Farm Animal Welfare Council, London. Available at: http://www.fawc.org.uk/reports/.

Food and Agriculture Organization (1998) Village chicken production system in rural Africa – household food security and gender issues. FAO Animal Production and Health Papers 142: 81 pp

Gregory, N.G. and Austin, S.D. (1992) Causes of trauma in broilers arriving dead at poultry processing plants. *Veterinary Record* 131, 501–3.

Haslam, S.M., Knowles, T.G. and Brown, S.N. (2007). Factors affecting the prevalence of foot pad dermatitis, hock burn and breast burn in broiler chicken. *British Poultry Science* 48, 264–75.

Knowles, T.G., Kestin, S.C. and Haslam, S.M. (2008) Leg disorders in broiler chickens, risk factors and prevention. *PLoS One* 3 (2), e1545.

Weeks, C.A. and Butterworth, A. (eds) (2004) *Measuring and Auditing Broiler Welfare*. CABI Publishing, Wallingford.

Goats

ALAN MOWLEM

Management and Welfare of Farm Animals: The UFAW Farm Handbook, 5th edition. John Webster
© 2011 by Universities Federation for Animal Welfare (UFAW)

9.1 Introduction

Archaeological evidence confirms that the dog and the goat were the first animals to be domesticated. Remains from sites in Jericho show that the goat was kept by humans in settlements dating back some 8,000 to 10,000 years (Zeuner, 1963). The domesticated goat (*Capra hircus*) is now found throughout the world and is only absent from areas of extreme cold near the polar regions. It almost certainly derives from the so-called Persian wild goat or bezoar (*Capra aegagrus*) found in Turkey, Iran and Western Afghanistan. The total world population of goats is estimated to be almost 500 million.

The difference between goats and sheep is often discussed. In spite of similarities between breeds of sheep and goats, hybrids do not naturally occur. Fertile matings between the species can sometimes occur, but when this happens the embryo is reabsorbed at around 15 weeks. The most obvious difference, though not visible, is that goats have 60 chromosomes, compared with 54 in sheep. Visible differences are not obvious. Usually with most breeds the tail of a goat is raised up, whereas that of a sheep hangs down. The male of both species smells, particularly in the breeding season, but the smell is quite characteristic of the species and would allow them to be identified even if they were not visible.

The most obvious difference between goats and any other farmed species is their behaviour. Goats are active and inquisitive. This can make them hard work until their habits and behaviour are understood. They seem unable to ignore anything they have not seen before and this inquisitiveness can lead to escapes from seemingly secure paddocks and buildings and the destruction of any fitting or equipment that has been fixed or left within their reach. An American author, Robert Wernick, wrote: 'Sheep are conformists: goats are unpredictable, flighty, capricious – the word comes from the Latin *capra* meaning goat. In the words of a French goat breeder, they are capricious not lunatic. "Sheep with their heads usually down, are in general quite unaware of and uninterested in the external world. If a sheep hears a low-flying plane, for example, it will become frightened and is likely to run, whereas a goat will often stand and watch. Despite their friskiness and unpredictability, goats are basically down-to-earth creatures, with a genius for making the best of any situation they may find themselves in. Centuries of co-habitation with mankind have put them in all kinds of situations: they have learned how to survive them all."

It is almost a paradox that animals of such independent spirit take so well to the relatively intensive conditions found on most goat farms in the developed world, where they may be kept in straw-bedded yards all year round. This helps to control levels of internal parasites to which they are particularly susceptible. For large herds this can also make other aspects of their management easier, as will be explained later.

9.2 Farmed Goats

Particularly in the Western world, goats are unusual in that they are the only farm species kept in large numbers as a hobby by people with no commercial aspirations. The converse of this is the subsistence farmer in a developing country who only has a few goats but who depends on them for the livelihood of himself and his family. Goats may be farmed for their milk, meat or hair. The extremes of developed milk production can be found in the UK and some other European countries. Here herds of over 1,000 milking goats may be found, and milking is usually carried out using a sophisticated and complicated rotary milking parlour. The standard of milk production and storage found in these establishments will be as good as or even better than may be seen with dairy cow production. The processing of the milk for drinking or into other dairy products may be on the farm or, more typically, at a separate dairy. This may be independent of the production business or may be managed by a group of farmers in some kind of cooperative (Mowlem, 2002).

Milk production in the developing world is usually for direct consumption by small family units. If a surplus is produced, which is quite likely if improved goats are available, some may be sold or converted into other products such as cheese if local market opportunities exist. Throughout the world more goats are kept for their meat than for milk or fibre. Most of these will be kept extensively on improved pasture or, more likely, on scrubland considered unfit for other livestock. Improved dairy production in the developed world generates many surplus kids which are usually reared for meat.

9.3 Breeds

There are more than 200 identifiable breeds of goat in the world (Porter, 1996). The principal dairy breeds in the UK originate from breeds from other countries. The Saanen and Toggenberg are from Switzerland and the British Saanen, British Toggenberg and British Alpine are derived from crossbreeding Swiss breeds. The Anglo-Nubian is the result of crossbreeding goats from the Middle and Far East with the indigenous English goat. These eastern goats were brought to the UK by ships returning from what was then the British Empire. They provided milk on the journey and when they eventually arrived in the UK there were always people keen to buy them. Two other minority UK breeds that are kept for milk are the Golden Guernsey and the Old English. Of all these dairy breeds the Saanen or Saanen type, with its impressive milk yield and relatively placid nature, is becoming the breed of choice for most large commercial dairy farms.

Although more goats are kept throughout the world for their meat than for any other product, there are very few breeds that have been developed specifically for meat production. The best-known improved meat breed is the Boer from South Africa. This impressive breed has been selectively bred to improve carcass conformation and now good males can be seen in South Africa with live-weights exceeding 200 kg. A few Boer goats are now to be found in some European countries including the UK.

There are two types of goat hair that are produced commercially. Mohair is produced by Angora goats which originate from Turkey but are now to be found in the largest numbers in South Africa, the USA, Australia and New Zealand. Some are also farmed, albeit in comparatively small numbers, in European countries including the UK. Although large numbers of goats are kept in some countries for the production of cashmere, there is not a specific cashmere breed. Cashmere is harvested, by combing, from a number of breeds that have been improved for cashmere production, notably in the People's Republic of China. Meat is essentially a secondary product from fibre-producing goats.

9.3.1 Breed improvement

In many countries and in many cultures goats have not been part of mainstream agriculture and have never received the benefit of improvement programmes enjoyed by other species. Although artificial insemination is possible it is not a technique that has been used extensively to speed up genetic improvement as has been the case with cattle. The improvement of dairy goat production is largely due to pedigree breeders whose hobby is goat breeding and improvement through competition with others. Their efforts have not been without success. The world record for milk production comes from British Saanen that produced over 3,500 litres of milk in one lactation. This compares with undeveloped indigenous breeds in the developing world that would produce a few hundred litres per lactation. Improvement schemes developed by NGOs in some countries, involving the use of indigenous goats crossed with improved European breeds, has doubled milk yields in some cases (Peacock, 1996).

Selective breeding on farms has resulted in greatly increased mohair yields from Angora goats. For example, the average yield in South Africa is about five times greater than produced by the goats imported from Turkey more than 150 years ago. Over a shorter time span the South African breeders have transformed the performance and conformation of the indigenous Boer goat for meat production.

The interest in cashmere production, particularly in the UK, has focused attention on improving the yield of fibre. The labour-intensive methods of harvesting the fibre means that commercial production in countries such as the UK would only be possible if yields could be significantly improved.

9.4 Environmental Requirements

Goats are, by and large, tolerant and adaptable to a variety of environments. Kept extensively, the one thing they cannot tolerate is prolonged rain, particularly if it is cold. In such environments some form of shelter is a minimum. As already mentioned, most dairy farms in Western countries do not allow their goats to graze. They are kept in large groups in covered yards. In these conditions a minimum floor area of $12\,m^2$ per goat should be provided. This should be increased when unfamiliar goats are put together such as when establishing a new herd. When available, straw makes a suitable bedding, and in warm dry environments slatted floors can be used. A good level of ventilation is necessary for all housed goats if respiratory problems are to be avoided. A reasonably high roof with air outlets and openings at goat level will allow air to circulate from floor level and out through the roof (Figure 9.1).

It is becoming conventional, with large numbers of milking goats, to house them in sheds with a central feed passage bordered by feed barriers through which the goats can feed on their daily forage ration. Goats seem to prefer to feed upwards, and if the floor of the feed passage between the feed barriers is at a higher level this will allow this and will also reduce contamination of the forage with faeces (Figure 9.2).

Any goat building must be constructed with due consideration for their inquisitive behaviour. They can be quite agile and therefore anything that may be damaged by them must be at least 2 metres above the ground. They will also jump onto windowsills, feed racks, ledges and in fact almost any near horizontal surface. It is also important that electrical fittings, cables water pipes and taps are all out of

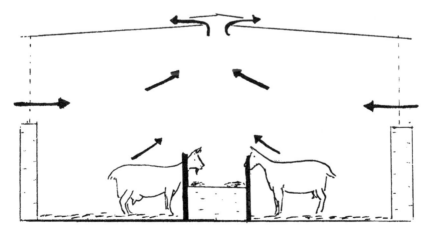

Figure 9.1 A simple naturally ventilated barn for dairy goats. Note the raised feed barrier.

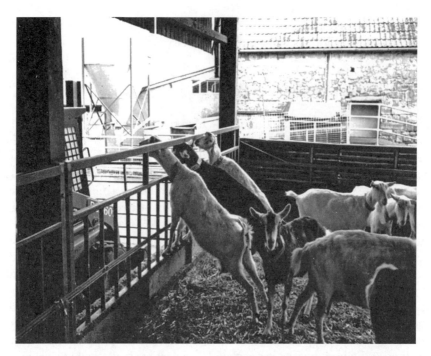

Figure 9.2 Feed barrier and restraining wall in a barn for agile, inquisitive goats.

reach. For those used to placid cows, goats can appear to be a nuisance but, if their behaviour is understood and buildings are provided that take this into account, most problems can be avoided. Goats are sociable animals and once a hierarchy has been established seem to be most content when housed together in groups. For those who just keep one pet goat, another animal will often provide sufficient companionship. Even chickens can fulfil this role. Without this, a single goat will always be calling for attention whenever it thinks anyone is about.

Non-dairy breeds are likely to be turned out to pasture as internal parasite infestations can be controlled by drenching with an anthelmintic without the problem of milk withdrawal. It will not be a great surprise to discover that fencing goats can be a problem. If sheep are turned into a fresh field or paddock they immediately start to graze. When goats are put into a fresh field they will run all round the perimeter, clambering up any available fences to reach any tasty herbage on the other side. This behaviour results in them quickly finding weaknesses in the fence and if they do they will escape. In fencing terms there is no such thing as goat-proof, but there are systems that will confine goats quite satisfactorily if well maintained. Any form of wire mesh will eventually fail but the clambering habit can be discouraged if an offset or hotwire is fixed. This is an electrified wire fixed just below the top of the wire mesh by supports that hold it 15 to 30 cm from the fence. Much the same result can be achieved if the offset is fixed at the bottom of the fence (Mowlem, 2001). Electrified high-tensile wire fences are effective but it is necessary to have at least five wires to prevent the goats escaping. Unlike sheep they learn very quickly if the electric fence unit is not working and, when they do, they will escape. It is thus very important that any electrified system is checked regularly.

Tethering is sometimes used as a simple alternative to fences. It should be considered only as a last resort. While undoubtedly it saves a lot of elaborate and expensive fencing there are many potential problems. As has already been described, goats are very active animals and there is a real risk of them becoming entangled in the tether. There have been cases when this has been fatal. If a tether is the only option then it should be made of lightweight chain rather than rope. There should be a swivel at either end and one in the middle. There should be no nearby bushes or trees on which the chain could be caught. The goat will need access to a shelter and care must be taken to ensure it cannot become caught on any part of it. In addition to the problems of being caught up, a goat on a tether will be vulnerable to dog worrying, vandalism and bad weather. All this suggests that the goat must be tethered where it can be checked a minimum of twice a day.

9.5 Nutrition and Feeding Systems

Goats are ruminants and as such have much in common with sheep and cattle. However, their choice of feedstuffs and their feeding behaviour is different to these two species. Goats are browsers and generally feed at a higher level from the ground than sheep. They prefer shrubs, tree leaves and woody material. Much of this is regarded as weeds and thus they can be useful in improving rough grazing. In sown pastures they eat grass-inhibiting weeds and do not eat much clover and thus they can be very beneficial when grazed before or with sheep. In terms of nutrient requirements the dairy goat is very similar to the dairy cow and the requirement for energy to produce a litre of milk from a given weight of animal is virtually the same for the two species (Agricultural and Food Research Council, 1998). The actual values for a dairy goat's energy needs are shown in Table 9.1.

The figures shown in Table 9.1 are only a guide because various factors will affect the requirement for energy. If a goat is outside grazing it will need more energy than a housed goat that has its food brought to it. Milk quality also influences the energy needs; goats producing particularly rich milk with a high fat content will require a higher energy intake.

When free to graze, goats are quite selective and seem to pick out preferred plants which are often the most nutritious in terms of protein and trace element content. Metabolic problems are rare in goats that have free access to natural grazing and browse material. This ability to select can be used in an intensive farming system. It has been shown that goats fed poor-quality forage at amounts equivalent to 50% more than appetite do better than sheep in similar conditions. It is interesting to note that when maize silage is fed to dairy goats the make-up of the silage changes as the day progresses. They initially select the parts of the maize they prefer and will only eat

Table 9.1 Daily energy requirements for dairy goats.

Maintenance 0.5 MJ ME/kg of metabolic bodyweight ($kg^{0.75}$)
Pregnancy 0.5 MJ ME/$kg^{0.75}$ rising to 0.7 MJ ME/kg $^{0.75}$ for the last month
Lactation maintenance needs +5 MJ ME per kg of milk produced

all of it if they are not offered any more silage or other material. Goat farmers who keep cattle may feed the silage refusals collected from the goats in the afternoon to their cattle and will then give the goats some fresh silage. Apart from this helping towards the quality of the goats' intake of nutrients the new silage will encourage them to eat more, thus increasing their dry matter intake (DMI). The greater the DMI the greater the potential for maximizing performance in terms of milk yield.

Dairy goat farmers, like their cattle counterparts, have the same aim, i.e. to feed their goats enough nutrients for them to be able to perform to their full genetic potential. It is not possible to achieve this with forage alone. High-yielding dairy goats will be fed up to 2 kg/day of concentrate feed containing about 18% protein. Daily feed intake, best described according to DMI, will be between 3.5% and 5% of their live-weight. Breeders of high-yielding pedigree goats sometimes achieve DMIs of around 7% live-weight/day by feeding their goats often throughout the day and by introducing different feeds. While this level of feeding would not be realistic in a farming situation, the achievements of these breeders does show what the genetic potential of goats can be.

The principles for increasing or optimizing production are the same for goats in any environment. Even in poorer countries much can be done by selecting the best goats and then doing all that is realistically possible to increase their intake of nutrients. This may create a slight conflict of considerations with some fibre-producing goats. These also need a reasonably high plane of nutrition if they are to perform well. However, particularly with Angora goats, there is some evidence to suggest that if the quality of their feed is too good the fibre will be coarser and thus less valuable. It should be borne in mind that the return from these animals is dependent on the weight of mohair produced as well as the quality, and thus the right balance must be achieved if they are to be profitable. The level of nutrition and feeding is not only related to productivity. For goats to remain healthy a good supply of all essential nutrients is necessary. Water must be available at all times. Dairy goats in particular must have a good supply if they are to be able to maintain a high milk yield. They need to drink about 1.5 litres of water per day for each litre of milk produced.

9.6 Reproduction and Breeding

Goats are seasonally polyoestrous, with females coming into heat or oestrus at regular intervals during the breeding season which, in the northern hemisphere, extends from about August to February. However, it is not safe to assume that females will not exhibit oestrus or conceive at other times of the year. Males are generally capable of breeding throughout the year but libido and sperm production are likely to be poorer during the summer months. Female kids become sexually mature and show oestrus for the first time at about 6 months of age. Male kids are usually reported to be sexually mature at 6 months but in fact fertile matings can occur as early as 3 months of age. Therefore if entire kids are kept it is important to separate them before unplanned matings occur. Hobbyist goat breeders often do not mate their young females until they are 18 months of age. Most commercial farmers would consider this wasteful and would normally expect to mate their goats when they have reached about 75% of their expected mature bodyweight. In practice this means spring-born kids that have grown well should be fit for mating by the end of the year in which they were born.

The length of the oestrous cycle is about 21 days and oestrus generally lasts for 2 to 3 days. Sometimes, particularly with females kept separately from others, oestrous activity may be delayed. The smell of a male may often stimulate the onset of oestrous cycling. If a male is not available a rag that has been rubbed over a male may have the same effect. Oestrus is readily detected by a range of behavioural changes including bleating, tail wagging, and staring in the direction of a male if there is one nearby. Often the vulva may be swollen and reddened. Where males are run with a herd of females one male can be expected to serve at least 40 females. However, it is common practice on large dairy farms to run one male with groups of several hundred females and he would be expected to mate with most of them over a period of 2 to 3 months. If he seemed to be working particularly hard and losing condition he would be rested while another male was used.

Artificial insemination can be used with goats (Mowlem, 1983). Goat semen freezes as well as cattle semen although the processing method is more difficult. The technique used to inseminate goats is more or less the same as that used with sheep. It is important to hold the female goat in a head-down, rump-up position. This is achieved by the handler straddling the goat's neck and then lifting her by her folded-back legs to present her rear to the inseminating technician (Figure 9.3). A duck-billed speculum, equipped with a light probe, is used to look into the vagina to locate the cervix. The appearance of the cervix indicates at what stage of oestrus the goat is, and this plus all the other behavioural sign helps to ensure the goat is inseminated at the correct time. The semen is deposited into and sometimes through the cervix. An experienced inseminator would expect to achieve a 60 to 70% conception rate for the first insemination.

Gestation lasts 146 to 156 days with an average of 150 days. Most females are bred annually although it is possible to achieve two kiddings per year. Dairy goats can have a prolonged lactation lasting 18 months and may be mated only once in two years. Some will even lactate without kidding and are referred to as maiden milkers. The number of kids produced varies with age and breed. Generally unimproved goats such as ferals average only one kid whereas most improved dairy goats average more than two, with twins and triplets being the norm.

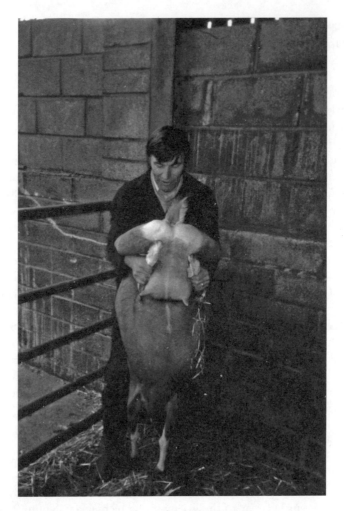

Figure 9.3 Restraining a nanny goat for artificial insemination.

Pseudo-pregnancy, false pregnancy or 'cloudburst', in which the female shows all the external and behavioural signs of pregnancy, without actually being so, can occur. This condition may last for the full term or longer and will end in a large release of fluid but no kid. Sometimes lactation will follow or sometimes it will be delayed with the goat coming into milk some months after the pseudo-pregnancy has ended. Ultrasonic scanning can be used to detect pregnancy and it should be possible to determine the number of kids or whether it is a false pregnancy.

9.6.1 Management of breeding males

Considering their importance, male goats often do not get the same level of care as breeding females. They have a very strong smell, especially during the breeding season, which means they tend to be kept away from, and out of sight of, the other goats. Even though they are rarely aggressive they will be much more amenable if they can be kept as part of, and with, the rest of the herd. They can work very hard for several months during the mating season and they often seem to lose interest in food. It is therefore important that they are allowed to improve their body condition by increasing their food ration before the start of the breeding season. The other aspect of male care that justifies special attention is housing. They require a dry, airy shed with adequate room for them to move around and it must be strongly constructed as they can sometimes be destructive for no obvious reason. This is also the case with fittings and fitments. The males can be just as inquisitive as the females but they are of course much stronger and when standing up on their hind legs can reach further.

9.6.2 Management of breeding females

Females in dairy herds should be so well cared for, to optimize milk production, that they are unlikely to need any special care for breeding. One possible problem may be a tendency towards fatness. When goats do get fat, most is deposited in the abdomen rather than subcutaneously or intramuscularly. For breeding females this may affect fertility and may cause problems at parturition. It is unlikely that a healthy farmed goat would ever be undernourished to a level that would affect its breeding performance.

Many European dairy farmers will be interested in controlling the breeding season in order to stimulate their goats into breeding all the year round to eliminate the problems of seasonal milk production. The two methods used most in a practical farm environment are intravaginal hormonal sponges or artificial lighting regimes. The sponge method involves implanting a sponge impregnated with the hormone progesterone, into the vagina, which remains in place for 11 days. Two days before it is withdrawn the goat is injected with pregnant mares' serum gonadotrophin (PMSG) and prostaglandin. The PMSG is a convenient source of follicle-stimulating hormone (FSH) and luteinizing hormone and the prostaglandin is given to cause regression of any corpus luteum that may be present, thus removing any source of endogenous progesterone. The goats will usually come into oestrus within 1 to 2 days of sponge removal. If artificial insemination is used, the goats will be inseminated 42 to 44 hours after sponge removal.

In temperate countries, such as the UK, the decreasing daylight and increasing dark period after the midsummer day triggers breeding activity in goats. The lengthening nights cause the release of the hormone melatonin which in turn triggers the release of the hormones which stimulate the ovaries to produce a follicle from which an ovum will be released. The onset of this sequence of events gives rise to oestrous behaviour, or heat, in the goat and the whole cycle of events is called the oestrous cycle. It is possible to mimic this effect by subjecting the goats to prolonged periods of light during the winter and then reverting to periods of increased darkness. Ashbrook (1982) has recommended an extended light regime, in which goats are exposed to 20 hours of light for 60 consecutive days during the period January to March. Oestrus will occur approximately 10 weeks after the return to ambient lighting. Melatonin implants are also used, in some cases in conjunction with an extended light regime. Such methods of controlling the breeding season are only really possible with housed goats and therefore are used mainly with dairy animals in which, as it happens, the need for all-year-round breeding is greatest.

9.6.3 Mating
Most goats are mated naturally, although artificial insemination is possible and in some of the major European goat farming countries is becoming more widely used. Where small numbers are kept, it is not always appropriate for the goat-keeper or farmer to keep a male. In these cases a female will be taken to the nearest male, of the correct type, when oestrous behaviour is observed. On large farms several males will be kept and one may be run with a large group. A male can successfully mate more than 100 females over a period of 2 to 3 months. If concentrated mating is required the male may be changed weekly. Sheep raddle harnesses may be used to time matings, although there have been instances of the female goats chewing the crayon to complete destruction! Regular ultrasonic scanning is often used in large herds to check on state and stage of pregnancy. Goat breeders with small numbers of goats may wish to take a female to a male some distance away. Unfortunately, the journey could well be a factor in the female not being in what is called standing heat when presented to the male, or it may simply be a case of the wrong time where the owner has not recognized the signs of heat or oestrus.

Artificial insemination, using either fresh or frozen semen, presents opportunities for extending the use of superior males. There are other advantages to artificial insemination even though it is not used widely in a number of countries. It reduces the risk of infection because it does not involve direct contact between the male and female goat. When goats are kept in small numbers it is hard to justify keeping a stud male, given all the problems associated with them, such as their strong smell and their superior strength. With small numbers there is always the problem of inbreeding, i.e. a male mating his own daughters. In some countries breeding groups have been set up where a high-quality male is shared by a number of goat-keepers, often by bringing their goats to him. There is also the possibility of semen being collected and diluted and used fresh. If kept cool this should allow use within 24 hours of collection and would be useful where it is difficult to move females to the male.

9.6.4 Feeding pregnant females
Whatever the goats are being farmed for, they will need good input of nutrients if they are to be fit for pregnancy and parturition. If they are dairy goats they will require feed to support milk production which will probably continue for the first 3 months of gestation. Whatever the type of goat, it is generally recommended that the energy and protein intake should be increased during the last month of gestation. Also goats that are encouraged to eat a high level of forage during gestation will be conditioned

for a high forage intake during lactation as this will benefit milk yield and quality. Conversely goats with a poor forage intake during gestation will have a lower intake during lactation even if the quantity and quality of the forage is increased. As a rough guide, an average dairy goat of around 65 kg live-weight should be offered a good-quality forage *ad libitum*, and, 2 months before parturition, 250 g of a dairy concentrate feed per day which should be increased to 450 g per day 1 month before parturition is due. Goats that are not kept for milk production will not require such a high plane of nutrition but they will require more than just forage in late gestation and early lactation. Goats require access to drinking water at all times but it is particularly important that they have a good clean supply during gestation and at parturition.

9.6.5 Housing pregnant females

It must be remembered that the abdomen of pregnant goats can become very large as multiple kids are quite common. Also the udder on a high-yielding female can become very swollen and sometimes pendulous to a point where it may drag on the ground (Figure 9.4). Goats in this condition require an unchallenging environment in which there is no risk of injury. All projections on which they could become caught must be removed or made safe. Goats with horns should not be housed with hornless ones. Even if they do not cause any injuries they will certainly dominate any feed racks or troughs, thus depriving some of their correct feed intake.

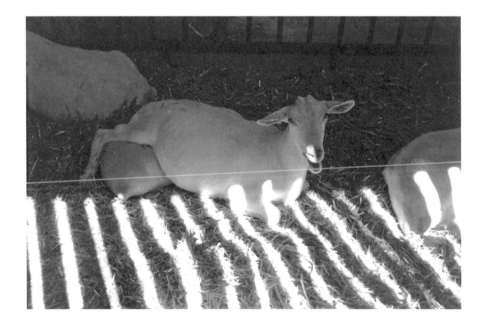

Figure 9.4 A nanny goat with a pendulous udder. These animals require special attention to housing and bedding.

9.6.6 Parturition and suckling

The ideal environment for a goat about to give birth is a separate, freshly bedded pen, possibly constructed at the end of the pen in which the rest of the herd is housed. This is not always possible and a compromise is to house those goats that are close to parturition together, separate from the main herd. The reasons for housing the goats in separate pens is to ensure the mother-to-kid bond is well established and to make sure the kid gets a good chance to suck its mother's udder. It is most important that newborn kids feed from their mother within a few hours of parturition.

When a female is close to parturition she will become restless, sometimes scratching the ground, and will usually stand away from the rest of the group. A sure sign that parturition is imminent is discharge from the vagina as the foetal sac ruptures. If the goat appears to be straining for several hours without any obvious progress it is best to call the veterinarian or someone else experienced with kidding or lambing. The first sign of a correct presentation is the appearance of front feet followed by a nose. If these can be seen, the goat should be able to kid without assistance. If one or, at worst, two feet are pointing back and/or the head is back, manual assistance will probably be required but it should be remembered that any interference does present some risk. If there is any chance the female will kid by herself she should be left to do so. Once the kid or kids have been born it is important that the mother has the opportunity to lick them. This stimulates the kids, strengthens the mother–offspring bond and the mother will normally dry and clean the kids very effectively. Goats with very pendulous udders will have difficulty feeding their kids but if the kid can be helped to feed for the first 24 h there is a good chance they will be strong enough to seek out and suck from even the most awkward teats. In all cases it is most important that the kids are fed on colostrum for at least the first 24 hours after birth. If the mother cannot do this then feeding the kid with a stomach tube may be the only option. These are available, often under the generic name of 'lamb reviver'. These are graduated plastic bottles of about 250 mL capacity with a small rubber stomach tube attached to a spout on the lid. With care, warm colostrum can be fed directly into the kid's stomach. This is a most effective way of reviving weak kids. Often a kid can be transformed from being too weak to stand to one that is running around looking for its next feed, after a single feed of warm colostrum.

9.6.7 Kid rearing

Kids from dairy herds will be artificially reared so that the milk can be sold. Those from meat- or fibre-producing herds are more likely to be reared naturally by their mothers. Milk replacers formulated for calves are quite suitable for kid rearing. This is not surprising as the gross composition of goat milk is very similar to cow milk. Table 9.2 shows a regime for feeding milk replacer to kids for either 6 or 8 weeks and Table 9.3 shows an alternative regime for restricted quantities of milk replacer. Some goat-keepers rear their kids on sheep milk replacer. The high fat level in this replacer makes it an expensive and unnecessary luxury. The kids will grow well on such a product but it will not be a cost-effective method. The most cost-effective method

Table 9.2 Feeding regime for artificial rearing of goat kids. (Figures in parenthesis show ages for a later weaning system.)

Age	Milk feeds
Weeks 1–4 (1–6)	Supplied *ad libitum*
Weeks 5–7 (7)	Half amount consumed end of week 4 (6)
Week 6 (8)	Half amount consumed end of week 5 (7)

uses a calf milk replacer which may be given initially *ad libitum* although a rationed system may be preferred and will certainly cost less (Mowlem, 1984).

Kids do not grow as well as comparable lambs when kept out on pasture. This is probably due to heavy endoparasite infestations and also to kids' behaviour. Young lambs seem intent on feeding and growing. Goat kids seem more intent on having a good time and spend a lot of time playing and investigating their environment. When doing this they are not only using up more energy but also eating less.

Kids reared for the more intensive dairy systems should be disbudded within a few weeks of birth. The longer the horn buds are left, the more difficult disbudding will become. With goats this is a veterinary procedure. It is virtually impossible to anaesthetize the horn buds using a local anaesthetic and general anaesthesia is therefore necessary. It is particularly difficult to completely disbud entire male kids and most of these will have some horn or scurs when they reach maturity (Buttle *et al.*, 1986). The main disadvantages of horns are the difficulty they present for goats going through a milking parlour and the injuries they can inflict on each other and their handlers. These will not be a problem where goats are kept extensively and go out to graze, and therefore it is unlikely the farmer will consider it necessary to go to the expense of having kids disbudded.

There are a number of ways of dispensing the milk feed. If relatively small numbers of kids are to be fed then bottles with teats placed in a rack are a labour-saving alternative to holding bottles while the kids feed. For large numbers of kids, as may be the case on large dairy farms, an automatic calf-feeding machine may be used. A more simple system is to use containers with a number of teats attached which allow several kids to feed at one time (these are often given the generic name of 'lamb-bar'). Open troughs can be used but they are best placed outside the pen with the kids

Table 9.3 A regime for feeding a rationed amount of milk replacer.

Weeks	Milk quantity	Number of feeds per day
1–7	1 litre/day	2
8	0.5 litres/day	1
9	No milk	

putting their heads through a hole or slot to gain access to the milk. This prevents the kids climbing into the trough and fouling the milk.

9.6.8 Housing kids

Kids are very adept at finding their way out of pens, and therefore solid partitions are preferable with sides about 1.2 m high. Approximately 0.5 m^2 of floor space should be provided per kid up to 2 months of age, increasing to 1.5 m^2 at 6 months of age. Care should be taken to ensure that there are no projections in the pens, or gaps where feet or legs may be trapped. Hay nets are not recommended because the kids will jump onto them and some will inevitably get their legs caught in the mesh.

Infection is likely to spread through groups of intensively reared kids and it is therefore important to maintain a high standard of hygiene and husbandry. Kids should be checked for signs of ill health and appropriate action should be taken if disease or infection is suspected.

9.7 Milk Production

9.7.1 Milking systems

The choice of milking system depends largely on the scale of the enterprise and the environment in which the goats are kept. A complicated, highly mechanized system would not be appropriate in countries where, for example, a reliable electricity source or the infrastructure for servicing milking machinery was not available. In this situation hand milking would be the only practical method. If milking by machine is an option then the choice of system ranges from a simple, small-scale and, usually, portable bucket unit to large sophisticated rotary or static milking parlours (Figure 9.5). The principles of machine milking goats are the same as for cows. Apart from the difference in size and the fact that goats have only two teats, much of the equipment is the same or similar.

The vacuum level is set lower for goats than for cows and the pulsation is faster (Table 9.4). As with other aspects of goat husbandry the goats' speed of movement and ability to learn means they quickly adapt to new and relatively complicated milking systems. With practice one person could milk about 150 goats per hour in a well-designed static milking parlour, whereas one person could milk about 400 goats per hour with a rotary parlour. Although the latter is expensive it is the only layout that can cope with really large numbers that may now be seen on dairy goat farms in a number of European countries. The fact that, with machine milking, the milk travels through a closed pipe system means that there is less chance for it to be spoilt or contaminated if good hygiene is observed. It is advisable, immediately before milking, to wash goats' udders with an approved disinfectant and then dry each using a disposable paper towel. A poor washing routine such as washing with plain water and using the same cloth to dry more than one udder is likely to cause more problems than no washing at all. In Europe, legislation is in place to regulate the

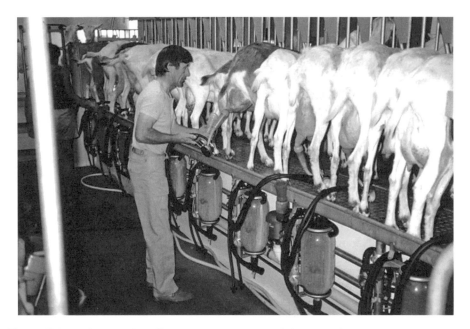

Figure 9.5 A large-scale milking unit on a commercial dairy goat farm.

standard of goat milk production. In the UK, goat milk production is regulated by the Dairy Products (Hygiene) Regulations 1995.

Goats are clean animals and their milk should have a very low total bacteria count (TBC), which means even after storage in a refrigerated bulk tank for several days it is still likely to have a lower TBC than relatively fresh cow milk.

For milk production in less controlled environments, as may be found in a tropical country, little can be done to reduce contamination of the milk. It is likely in these circumstances that the goats will be hand milked and if so this should be carried out on a clean surface on which the goat will stand. This may be, for example, concrete, a smooth rock or a wooden platform. Care should be taken to remove any visible dirt or faeces from the udder so that it will not drop into the milking vessel. If water is available, udders should be washed with a sanitizing solution. Clean cloths or paper towel should be used to dry the udder. If udders are not dried there is a very good chance that along with the first drop of milk will be a drip of washing solution containing all the contaminants that were on the surface of the udder. Mastitis seems to be much less of a problem with goats than with cows in a comparable environment.

Table 9.4 Mechanical settings for goat milking machines.

Vacuum	Pulsation rate	Pulsation ratio
37 kPa	70–90/min	50 : 50

9.7.2 Handling goat milk

The most important aspect of handling goat milk is keeping it as cool as possible immediately after milking. There are several reasons for doing this: for example, contaminating micro-organisms will work much more slowly if the milk is cooled and therefore the time the milk can be kept will be extended. In good hygienic on-farm dairies, where the milk will be stored in a refrigerated bulk tank with a temperature of 4 °C, it will remain in good usable condition for at least 4 days. When refrigeration is not available, standing the container of milk in cold water will be of some advantage. If the milk is not cooled immediately after milking, lipolytic enzymes break down the fat and fatty acids will be released. Two of these in goat milk, caproic and caprilic acid, will give the milk an unpleasant flavour which will taint any products made from it. This lipolysis can also be the result of too much agitation of the milk when the fatty acids will be released as a result of mechanical action. This may happen if the milk travels through a complicated pipe system, particularly if moved by centrifugal pumps. If goat milk is handled carefully and cooled quickly after milking it is difficult to differentiate it from cow milk by taste alone.

9.8 Fibre Production

Goats produce two types of hair. The primary hair follicles produce relatively coarse hairs which make up the main outer coat of most goats. Secondary follicles produce much finer hairs which usually grow as an undercoat beneath the outer hairs. This soft underhair is used commercially in the textile industry and is called cashmere. The Angora goat has evolved to produce its main coat from secondary follicles which, in the case of this breed, is soft and lustrous and any primary hairs in the fleece are regarded as a contaminant and are called kemp. The hair produced by Angora goats is called mohair. Mohair grows at about 2.5 cm a month and the ideal processing length is 12 to 14.5 cm. To achieve this, farmers shear their goats twice a year, ideally just before mating and before kidding. Good-quality Angoras may produce 10 kg of mohair per year, the most valuable being the very fine fleece produced by young goats. In the UK, farmers may add value to their mohair by processing it into fashion garments or they may sell it raw and in bulk to the processing mills, mainly in Yorkshire, which traditionally have been a world centre for processing animal fibres for hundreds of years. Mohair has many qualities that make it a valuable natural fibre. It is lustrous, hard-wearing and accepts and retains dyes, and when used for garments such as suits or skirts is extremely comfortable to wear. Its hard-wearing and non-fading qualities make it suitable for furnishing fabrics.

Cashmere is an insulating layer of fine hair that grows under the main outer coat of a number of types and breeds of goat. There is not a cashmere breed but there are a number of types that are bred specifically for cashmere production. The main cashmere-producing countries are the People's Republic of China, the Mongolian People's Republic, Tibet and parts of Northern India. In these countries the fibre is harvested by hand combing the goats when they are close to moulting and also by collecting the hair after moulting. A maximum of about 250 g per annum would be produced by a good goat.

As with mohair, the United Kingdom is a major importing and processing country which has generated an interest in home production. Feral goats from some of the more mountainous regions have been selected for this purpose and these have been crossed with improved cashmere-producing goats from other countries. Relatively poor yields and the costly labour-intensive harvesting methods have so far prevented profitable production in the UK, but small numbers of producers have been successful with small-scale added-value enterprises. Profitable fibre production is more likely if it can be underpinned by a good market for the meat. This is by no means the case throughout the UK.

9.9 Meat Production

Throughout the world more goats are kept for their meat than for any other product. However, there are very few developed meat breeds. One of the few breeds to have been improved for meat production is the Boer from South Africa. These have been selectively bred for carcass conformation and now some males have been produced with live-weights of well over 200 kg.

In some countries such as the UK cultural prejudices have been difficult to overcome to create a market for goat meat. In many other countries, however, the lean nature of the meat coupled with its unique flavour has pushed it to the top of the meat market. For meat production to be profitable, low-cost rearing systems are necessary which generally means kids are left to be reared by their mothers. In countries such as the UK it is difficult to achieve prices for the meat that will cover the cost of the artificial rearing of surplus dairy kids. As most developed breeds average at least two kids per year the large dairy herds that now exist generate large numbers of surplus kids which cannot be reared profitably, with the exception of the relatively small numbers reared for herd replacement.

Large numbers of surplus kids raise the question of euthanasia. Various methods are used and it is an aspect of goat farming that is under discussion. A light-weight captive-bolt humane killer or an overdose of barbiturates would be the preferred method at present although the latter may be considered too expensive for large numbers and of course would render the meat inedible.

9.10 General Care and Handling

In general the care of goats is similar to that of other farmed ruminants. Their independent and inquisitive nature, however, is different from other livestock and it is only after much experience that the understanding necessary for successful management is acquired. Anyone contemplating starting a goat enterprise, however small, is advised to visit other farms and even to arrange for a few weeks' working experience to help understand what is required to farm them successfully.

9.10.1 Handling and restraint

Most dairy goats will have been artificially reared and therefore will have grown up used to a lot of human contact. This means they will be confident and inquisitive and will generally crowd round their handler, seeking attention or, if on offer, food! This friendly behaviour makes them easy to catch and restrain because by and large they seem to enjoy it. However, they are intelligent and if they feel threatened they will become suspicious and uncooperative and will be difficult to catch. Once caught, they can be restrained by being gently but firmly held around the neck, just behind the ears. This is easier if the goat has a collar and if they need to be moved they will usually walk on a lead. If a procedure such as an injection is necessary the goat can be tied to a gate or hurdle by way of its collar. If another person is available it can be gently but firmly held.

Unlike sheep, groups of dairy goats are not easy to drive and are more easily moved by being led, particularly if the person in front is carrying a bag or bucket of food. It is advisable to have a second person walking behind the group to move along those stopping to investigate points of interest. Goats that have been used to a fair degree of freedom and little human contact, such as ferals, are a much more difficult proposition. They will be faster and more agile than sheep and will jump out of most sheep-handling systems, which therefore need to be higher and with no surfaces on to which the goats can jump. They do not usually respect a trained dog and in fact will often face up to a dog, which may create a difficult situation for both goat and dog. A little time spent on training goats to recognize a bag or bucket of food will be time well spent. Once kept in more confined conditions, they will settle down and kids that are hand reared will be as tractable as dairy goats.

9.10.2 Routine procedures

Goats, like sheep, need their hooves to be regularly trimmed. They do not seem to suffer from foot rot nearly as much as sheep but occasional chronic infection may occur, with some animals not responding to treatment. Overgrown hooves can be the cause of severe lameness. Ideally they should be trimmed three or four time a year unless, as in some countries, they are constantly out on hard dry ground. It is important to make sure the feet of heavily pregnant goats do not need trimming.

With the exception of Angora goats, foot trimming is carried out with the goat in a standing position tethered to a convenient fence or hurdle. With their thick fleece and rounder conformation Angoras can be cast and all four feet trimmed with the goat restrained between the handler's legs. Handling crates, in which a goat can be restrained and raised up on its side, are available for foot trimming and these can speed up the procedure and reduce back strain for the operator.

Male kids to be kept for reasons other than breeding should be castrated, and the simplest way is to use the rubber rings available for castrating lambs. This procedure must be carried out within 1 week of birth. The problems of disbudding have been mentioned earlier in the chapter (section 9.6.7) but it is perhaps appropriate to reiterate that the earlier this is carried out the easier it is. De-horning mature goats is a difficult and unpleasant procedure that is very traumatic for the goat and should only be carried out as a last resort.

In the UK it is now a requirement by law that goats are tagged for identification in both ears. The tags need to identify the animal by number and they must show the herd number and an identification code to show the farm of origin. Pedigree goats registered with a breed society are normally tattooed and it is possible this may eliminate the need for tags as long as the correct information can be seen. A number of marking systems are available for the farmer to identify individual goats. Numbered collars are useful and have the added advantage of being something to hold on to when restraining or leading goats. Leg bands are available for identifying goats from the rear, which is useful in many types of milking parlour.

Oral drenching of goats is the same as for sheep and the same equipment can be used. Vaccinations are relatively straightforward because of the very small subcutaneous fat deposits on a goat. The jugular vein is particularly easy to locate compared with a sheep. It is, however, quite difficult to find in very young kids.

Goats are able to reach almost all parts of their body with their mouths and it is difficult to apply dressings in such a way that they will not be pulled off. The only way this can be avoided is to restrain the goat so that it cannot turn round. This can be achieved by short tying the goat using a halter or by confining it in a narrow pen which restricts movement.

9.10.3 Transport

If goats have to be moved long distances a suitable vehicle should be used. Goats generally travel well, being able to maintain their balance easily, provided they do not slip on the floor. The ideal floor covering for a truck or van is a rubber mat covered with a thin layer of straw. Space should be adequate but not excessive, otherwise they may fall when the vehicle turns or brakes sharply. In the interest of safety a partition should separate the driver from the area occupied by the goats.

9.11 Health and Disease

The maintenance of a healthy herd in any environment demands a high standard of stockmanship and the ability to recognize diseases and disorders in the early stages so that proper attention and treatment can be given promptly.

9.11.1 Parasites

Whatever environment the goats are in, internal parasites will be a major issue. Goats are particularly susceptible to intestinal parasites (generically called worms). They do not build up the same level of resistance as sheep and, although they may not show obvious signs of infestation, if uncontrolled it is likely that production performance will be considerably reduced. One possible explanation for the different suscepti- bility of sheep and goats is that sheep graze close to the ground whereas goats feed on shrubs and tree leaves (browse). These different feeding habits mean that sheep have always ingested worm larvae whereas goats have not. This has possibly resulted in sheep evolving with a greater resistance or tolerance. This problem of high worm burdens is the main reason why dairy goats in many countries are permanently housed. If they do not graze they will not ingest worm larvae and therefore with suitable medication can be cleared of internal parasites. It has been estimated that heavy worm infestations can reduce milk yield by as much as 18% (Lloyd, 1982).

Parasite infestations can be controlled by regular oral drenching with an anthel- mintic, in severe cases as often as every 3 weeks, but this will mean milk withdrawal for up to 3 days each time and therefore will not be used in large dairy herds. This is not a problem with goats kept for meat or fibre and consequently these goats will be turned out to graze during spring through to autumn in the northern hemisphere and anthelmintics will be used to reduce the worm burden. Parasite resistance is an increasing problem and it is vital that the correct dose of anthelmintic is given; it is recommended to change the drug on a rotational basis.

Goats, like most animals, can be infested with external parasites. Lice are common; goats can also be infested with various types of mange mites. The ivermectin group of drugs are effective against both ecto- and endoparasites but, again, there will be the problem of milk withdrawal in dairy herds. It should be noted that in the UK very few veterinary products are licensed for use with goats. If unlicensed products are used it is a statutory requirement that milk should be withdrawn from sale for human consumption for 21 days.

9.11.2 Bacterial and viral diseases

The *Clostridium* bacteria are a group which thrive in anaerobic conditions. They produce very powerful toxins and are well-known for the diseases they cause which include tetanus, botulism and gangrene. In ruminants, specific types exist in the gut and normally do not cause problems. However, if conditions are favourable they multiply and the toxin they produce will be fatal. The clostridial diseases most commonly seen in goats, caused by *Clostridium perfrigens* type D, are enterotox- aemia in adults and pulpy kidney disease in kids. These are most usually seen after an abrupt change in diet which often results in a period of incomplete digestion and when conditions in the gut encourage the bacteria to multiply. Goats would be particularly at risk when turned out to grass after being housed through the winter months. It is possible to vaccinate goats to protect them from these diseases. Many vaccines are available which give immunity to a wide range of *Clostridium* species but it is recommended that those that are most effective are those that protect against the specific types that affect goats. Adult goats should be vaccinated twice a year, not once yearly as with sheep, and if one vaccination takes place during late pregnancy some immunity will be passed to the kids. Kids from vaccinated mothers should be vaccinated at 8 weeks of age and those from unvaccinated mothers at 3 to 4 weeks of age. In both cases they should receive a booster vaccination 4 to 6 weeks later.

9.11.2.1 Johne's disease

Johne's disease, otherwise known as paratuberculosis, is caused by the bacterium *Mycobacterium avium* ssp. *paratuberculosis* and can be a problem in all ruminants. In goats, clinical disease seems to be seen more in large commercial herds and is thought to be initiated by low levels of stress. Typical signs are a short period of diarrhoea followed by a rapid loss of condition and, in the case of dairy animals, loss of milk. There is no cure or treatment and, if left, the infected goats will usually die 2 to 3 months after the first clinical signs. To control the disease it is necessary to eliminate all those animals showing signs and to vaccinate all kids within 1 month of birth. It is possible to test for the organism in blood and faeces and a skin test is also possible. None are 100% reliable as false-negatives can occur with all three tests. However, if all are positive, it is highly likely that the mycobacterium is present.

9.11.2.2 Caprine arthritis and encephalitis

Another disease that has become economically important is caprine arthritis and encephalitis (CAE). This disease is cased by a lentivirus closely related to the one which causes Maedi-visna in sheep. The signs of the disease are varied, with adult goats usually showing signs of arthritis with inflamed and swollen knee joints which will make walking painful. There will be loss of condition with extreme cases becoming emaciated and very weak. There is no cure and, if a high incidence is to be avoided, it is important to test goats regularly and to cull any positive reactors. In some European countries, the USA and Australia around 80% of goats tested are reactors. In the UK an effective testing and culling scheme has resulted in an incidence of around 2%.

9.11.2.3 Mastitis

The prevention and treatment of mastitis is a major issue with dairy cow farmers. The importance of this disease has generated a lot of good advice, and a wide array of treatment and preventive drugs are available for the dairy cattle industry. As mentioned earlier (section 9.11.1) there is a problem with so few drugs licensed for use with goats, and if unlicensed products are used farmers in the UK are faced with a 21-day milk withdrawal period. However, mastitis is much less of a problem with goats. One factor may be the fact that a goat's udder is rarely dirty and because of their dry faeces the milking parlour is much less dirty and wet than would be the case with cows. If sensible precautions are taken, such as teat dipping with an approved bactericidal dip and if a clean environment for milking can be created, mastitis should not be a problem. It is worth noting that goat's milk contains a high level of cellular debris that may have nothing to do with infection. It has been shown that 65% of goat milk samples will have a somatic cell count greater than 10^6 cells/mL. In the case of cow's milk this would be indicative of mastitis. To get a more accurate picture it is necessary to do a much more specific differential cell count.

9.11.2.4 Listeriosis

A disease that is becoming more prevalent, particularly on large dairy farms, is listeriosis. It is caused by the soil-borne bacterium, *Listeria monocytogenes*, which can occur almost anywhere. The main reason for its increase in larger dairy herds is because of the increased feeding of silage. It has been alleged that *Listeria* bacteria are not able to survive when the pH is below 4, yet the disease can occur in goats fed on maize silage at pH values less than 4. As with any other silage it is assumed the bacteria survive in pockets of the material where fermentation is not so good, in some cases because there is contact with air. This is more likely with bagged or wrapped silage where damage to the wrapping can occur. This is such a problem with goats that it is probably appropriate to advise that they should never be fed wrapped or bagged silage.

9.11.3 Metabolic diseases

Goats rarely suffer from metabolic diseases. This is surprising in the case of the high-yielding dairy goat which, as already mentioned, on a live-weight (or metabolic bodyweight, $kg^{0.75}$) basis produces as much milk as a high genetic-merit Holstein cow. Milk fever (hypocalcaemia) and grass staggers (hypomagnesaemia) are rarely seen. The one metabolic disease that is seen in dairy goats is ketosis or acetonaemia. When a goat becomes fat most of the fat is deposited in the abdomen; if the goat is pregnant at the same time, bearing in mind that she could be carrying three or four kids, there will not be much space for normal digestion. In this situation it is necessary for the goat to have frequent small meals; if not, the goat may draw on its own fat reserves to get enough energy. When this happens chemicals called ketone bodies are produced and these can poison the system, giving rise to the disease ketosis or acetonaemia. A goat suffering from this disease will be listless and will not be interested in its food and its breath may smell like 'pear drops', or acetone. Treatment is difficult; an injection of corticosteroids and a multivitamin preparation may restore normal metabolism in about 30% of cases. This is a very good example of prevention being the best solution. Goats should not be allowed to get fat, particularly when pregnant, and at this time they should be given at least four feeds a day so that they are able to obtain enough energy from their feed. Exercise also helps so they should be turned out into a yard or paddock where they can run around.

9.11.4 Zoonotic diseases

All people working with goats, particularly veterinarians, should be aware there are some diseases that can be transmitted to humans. These include enzootic abortion, toxoplasmosis, ringworm, orf (contagious pustular dermatitis), anthrax, listeriosis, louping ill, pox virus, brucellosis and leptospirosis. Precautions against some of these can have a serious affect on work routines; for example, it is generally advised that women of child-bearing age and certainly women who are pregnant should not work with kidding goats. Some of the diseases that cause abortion can have teratogenic effects on unborn children.

As with any animal, there are many diseases that can affect goats, but a large number are only seen rarely; therefore only the more common diseases have been included in this chapter. More information can be found in the publications listed at the end of the chapter.

References and Further Reading

Agricultural and Food Research Council (Great Britain) (1998) *The Nutrition of Goats.* ARC Technical Committee on Response to Nutrients. Report No 10. CABI Publishing, Wallingford.

Ashbrook, P.F. (1982) Year-round breeding for uniform milk production. In: *Proceedings of 3rd International Conference on Goat Production* pp. 153–4. Dairy Goat Journal, Scottsdale, AZ.

Buttle, H., Mowlem, A. and Mews, A. (1986) Disbudding and dehorning goats. *In Practice* 8, 63–5.

Lloyd, S. (1982) Parasite control. *Goat Veterinary Journal* 3(1), 91.

Mowlem, A. (1983) The development of goat artificial insemination in the United Kingdom. *British Goat Society Yearbook*. British Goat Society, Newton Abbot, UK.

Mowlem, A. (1984) Artificial rearing of kids. *Goat Veterinary Journal* 5(2), 246.

Mowlem, A. (2001) *Practical Goat Keeping*. Crowood Press, Marlborough, UK.

Mowlem, A. (2002) Current state and future prospects for dairy goats in England. *Journal of the Royal Agricultural Society* 163, 132–40.

Oldham, J.D.and Mowlem, A. (1981) Feeding goats for milk production. *Goat Veterinary Journal* 2(1), 97.

Peacock, C. (1996) *Improving Goat Production in the Tropics*. Oxfam-Farm Africa, Oxford.

Porter, V. (1996) *Goats of the World*. Farming Press, Ipswich.

Zeuner, F.E. (1963) *A History of Domesticated Animals*. Hutchinson, London.

General reading

Department for Environment Food and Rural Affairs (1989) *Codes of Recommendations for Welfare of Livestock: Goats.*

Dunn, P. (1994) *The Goatkeeper's Veterinary Book*. Farming Press, Ipswich.

Matthews, J. (1999) *Diseases of the Goat*. Blackwell Scientific Publications, Oxford.

Mackenzie, D. (1993) *Goat Husbandry*. Faber & Faber, London.

Mowlem, A. (1992) *Goat Farming*. Farming Press, Ipswich.

Mowlem, A. (2001) *Practical Goat Keeping*. Crowood Press, Marlborough, UK.

Porter, V. (1996) *Goats of the World*. Farming Press, Ipswich.

Red Deer

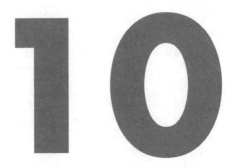

ALISON HANLON

Management and Welfare of Farm Animals: The UFAW Farm Handbook, 5th edition. John Webster
© 2011 by Universities Federation for Animal Welfare (UFAW)

10.1 Introduction

Parkland deer have been kept for centuries for venison production. In contrast, venison production from farming deer only started in the United Kingdom and New Zealand in the 1970s. One of the main objectives of the deer farming initiative was to find an alternative land use for poor-quality hill pasture and to exploit the large populations of wild red deer. From an ethical perspective, capturing and keeping wild animals in captivity could be considered as largely beneficial, utilizing an abundant resource and generating income from poor-quality land. However, during the early days of deer farming there were also costs to animal welfare such as the stress associated with capture and captivity of wild animals. Deer farming has progressed over the last 40 years and adopted extensive managements systems, balancing the benefits with the costs.

Red deer (*Cervus elaphus*) and fallow deer (*Dama dama*) are the most common species farmed in England, Scotland, Wales and Ireland. Other species of deer are farmed worldwide including sika deer (*Cervus nippon*) and rusa deer (*Cervus timorensis russa*).

In Europe, red deer are farmed for venison; elsewhere in the world, antler velvet is also harvested (removing the antlers while still 'in velvet'), a practice that is prohibited in England, Scotland, Wales and Ireland and across continental Europe. Historically, venison production has not been subsidized by the EU, although deer farmers in some EU countries are now eligible for the Single Farm Payment. Because of the lack of subsidy, deer farming has been open to market forces, which is reflected by the trends in the number of deer farms in England, Scotland and Wales. The 2008 Agricultural Census indicates that the farmed deer population decreased between 2006 and 2008 in England and Scotland (Table 10.1).

Table 10.1   Current trends in deer farming: agricultural census – number of deer in England and Scotland.

Country	2006	2007	2008
England[1]	26,000	22,000	22,000
Scotland[2]	6,500	6,380	5,960

[1]DEFRA (2008).
[2]The Scottish Government (2008).

There are two basic farming systems for venison production:

1. *Deer farms*: – deer are managed in artificial groups, enclosed in fenced paddocks. Some stock, especially calves, may be housed over winter. Management of the herd is according to a calendar of events (Figure 10.1). Farming involves the management of breeding and weaning, administration of routine veterinary treatments, supplementary feeding and some husbandry procedures to optimize productivity.
2. *Deer parks*: – present a more extensive form of deer management and involve less direct human contact and intervention. In contrast to a deer farm, park deer form natural social groupings throughout the year. Management may involve providing supplementary feed.

This chapter will focus on farming red deer. Similar principles apply to farming fallow deer, except that fallow deer are smaller and have a reputation for being more nervous and flighty than red deer.

10.2 Structure of the Industry

Deer farming may be divided into four husbandry systems:

1. calf rearers;
2. calf finishers;
3. breeder, finishers;
4. producers, processors.

Deer farmers may focus on one or more of the above husbandry systems, depending on the location of the farm, the type of land and its suitability.

10.2.1 Meat quality

Farmers produce prime venison from deer slaughtered at 1 to 2 years of age (maximum 27 months). Venison has a reputation for being a low-fat, low-cholesterol meat and has a higher lean to bone ratio in comparison with beef, lamb and chicken.

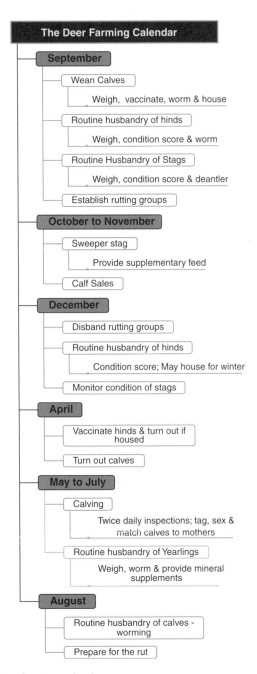

Figure 10.1 The deer farming calendar.

The proportion of fat is higher in hinds than stags (except pre-rut) and in older animals. As with other livestock species, poor-quality handling immediately pre-slaughter can have a detrimental effect on carcass quality.

10.3 Natural History and Behaviour of Wild Red Deer

Wild red deer evolved as forest dwellers inhabiting open woodlands and forest margin and have adapted to survive on open moorland. Being a prey species, they are vigilant and agile animals, which are easy to excite or frighten. For most of the year wild red deer form single-sex groups, only coming together during the mating (rutting) season. Adult females (hinds) form family groups comprising related adult hinds and their offspring from the current and previous years. Group size varies, depending on habitat and season and may range from two to more than 50 individuals per group. Stags form all-male 'bachelor' herds, which are smaller and less stable than the female herd, comprising adult and juvenile stags.

10.3.1 Feeding

In temperate climates red deer show seasonal variations in feeding behaviour. Photoperiod and the quantity and quality of food available determine seasonal feeding activity. Under natural conditions, red deer have five to eleven grazing bouts per day, the majority occur during daylight, with peaks in activity at dawn and dusk. Feeding behaviour varies with sex; hinds tend to select areas with higher-quality forage than stags. In addition both stags and hinds modify their feeding strategy to optimize their nutrient intake. For example, stags and hinds on poor-quality grazing will extend their feeding time to increase nutrient intake.

10.3.2 Life cycles: the rut

The annual breeding period, known as the rut, occurs in the autumn. However, changed behavioural patterns are evident in stags in the late summer, as they start to compete for hierarchical status, associated territories and access to females. The initiation of aggressive behaviour in males during the pre-rut period corresponds to increasing levels of testosterone. Stags typically perform dominance displays to establish or reinforce their position in the hierarchy. Typical behaviours include roaring, sparring (frontal fighting) with interlocking antlers and scent marking. Mating strategies differ between different species of deer. Red deer stags commonly compete for a territory, for example the area surrounding an oak tree, providing acorns or browse for passing hinds. Stags in possession of a territory are extremely aggressive, instigating fights against trespassing stags and those on neighbouring sites.

After establishing a territory, stags then focus on attracting hinds and gathering a 'harem' onto their territory. Apart from mating, stags have no other investment in their offspring, thus to maximize their reproductive success it is important for each stag to mate with as many hinds as possible. Stags therefore devote most of their time and energy to defending territory, attracting, guarding and mating with hinds. As a consequence, stags spend significantly less time feeding, losing up to 20% in live-weight and 80% of their fat reserves. Under natural conditions, stags maintain their harems for approximately 3 weeks, abruptly terminating rutting behaviour once a critical lower live-weight is reached.

Sexual behaviour manifests in early October, coinciding with the onset of oestrus in hinds. Mounting by hinds is indicative of oestrous behaviour. To assess oestrus and sexual receptivity, stags periodically sniff and lick the anogenital area of hinds. Stags also chase and attempt to mount hinds, but unless the hind is sexually receptive, she will not stand for the stag. Standing immobility or standing oestrus in response to tactile stimulation by the stag is a key sign that a hind is ready to be mated. Copulation comprises a true mount with simultaneous intromission and a single ejaculatory thrust. The stag dismounts and enters a brief refractory period before resuming guarding and mating of his harem. In the wild, normally only adult stags are strong enough to compete for territories and harems, precluding younger juvenile stags from mating. However, observations have shown that young stags may mate with hinds when the territory holder is busy!

10.3.3 Life cycles: calving

Red deer produce singleton calves, although twins have occasionally been reported. The gestation length in wild hinds is on average 235 days. Farmed hinds have been reported to have a slightly shorter gestation period of 231 days. The shorter gestation in farmed than wild hinds is most likely indicative of a higher plane of nutrition. Calving normally starts in May and continues until the end of June. Shortly before calving, hinds move away from the herd to give birth in isolation. As parturition approaches, the udder begins to swell and redden. The stages of parturition are not well defined in red deer. The onset of parturition and uterine contractions often manifest as restless behaviour, characterized by the hinds repeatedly touching and grooming their flanks, running in a high-stepped gait with neck outstretched and fence pacing. As parturition progresses hinds become increasingly restless, alternating between lying and standing. Hinds typically stand as the calf is delivered, to ease the calf's delivery and most likely to facilitate the severing of the umbilical cord. Calves are normally born in the anterior-dorsal position, although breech births may also occur. The duration of calving varies depending on factors such as the size of the calf and the ease with which the calf passes through the pelvis.

10.3.3.1 Mother–infant interactions

Following parturition, the hind consumes all traces of the foetal membranes from the calf and the birth site. In farmed red deer, newborn calves normally stand within 30 minutes and suck within 40 minutes. After the hind has nursed the calf, she moves away from the birth site, followed by the calf. At this stage the calf is not strong enough to run with the maternal herd, so after a short distance it lies down and remains at this location until the hind returns to nurse it. In terms of behavioural development, although calves are precocious, i.e. born in an advanced neural and motor state, they are considered to be a 'hider' species. This is because neonatal calves lack the strength and stamina to follow the herd and remain hidden for the first few days, and are periodically nursed by their dam in the hideout. Hinds nurse their calves for the first few days at 2 to 3 hour intervals. As the calf suckles, the hind licks the calf's anogenital area to stimulate defecation and urination, which is involuntary in neonatal calves. The hind ingests the meconium (first faeces) to remove all traces of the presence of the neonatal calf.

Peak lactation occurs at approximately 40 days postpartum (Loudon *et al.*, 1984). Under natural conditions, weaning is a gradual process. Suckling bouts decrease as lactation progresses and by 3 months of age calves suckle on average three to four times a day. The hind rejects up to 50% of suckling attempts by the time calves are 6 months old. At this stage the suckling bout lasts for approximately 30 seconds. The timing of weaning depends on the reproductive state of the hind. Pregnant hinds will gradually stop lactating in the winter, although barren hinds may continue to nurse their young until the following summer.

10.3.4 Life cycles: breeding

10.3.4.1 Reproductive biology
Red deer are seasonal 'short day' breeders such that breeding occurs during the autumn, corresponding to shorter daylength. Weight largely determines the onset of puberty in both hinds and stags. Stags normally reach puberty at approximately 16 months old. However, the presence of mature stags will preclude yearlings from mating. Thus stags do not successfully mate until they are able to compete for territories and gain access to hinds.

In the wild, red hinds reach puberty at 2 to 3 years of age. Red deer are seasonally polyoestrous and come into oestrus every 19 days for 12 to 24 hours until they have successfully mated and conceived. Research suggests a 'stag effect'; as with other livestock species, presence of a sexually mature male can stimulate the onset of oestrus. Farmed hinds normally conceive in their first oestrous cycle, although may continue to cycle two or three times before conceiving. Wild hinds have a lower live-weight and reproductive success than their farmed counterparts, corresponding to the poorer quality of forage and the lack of shelter.

10.3.4.2 Antler development
Antlers are a unique anatomical structure and are not equivalent to horns of other ungulates. Horns are permanent, with growth developing from the base of the horn; in contrast, antlers are not permanent and are grown and shed annually by red deer stags (antlers develop in both sexes in some species of deer). Antlers grow from the tip and form new branches after the first year of growth. Stag calves develop pedicles, circular bony 'stalks', on frontal lobes of the skull, which later act as a platform for

antlers. The antler growth cycle begins in spring, between April and May. Growing antlers are covered with a thick velvet skin, which contains a network of blood vessels and nerve endings. Growth is complete by August. In the final stages of growth, a ring, the coronet, forms around the antler base, constricting blood and nutrient supply to the antlers. As a consequence, the velvet starts to shrivel and peel off, assisted by the stag actively rubbing the antlers against trees and bushes. At this stage strips of velvet hang from the antlers, exposing the hard calcified bone of the antler. This process is referred to as antler cleaning and is associated with an increase in testosterone levels.

Once the velvet has been shed, the stag remains in hard antlers during the rut and over winter and casts them during the early spring, coinciding with a decline in circulating testosterone concentrations. Before casting, stags typically leave the herd and each antler is cast separately within a day or two. New antler growth begins shortly after casting, thus completing the cycle. The complexity of antler architecture increases with age; the number of points on an antler is related to the age of the stag. For example, the antlers of yearling stags are simple spikes.

10.4 Management of Farmed Red Deer

10.4.1 Mating

The deer farming year begins in the autumn, with the rut. One month before the rut, stags are routinely de-antlered as a safety measure, weighed and prophylactic treatments such as anthelmintics may be administered. From a management perspective, the main objectives are to achieve a high conception rate and manage groups to ensure early and compact calving. To achieve the first objective, both stags and hinds must enter the rut in good body condition. Audigé and his colleagues have conducted large-scale studies on the reproductive performance of farmed red deer yearlings and hinds in New Zealand (1999a) and identified a number of risk factors influencing reproductive success (Table 10.2). As expected, body condition score (BCS) is very important, together with achieving a certain weight threshold. The nutritional demands of lactation have a direct impact on BCS and thus reproductive success, especially on yearlings. Hinds should have a minimum BCS of 2 and the odds of conception are further increased for hinds with a BCS of 2.5. The timing of weaning influences the date of conception and conception rate. Late weaning delays oestrous cycling and recovery of BCS before the rut. In some herds, hinds are weaned after the rut.

Stags are allocated to rutting groups in mid- to late September or immediately following weaning. Research has shown that it is beneficial to form rutting groups in advance of the mating season. In addition, early introduction of the stag to the rutting groups has been reported to advance the first oestrus by 6 days. Deer farms commonly adopt single-sire mating systems – allocating one stag to a group of hinds. The stag to hind ratio depends on the age of the stag (Table 10.3). Stags are

Table 10.2 Risk factors effecting conception rate in farmed red deer hinds and yearlings. Modified from Audigé *et al.* (1999).

Risk factors	Hinds	Yearlings
Wean calves early	✓	—
Exclude or cull hinds that fail to rear a calf to weaning	✓	—
Exclude hinds with a BCS <2 at mating	✓	✓
Form rutting groups early	✓	✓
Only use proven stag sires	✓	✓
Limit the hind to stag ratio	✓	✓
Use a sweeper stag after the peak of mating	✓	✓
Maintain sward heights at <5 cm	✓	✓
Avoid disturbing rutting groups	✓	✓

removed from the rutting group after peak mating at approximately 6 weeks and commonly replaced by a 'sweeper stag', to ensure that all hinds have been mated.

Yearling hinds have a lower bodyweight and consequently a longer latency to their first oestrus than adult hinds and thus yearlings should be managed in a separate group from adult hinds. Similarly there are management differences between yearling and adult stags during the rut. Yearling stags are not commonly used for breeding because they have a lower fertility and are inexperienced compared with adults. In addition, the presence of adult stags can suppress the libido of yearling stags and therefore it is advisable to ensure that, when yearling stags are allocated to rutting groups, they are not situated in close proximity to adult stags.

10.4.2 Calving

Calving normally starts in mid-May and continues until early July. As already stated, the mating period should be designed to support early and compact calving. Research has shown that calves born early in the calving season have higher weight gains than later-born calves. In addition, late-born calves have a higher risk of contracting bacterial diseases in the immediate postnatal period.

Table 10.3 Stag to hind ratios. Modified from Haigh and Hudson (1993).

Age of stag	Number of hinds
16 months	10
2 years	20
3 years	>30
4 years	>40
5–8 years	50
>9 years	<50

Adult and yearling hinds are allocated to calving groups in early May. Most hinds calve unassisted. As previously mentioned, hinds tend to move away from the herd shortly before calving. They show a number of characteristic behaviours at this time including restlessness, alternating between lying and standing; touching, sniffing and grooming their flanks and anogenital area; running in a high-stepping gait with neck outstretched, and fence pacing. Wass *et al.* (2003) studied calving behaviour and reported that the duration of calving, from the appearance of the foetal sac to the expulsion of the calf, takes on average 84 minutes. Immediately postpartum the dam normally initiates grooming, removing the foetal fluids from the calf. Thereafter the calf attempts to stand and teat-seek. Calves are able to stand on average 24 minutes after birth and suckle within 30 to 40 minutes of birth. The latency to suckle was reported to take longer for calves born to yearling than adult hinds.

It is advisable to locate calving paddocks close to the home farm and/or a handling area in the event of dystocia or other calving problems. By monitoring the behaviour of hinds and the relative duration of calving it is possible to identify hinds with calving difficulty. Detailed advice on handling and assistance at calving is available from Haigh and Hudson (1993). Farmers normally tag and weigh calves from 12 to 36 hours after birth. Handling calves during the first 12 hours may increase the risk of abandonment and mismothering. The stockperson should be aware that hinds can become aggressive at this time.

10.4.3 Weaning

Hinds can be weaned before or after the mating season. Commonly weaning takes place before hinds are allocated to rutting groups, when calves are approximately 100 days old. Weaning pre-rut enables hinds to recover body condition, which has a direct effect on the conception rate. At weaning, farmers weigh calves and typically commence a vaccination programme against clostridial diseases. Calves are then either housed or allocated to a paddock away from the maternal herd. Abrupt weaning is considered to be stressful for many food animal species, because it is associated with a number of sudden changes in both social and physical environment. At weaning, deer calves are separated from the maternal herd, vaccinated, weighed and allocated to groups. Calves at this stage may also be housed over winter and until the following spring. Calves lack experience of both housing and handling and together with new social groupings this can culminate in stress.

10.5 Environment and Housing

10.5.1 At pasture

Deer farmers generally maintain adults on pasture throughout the year. The number of paddocks depends on the production system. Location, access to paddocks and integrated raceways to handling facilities are important considerations, especially during calving. Calving paddocks are often situated close to the farm, to enable farmers to monitor calving without disturbing the deer. Trees, although not essential, can improve both physical and mental welfare. They provide natural shelter from wind and rain, a more secure natural environment and help to improve calving success.

The stocking rate depends on the type of land and quality of grazing. Deer should be stocked at a rate that maintains an adequate body condition in winter, otherwise supplementary feeding will be necessary (DEFRA, 2007). Overstocking during calving can lead to abnormal behaviour in hinds such as hinds showing aggressive behaviour towards calves.

10.5.2 Housing

In temperate climates, producers usually group-house weaned calves over winter, because they possess proportionally less body fat than adults and are therefore less able to cope with climatic stress. Some producers also house breeding hinds over winter, to prevent poaching of grass. Calves are housed on deep bedded straw and should have a minimum space allowance of 2.25 m^2/head at weaning. Bullying may occur during housing and can be reduced by providing forms of environmental enrichment such as placing a wheel of straw in the pen.

The same principles of housing apply to deer as other farmed livestock. Pens should be constructed with non-harmful material that can be disinfected when the animals are turned out. The pen walls should be at least 2 m high, to discourage escape. Individual deer may respond aggressively to stockpersons during handling (and routine feeding). It is therefore important to be able to recognize threatening behaviour that precedes an attack, such as prolonged eye contact, ears flattened back, grinding teeth, stamping and snorting.

10.5.3 Handling

During the early years of deer farming when wild deer were being used to stock farms, stress at handling was reported to cause capture myopathy (also known as white muscle disease), which is characterized by myodegeneration and necrosis of skeletal and cardiac muscle. In acute cases, clinical signs include respiratory distress, increased heart rate and hyperthermia; the deer may be reluctant to move, and suddenly collapse. Death may occur within hours, days or weeks of the stressful event. Capture myopathy is a complex syndrome and poorly understood. Dietary deficiencies in vitamin E, selenium or both have been indicated in the development of capture myopathy. Overall the agility of deer and infrequency of handling can combine to elicit fear-related behaviours. There is no treatment for capture myopathy and therefore special consideration should be given to minimizing stress during handling and restraint.

Depending of the type of production system, farmed deer may be handled less than four times a year. The age and experience of the deer, as well as the skill of the stockperson and the type of handling facilities available, determine ease of handling. New stock and calves at weaning are generally difficult to handle because they are unfamiliar with the stockperson and the layout of the handling facilities. At weaning calves may attempt to escape through fencing or underneath gates. Pollard *et al.* (1992) suggest that including a tame hind in the weaning group can reduce panic among calves. The same principle applies to new stock.

Stags during the rut and, to a lesser degree, hinds during calving may behave aggressively towards the stockperson. Ideally, handling stags during the rut should be avoided. However, if it is necessary e.g. moving a stag into a new rutting group), special precautions should be taken. During this time stags should be handled individually and not in a group, especially when in hard antler, because of the risk of fighting and associated injury. Except for stags during the rut, it is better to gather or muster deer as a group. If an individual becomes separated from the group, it may panic and try to escape. In this situation it is easier to allow the separated animal to rejoin the group by moving a small group towards the separated animal.

10.5.3.1 Handling facilities

Besides good stockmanship it is possible to reduce stress during handling by incorporating specific features into the design and layout of handling facilities. The system should enable animals to move continuously from the home paddock or pen through the raceway(s) to the handling area with minimum stress and risk of injury.

All deer farms should have handling facilities so that deer can be restrained for veterinary treatments. The most important requirements are a drop floor or pneumatic crush, weighing crate and at least one holding pen (and ideally several holding pens of different sizes). Some procedures such as body condition scoring and administration of anthelmintic treatments can be conducted in holding pens, when animals are grouped. In contrast, de-antlering will require physical restraint in a drop-floor crush, short-term sedation or anaesthesia.

Paddock design and access to handling facilities are important considerations. Some farms have an integrated system of raceways linking paddocks with the handling facilities. Where this is not possible, paddocks should be long and narrow or tapered towards the gate. Deer, like other livestock, move faster along curved raceways. Walls in the handling facility and fences should be sufficiently high, to prevent deer from attempting to jump and escape. Most accidents occur between the home paddock and handling facilities. Deer should be gathered and moved in a group at a walking pace. Raceways need to be sufficiently wide to enable group movement. Deer can be effectively trained through feed rewards to come to the stockperson's call.

10.5.4 Fencing

Deer farmers use three main types of fencing: strained wire (horizontal wires), mesh and wire and baton. They also use electric fencing for controlling grazing or to prevent fighting between stags in adjacent paddocks. Fencing requirements differ for perimeter and internal use. Perimeter fences need to be approximately 2 m high to prevent deer from escaping and other wildlife entering. Some areas of internal fencing, such as raceways, need to be stronger as they will be under greater pressure. At pressure points, fencing needs to prevent escape, entanglement and injury and to be visible, to prevent deer, especially weaned calves and new stock, from accidentally running into it. To prevent entanglement and injury, wire spacing needs to be sufficiently small to prevent deer from pushing their heads through, otherwise it can lead to damage to ears, as tags are pulled out, and damage to antler buds. Calves are most at risk from entanglement in fencing; this can be minimized by using small mesh netting on the lower portion of fence. It is inadvisable to use electric fencing in calving paddocks, because of an obvious risk of electrocution to calves.

10.6 Nutrition

Farmed red deer have a higher basal metabolic rate than sheep and require approximately one-third more energy. Adult hinds have a maintenance requirement of approximately $0.57\,MJ/kg^{0.75}$ (Adam, 1994). Their requirement varies with live-weight and reproductive status. For example an 80 kg hind requires approximately 17 MJ ME/day for maintenance, increasing to approximately 20 MJ ME/day during late pregnancy, and a further increase to 32 MJ ME/day at peak lactation. Digestion is similar to that of other ruminant livestock given the same diet.

10.6.1 Nutrition of breeding hinds

Nutrition and corresponding live-weight and body condition can dramatically increase the reproductive success of red deer hinds by:

- reducing the age of first calving;
- increasing the rate of conception;
- increasing calf survival.

Live-weight is an important determinant of the age at first calving. By improving the nutrition of red deer hinds, producers have advanced the onset of puberty to 16 months, compared to 24 to 36 months in their wild counterparts. Body condition also influences the subsequent reproductive success of hinds. In the wild, lactating hinds have a 50% chance of calving in the following season. Conception rate positively correlates with the pre-rut weight of hinds: those over 70 kg have a 90% rate of conception compared with only 50% of hinds less than 65 kg (Hamilton and Blaxter, 1980). For example, yearlings on heather-dominant pasture conceive approximately 17 days later than those on good-quality pasture; similar trends occur in adult hinds.

To provide adequate forage to grazing hinds during lactation, farmers need to maintain sward heights of grass at 6 to 8 cm. Stocking rates depend on the quality and growth of pasture. For example, poor-quality grazing such as heather moorland can only maintain 0.66 lactating hinds per hectare; in contrast, cultivated upland and lowland pasture can support 10 to 12 and 12 to 16 hinds per hectare, respectively.

Maintaining body condition during pregnancy is critical to ensure prenatal development and neonatal survival. As with other livestock species, poor nutrition during gestation influences birth weights of calves, thereby increasing the risk of calf mortality. Overfeeding is also undesirable because of the risks of dystocia. The constant provision of supplementary feed has been reported to lower the muscle tone and fitness of hinds, due to lack of exercise associated with the reduced need to forage.

10.6.2 Nutrition of calves

The weight and body condition of hinds during gestation determines the birth weight of calves and influences growth rate. Stag calves are approximately 1 kg heavier at birth than hind calves and have a higher growth rate from birth until weaning. Birth weight is correlated to calf survival such that 4 kg calves have 100% mortality. In contrast, 5% mortality has been recorded in calves of 6 to 7 kg at birth (Blaxter and Hamilton, 1980).

Calves are totally dependent on milk for their energy requirements during the first 30 days. They consume between 200 and 600 g of milk per suckling bout and a maximum of 2000 g/day (Arman *et al.*, 1974). As lactation progresses, dependency on milk gradually decreases. By the time calves are approximately 3 months old, milk account for only 10 to 20% of energy intake.

The ME requirement for growth varies with season and live-weight gain (Table 10.4). The weight of calves at weaning depends on the production system and may vary from 25 to 45 kg. Live-weight gain falls as the quality of pasture decreases in late summer. Seasonal inappetance over winter also greatly affects live-weight gain, although skeletal growth continues at a slower rate. In many circumstances, particularly on hill and upland farms, supplementary feeding and housing may be necessary to achieve target live-weights at 15 months of age. Weaned calves that are housed and fed maintenance rations over winter have a lower live-weight gain than those on *ad libitum* diets. However, the rapid growth of calves following turnout on pasture in late spring partly compensates for this differential growth.

Table 10.4 Approximate metabolizable energy (ME) requirements (MJ) for growing calves. Modified from Adams (1994).

Season	Growth (g/d)			
	50	**100**	**150**	**200**
Autumn	2.8	5.5	8.3	11.0
Winter	4.4	8.7	13.1	17.4
Spring/summer	2.4	4.9	7.3	9.7

At weaning, the target live-weights for hind and stag calves on good quality pasture are 43 and 46 kg, respectively. Farmers need to maintain a sward height of 8 to 10 cm for calves at pasture following weaning, to maximize growth before winter. Growth rates can vary by up to 100 g/day, depending on the quantity and quality of pasture and the weather conditions. Supplementary feeding of calves on poor-quality pasture is necessary to achieve mid-winter live-weights of 56 and 60 kg for hind and stag calves, respectively (Adam, 1994).

10.6.3 Nutrition of stags

Farmed red deer stags of 150 and 250 kg have maintenance requirements of 24.4 and 35.8 MJ ME, respectively (Table 10.5). Stags have similar maintenance requirements in summer and winter. During the rut, stags may lose up to 30% of weight due to spending a large proportion of time guarding, mating or competing for hinds and a corresponding decrease in the amount of time spent feeding. By the end of the rut, stags can typically be in poor body condition and this problem can be compounded by the onset of winter inappetance. It is therefore important to ensure that stags enter the rut in good body condition and are removed after a 4- to 6-week period to reduce the detrimental impact of rutting on body condition before the onset of winter.

10.6.4 Mineral requirements

Calcium, phosphorus and magnesium are essential components in the diet. Deer can to some extent counteract short-term dietary deficiency in the major minerals by mobilizing body reserves, although this may impair skeletal growth and development in calves. Mineral requirements are normally high during growth and lactation. Hinds lose approximately 2.2 g calcium and 1.9 g phosphorus per kg milk (Adam, 1994). Phosphorus deficiency may reduce fertility. Deer require other minerals such as copper, cobalt, selenium and iodine in trace quantities. Deficiency in all except iodine can cause subclinical problems; clinical signs may only become evident when compounded by other factors.

Table 10.5 Approximate daily metabolizable energy (ME) requirements for maintenance in weaned calves, hinds and stags.

	Live-weight (kg)	ME requirement (MJ)
Calves (3–16 months)	40	7.2
	50	8.5
	60	9.7
Hinds	80	15.2
	100	18.0
Stags	150	24.4
	250	35.8

10.6.5 Body condition scoring

Body condition scoring (BCS) is an important management tool for ensuring that the nutritional intake of animals is sufficient to support good health and productivity, especially of breeding females. Audigé *et al.* (1999b) have developed a scoring system for farmed red deer hinds and yearlings, based on a scale of 1 (lean) to 5 (fat) with half-unit increments (Table 10.6). Assessment is based on the muscle and fat coverage over three distinct areas: the wings of the pelvis, the tuber coxae and the spinous processes. Minimal or mild restraint is required for BCS. A group of deer should be moved into a small holding pen, which will allow the stockperson to move among the deer and gently palpate the pelvic area, spinous processes and rump.

10.7 Health and Disease

This section provides an outline for the most common diseases reported in farmed red deer. For a comprehensive review of diseases, refer to Alexander and Buxton (1994).

10.7.1 Tuberculosis

In 2008 the European Food Safety Authority (EFSA) published a review on tuberculosis testing in farmed deer. An outline of the main points is provided below. Tuberculosis (TB) in deer is caused by infection with species within the *Mycobacterium tuberculosis* complex. The complex members include *M. tuberculosis*, *M. canetti*, *M. africanum*, *M. pinnipedii*, *M. microti*, Dassie bacillus, *M. caprae* and *M. bovis*. The *Mycobacterium tuberculosis* complex also includes the vaccine strain, *M. bovis* bacille Calmette Guerin (BCG). The disease has a slow progression in deer and infected deer can appear to be clinically healthy, even in the advanced stages of the disease.

A number of diagnostic tests are available to detect TB in deer; however, it is unlikely that all infected deer in a herd will be detected at the same time. Therefore testing should be repeated in order to provide any degree of certainty about whether a herd is TB free. Moreover, farmed deer are also susceptible to other mycobacterial diseases such as paratuberculosis (or Johne's disease) and avian tuberculosis. Some of the pathological lesions present in deer infected with the latter can be similar to those caused by *M. bovis*, thus confounding slaughterhouse surveillance of TB.

10.7.2 Johne's disease

Johne's disease or paratuberculosis, caused by *Mycobacterium avium* ssp. *paratuberculosis* (MAP) is more commonly seen at a younger age in deer than happens in other susceptible ruminants and is transmissible *in utero*. The clinical signs include loss of condition, retention of the winter coat and, as the disease progresses, diarrhoea. It is advisable to isolate infected animals because bacteria are shed in the faeces. There are no effective treatments available and death will occur in weeks

Table 10.6 Body condition scoring chart for farmed red hinds and yearlings. Source: Audigé et al. (1999).

Body condition score	Wings of the pelvis	Spinous processes	Rump area
1. Very poor condition	Extremely prominent and sharp	Very sharp	Little muscle or fat cover; concave on palpation
2. Poor condition (lean)	Prominent, but rounded and easily felt by palpation with slight finger pressure	Slightly rounded and not prominent	Flat
3. Moderate condition	Prominent, but rounded and easily felt by palpation	Slightly rounded and not prominent	Flat
4. Good condition	Rounded and easily felt by palpation under a thin layer of fat	Rounded and felt by palpation only with firm pressure	Slightly convex
5. Very good condition (fat)	Concealed under a thick layer of fat and cannot be felt with firm pressure	Well rounded and not felt on palpation	Convex

or months. Bovine vaccines against MAP are effective in deer, although they may confound subsequent tests for *M. bovis* and are therefore not routinely used.

10.7.3 Yersiniosis

The bacterium *Yersinia pseudotuberculosis* causes Yersiniosis. Both wild and domestic animals can be carriers and it can occur in the faeces of healthy deer. Infected deer shed large quantities of the organism in their faeces and so infection can rapidly spread within a group. Deer commonly encounter Yersinia in their first winter, but may not show any clinical signs of infection. Clinical disease is triggered by stress such as weaning, under-feeding, over-crowding, rough handling and transportation. The clinical signs include weight loss, green diarrhoea, dehydration and prolonged inactivity before death. Yersiniosis can be successfully treated with antibiotics, combined with non-specific diarrhoea treatment and fluid replacement therapy. Some countries have a vaccine available for Yersiniosis.

10.7.4 Clostridial diseases

Species of *Clostridium* cause a variety of disease. For example, *C. perfringens* (also called *C. welchii*) causes enterotoxaemia. Clostridial infection can occur when the diet changes suddenly, effecting a change in the gut flora supporting clostridial growth, which produce a lethal toxin. Other examples include blackleg and malignant oedema, caused by infection of open wounds by clostridial species, and results in septicaemia. The condition is fatal unless diagnosed in time. Commencement of a vaccination programme (usually at weaning) followed by re-vaccination at yearly intervals using multivalent vaccines can reduce clostridial infections.

10.7.5 Bluetongue

Bluetongue (BT) is caused by a virus within the Orbivirus genus of the Reovirus family. According to DEFRA (2008) it affects all ruminants, including deer. In the UK and elsewhere, it is a notifiable disease and therefore its occurrence should be reported to the competent authority, e.g. DEFRA in the UK. The clinical signs reported in sheep and cattle include changes to the mucous linings of the mouth and nose and the coronary band of the foot. No clinical signs have been reported in deer. The disease is spread by the Culicoides family of biting midges. Culicoides, and therefore the risk of bluetongue transmission, is most common in the late summer and autumn. However, according to DEFRA the likelihood of mechanical transmission of the virus between herds/flocks and within a herd/flock by unhygienic practices (e.g. use of contaminated surgical equipment or hypodermic needles) cannot be excluded. A vaccine against BT serotype 8 is available but is not licensed for use in deer (though could be used under the cascade system in the UK).

10.7.6 Malignant catarrhal fever

Malignant catarrhal fever (MCF) has been a major cause of mortality in farmed deer in New Zealand. It is caused by two viruses, alcelaphine herpesvirus-1 (AHV-1) and ovine herpesvirus-2 (OHV-2). Wildebeest and sheep are hosts of AHV-1 and OHV-2, respectively. The viruses become pathogenic once they are transmitted to another species. Susceptibility to MCF varies with deer species and the disease can be fatal. Stress can trigger the onset of clinical disease in deer. Clinical signs include inappetance, dysentery, enlargement of lymph nodes, bilateral corneal opacity, mucosal secretions and skin ulcers. There are no vaccines available. As part of a herd health strategy it is important to reduce the risk of disease transmission by ensuring that farmed deer are not kept in close proximity to sheep or wildebeest. Biosecurity measures should be taken on farms containing both sheep and deer, for example separate stockpersons should be responsible for managing each species.

10.7.7 Parasites

10.7.7.1 Ostertagia

Ostertagia species are the main gastrointestinal parasites, although others may also be present in the gut, but at such low numbers that they are effectively non-pathogenic. Clinical infestation with *Ostertagia* causes the same symptoms as in other livestock, namely, weight loss, poor coat condition, soft faeces and a soiled tail. Treatment depends on the degree and spread of infestation and grassland management. The most effective strategy is to combine anthelmintic treatment with pasture rotation.

10.7.7.2 Cryptosporidiosis

Cryptosporidiosis is caused by a coccidial parasite, *Cryptosporidium parvum*, which infects the small intestine. The disease is transmitted through ingestion of *Cryptosporidium* eggs shed in the faeces of infected animals. It is highly contagious and can spread rapidly in a group of young calves either at pasture or in a pen. Clinical signs occur within 5 to 6 days and include inappetance and diarrhoea. Infected animals should be immediately isolated to prevent further spread. Anticoccidial vaccines are ineffective and most farmers treat infected calves for dehydration. *Cryptosporidium* is also a zoonotic disease, causing acute gastroenteritis in humans.

10.7.7.3 Lungworm

Lungworm, *Dictyocaulus viviparus*, can have a significant impact on health, welfare and productivity. Calves are the most vulnerable age group, particularly in autumn and winter. In addition to *D. viviparus*, deer are also susceptible to bovine strains of *Dictyocaulus*. Clinical signs include inappetance and weight loss. Heavy infestations can lead to sudden death. Deer may also show signs of respiratory difficulty, culminating in suffocation if the condition is not treated. Faecal egg counts should be part of a herd health strategy. Prophylactic treatment with anthelmintics should be considered for hinds on farms with a history of calves infected with lungworm.

10.7.7.4 Nasal bot flies

Nasal bot flies, *Cephenemyia auribarbis*, may cause respiratory distress in red deer. From May to July female bot flies inject larvae into the nostrils of deer. Initial growth occurs in nasal cavities; by April or May the larvae migrate to the pharyngeal pockets until they develop fully. Before pupating, larvae drop out of the nose and onto the ground. Heavy infestation with bot fly larvae may cause suffocation or secondary infections at the site of attachments following inhalation of larvae. Warbles (*Hypoderma diana*) and headfly (*Hydrotaea irritans*) can also cause problems.

10.7.7.5 Liver fluke

Liver fluke (*Fasciola hepatica*) infection in red deer commonly occurs at a subclinical level. However, it is an important cause of liver condemnation postmortem. Treatment with flukicides is more effective for adult (90–100%) than immature fluke. To ensure effective treatment, application of flukicides should be repeated approximately 1 month after initial treatment.

10.7.8 Management-related problems

In the past, problems related to the stress of wild deer in captivity. Although farmed red deer may not yet be considered domesticated, selective breeding over the past 40 years is likely to have selected deer best suited to a farm environment. As with most livestock, stressors such as handling, housing and transportation have the potential to reduce the health and wellbeing of farmed red deer. Handling in particular needs to be performed with skills. Haigh and Hudson (1993) have developed the '3 T rule': Training, Taming and Tempo, which if adhered to can minimize difficulties during handling.

Metabolic disorders such as acidosis may arise from inappropriate supplementary feeding. Excess lactic acid is produced during fermentation in the rumen, following the consumption of large quantities of concentrated feed. The consequent increase in acidity can destroy the tissue lining and microflora of the rumen. Once the lactic acid enters the circulation it can cause damage to other tissues and organs. Dominant animals are more likely to suffer from acidosis because they have priority of access to feed. The clinical signs include inappetance and reduced activity, eventually resulting in an inability to stand and in severe cases leading to death. The treatment for acidosis is to wash out the rumen, a procedure which must be conducted by a veterinary surgeon. The condition can be prevented by the gradual introduction of concentrate feed and spreading the distribution over a wide area to stop individuals from gorging.

Neonatal mortality is reported at 10 to 12% in New Zealand (Wass *et al.*, 2003), with yearling hinds having a higher rate of loss than experienced adult hinds. Similar differences are seen in other livestock species and may be partly related to lower levels of maternal care observed in first-time mothers. However, management and environment also play a role. The environment should facilitate the behavioural ecology of red deer at calving, in particular to have areas of cover to enable calves to hide, as described earlier. Wass *et al.* (2003) suggested that yearlings experience greater interference from adult hinds at calving and this is associated with an increased latency to nurse their calves. Managing young hinds in separate groups from adult hinds may also be important to reduce the risk of bullying or mismothering.

10.8 Transportation

The regulations on the welfare of animals in transport change over time. Updates are published on the DEFRA website (and national counterparts in the EU). General regulations from the EU Welfare in Transport Regulation (EC) No 1/2005 apply to farmed deer. The main provisions of the regulations are intended for commercial transport of livestock >65 km. For journeys <65 km there remains a duty of care on the person transporting animals to avoid injury and undue suffering to the animals. According to DEFRA, all persons transporting livestock should adhere to the following guidelines on good transport practice:

- Journey planning to ensure that the journey length is kept to a minimum.
- The animals are fit to travel.
- The vehicle, loading and unloading facilities are designed and maintained to avoid injury and suffering to the animals.
- A competent person handles the animals.
- Providing for the animals' needs including water, feed and rest, as appropriate, sufficient floor space and height to allow the animals to lie and stand, respectively, without impediment.
- Monitoring animals during the journey.

Stags in velvet are specified in the regulations as not fit to travel. This is due to the risk of pain and injury to the antlers during this stage of development. In certain conditions, deer may not be considered 'fit to travel' and transportation under these circumstances should only be conducted in emergency. Hinds in late pregnancy and sick or injured deer are generally considered not fit to travel. In addition the transportation of entire adult stags during the rut should be avoided due to their aggressive behaviour. For stags in hard antler, it is advisable to remove the antlers several days before transportation. De-antlered stags should not be grouped with stags in antler, due to an increased risk of injury.

In addition to the above, a number of technical rules involving authorization apply to journeys >65 km. The level of authorization depends on journey length and duration.

10.9 Slaughter

In contrast to other farmed livestock, deer can be humanely slaughtered either in an abattoir (which may be purpose-built) or by shooting by a trained marksperson at the home farm (field slaughter). Field slaughter has the advantage of being conducted in a familiar environment with minimal stress. DEFRA provides a code of recommendation for field slaughter. Deer should be quiet and inactive at the time of field slaughter and this can be achieved by providing lines of concentrate feed for the deer. Tame or inactivate deer can be shot at close range (10 to 20 m) using a head shot. Less tame deer can be dispatched up to a range of 40 m using a high neck shot. Ranges beyond 40 m should only be undertaken by proven markspeople but should be unnecessary for farmed deer. In addition to the skill of the marksperson, a suitable rifle and ammunition should be used.

Limitations to field slaughter include the need for antemortem inspection in relation to killing a small number of animals at any one time, throughput, human safety and poor marksmanship. In terms of throughput, only a limited number of deer can be shot at any one time, before the noise of the shooting starts to agitate other deer on the farm. A prerequisite for humane field slaughter is that the marksperson is properly trained and has sufficient experience to ensure that the deer are humanely dispatched with a clean shot. Public safety is an issue for farms that adjoin areas accessible to the public. DEFRA recommends that farmers should:

- walk the fence perimeter of the farm to check that there are no members of public in the vicinity;
- conduct field slaughter early in the morning;
- shoot away from roads, house and garden.

Humane slaughter in an abattoir normally includes a series of potentially stressful events including handling, loading, transportation, unloading and lairage before the deer are slaughtered. Conventional slaughter of farmed deer is the same as for other livestock species and is described in the preceding chapters.

10.10 The Way Ahead

Deer farming is more extensive than other forms of conventional livestock production. The underlying ethos has been to adapt management systems and environs to the nature of deer, facilitating normal patterns of behaviour such as rutting and calving. As a consequence it is more naturalistic. From an ethical perspective it may be considered to be more acceptable than intensive production systems, which are associated with production diseases and stereotypic abnormal behaviours and other indicators of poor animal welfare. In the future it is important that deer farmers continue to demonstrate a good understanding of the behavioural and physical requirements of deer and to avoid the mistakes made by intensive agriculture. Furthermore, by adopting welfare-based quality assurance schemes, deer farmers have a unique opportunity to market venison as a natural and high-welfare product.

Acknowledgements

I would like to express thanks to Mr Kevin Blurton and Dr Pete Goddard for therir assistance.

References and Further Reading

Adam, C.L. (1994) Feeding. In *Management and Diseases of Deer: a Handbook for the Veterinary Surgeon*, 2nd edn., Alexander, T.L.and Buxton, D. (eds), pp. 44–54. Veterinary Deer Society, London.

Alexander, T.L.and Buxton, D. (eds) (1994) *Management and Diseases of Deer: a Handbook for the Veterinary Surgeon*, 2nd edn. Veterinary Deer Society, London.

Arman, P., Kay, R.N.B., Goodall, E.D. and Sharman, G.A.M. (1974) The composition and yield of milk from captive red deer (*Cervus elaphus L*). *Journal of Reproduction and Fertility* 37, 67–84.

Audigé, L.J.M., Wilson, P.R., Pfeiffer, D.U. and Morris, R.S. (1999a) Reproductive performance of farmed red deer (*Cervus elaphus*) in New Zealand: II. Risk factors for adult hind conception. *Preventative Veterinary Medicine* 40, 33–51.

Audigé, L.J.M., Wilson, P.R. and Morris, R.S. (1999b) A body condition score for use in farmed red deer. *New Zealand Journal of Agricultural Research* 41 (4), 545–53.

Blaxter, K.L. Hamilton, W.J. (1980) Reproduction in farmed red deer: 2. Calf growth and mortality. *Journal of Agricultural Science, Cambridge* 95, 275–84.

Blaxter, K.L., Kay, R.N.B., Sharman, G.A.M., Cunningham, J.M.M. and Hamilton, W.J. (1988) *Farming the Red Deer*, 2nd edn. HMSO, Edinburgh, UK.

British Deer Farmers Association (2008) The Deer Farming Year. Available at: http://www.bdfa.co.uk/deerfarming/.

Clutton-Brock, T.H. and Albon, S.D. (1989) *Red Deer in the Highlands*. BSP Professional Books, Oxford, UK.

Clutton-Brock, T.H., Guinness, F.E. and Albon, S.D. (1982) *Red Deer: Behavior and Ecology of Two Sexes*. University of Chicago Press, Chicago.

DEFRA (2007a) *Animal Welfare: Codes of recommendations for the welfare of livestock – Deer*. Available at: www.defra.gov.uk/animalh/welfare.

DEFRA (2007b) Veterinary surveillance: Deer. Available at: www.defra.gov.uk/animalh/diseases/vetsurveillance.

DEFRA (2008) *Survey of Agriculture and Horticulture: England*. Available at: https://statistics.defra.gov.uk.

European Food Safety Agency (2008) Scientific Opinion of the Panel on Animal Health and Animal Welfare on a request from the European Commission on 'Tuberculosis testing in deer'. *EFSA Journal* 645, 1–34.

Farm Animal Welfare Council (1985) *Report on the Welfare of Farmed Deer*. FAWC, Surbiton, UK.

Haigh, J.C. and Hudson, R.J. (1993) *Farming Wapiti and Red Deer*. Mosby, St Louis, MO.

Hamilton, W.J. (1989) Farming red deer – the keys to good management. In *Deer Farming: a Handbook for the 1990s*, Gould, J. (ed.), pp. 21–3. British Deer Farmers Association, Matlock, UK.

Hamilton, W.J. and Blaxter, K.L. (1980) Reproduction in farmed red deer: 1. Hind and stag fertility. *Journal of Agricultural Science, Cambridge* **95**, 261–73.

Hanlon, A.J. (1997) The welfare of farmed red deer. *Deer Farming* **53**, 14–16.

Pollard, J.C., Littlejohn, R.P. and Suttie, J.M. (1992) Behaviour and weight change of red deer calves during different weaning procedures. *Applied Animal Behaviour Science* **35**, 23–33.

Putman, R.J. (1988) *The Natural History of Deer*. Christopher Helm, London.

Scottish Government (2008) Final results of the June 2008 agricultural census. Available at: www.scotland.gov.uk/Publications/2008/10/agriccensus2008.

Wass, J.A., Pollard, J.C. and Littlejohn, R.P. (2003) A comparison of the calving behaviour of farmed adult and yearling red deer (*Cervus elaphus*) hinds. *Applied Animal Behaviour Science* **80**, 337–45.

Whitehead, G.K. (1993) *The Whitehead Encyclopedia of Deer*. Swan Hill Press, Shrewsbury, UK.

Horses and Donkeys

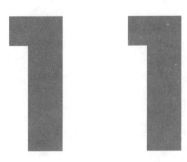

11

HELEN (BECKY) WHAY

11.1 Introduction

11.1.1 The domestication of equids; uses and worldwide distribution

The wild ancestors of today's horses and donkeys (equidae) had unique qualities which led to their domestication; indeed it was the use of horses and donkeys, not wheels, which marked the first significant step in land-based transportation and trading over long distances. Their speed, strength, stamina and ability to cross

Management and Welfare of Farm Animals: The UFAW Farm Handbook, 5th edition. John Webster
© 2011 by Universities Federation for Animal Welfare (UFAW)

difficult terrain while carrying loads or being ridden became pivotal in human evolution. They allowed travel over greater distances, more effective hunting, aiding warfare and trading, changing agricultural practices and social organization. In Central Asia there is a saying: 'the horse is the wings of the human being'. Horses and donkeys appear to have been amenable to domestication, prepared to live in close proximity to humans, showing a versatility and adaptability which probably underpins their unique position in human society today where they straddle the boundary between a working animal and a pet.

The process of domestication began with the use of both horses and donkeys for meat. It is likely that humans began capturing and breeding wild equidae so that their meat supply could be farmed rather than chased. Although it is still not clear how the process of domestication took place, at some point their potential to help with work and transportation must have been recognized. There would have been a transition from capturing and keeping wild animals to selecting and breeding animals most suited to specific tasks such as carrying packs or being ridden. Recently, 5,000-year-old ass skeletons were discovered in tombs adjacent to the mortuary complex of an early Egyptian king (Rossel et al., 2008). Archaeological evidence showed that, although the process of domestication began 6,000 years ago, these ass skeletons still had many characteristics of the wild ass, from which modern donkeys are descended, but showed pathologies and skeletal wear consistent with load carrying. This implied that 1,000 years on from the start of domestication, the selection strategies that led to the emergence of what we now recognize as the donkey were far from complete. It is also worth noting that these asses were buried near an Egyptian king. Archaeologists interpret this as an indication of the ass's importance and status in Egyptian society. The greatest density of archaeological evidence for the process of horse domestication comes from the Ukrainian steppes, again dating from 6,000 years ago. Skeletal remains from as far back as the Copper Age have provided evidence of tooth wear in horses, indicative of the use of bits (Anthony and Brown, 1991).

Domestication occurs when humans take control of animal breeding. Selective breeding describes the practice of identifying particular traits in individual animals which the breeder would like to keep and even enhance in future generations. These qualities might be physical attributes such as strength, height or colour or behavioural characteristics such as a quiet temperament, being amenable to human company, or competitiveness. Not all desirable traits are particularly heritable, and some may have negative relationships with other traits. For example, selecting a mare for good maternal ability might result in the diminution of another desirable trait in the offspring. Early attempts at selective breeding would have been carried out on a trial-and-error basis and learning by experience. However, it is possible to see the routes which have led to the huge diversity of breeds that we see today, with horses (especially) selected for many specific purposes; e.g. pulling, speed, stamina, manoeuvrability, agility and aesthetic appearance.

Figure 11.1 illustrates some of the different types of use to which modern equines are put. It can be seen that these uses range from leisure and sport, predominantly in

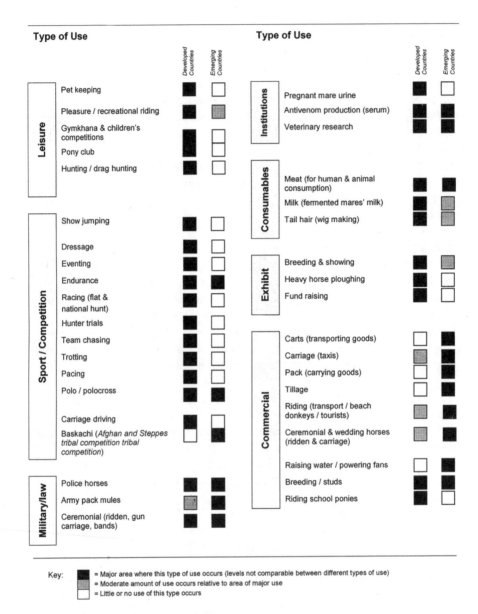

Figure 11.1 Summary of the diversity of uses for domesticated equidae.

developed countries, through to the military and traction work still widely relied on in the developing world. In 1998 the US Congress estimated that 75% of all traction energy in the developing world was provided by animals, rather than lorries, tractors and vans. In times of high global fuel price rises and restrictions on power generation capacity, dependence on animal power is likely to grow and horses are the fastest

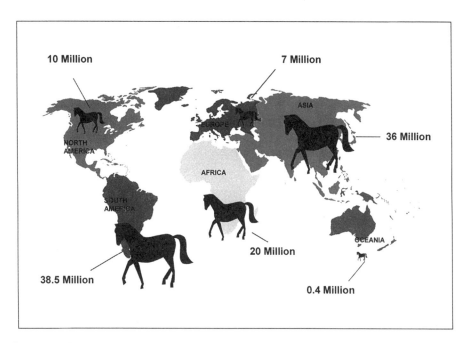

Figure 11.2 A pictorial summary of the distribution of equines (horses, donkeys and mules) across the world calculated from the 2005 Food and Agriculture Organization (FAO) statistics (courtesy of Dr Charlotte C. Burn).

transporters available. Figure 11.1 also lists some more unusual and less widely recognized roles of the horse, such as antivenom production and the harvesting of horse hair for wig making.

The Food and Agriculture Organization (FAO) estimated that in 2005 there were over 112 million equids in the world, the vast majority of which are domesticated. Of these 112 million, nearly 95 million (85%) are to be found in the developing world. Their distribution throughout the world's continents is illustrated in Figure 11.2 where it can be seen that the greatest numbers (38.5 and 36 million) are in Central/ South America and Asia, respectively, while the smallest numbers (0.4 and 7 million) are found on the continents of Oceania and Europe. Table 11.1 divides the count of equidae into horses, donkeys and mules and examines their distribution across continents.[1] From the table it is possible to see that different species predominate in different regions of the world. For example, in Africa there are more than twice as many donkeys as horses (15 million vs 4 million); donkeys being very well adapted to living in the arid environments of this region where water is scarce. In Central and South America 24 million horses predominate over roughly equal numbers of donkeys and mules (approx 7 million of each). These figures clearly illustrate that equids are not only a feature of the developed world but are extremely important in

[1] No count of mules was available for Oceania.

Table 11.1 The numbers of horses, donkeys and mules in the world and their distribution between developed and developing regions in 2005. Source: FAO statistics (http://www.fao.org/corp/statistics/en/).

	Horses	Donkeys	Mules
Oceania	374,657	9,000	-
Europe	6,298,202	653,244	228,503
North America	9,586,060	52,005	32,001
Africa	4,177,841	15,014,947	1,086,771
Central & South America[1]	24,112,558	7,769,956	6,596,912
Asia	14,234,985	17,455,571	4,501,463
World population	58,784,303	40,954,723	12,445,650

[1] Central & South America data includes equids from the Caribbean.

the developing world. In developing countries the majority of horses, donkeys and mules are owned and worked by poor, marginalized and vulnerable people. The harsh position in which people find themselves means that they are often compelled to overwork their animals, leading to many animal welfare compromises and considerable suffering. However, the ways in which we use horses in the developed world can also present considerable challenges to their welfare. It is perhaps for horses in the developed world where there is the greatest opportunity for change and welfare improvement. Far more attention has been paid to the welfare of horses in developed countries compared to the developing world in terms of funded research, scientific publications and textbooks. Very few texts address the special problems in developing countries, still less the special problems of donkeys. This means that much of the information available refers to horses in the developed world. However, throughout this chapter equids from all around the world, performing all sorts of different types of work, will be considered as far as possible.

11.1.2 Equidae in the wild; a reference point for considering equine welfare

In order to consider the welfare of domesticated equidae it is useful to understand something about the behaviours, social structures, feeding and breeding habits of their non-domesticated relatives. This allows us to infer something about how they have been adapted to meet the needs of humans through domestication. It can also highlight areas where the lives of modern domesticated equidae differ so dramatically from the lives of feral animals that we would want to consider what implications these changes might have for their welfare.

The success of horses and donkeys as domesticated animals and the methods by which humans carried out domestication mean that the majority of equine species we see today, with the possible exceptions of zebras, African and Asian asses and Przewalski horses, are descended from previously domesticated animals. The obvious limitation of this is that the wild horses that we might use as our reference point for a 'natural animal' have themselves been modified in some way by domestication. However, observing modern-day herds of wild, feral and free-range horses does give us some insight into how, given some free choice, horses and donkeys might organize their social structures. We can see how they budget their time, protect themselves against predators, communicate with their peers and organize their breeding.

11.1.2.1 Social organization

Horses are extremely social animals that organize themselves into herds, sometimes containing hundreds of individuals. Herds organize themselves into social subgroups known as 'bands' that allow for protection of the young and the breeding mares while ensuring a place within their society for groups of sexually mature males. There is a band which consists of one breeding stallion, some breeding mares and their young. This band used to be called the harem band, implying that the stallion was in total charge of the mares. More recently it has become understood that some mares within the group have leadership roles, so to recognize this sharing of responsibility these bands are now more commonly referred to as natal bands. The natal band is where the main reproductive activity of the herd takes place. The stallion and lead mares have an important protective role within the band, defending the remaining mares and their offspring against other stallions, bands or predators. The young stay within the natal band for between 1 and 3 years, during which time they participate in a considerable amount of play behaviour with their young relatives. As they grow older the young male and female horses begin to form affiliations with yearlings and 2-year-olds from other bands. Eventually, the young females will leave the natal band into which they were born to join or form new ones. Obviously this leaves considerable numbers of males outside these reproductive bands: these males form themselves into bachelor groups which stay on the margins of natal groups. Existing wisdom from the domesticated horse world assumes that stallions cannot be kept within this type of social order without vicious conflicts occurring between the males. There are undoubtedly lots of agonistic and competitive interactions within the bachelor groups but serious injuries are uncommon. Indeed, there is evidence that within the bands, including the bachelor groups, individuals form close relationships with some of their peers, which may involve co-operation to control or manage resources.

The social structures of feral donkey groups are far less rigid and, while they can form family structures similar to those described for horses, if resources are limited then they are equally likely to break away and function as individuals.

11.1.2.2 Feeding and drinking behaviour

Horses and donkeys are by preference grazing animals but they do have the capacity to browse trees, shrubs and woody plants when grazing is sparse or unavailable. Free-ranging populations of horses typically spend between 16 and 17 hours a day grazing, but this may go above 19 hours when forage becomes scarce, and grazing activity occurs at night as well as during the day. In contrast to ruminants, horses can graze for long periods of time without stopping; they can exploit shorter grass than cattle and have also been shown to increase their bite rate when grazing material is in limited supply. Horses move continuously when grazing so that they take a few bites and then move forward to the next piece of sward. These grazing strategies are important as horses are driven to maintain a high level of gut fill. During grazing horses are able to be selective about what they eat; this is important for avoiding the accidental ingestion of contaminated or toxic plants. It also appears that in free-ranging herds of horses social facilitation, or eating in company at times determined by herd leaders, is a cue for eating to take place. The frequency and volume of water drunk by free-ranging horses is determined by the climate in which they are living, the distance between forage and water supply and the amount of work or exercise undertaken. Where water is easily accessible and freely available then horses will tend to drink once or twice a day. Where access and availability of water are limited then drinking bouts may become as far apart as 3 days. Drinking is again a social activity and is also a time when individuals are at high risk of predation. Donkeys are particularly efficient at drinking and then departing rapidly from the watering site.

11.1.2.3 Communication

Much of the communication that takes place among horses is subtle and non-vocal. This is a good strategy for predated animals where efficient passing of information is essential for protection but loud or obvious communications would either draw attention to the group or forewarn predators of their intentions. In addition, many of the behaviours of horses are highly coordinated, for example in observations of Przewalski horses the behaviour of the whole herd was synchronized up to 89% of the time (Dierendonck et al., 1996). These subtle forms of communication are based around body language, olfaction, touch and posturing.

The ears and tails of horses appear to be very important for communication through body language but sounds made by the hooves, such as pawing and stamping, are also mediums for transferring information. Vocal communications such as neighs, grunts, snorts etc are also very valuable tools, although as previously highlighted not always appropriate. Urinary and faecal marking are both used as a means of communication between horses and as a threat to potential predators. Males in particular devote considerable time to this form of communication and the way in which marking is carried out can have ritualized components. Both male horses and donkeys can build up large mounds of faeces as a means of marking territories. Touch between equids possibly serves multiple purposes; mutual nibbling, biting and swatting of flies serve a useful function but they may also communicate bonding and trust between adults or between a mare and foal. Finally, displays and posturing, and approaches and retreats allow hierarchies to be established within groups without resorting to fighting.

The large array of communication tools used by horses and donkeys highlights the social nature of these animals and the importance of communication within their social groupings. This may suggest how much communication domesticated equids offer to their owners who are then not able to respond in an appropriate way.

11.1.2.4 Reproduction

Mares have a gestation period of just over 11 months and in wild or free-range herds the time of foaling would usually coincide with the time of year when the best and most appropriate vegetation is available to support the new foal. Thus most foaling occurs in the spring time. A mare would normally have one foal a year so would come back into oestrus shortly after foaling and need to be pregnant again within 1 month. During oestrus the mare will offer an array of signals to the stallion, who will stay close by, to indicate that she is receptive to mating. Regular repeated mountings occur while the mare is in oestrus; each mounting would be unlikely to last for more than 1 minute and should be a relatively quiet event. In free-range groups parturition will be rapid and the mare will show few signs that she is preparing to give birth until just before delivery begins. Although a foaling mare is likely to be kept away from other herds she may well be attended by other members of her family or horses from her own natal band. Newborn foals quickly rise to their feet and are often ready to run with the herd within half an hour of being born. By the end of the first day of life the foal will already be performing many of the basic behaviours needed for successful integration and communication within a herd; grooming, foraging, vocalizing and playing.

What we see from observing free-ranging herds is that stallions retain involvement in the care and upbringing of foals they have sired. Mares do not necessarily give birth in total isolation, and early and rapid communication is learnt and used by the foal as a necessary means of integrating into the herd.

11.2 Good Husbandry of Domesticated Horses and Donkeys

In broad terms, good husbandry requires meeting the behavioural and physiological needs of animals. This section considers how to meet the needs of domesticated equidae: horses, donkeys and mules. Since most of our knowledge, at least in the developed world, relates to the horse, and many of the principles are common to all equidae, the word horse (rather than equid) will be used hereafter except in cases where the needs of donkeys or mules call for special attention. Horses owned and managed in captivity are completely dependent on humans for the delivery of their needs. This means that there is a requirement to balance the constraints imposed by particular types of animal use against the animals' welfare needs. The equine industries that we see today have grown out of humans identifying a purpose or use for horses (see Figure 11.1) as a result of their adaptability and versatility. This presents us with the challenge of examining their needs and determining whether, in the multitude of 'unnatural' situations in which horses find themselves, these needs are being met.

The first step is to use some form of structured approach to consider the general welfare needs of equids and then to extend this knowledge to consider welfare in the context of specific examples of equine use. A helpful general structure to use is the 'five freedoms' (Chapter 1). In the following sections welfare will be considered using this framework but with specific reference to particular types of equine use.

11.2.1 Nutrition and digestion

Horses need to eat to provide themselves with nutrients to sustain maintenance, work, growth and reproduction, to maintain their overall health and that of their digestive tract; and to provide the behavioural satisfaction that the process of eating delivers. The essential constituents of any diet are water, energy (principally as carbohydrates and oils), proteins, minerals and vitamins. Horses evolved as herbivorous grazing animals but, unlike most other domestic grazing species that obtain much of their energy from the fermentation of plant fibre, they are not ruminants. Their digestive system is described as monogastric. Fermentation of fibre (principally cellulose) takes place in the large hindgut (caecum and colon).

The stomach is surprisingly small considering the large volumes of forage that these animals consume each day. Only a minimal amount of nutrient absorption occurs while food is in the stomach; its main role is to mix the food, begin the process of enzymatic digestion, then rapidly pass the food along to the small intestine. The horse is physiologically adapted to maintain a full (albeit small) stomach, which helps explain why in their wild state horses spend so much time consuming food. The small intestine is largely responsible for the enzymatic digestive process. This allows absorption of proteins and soluble carbohydrates (e.g. sugars and starch) which would destabilize the hindgut. Again the rate of food passage through the small intestine is rapid, moving the indigestible fibrous materials containing insoluble carbohydrates along to the hindgut. The large intestine, also known as the hindgut, makes up about 60% of the horse's digestive tract and comprises the caecum and the colon. It acts as a fermentation vat allowing microbial digestion of the fibrous plant material which leads to production of volatile fatty acids along with vitamins and microbial protein, some of which may be absorbed into the bloodstream as amino acids, although this is not proven. The hindgut also acts as a reservoir and the main absorption route for water and electrolytes which are needed for the maintenance of homeostasis. The water in the hindgut is also important in regulating the transit of solid materials.

Horses are well adapted to utilize forage-based diets and in a domestic situation these are usually presented in the form of grazing or conserved plants such as hay, silage or haylage which is a form of ensiled long-fibre grass. Horses and donkeys can survive very well on forage as a basic ration as long as they have access to water. Stabled horses that have limited access to fresh pasture may also require some form of mineral supplement. When grazing is not available or adverse weather conditions make it inaccessible, then conserved forages are offered in hay nets, mangers or, less commonly, on the ground. Supplying forages off the ground in hay nets and mangers is contrary to the normal grazing posture seen in horses and donkeys, and may have implications for both the behavioural satisfaction an animal derives from eating forage and the efficiency with which the digestive tract is able to receive and utilize the food. There is now a wider acceptance that whenever possible confined horses should be offered continuous access to forage. This is not always easy; in some cases either through tradition, received wisdom, or lack of resources animals still have limited or restricted access to forage during the course of a day. In other situations, owners of animals that are stabled or particularly prone to putting on weight find that they have to restrict access to forage to prevent their animals becoming obese.

Concentrate feeds are introduced into the diets primarily as a source of readily digestible, soluble carbohydrate, i.e. energy. This is sometimes done because the horses are being worked to such an extent that their energy requirements cannot be fully met by the provision of forage alone; in other circumstances limited supplies of forage may mean that it is more practical to feed concentrates. Most concentrates are based on cereals (maize, oats, barley or wheat) mixed with other ingredients such as soya bean meal to provide extra protein, beet pulp or dried grass to provided digestible fibre, vitamins and minerals. They may be sold as simple mixtures ('coarse mix') or in pelleted form. When offered concentrate feed most horses consume it rapidly and there is concern that they derive little behavioural satisfaction from eating concentrates and that such feeds deliver too much energy too quickly.

The most visible signs of inadequate nutrition are weight loss and loss of body condition. When this reaches extreme levels it is accompanied by deterioration in coat condition, a loss of skin elasticity, weakness, depression and compromised immune function. The term 'inadequate' may simply mean a shortage of feed or an imbalance between nutrient input (energy, protein, etc.) and requirements (maintenance, growth, work and reproduction). An entirely appropriate diet for a leisure horse living in a temperate climate doing a limited amount of work would be totally inadequate for a carriage or 'tonga' horse working for 12 hours a day in extremely hot conditions in Asia. Indeed, in some circumstances the level and duration of work performed by these animals so far outstrips their capacity to take in the nutrients they need that owners are advised to feed their animals supplements of oil, milk or cream as a source of energy-dense fats.

Problems can arise from inappropriate nutrition as well as from inadequate nutrition. In common with the modern disease of humans in the developed world, many horses and (especially) ponies can suffer from obesity resulting from a combination of lack of exercise and excessive nutrient intake. This may be coupled with the syndrome that afflicts many leisure horses, a perception by their owners that fat horses are happy, well-cared-for horses and a belief that treats such as polo mints, sugar cubes and carrots will make them happy. The consequences of obesity can be very serious and harmful. Overweight animals are prone to joint, heart and lung problems and it has been speculated that there may be a link between equine obesity and laminitis. Laminitis is an inflammation of the delicate structures that line the inside of the hooves suspending the internal apparatus of the hoof in its position. Laminitis it can cause extreme pain to the animal, may result in lifelong unsoundness and can often reoccur. Obesity in horses and particularly donkeys is also associated with an often-fatal condition called hyperlipemia, where the animal's fat reserves rapidly enter the bloodstream and overstress the liver.

The introduction of concentrate feeds into the diet poses some risk to digestive health. The nature of concentrate feeds means that they can be rapidly consumed rather than 'grazed' in the way that forages are eaten. Concentrate feeds increase the risk of creating an acidic environment in the stomach and have been linked to impaction colic. Colic is a generic term describing signs of abdominal pain, all too commonly associated with domesticated horses. The very long and convoluted forms of the small and large intestines have been implicated as a risk in themselves for colic; in fact, at one point the large intestine folds right back on itself. Colic can take the form of mild through to severe bloating resulting from a build-up of gas (usually from microbial fermentation within the intestines) through to very serious and life-threatening impactions (blockages) or twists in the intestine. Feeds containing large amounts of easily digestible soluble carbohydrates or which break down into very small particles which then have a tendency to clump together are often implicated in colic. Such characteristics can be easily attributed to concentrate feeds. Other well-recognized risks to digestive health include problems with teeth, most commonly overgrowth, as horses' teeth continue to grow throughout their life. The rate of wear of teeth is affected by the horse's diet and overgrown teeth can ultimately cause pain and difficulty in eating. Choke is not as commonly seen as colic but is extremely serious. Horses do not have the vomiting reflex that humans are familiar with; this means that they find it difficult to expel food which becomes lodged in their oesophagus. Insufficient chewing of feed, rapid eating and lack of water have all been suggested as causes of choke.

Welfare is as much about behavioural satisfaction as physical wellbeing. Behavioural satisfaction associated with eating and drinking is likely to have multiple components. As already discussed, the common practice of offering horses forage in hay nets or mangers asks the animal to 'graze' in a manner that does not mirror how it would be grazing in a free-ranging situation. Locomotion while eating and the process of selecting food are also both very important components of the grazing process which are not available to the housed animal. It is difficult to gauge how significant these deviations from the natural grazing behaviours are to horses and donkeys but they may lead to frustration, anxiety or perhaps reduced satisfaction from eating. Observations of horses in the wild show that they expend considerable amounts of their daily time budget on grazing, including time spent grazing during the night. Restricted access to forage will reduce the amount of time the horse is able to devote to grazing each day, so perhaps not surprisingly feeding practices have been implicated both directly and indirectly in the development of behaviours that owners describe as undesirable. One example of an undesirable behaviour is the eating of bedding at night. Greet and Rossdale (1987) suggest that this behaviour may arise from restrictions in the availability of food and fibre, leading to horses consuming their straw bedding, which itself becomes a risk for colic. Owners often seek to ameliorate this problem by changing the type of bedding rather than addressing the underlying reason for the initiation of the behaviour. McDonnell (2002) suggests that the reduction in feeding duration imposed on many domesticated horses is a primary cause of behavioural problems, arising from inactivity or boredom. A final point to consider when looking at behavioural needs of equids, in particular horses, associated with feeding and drinking is the importance of having their herd around them. Many domesticated horses are stabled or tethered in isolation from other animals, and when they do live in groups these can be unstable and not constructed in the way that the bands of a herd would be, for example, mature females and castrated males housed collectively, or breeding-age females housed without a stallion. From the perspective of offering behavioural satisfaction associated with nutrition to horses, it is worth remembering that they are social eaters and drinkers; the presence of their group members offers them protection and security and may also offer cues, i.e. 'social facilitation' indicating when and where to begin eating.

Case study: Elite performance horses: how concentrate feeds affect their lives

Elite performance horse is the collective term describing top-level race horses, show jumpers, event, endurance and dressage horses. They belong to an industry of the developed world and are often worth huge sums of money and represent enormous investments of time and skill on the part of their owners and trainers. The nutrient requirements of performance horses cannot be met from forage alone and so the normal practice is to feed high-quality, highly palatable concentrate diets in conjunction with limited but high-quality, low-fibre forages. There are a number of reported consequences associated with this particularly intensive form of dietary management (Henderson, 2007). It is believed that high-concentrate, low-forage diets make horses vulnerable to gastric ulcers as a result of high gastric acidity. Stomach acid is buffered by saliva which is produced in response to eating forage and consistent gut fill. An endoscopic examination of US race horses in 1996 revealed that 93% had gastric ulcers (Murray et al., 1996). Gastric ulcers are probably painful; they are associated with weight loss, inappetance, reduced performance and colic. The speed with which concentrates are consumed can also present problems for the horse. Despite meeting the biological needs of the animal, the rapid completion of feeding will not address the horse's strong drive to forage over extended periods of time. Simply increasing the frequency of feeds rather than providing continuous foraging substrates does not appear to succeed in meeting horses' psychological needs. A further problem associated with such highly nutritious diets is that they provide horses with greater energy reserves, which often manifests in explosive and volatile behaviour. Not only can this be a problem for the handlers of these animals, but it leads to a reluctance to allow elite horses to mix with other horses because of the increased risk of injury. It is ironic that the management that helps these horses towards their 'elite' status in fact makes them less horse-like than their wild contemporaries.

11.2.2 Environment

Many horse management texts acknowledge that, from a behavioural perspective, horses and donkeys would be better off left outside all year round. This is obviously inconsistent with our aims for these domestic animals. In most practical circumstances it is also unlikely to be conducive to good welfare, since the quality and quantity of the pasture is likely to range from insufficient (leading to hunger and loss of condition) to dangerously rich (leading to obesity and laminitis). For practical reasons, enormous numbers of domesticated horses and other equine species are kept in stabling, or housing, or are restrained in some way as part of the management routine that surrounds them. This is an artificial environment which increases the animals' dependency on external provision of resources; food, water, bedding, light and companionship all have to be brought to them. When considering the welfare of horses kept in these artificial environments, it is useful, first, to consider why this management practice has gained such universal acceptance and then to look at how these environments perform in delivering needs such as comfort, protection and social contact.

In many urban areas of Asia owners can hire a space in a communal stable where the animals are tethered by the neck and/or forelimb and hindlimb in rows, rather like stalls without the divisions. All over the developing world the practice of tethering horses or donkeys, with or without shade, grazing or water, is extremely common. This is in part because many owners are very poor and have no land of their own. Traditional European and North American horse housing designs include single, high-walled loose-boxes with split doors that allow the horses to look out, or stalls in which they are tethered, usually by their halter. There are also more open designs emerging where a group of horses might be kept in a barn with divisions between animals created using bars or poles. The question to ask is: why are horses housed in this way? Eileen Gillen from World Horse Welfare (formerly ILPH) put it very well when she asked: '*Is it because they are in work and clipped out, so that they do not lose condition? Is it because they will poach the ground, causing more work and expense for the human to reclaim good grazing for the summer? Or is it because we feel sorry for them, as they cannot come into the house to sit by the fire so we stick them into a box to make us feel better?'* To add to Eileen Gillen's list, other common reasons given for housing or tethering animals include:

- to make their capture easier or to stop them from wandering off (in Guatemala there are reported incidents of horses breaking free from their tethers and damaging neighbouring farmers' crops, resulting in these animals receiving slash wounds from machetes);
- to bring them closer to make inspection easier;
- to permit controlled feeding;
- to avoid having to carry resources (feed, water, saddles) out to their fields;
- to keep them clean, so they are not wet and muddy when they are wanted for work;
- to prevent conflicts between individuals and to reduce the risk of theft.

The important point to consider here is whether this list of reasons for stabling represents genuine benefit for the animals or greater expediency for the owners.

The comfort of the housed or tethered horse has multiple components. The most immediately obvious is to ensure an appropriate lying surface. A common and popular substrate is straw, but owners also use materials such as wood shavings, wood chips, peat, paper and mattresses. In dry areas, sand or dust is considered satisfactory. In some parts of the world very traditional stable practices are followed whereby horses are tethered by fore- and hindlimb on brick or paved floors during the day and only offered bedding at night. The selection criteria for bedding materials are influenced by their local availability and the ease with which the stable can be cleaned or mucked out. Horses seem to have a preference for straw and, as has already been discussed, they can also eat it. There is relatively little information available about the optimum depth of bedding but it has been observed that, when bedding material is sparse, horses will lie down as soon as new material is added (Houpt, 2001). Comfort for the confined animal is also likely to be influenced by the space available and freedom of movement. Again, reflecting back to the evidence from wild and free-ranging herds of horses, much of their day is spent engaged in locomotor activity, in particular when they are eating. Both tethered and loose-housed horses have their capacity for movement severely restricted. A combination of space allowance and bedding substrate will also affect their capacity to roll. Both horses and donkeys are very strongly motivated to roll and they will try to establish a dusty area specifically to service this need. In stabled animals there is a risk of them becoming cast (stuck too close to a wall and unable to stand up) which can be associated with attempting to roll in a confined space. Further elements of comfort to be considered in a stable, stall or barn are the level of ventilation and lighting, both of which are likely to be altered in some way by the construction of a building.

The tethered horse is obliged to remain in the same space as its own faeces and urine. There are three potential issues arising from this: living among faeces and urine may be unpleasant and have health implications for the animal in terms of parasitic

transmission, raised stable humidity and build-up of ammonia. Stallions in particular use faeces and urine as territorial markers and although it is not proven it must be
considered that they may become confused or frustrated at being unable to position
their markers and move away from them once placed, or alternatively may feel
thwarted by having their carefully placed marks of territory regularly cleaned away.
Finally, horses may perceive that strong concentrations of urine act as an olfactory
indicator of their presence to potential predators.

From a human perspective we see stables as affording protection: from the
weather, from theft, from agonistic interactions with unfamiliar conspecifics and
from potentially injurious grazing environments. These are legitimate concerns
when looked at from a purely human viewpoint. What we also need to do is look
at them from the point of view of the horse. Horses appear to cope better with
inclement weather than we think they do, they are unaware of the risk of theft, and
when faced with any situation they perceive as threatening their instinctive response
would be to initiate flight (run away) and seek the protection of other horses (if
possible). Horses frightened into bolting while out on a hack will attempt to return to
their field mates (Summerhays, 1975). What the stabled or tethered horse seems to
experience is the opposite of what we think we are offering. The confined
and isolated horse is unable to follow its natural instincts for self-protection. At
best it may feel fearful when under immediate threat; at worst it may experience
chronic frustration and anxiety at having its protective mechanisms compromised to
such a degree.

A major welfare consideration for the housed and even paddock-grazed horse is
social contact. It is very clear that horses and donkeys are social animals. Their social
structures help keep them feeling secure and allow them to establish permanent
societies, afford them companionship and facilitate relationships between individuals. Bearing this in mind, it can be seen that keeping a single horse isolated for long
periods in a stable is a complete contradiction of its normal social situation. Mares
held either in confinement with some social contact or in stalls allowing no social
contact whatsoever demonstrated physiological changes indicative of stress
(Mal et al., 1991). Many loose-box stables on yards are designed with split doors
which allow horses to look out and may still affords horses some stress. This may be a
consequence of knowing that others are close by but being thwarted from performing
social activities such as mutual grooming and mutual, head to tail, fly swatting.
Ironically, the converse may also be a source of stress to confined horses; they may
find themselves housed next to animals with which they have no established social
bonds or even have outright animosities towards. Many yards position horses in
ways that offer greatest convenience and access for those looking after them, horses
and ponies come and go regularly and are often popped into one another's stables
when they are unoccupied. Similar problems may be experienced by horses during
periods of turn-out to pasture; there may be a dynamic and changing group of
animals and the balances of males, females and young may be inappropriate for
forming social subgroups.

Stabling is recognized as one of the most commonly occurring risk factors for unwanted behaviours. Unwanted behaviours ranged from 'bad manners', pushing through doorways and fidgeting during mounting, through nipping and biting, to stereotypies. The problem with unwanted or undesirable behaviours is that because the human defines them as a problem they can elicit reprisals, attempts at discipline and even result in equids being frequently passed from owner to owner. These behaviours may or may not be of significance to the animal's welfare in their own right, but how they are perceived by owners can have a very great impact on their welfare.

Case study: Donkeys, horses and mules pulling carts around Delhi, India

There are an estimated 5,000 horses, donkeys and mules working in and around Delhi in India. These animals either pull carriages used for carrying people or carts used for transporting commercial goods; these may be loads of scrap metal, bricks, hides, sanitary ware such as sinks and baths, fruit and vegetables, plastic chairs, filing cabinets or piles of refuse. They are also used to work in brick yards such as the one shown in Figure 11.3. It has been suggested that dense populations of working equidae provide a social environment that

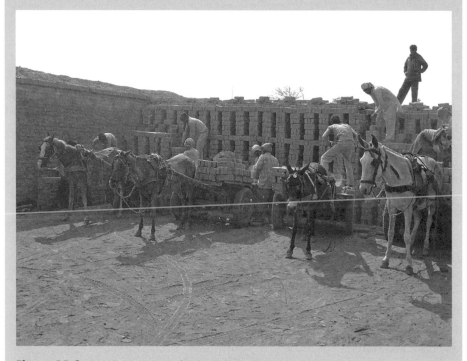

Figure 11.3 Loading carts at a brick works, Delhi, India.

elevates their welfare above that of their European and North American counterparts. Many of these animals work up to 12 hours each day and, although there may be many periods during the day when they are waiting for loads, they are rarely released from the cart. In this type of environment the animals have many, many fleeting interactions with other horses, donkeys or mules each day and will regularly find themselves parked or pulled up beside an animal they have never met before. This constant interaction with strangers may well be stressful in itself. In such circumstances it would be normal for two animals to offer some behavioural signals to one another, take the opportunity to smell each other and generally size one another up. None of this is possible while restrained between the shafts of a cart. In this circumstance some animals may be experiencing regular bouts of fear and anxiety at being presented with strange and potentially threatening animals, many of which are stallions, or the more gregarious may be constantly frustrated at being unable to initiate communication with new animals, or even old acquaintances, that they meet. During the time the horse or donkey is held between the shafts of a cart, this defines its environment and largely reduces its capacity to make choices: to meet other animals, to stand in the shade, to scratch or swat flies, to eat or drink, or to lie down.

11.2.3 Health

The physical condition of an animal is obviously an extremely important component of its welfare. It is the horse owner who has the greatest influence and responsibility in keeping their animal healthy because they spend the most time with it and make all the management decisions that affect its life. When considering animal health from a welfare perspective it is the management decisions that horse owner makes that are of particular interest, although of course, many other groups are involved in and advise on the health care of domesticated equidae including veterinary surgeons, farriers, alternative practitioners, feed suppliers, ayurvedic compounders (traditional healers) and even welfare charities.

In this section the issues that will be discussed are:

- preventive health care (stopping a problem before it starts);
- how modern management and animal use may lead to increased health risks.

To illustrate these points only four 'health themes' will be discussed here although in reality this topic is vast. The themes to be discussed are vaccination; parasite control; lameness; and skin lesions associated with work.

Vaccinations are used to protect individuals against specific infectious diseases, both viral and bacterial. When they are used widely within the population they can help prevent diseases spreading and in some cases have been used to eradicate diseases, such as human smallpox, from regions of the world. Vaccinations are particularly important for preventing infectious diseases for which treatment has poor success. They are made from a killed or weakened form of the bacterium or virus to be vaccinated against. When this is injected into a healthy horse, the horse's own immune system will learn to recognize the virus or bacteria and be able to mount a rapid and strong defence against it if the horse becomes infected at a future date. The most common diseases against which horses are vaccinated in the UK and Europe are tetanus, caused by the bacterium *Clostridium tetani* which lives in soil, and equine influenza, a contagious virus spread in an aerosol by coughing and sneezing animals. Worldwide, there are many other diseases for which vaccines are now available; e.g. equine encephalitis, herpes, strangles, botulism and Potomac horse fever. Clearly vaccination is a critical element of preventive health care. It is relatively easy to implement and does not require drastic changes in management routine. Some objections have been raised against the use of vaccinations on ethical and health grounds and there is a low risk of adverse reactions associated with vaccination, both at the injection site and systemically.

What cannot be in doubt, however, is the principle that preventing a disease or injury before it occurs is always preferable to presenting a suffering animal for treatment. However, it is also important to consider the reasons why a problem is sufficiently severe that preventive action, in this case vaccination, is required. Equine influenza is not a modern disease; reports of horses with flu-like signs have been traced back as far as 400 BC. However, as equine influenza is highly contagious and transmitted via aerosol it is worth considering whether management of the modern domestic equids facilitates transmission of the disease. In other words, is equine influenza a disease that has been allowed to flourish as a result of the way we use and keep domesticated horses? If this were the case then it would spark an ethical debate about the use of preventive steps, such as vaccination, to mitigate for poor animal management practices. In a wild or free-ranging situation, animals would be grouped in herds and would take steps to keep themselves segregated from other herds that would be considered a potential threat. Ever since horses have been domesticated it has been the practice to encourage mixing of animals, to move them from place to place, or even between countries, through competition, work or sale. The ways equidae are now used means that the giving of an equine influenza vaccine is a sensible measure to protect animal health because the way we choose to frenetically move and mix equids seems ideal for encouraging a disease like equine influenza to flourish.

Horses are at risk from many parasites including flies and ticks; however, a particular problem are endoparasites that live in the large intestine, including large and small red worms, tapeworms, roundworms and pinworms (collectively classified as helminths). Roundworms are perhaps the most commonly experienced problem; once in the horse's gut they lay eggs that are flushed out in the faeces onto the grazing pasture where they can survive for a considerable time and infect or reinfect animals that graze the pasture. Roundworms can cause colic, loss of condition and in severe cases can be fatal. Older animals can develop a partial immunity to the worms but young foals are particularly susceptible.

The restrictions placed on domesticated equids increases the risk of picking up parasites (eating grass infected with worm eggs and larvae) because they are not continually moving onto new, fresh grazing land but are often kept on unchanging pasture which can become overburdened with parasites. For a considerable time now a cornerstone of worm management has been the use of anthelmintic drugs (de-wormers), the idea being that the drugs clear the animal of parasites and interrupt the cycle of shedding worm eggs into the environment via faeces. If de-worming is accompanied by separation of the animal from likely areas of worm burden, for example the pasture they have just occupied, this should prevent reinfection and allow time for the pasture to become 'clean' of worm eggs. In many instances it appears that anthelmintic use has not been paired with careful pasture management, perhaps through lack of available land, and a heavy dependence on anthelmitics has developed. There is now evidence that this heavy, and somewhat irresponsible, use of de-wormers has led to parasites developing resistance to some classes of drugs. In a study of equines working in Moroccan souks (markets) it was found that there was no significant difference in faecal egg counts between animals that had been receiving routine anthelmintic treatment and control animals from a separate souk that were not part of the worm control programme. There was also no difference in the body condition score of the two groups, although the raw data showed a trend towards the control animals being in better condition (Wallace, 2003). It is evidence such as this that has led to the suggestion that in some situations animals are able to live in equilibrium with their gut parasites (a form of endemic stability); it is worth considering whether continuous attempts to scour away these parasites make animals more vulnerable to spikes in worm burden when they become reinfected.

Lameness seems to be a curse of domesticated horses. There is plenty of evidence that it is a painful condition, not least because it has been shown to improve following administration of analgesics or local anaesthetic. Lameness is the most commonly reported health problem in horses (Kaneene et al., 1997) and the risk increases with particular work types. Horse racing has long been recognized as being a high risk for limb injuries, a proportion of which are fatal. Among both horses and donkeys working in developing countries such as India and Pakistan, a lameness prevalence of 100% has been recorded, with most animals lame in all four of their limbs (Broster et al., 2009). Horses' feet and legs were well designed for their original purpose but the range of demands that have come with domestication have overwhelmed the initial design specifications of the limbs. Both carrying riders and pulling carts have changed the stresses and strains that act on the limbs. Activities of domesticated horses now include running and jumping to exhaustion when racing, using incredible agility and lift in show jumping, needing extremely controlled and fine movement in dressage, maintaining speed over very long distances in endurance riding, and pulling and turning during traction work. In addition, leisure horses are often worked infrequently and erratically so are unprepared for the sudden strain of enthusiastic exercise. In addition to the problems of pain and locomotor impairment associated with lameness, when treatment is offered the regimens often involve 'box rest', where the horse is kept shut in a loose-box for several weeks to restrict movement and exercise as much as possible. Rest is indeed extremely important for the healing of limbs but, as discussed previously, imposes the stress, frustration and anxiety of isolation on the patient and, ironically, some of the physiological responses associated with stress may in fact slow down healing.

The last health theme to be discussed in this section is skin lesions associated with work. Although not a very widely recognized problem in Europe and North America, it is very much a problem for equines working in developing countries in Central and South America, Asia and Africa. Historically, skin lesions were referred to as harness lesions, inferring that the cause was well understood and related to harnessing alone. This implies that the cause of these lesions is straightforward and consequently so too should be the solution. Although harness design and maintenance are very important, they are part of an interaction with the way in which the animal is driven, the weight of the load it is pulling, the standard to which the cart is maintained, the temperature, humidity and dustiness of the working environment and the general health and condition of the animal. In a recent communication with members of the Brazilian Mounted Police who use well-maintained, well-designed saddles and harnesses, they stated that they found it virtually impossible to prevent their horses developing skin lesions; such is the complexity of the problem. The results of recent work looking at risk factors for tail-base lesions in donkeys carrying tourists in Petra (Burn *et al.*, 2008) indicated rather counter-intuitively that wide, well-padded rump straps posed the greatest risk for causing lesions. Skin lesions are likely to be painful for the animal, they seem to escalate over time if the animal continues to work and have the added annoyance of being very attractive to flies. Skin lesions are not only a function of poorly designed and maintained harnesses but a problem of animals being asked to work in difficult environments and beyond the point where they are able to maintain their own physical wellbeing. This clearly reflects the poverty and desperation of the owners who use these animals, but none the less represents an enormous preventive challenge to be resolved.

Case study: Endurance and performance horses – a problem associated with overexertion?

For a long time it has been recognized that, following bouts of strenuous exercise for training and competition, human athletes become more susceptible to common infectious diseases, particularly upper respiratory tract infections. This problem is attributed to the stress of strenuous exercise having a negative effect on immune function. The levels of exertion demanded of endurance and performance horses and working equidae are comparable to that of human athletes such as marathon runners and sprinters. Many researchers have reported an apparent link between strenuous exercise and the development of pleuropneumonia in horses and these findings have led to further studies of equine immune function following exercise. A study of the effect of exercise intensity using Standardbred horses found evidence of improved neutrophil function following moderate-intensity exercise but a reduction in neutrophil function following high-intensity exercise; a reduction which persisted across 17 weeks of training (Riadal *et al.*, 2000). Neutrophils are phagocytic white blood cells which can consume harmful infectious cells which invade the body. They are part of the first line of immune defence and, although short lived, are very important in protecting against adventitious infections. The implication of this research is that horses' immune function may benefit from moderate-intensity exercise, but high-intensity exercise, which was described as a run to fatigue, exposes horses to an increased risk of infection. This knowledge can now be translated into examining the types of use to which horses and donkeys are put and asking ethical and welfare questions about the level of harm and risk animals should be exposed to, and how this risk can be controlled.

11.2.4 Emotion

It is safe to state, without recourse to anthropomorphism, that emotion – the internal experience of a sentient animal, how it 'feels' – has a significant *direct* influence on welfare. For example, a physical problem such as a fractured limb will be translated into an internal experience. The animal must experience the pain associated with the fracture, finds itself unable to move and then considers the implications of being unable to run if danger approaches. It is also important to bear in mind that in the context of welfare we are not only concerned with negative emotions such as fear, distress, pain and anxiety but also with positive emotions such as happiness, anticipation and contentment. Three illustrations of components of domesticated equine lives that are to be considered here in the context of emotional welfare are the fulfilment of purpose (telos), isolation and human–animal interactions.

Telos is a term derived from the Greek word for purpose and refers to animals being allowed to live out the purpose for which they themselves evolved. The philosopher Bernie Rollin borrowed a line from a popular 1920s musical to explain telos as an animal welfare concept: 'Fish gotta swim, birds gotta fly'. The ethical principle of respect for autonomy (Chapter 1) requires us to allow a horse to be a horse and to 'do horsey things'. This raises some obvious conflicts between the concept of telos and domestication and animal use. Even a horse being galloped across the downs by its rider is being ridden by a human and therefore is less of a horse than a wild animal galloping with its herd. The ethical principle of justice requires us to seek a fair compromise between our needs and theirs. In relation to a horse's emotions it is worth looking at the myriad of constraints placed on their lives by humans and questioning how these constraints (stabling, environment, companionship and nutrition) might affect the animal's emotional state. David Fraser and co-workers (1997) have illustrated the problems faced by animals when they move from a wild state into a domesticated environment. They pointed out that there are some adaptations (physical or behavioural) which were useful in a wild environment but do not serve an important function in their new domesticated role; there are some adaptations that serve the animal equally well in both a wild and domesticated context; and there are demands of domestication for which the animal does not have adaptations. What this suggests is that animals, in this case horses, are likely to experience problems of unwanted adaptations and may well experience frustration and confusion at being unable to use these attributes. At the same time they may also be experiencing a lack of physical or behavioural skills needed to be able to cope in the domesticated environment and with the work given to them. This could not only lead to physical harms but emotional distress at not being able to understand, cope with or adapt to the demands being made.

Periods of isolation appear to be an integral part of the life of many domesticated horses and donkeys, whether this involves living alone in a stable or field, or being surrounded by other animals but isolated by the shafts of a cart or the walls of a stall. We know from their behaviour in the wild that horses are herd animals and would not normally spend prolonged periods in isolation. They also establish relatively stable social groupings so would not normally be subject to constantly changing or multiple transient interactions. Even short periods of isolation (6 hours) appear to evoke behavioural and physiological responses in mares separated from their established social groups. There is most evidence of the harm caused by isolation in young animals. Foals that are kept in isolation from conspecifics run the risk of failing to develop the social skills they will need throughout their lives, potentially leading to undesirable behaviours such as aggression, stereotypies or self-mutilation. In a study looking at the weaning of foals either as groups in paddocks or individually in solidly partitioned stalls, it was found that the weanlings kept in stalls spent more time engaged in aberrant behaviours such as licking or chewing the stall walls, kicking the walls, pawing, bucking and rearing, whereas the paddock-housed groups budgeted their time similarly to feral horses, including showing strong motivations to graze and spend time close to their colleagues (Heleski et al., 2002). A further risk of isolating young animals from their conspecifics is that they form strong attachments to their human owner. This can even reach the level of mal-imprinting where a foal may perceive a human to be its mate. This is potentiallly dangerous for the human but it also prevents the young foal from developing into a truly horsey horse. It is salutary to point out that the two domestic species most prone to behavioural disorders are the horse and the dog, the species that we have forced to become most emotionally dependent on ourselves.

The interaction between humans and their horses is a very important element of equine welfare. Many horses and donkeys are kept as pets and their human owners are looking for an emotional connection and a reciprocation of affection from their animal. This apparent return of affection from animals secures their status within a household and helps ensure their care and protection. Dogs have been particularly successful at learning to offer behaviours that humans interpret as emotions such as adoration, devotion and dependency. Horses and (particularly) donkeys are perhaps less adept than dogs with this skill but clearly form personal relationships with their owners. Humans, however, are inclined to anthropomorphism and attribute complex emotions and thought processes to their animals, who may view their owners simply as a resource and are trying to work out how best to extract offerings such as food, exercise and treats. An example of where this over-attribution of human characteristics can be problematic is in the training of horses and donkeys. Trainers will often make statements such as '*He did that wrong just to annoy me*' when an animal has simply misunderstood the question, or its consequences. Training succeeds when it is consistent, conducted in a minimally stressful environment and is based on an understanding of the way horses learn and communicate. Training exploits the animal's willingness to learn and adapt. It is a good survival strategy for a domestic animal to offer what is asked of it; however, the risk is that humans are inconsistent both in what they ask for and sometimes in what they give in return, both in terms of physical resources and behaviour. A human who demands an emotional relationship with their horse or donkey and then sells it on when it is outgrown, unable to perform at the level demanded or is chronically unwell betrays their side of the bargain.

Case study: Riding school horses and ponies

Riding schools are establishments where a number of horses (and ponies) are kept and hired out to people who would like to ride a horse but may not have the money, resources, time or expertise to keep an animal of their own. Some people will hire an animal to ride out (hack) into the countryside and enjoy the experience of riding; others will have riding lessons where they learn the skills and signals needed to be a successful rider. Riding school horses often work long hours, working for a number of sessions each day. The horses will be ridden by a whole variety of people, with varying levels of competence. The variation in competence of riders means that on some occasions the horse will have a rider who gives very clear signals and directions, while at other times a less competent rider may give very unclear and contradictory signals to the horse. While at work the horse will find itself mixed with different groups of animals for each lesson or hack, and during rest it may not have one fixed stable which is its own domain. It is quite common for riding stables to have fewer saddles and harnesses than they have horses, so that animals will sometimes find themselves wearing a harness that smells of other, possibly unfamiliar, individuals. Clients of riding schools often feel a strong affection for a particular horse within the school and will either request a particular individual for their lessons or ensure that they visit their favourite horse to give it a treat before they leave. The objects of this favouritism are quite likely to find these gifts of affection unpredictable and confusing as they are not necessarily able to recognize the pattern which determines who will offer treats and attention and when this might occur, this can escalate into horses beginning to demand attention from everyone who visits the stable – these horses are then classified as badly behaved.

11.2.5 Behaviour

It is important to understand that animal behaviour results from an interaction between genotype and environment. Genotype may predispose towards certain behaviours but this will only be part of a complex which includes learning, environment and context. For example, a nervous and fearful horse may have had a genetic disposition towards fearfulness but this would not necessarily have resulted in a fearful animal had its training and life experiences acted to build up its confidence. Observation of behaviour is essential for gaining insight into an animal's experiences; it allows us to see what choices they make, what preferences they have, how they spend their time and with whom. However, interpreting behaviour is not always straightforward and sometimes humans can misunderstand animal behaviours. Male donkeys often display a reciprocal biting or nipping behaviour which can be accompanied by quite a lot of squealing and foot stamping. Humans often interpret this as aggression and rush to separate the protagonists. However, if left to themselves the donkeys will carry on with this behaviour for hours, either one reinitiating the activity when it has broken off. They do not cause injuries or retreat from each other and in fact the behaviour is much more akin to play than aggression. Humans often try to stop behaviours as a result of either not understanding their purpose or of classifying them as undesirable or inappropriate (from the human point of view); a playful young horse, excited about getting exercise, might be described as bad mannered as it fidgets and skips about in anticipation of going out. This chapter has used behavioural evidence in many of the welfare problems discussed, illustrating how important a knowledge of behaviour is when considering animal welfare. However, one huge topic of equine behaviour remains to be addressed: stereotypic behaviours.

Stereotypies are defined as repetitive behaviours that have no apparent purpose or function. However, in the context of the equidae, they have also been defined as 'variations on "normal" behaviour, developing as a result of a deficient environment, in which movement, diet, and social contact are restricted'. In this case they serve the very important function of signalling that something is wrong. The topic of stereotypic behaviour is extremely complex and this chapter can do no more than offer some uncertain generalizations taken from research into equine stereotypies, nearly all of which has involved the horse.

A substantial range of behaviours are classed as stereotypic (McGreevy, 2004): these include:

- *oral and head-related behaviours* such as chewing, lip licking, licking the environment, wood-chewing, crib-biting, wind-sucking and head-nodding, shaking, tossing and circling.
- *locomotor behaviours* such as box (or stall)-walking, weaving, pawing, door-kicking with the front feet and box-kicking with the hind feet; and self-directed behaviours such as rubbing and self-biting.

The most commonly discussed and researched stereotypic behaviours are crib-biting, wind sucking, weaving and box-walking. Stereotypic behaviours are often colloquially termed 'stable vices' or 'abnormal behaviours' – terms that reflect how horse owners view them. Traditionally, owners report concern about horses with stereotypies because of reduced performance or work output, reduction in the financial value of the animal and possible associations with health problems including hoof damage, musculoskeletal problems and loss of condition. These repetitive behaviours can also be distressing to watch and can cause costly damage to stabling or fencing. However, the most important reason for concern should be that in some way, either directly or indirectly, these behaviours indicate that the horse is being subject to adverse management factors.

The reported prevalence of crib-biting, wind sucking, weaving and box-walking is between 0.4% and 5% among domesticated horses in developed countries. However, in Thoroughbred horses the prevalence of these stereotypies is as high as 11%. The majority of Thoroughbred horses are employed in the racing industry and are subject to intensive management practices specific to racing yards, so it has not yet been possible to determine whether this higher prevalence is a function of breed or management (or both). It has also been shown that the prevalence of stereotypic behaviours in horses increases with age, which suggests that stereotypies persist over long periods of time, and with time the behaviour may become detached from the original reason it first started. This has implications for curing stereotypic behaviours; despite changing a horse's environment or removing factors that are believed to contribute to the behaviours, the stereotypic activity may not stop because it is no longer linked to the original cause. This is borne out by the evidence that stereotypic behaviours are rarely cured.

Weaving and crib-biting/wind sucking are examples of stereotypies which demonstrate that the underlying causation is not straightforward or universal for all stereotypies. A weaving horse sways its head from side to side, often over the top of its stable door. In some cases the whole body can become involved with the swaying and it is not uncommon to see the horse stepping from one front foot to the other as it sways. This behaviour, along with other locomotor stereotypies, often coincides with feeding time or with a view of other horses being taken out for exercise. This suggests that, rather than a consequence of boredom, weaving is a consequence of frustration; as the horse anticipates walking forward and greeting a passing horse or moving towards a source of feed it is blocked by the stable door. This scenario associated with the onset of weaving is so common that it begs the question: 'Why don't all horses weave?' In a study of foals, Waters *et al.* (2002) found the median age at which weaving began was 60 weeks, long after the usual age for weaning foals. In fact 60 weeks coincides with the time when foals are sold from or moved away from the studs where they were born. This suggests that young horses are vulnerable to 'social disturbance', i.e. leaving behind familiar animals and being put into a new environment where they may feel vulnerable and need to rapidly form a new network of social support (make new friends). This then ties in with these young animals feeling a strong desire to greet other animals on their new yard but being thwarted from doing so by the constraints of being stabled or held in a distant paddock. The 'treatment' of stereotypies often centres on taking steps to physically prevent the activity. In the case of weaving, this involves restricting the space above the stable door to inhibit the side-to-side movement of the horse's head. In practice this is rarely successful as the horse simply withdraws inside the box to weave there instead. In fact, this idea of preventing the stereotypic behaviour as a form of treatment is a matter of considerable controversy. Put very simply, thwarting an 'unnatural' behaviour that arose as a consequence of thwarting a natural behaviour does not make much sense; two wrongs don't make a right.

It has been suggested that stereotypic behaviours are part of a coping strategy designed to reduce stress in circumstances where welfare may be compromised by environment or management. If so, then forcibly stopping an animal from using a strategy designed to cope with problems in the environment, rather than removing the cause of the behaviour, could be exceptionally cruel.

Crib-biting and wind sucking are believed to be closely related stereotypic behaviours. Crib-biting describes a horse which uses its front teeth to grab hold of a fixed object such as the top edge of a stable door, a manger or a fencing rail. The horse then leans backwards while holding on to the object and makes a grunting noise as air passes into the oesophagus. Wind sucking is thought to be an extension of crib-biting where the horse is able to take air into the oesophagus without having to hold onto any kind of fixed object. The environmental risk factors identified for crib-biting include feeding high concentrate diets with associated reductions in provision of forage, and housing horses in stables that do not allow communication with their neighbours. However, this may not be the entire story. Unlike weaving, which begins around about 60 weeks, crib-biting can begin as early as 20 weeks of age (Waters *et al.*, 2002). This puts the timing of crib-biting development much closer to the time of weaning. Weaning, especially abrupt human-mediated weaning, is a stressful time for all young animals and foals are no exception. It is possible that crib-biting emerges as a redirected suckling behaviour, but it has also been linked to the feeding of concentrates at the time of weaning, a food source that would never be available to foals in wild herds. The role of concentrate feeds in the development of crib-biting may be through the increased risk of animals developing gastric ulcers. Over 50% of Thoroughbred foals aged 3 months or less have gastric lesions (Murray *et al.*, 1998) and it is the feeding of concentrates with an associated reduction in forage provision or intake which has been identified as leading to increased gastric acidity and gastric ulceration. Saliva is used to buffer against gastric acidity and in horses this is produced by the process of chewing food. Horses and foals fed concentrates and offered only limited access to forage may not be able to produce sufficient saliva to adequately buffer against acidity in the stomach. So, one hypothesis for the initiation of crib-biting behaviour is that it acts to increase saliva flow, thus helping to counter gastric acidity. As with weaving, a physical means of preventing crib-biting is available. A tight metal collar can be fitted high up on the neck of the horse, which makes the act of crib-biting at best uncomfortable or at worst physically painful. This collar does often succeed in inhibiting the crib-biting behaviour, but as soon as it is removed horses will begin crib-biting again at a higher rate than before the collar was fitted (McGreevy and Nicol, 1998). This suggests that the horse's motivation, or need, to crib-bite was increasing during the time that the behaviour was being thwarted by the collar. This strong motivation to crib-bite also explains the relative lack of success of other radical treatments such as electric shock collars and surgical removal of neck muscles and nerves.

There is also a widely held belief that horses learn to perform stereotypies through observation of each other, although the research evidence in this area is conflicting. The consequence of this belief is that horses with stereotypies may be isolated and kept out of visual contact with their conspecifics. This is a matter of considerable welfare concern, since isolation itself is a major source of distress.

It is clearly better to avoid stereotypic behaviour than to try to treat the problem once it has started. A greater understanding of the risk factors that predispose horses to develop stereotypies and knowledge of the high-risk periods in the horses' life will allow better targeted preventive activities. Once a horse has developed a stereotypy there are alternatives to imposing physical constrains on the animal to try to control the behaviour. Examples include managing the schedule of the stable so that weaving horses are fed first or taken out to exercise first in order to compensate for the factors that trigger a bout of weaving. Horses which crib-bite may be given diets and have forage delivered throughout the day to promote production of saliva. These are not cures, nor are they easy answers, but it is important to remember that wild horses do not have stereotypies. Whether they are indicators of coping or distress, they are unequivocal signs of human failure to match our husbandry to their physiological and behavioural needs.

Case study: Stereotypic behaviour in working equids

There is a general belief that horses and donkeys working as traction or pack animals in developing countries do not develop stereotypic behaviours. If this is true then investigating the reasons for this might shed further light on the causes of the problem in equines living in developed countries. It has been variously suggested that the reasons for this might be that they have considerable contact with other animals, they work long hours so are not subject to boredom or perhaps are simply too exhausted to go to the trouble of performing stereotypic behaviours.

During a research trip to Lahore, Pakistan, in September 2006 to study the behavioural repertoire of working donkeys, a young, 2-year-old, cart donkey was released into a 4 m by 4 m sand-filled pen enclosed with wooden post-and-rail fencing. From the moment the donkey was released into the pen it put its head between a set of horizontal railings and began to weave frantically. After waiting for a while to see whether the behaviour was transitory, it became clear that the weaving was not going to stop. It was not possible to keep the donkey on the study as the weaving masked all other behavioural activity. It was extremely distressing to see an already tired, thin donkey weaving with such vehemence. On talking to the owner of the donkey he confirmed that whenever it was released from the shafts of its cart it weaved continuously; unfortunately this meant it was rarely let out of the shafts. This was a one-off observation and one cannot construct a case around a single event; however it does illustrate two points: (1) that at least one working donkey shows signs of extreme stereotypic behaviour; (2) that researchers, veterinarians and welfare scientists working in developing countries should remain open to the possibility that working equids do show stereotypic behaviours and, if this is the case, we certainly need to know more about them and how equine owners are currently managing the problem.

11.3 Assessing Welfare in Practice

Welfare assessment is a tool used to capture data that can lead to judgements about the welfare of a single animal, a group of animals or even a population. Such judgements are made on the basis of both scientific knowledge and ethical reasoning. In reality an animal's welfare is private and internal to itself. We as welfare assessors cannot know for certain how an animal feels and what it is experiencing so we use indicators of welfare, sometimes referred to as 'proxy indicators' because we are using them as a substitute for actually knowing what the animal is feeling. This section will look at the purpose of welfare assessment and how this can determine assessment structure. It will consider the components to be included in a welfare assessment and how these can be brought together to create a protocol for monitoring equine welfare in practical situations, whether for Thoroughbred racehorses or donkeys working in a brick factory. Finally, it will look at how welfare assessment can link with action for improvements in equine welfare.

The principles that underpin welfare assessment are described in Chapter 18. It is now widely believed that in order to know about an animal's welfare the assessment has to be carried out in the animal's own environment, and that all aspects of its life and welfare should be considered, not just single components. For example, to assess the welfare of a racehorse (or population of racehorses) we need measures to reflect the different elements of its life: yard or stable routine, training and exercise activities, travelling to and from racecourses, and time at the racecourse. We should also review the management decisions that surround the animal: who takes care of the animal and how, what veterinary services are provided and how, who decides what the horse eats, what social contact it is allowed, and on what basis are these decisions made. In addition we should look at the history of the animal: where it has been before, previous injuries, times when behavioural problems began to emerge. The assessment should also give some insight into future welfare and identify future risks. This is clearly a huge task; to make welfare assessment possible some rationalizing of objectives is needed.

If a protocol for assessing the welfare of a horse or population of horses is to succeed, it has to be feasible, practical and avoid infuriating owners and trainers. An essential first step is to ask the question: 'What is the purpose of this welfare assessment, what do we need the information for and how may it be put to use?' The aims may be general or specific. They include:

- Better understanding of the welfare needs of horses and how we can promote them in a domestic environment. Here the assessment would be directed towards consequences of domestication, looking at the lives of domesticated horses compared to their free-ranging counterparts.
- Provision of information for an equine industry, regulating body or policy-maker about specific problems associated with a specific type of use.
- Provision of information for owners about the welfare of their animals. This type of assessment would focus on individual horses or donkeys and the data collected would need to be useful and relevant to the owner, showing them opportunities for improving their animals' lives.
- Assessment of welfare in novel and little-known circumstances of domestication.

An example of this fourth case is provided by the industry to harvest pregnant mare urine, which has grown rapidly in the United States and Canada. The urine of pregnant female horses contains hormones that can be used in the production of hormone replacement therapies for menopausal women. Mares are kept in tie stalls in large barns and their movements are restricted in order to keep them attached to the urine collection apparatus. There has been huge debate about the ethics of this industry and the concerns about the welfare of these mares. In a case such as this, an initial welfare assessment is necessary in order to identify the main welfare issues and this might then become more focused and detailed once the main issues had been discovered.

Any welfare assessment on a specific establishment, be it a racing stable or a pregnant mare serum (PMS) 'ranch' needs to be built into a dynamic programme of welfare control that allows monitoring of a problem over time. The assessment should be sensitive enough to detect changes in welfare and broad enough to monitor whether improving one welfare parameter impacts positively or negatively on others.

Indicators of different types can be included within a welfare assessment. Measurements of the environment can be made; the dimensions of a stall, the thickness of the bedding, the visual range available to the horse, the levels of ventilation and airflow in a loose box, quantities and frequencies of feed given and so on. These are commonly referred to as measures of resource or provision and they help to build up a picture of the life the horse (or donkey) leads. From this the welfare assessor would have to infer how the animal feels about its situation. Further information could be added by interviewing the owner to bring in information about routines, how much exercise it receives, when it has access to companions, problems the owner might be concerned about and so on. Having obtained a record of husbandry (resources and management) it is then necessary to look at the animal itself, using direct or animal-based observations. This will involve measures of the animals' physical state including body condition scoring, counting the number of lesions on the body, examining the colour of the mucous membranes, checking for nasal discharge, looking for signs of limping, and so on. It might involve physiological measures such as measuring heart and respiratory rate, taking blood samples to test for cortisol and catecholamine concentrations, or collecting faecal samples to carry out faecal egg counts to check for endoparasites. The interpretation of these measures should be relatively straightforward. However, the measures that are likely to give the most direct insight into the horse or donkey's internal experiences are measures of behaviour since they are a result of the animal's own decision-making processes. Measures of behaviour might include observing the responsiveness of a horse or donkey to its environment, observing whether stereotypic behaviour is present, testing how a horse responds to a familiar and unfamiliar person, or observing how a donkey responds to being touched. Often a combination of approaches brings the most useful information.

Table 11.2 describes a set of welfare assessment measures made up entirely of animal-based observations. This welfare assessment was used among horses, donkeys and mules working in five developing countries: India, Pakistan, Egypt, Jordan

Table 11.2 Examples of welfare parameters used to assess working horses, mules and donkeys. Source: Pritchard *et al.* (2005).

Observations of behaviour	Observations of health
Alert/apathetic/severely depressed	Mucous membrane colour
Response to observer approach	Lesions at commissures of lips
Response to walk down side of animal	Molar hooks or sharp edges
Tail tuck (donkeys only)	Eyes
Accept/avoid chin contact	Coat staring/dry/matted/uneven
	Ectoparasites
General observation	Diarrhoea under tail
Body condition score (scale 1–5)	Heat stress
	Firing lesions or scars
Lesions of skin and deeper tissues	Tether/hobble lesions or scars
Head	Carpal lesions or scars
Ears	Hock lesions or scars
Neck	Swelling of tendons and joints
Breast and shoulders	Limb deformity
Withers	Cow-hocked conformation
Spine	Hoof walls length
Girth	Hoof horn quality
Belly	Sole surface
Ribs and flank	Gait
Hindquarters	
Tail and tail base	
Forelegs (except carpus)	
Hindlegs (except hock)	

and Afghanistan. The criteria which determined the design of this assessment were that:

- a large number of animals needed to be assessed (just under 5,000) so time per assessment was limited;
- it was not culturally appropriate for observers to visit animals at home so observations of animals were made during work;
- stopping animals during their daily work would affect their owners' capacity to earn money so the assessment had to be for the minimum time possible;
- owner interviews were not possible because too many languages and dialects were involved to get reliable and consistent translation;
- the working animals led such complex lives that the assessment of their environment could not be comprehensive.

The animals in this study were involved in a number of different work types: pulling carts which carried goods or people, carrying packs or being ridden by tourists. From the data it was seen that in all three species 90% or more of the animals observed walked abnormally, between 18 and 28% had serious skin lesions in the region of the girth, up to 88% of donkeys had lesions associated with hobbling or tethering (79% in mules and 62% in horses) and the majority of animals were of low body condition score (either thin or very thin). Behavioural measures revealed that around 10% of all animals showed signs of apathy or severe depression, significantly more animals of all species showed aggressive or avoidance responses to the observers than friendly responses, and around 20% of all the animals avoided being touched on the chin.[2]

These data dramatically illustrate the many problems faced by horse, donkeys and mules working in developing countries. However, expensive horses in developed countries also have their problems, which include high prevalence of lameness and stereotypic behaviours. Many horses and donkeys live in social isolation, exercise is often limited or so excessive that immune function is compromised, and feeding regimes no longer reflect the patterns and time budgets of horses still living in the wild.

Addressing welfare problems of domesticated equidae is a considerable challenge. The result of domestication is that welfare problems, and remedies, are all mediated by humans. So resolving equine welfare problems is about changing human behaviour. The way that humans manage their animals, wherever they are in the world, is a synthesis of cultural norms, experience, learning, received wisdom and trial and error (and is, of course, dependent on income and access to resources). Many aspects of horse and donkey management are based around routines and these routines are often planned to deliver convenience for humans rather than to address the complex needs of the animals. Once routines are established they can be difficult to change, as the following, rather simplistic, example shows. The owner of a horse kept for recreational riding at weekends offers it food twice a day, morning and evening, because he or she has to work during the day to earn money to keep the horse. However, the horse is behaviourally driven to eat forage steadily for between 17 and 18 hours each day, and twice-a-day feeding does not allow this. To accommodate the horse's need the owner might have to travel home at lunchtime to provide more forage and go out late each night to give one last hay-net, hire pasture and spend extra time each day turning out, checking or grooming the horse, and extra time at weekends maintaining the pasture, or employ someone to offer additional forage to the horse during the day. Although all these options would improve the horse's welfare, none are as convenient for the owner as the current routine.

Owners should be aware of the inadequacies of such a routine and consider ways in which it might be improved. They must consider possible alternative strategies, perhaps talking to other owners to see how they have addressed the problem, and

[2] This work was carried out on behalf of a working equine welfare charity, 'The Brooke'; Brooke Hospital for Animals, 30 Farringdon Street, London EC4A 4HH, UK.

imagining how they might find the space in their daily schedule to introduce the new elements to the routine. This should be recognized as a fundamental responsibility of all owners to fulfil their duty of care. For people in developing countries, using horses and donkeys as a means to earn a meagre living, making changes to improve the welfare of their animals may represent the difference between earning enough money to buy food or not.

Figures 11.4 and 11.5 illustrate a project to help working donkey owners in Lahore, Pakistan, make changes to their working practices and routines to improve the welfare of their donkeys.[3] The condition of many of these donkeys is very bad and donkey owners are extremely poor, marginalized and vulnerable. In order to promote improvements in the welfare of these working donkeys, meetings were held with a group of donkey owners who attended on behalf of the other donkey owners living in their communities. The owners identified a set of needs for their donkeys (Figure 11.4). These included provision of resources including food, water, veterinary treatment and opportunities to roll; animal care activities including grooming, washing and hoof picking; guidelines for the working day including maximum cart loads, driving adjustments for poor road surfaces and driving speeds; and guidance on owners' behaviours such as no beating, not putting donkeys in to work until 4 years of age, and resting female donkeys in late pregnancy. Although these needs failed to include such things as behavioural freedom, they became the priorities in order to give control of the project to the donkey owners themselves and allow them to take actions which they perceived as achievable within their own context.

The donkey owners in communities participating in the project were asked to assess how well each of the needs shown in Figure 11.4 was being met for each donkey in their community. To do this a welfare monitoring chart (see Figure 11.5) was set up and the whole community was invited to join in the process of allocating red, yellow or green dots for each donkey in their community to indicate how well each need was being delivered. A red dot indicates that the need is not being met at all; a yellow dot indicates that the need is almost being met; and a green dot indicates that the need is being met completely. This process is repeated on a monthly basis so that all donkey owners can join in and owners who receive green dots can tell others how they have achieved this.

Processes such as the welfare intervention with the Lahore donkey owners are still experimental but they illustrate the effort and imagination needed to bring about welfare change. Although some of the changes identified by the donkey owners may seem modest, once the habit of making changes becomes familiar and the benefits to the donkeys can be seen, the owners will then be more likely to initiate further changes for themselves.

---

[3] This project was commissioned by The Brooke and carried out in conjunction with an Indian development organization called Praxis; Praxis Institute for Participatory Practices, 1st floor, Maa Sharde Complex, East Boring Canal Road, Patna 800001, India.

WATER	The donkey should be offered water 5 times per day and given sufficient time to drink as much as it wants	
FOOD (per day)	10kg green fodder 2kg dry fodder 2kg grain (barley or wheat) 1kg wheat bran	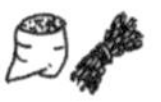
SUPPLEMEMENTS (per week)	50g ghee 25g salt 125g molases	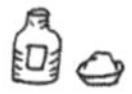
ROLLING	Rolling should be allowed twice a day, morning and evening	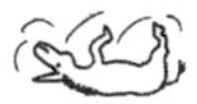
GROOMING	Grooming should be done gently, twice a day, morning and evening	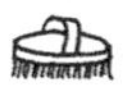
WASHING OF EYES & FEET	Washing of the donkey's eyes, muzzle, face and feet should be done at least once a day in the morning	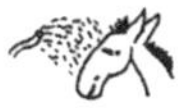
SHADE	When there is spare time during and after work the donkey should be in the shade	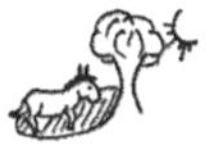
HOOF PICKING	Hooves should be picked out twice a day, morning and evening	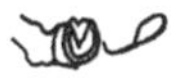
TREATMENT	All problems should be treated in a timely (early) manner	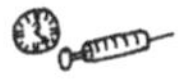
FARRIER	Shoes should be fitted immediately when needed	
HARNESSING	Harnesses should be repaired immediately, should be kept soft and fitted according to the size of the donkey	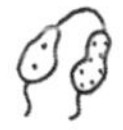

Figure 11.4 Welfare needs of donkeys working in Lahore, Pakistan; identified by owners' groups representing their communities.

11.4 Final Notes

Today's domesticated equidae are important to humans for economic and commercial reasons as well as for providing pleasure to people who use them for leisure and view them as pets. The individual horse or donkey may find itself anywhere

TYRES	14inch tyres should be kept at a pressure of 50psi and 16inch tyres should be kept at a pressure of 60psi 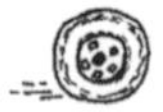
CART MAINTENANCE	Carts should be repaired in a timely manner by an expert cart repairer. Carts should be regularly greased and nuts kept tight 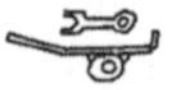
LOADING	Carts pulled by small donkeys should not be loaded with more than 400kg and carts pulled by big donkeys should not be loaded with more than 6-700kg 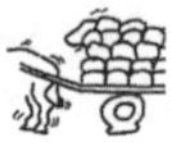
BEATING	Donkeys should not be beaten. Voice or rattle (stones in bottle) should be used instead of beating 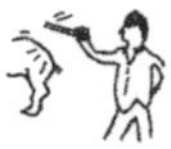
ROAD CONDITION	If the road is in a poor state the cart should be driven slowly and the donkey allowed free movement to pick its own route 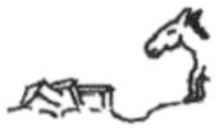
RESTRAINT	No tethering. The donkey should be controlled humanely with no ear twitching, beating or tying up (casting) 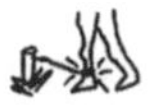
AGE OF STARTING WORK	Donkeys should not start work until 4 years of age 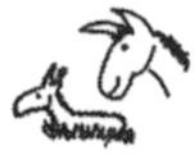
STABLING	The stable floor should not be cemented (katcha), provide space to roll, be clean and have bedding. 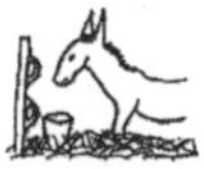
PREGNANCY	Donkeys should not work in the last 3 months of pregnancy and for 1 month after giving birth 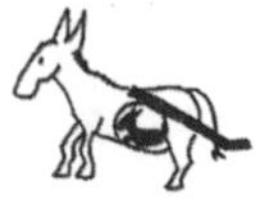
DRIVING SPEED	Drive slowly – Donkeys are not suitable for racing 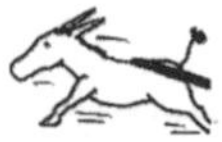
MUTILATIONS	No firing, no nostril slitting, no tail amputation, no ear cutting 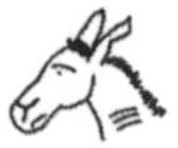
COMPASSIONATE OWNER	Owners should take care of the needs of their donkeys 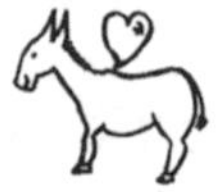

Figure 11.4   (Continued)

	Jugnu		Rocket		Rani		Hira	
Food (fodder plus grain)	◆	○	◆	○	○	○	◆	◆
Water (5 times daily)	✕	◆	✕	✕	○	○	◆	○
Washing (daily, AM)	○	○	✕	✕	○	○	◆	◆
Hoof picking (twice daily)	◆	○	◆	◆	○	○	◆	◆
Loading max 400 kg for small donkeys max 600–700 kg for large donkeys	✕	✕	◆	✕	◆	○	✕	◆
Rolling (twice daily)	✕	○	○	○	○	○	◆	○
Tethering No tethering, twitching or casting	◆	○	◆	○	✕	○	✕	✕

Key: Donkeys (Jugnu, Rocket, Rani and Hira) are monitored each month for welfare according to the needs described in Figure 11.4, and rated using a 'traffic light' system, where green is good, yellow is intermediate and red is bad. In this table red = ✕, yellow = ◆ and green = ○. Owners are given a clear explanation of the reasons for unsatisfactory ratings and advice as to appropriate action.

Figure 11.5 Example working donkey welfare monitoring chart for use on a monthly basis by owners of working donkeys in Lahore, Pakistan.

within a spectrum that ranges from that of loved companion to a mere commodity ('workhorse'). To the horse, donkey or mule, what is important is how our differing perceptions of their use and role are translated into actions that affect their welfare. Across the wide range of uses we find for our horses, ponies and donkeys, a common theme seems to be a continual demand for them to deliver and achieve more. They are expected to run faster, jump higher, live at greater convenience to their owners, pull heavier loads or work longer hours. Domestication is an ongoing process and there is a danger that it is being driven entirely by our needs, not theirs. People who care about horses and donkeys need to have both knowledge of the principles of animal welfare *and* a thorough understanding of how they live. Welfare themes that recur time and again include thwarting of normal behaviours, problems of isolation, risks of inappropriate feeding, unstable social groupings, and health problems associated with overwork. To make judgements about the welfare of horses or donkeys we must integrate information from all aspects of their lives. The huge diversity of roles and uses that they fulfil means that there is no simple single formula for assessing their welfare.

This chapter has considered equidae from all around the world, in acknowledgment of the fact that 85% of the world's horses, donkeys and mules can be found in developing countries. Each region and each task we set our equidae presents particular challenges. Nevertheless, the animals are equally important wherever they come from and all are vulnerable to compromises in their welfare. What domesticated horses, donkeys and mules give to humans through their versatility, adaptability and capacity to endure is truly amazing.

References and Further Reading

Anthony, D.W. and Brown, D.R. (1991) The origins of horseback riding. Antiquity **65**, 22–38.

Broster, C.E., Burn, C.C., Barr, A.R.S. and Whay, H.R. (2009) The range and prevalence of pathological abnormalities associated with lameness in working horses from developing countries. *Equine Veterinary Journal* **41**, 474–81.

Burn, C.C., Pritchard, J.C., Farajat, M., Twaissi, A.A.M. and Whay, H.R. (2008) Risk factors for strap-related lesions in working donkeys at the World Heritage Site of Petra and Jordan. *Veterinary Journal* **178**, 261–9.

Fraser, D., Weary, D.M., Pajor, E.A. and Milligan, B.N. (1997) A scientific conception of animal welfare that reflects ethical concerns. *Animal Welfare* **6**, 187–205.

Greet, T.C.R. and Rossdale, P.D. (1987) The digestive system. In *Veterinary Notes for Horse Owners*, Hayes, M.H.and Rossdale, P.D. (eds), pp. 5–24. Stanley Paul, London.

Heleski, C.R., Shelle, A.C., Nielsen, B.D., Zanella, A.J. (2002) Influence of housing on weanling horse behaviour and subsequent welfare. *Applied Animal Behaviour Science* **78**, 291–302.

Henderson, A.J.Z. (2007) Don't fence me in: managing psychological well being for elite performance horses. *Journal of Applied Animal Welfare Science* **10**, 309–29.

Houpt, K.A. (2001) Equine welfare. In *Recent Advances in Companion Animal Behaviour Problems*. International Veterinary Information Services, Ithaca, NY. Available at: http://www.ivis.org/.

Kaneene, J.B., Whitney, R.A. and Miller, R.A. (1997) The Michigan equine monitoring system. II. Frequencies and impact of selected health problems. *Preventive Veterinary Medicine* **29**, 277–92.

Mal, M.E., Friend, T.H., Lay, D.C., Vogelsang, S.G. and Jenkins, O.C. (1991) Physiological responses of mares to short term confinement and social isolation. *Journal of Equine Veterinary Science* **11**, 96–102.

McDonnell, S.M. (2002) Behaviour of horses. In *The Ethology of Domestic Animals: an Introductory Text*, Jensen, P. (ed.). CABI Publishing, Wallingford.

McGreevey, P. (2004) *Equine Behavior: a Guide for Veterinarians and Equine Scientists*. W.B. Saunders, Philadelphia.

McGreevy, P.D. and Nicol, C.J. (1998) The effect of short-term prevention on the subsequent rate of crib-biting in Thoroughbred horses. *Equine Veterinary Journal* Supplement **27**, 30–34.

Murray, M.J., Schusser, G.F., Pipers, F.S. and Gross, S.F. (1996) Factors associated with gastric lesions in Thoroughbred racehorses. *Equine Veterinary Journal* **28**, 368–74.

Pritchard, J.C., Lindberg, A.C., Main, D.C.J. and Whay, H.R. (2005) Assessment of the welfare of working horses, mules and donkeys using animal-based measures. *Preventive Veterinary Medicine* **69**, 265–83.

Riadal, S.L., Love, D.N., Bailey, G.D. and Rose, R.J. (2000) Effects of single bouts of moderate and high intensity exercise and training on equine peripheral neutrophil function. *Research in Veterinary Science* **68**, 141–6.

Rossel, S., Marshall, F., Peters, J., Pilgram, T., Adams, M.D. and O'Conner, D. (2008) Domestication of the donkey: Timing, processes, and indicators. *Proceedings of the National Academy of Sciences* **105**, 3715–20.

Summerhays, R.S. (1975) *The Problem Horse*. Allen & Unwin, London.

van Dierendonck, M.C., Bandi, N., Batdorj, D., Dügerlham, S. and Munkhtsog, B. (1996) Behavioural observations of reintroduced Takhi or Przewalski horses (*Equus ferus przewalskii*) in Mongolia. *Applied Animal Behaviour Science* **50**, 95–115.

Wallace, A.G. (2003) *Assessing the Efficacy of an Anthelmintic Programme on the Health and Welfare of Working Equines in Morocco*. Available at: http:www.taws.org (accessed 28 October 2008).

Waters, A.W., Nicol, C.J. and French, N.P. (2002) Factors influencing the development of stereotypic and redirected behaviours in young horses: findings of a four-year prospective epidemiological study. Equine Veterinary Journal **34**, 572–9.

Farmed Fish

12

TONY WALL

Management and Welfare of Farm Animals: The UFAW Farm Handbook, 5th edition. John Webster
© 2011 by Universities Federation for Animal Welfare (UFAW)

12.1 Introduction

Controlled fish culture probably originated many centuries ago in China and the Far East. The culture of salmonid fish is relatively more recent, beginning during the nineteenth century to enable the stocking of fish into rivers for anglers. The farming of rainbow trout (*Onchorynchus mykiss*) for human consumption was pioneered in Denmark. This practice has developed throughout the United Kingdom during the twentieth century, resulting in the relatively stable production we see today. Atlantic salmon (*Salmo salar*) farming using sea cages to on-grow fish to market weight is a relatively recent development that has grown rapidly over the last 40 years, and continues to expand. Chile is now the biggest producer of farmed salmon (both Atlantic and coho) followed by Norway, Scotland and Ireland, all of which produce only Atlantic salmon.

The development of these industries in the UK has corresponded with a demand for the relatively high-value fresh and smoked products, both within the UK and in northern Europe. Increasing production and more widespread availability, coupled with public demand, has led to a gradual but substantial reduction in the market price. Although the European market has continued to increase steadily, the rapid increase in production, particularly in Atlantic salmon, has led to a search for new markets, mainly in North America and Japan. Production methods and efficiencies have improved dramatically in tandem with reducing market prices, in order that the industry maintains its profitability.

12.2 UK Farmed Fish Production

While rainbow trout production in the UK remains relatively stable, Atlantic salmon production is predicted to grow at an annual rate of 7% until 2011. Further increases in production will be achieved, mainly by improved survival and performance, rather than a straightforward increase in numbers of fish. The majority of salmon and trout production in the UK is sold fresh or smoked. Rainbow trout, brown trout and sea trout are also grown for restocking (put-and-take fisheries) as well as for rivers and lakes. Pilot schemes and small-scale projects for the farming of other species, such as cod, turbot, halibut, carp, barramundi and tilapia, are also part of the UK aquacultural effort. With the exception of cod, which is slowly increasing, they do not contribute significantly to national aquacultural output in terms of tonnage. Farming some of the marine species such as cod and halibut can be challenging because the small size of the egg with a limited yolk sac reserve makes it difficult to establish the free-living larvae.

With the constant pressure on market prices, more effort to improve quality of the final product has been focused on fish husbandry and feeding. Maintaining high standards of water quality has led to improvements in the environment of the fish. Some selection and stock manipulation programmes are in use, to improve health status and production efficiency. These include:

- programmes to select stock lines for particular purposes (e.g. low or late sexual maturation, increased growth and efficiency of food conversion);
- the use of all-female stocks, especially in the rainbow trout industry. Females tend to become sexually mature later than their male counterparts so the use of all-female fish will delay this maturation that can cause a deterioration in flesh quality and is to be avoided;
- manipulation of photoperiod and temperature regimes, in order to allow extension of the spawning season, accelerated egg incubation and in Atlantic salmon to induce early or late smoltification;
- initiatives looking at disease resistant stocks. These are at an early stage.

These programmes will allow the industry to exert greater control over production targets so that fish of appropriate size and quality can be supplied to the market all year round. The life cycle of most fish (from egg to mature broodstock) is usually about 2 to 3 years. This relatively long cycle will necessarily mean that selecting for specific traits will take some time.

12.3 Biology and Reproductive Physiology

12.3.1 Atlantic salmon: in the wild

Atlantic salmon can be found occurring naturally in most rivers bordering the Atlantic in the northern hemisphere. The majority of populations are migratory – hatching in fresh water, migrating to the sea and back to fresh water in order to complete their (anadromous) life cycle. Because the natural range of Atlantic salmon is so great, conditions under which they develop in fresh water also varies, particularly with respect to light and temperature. This results in very different growth rates and times spent in fresh water before migration to the sea. In the wild, at the onset of sexual maturity salmon return and collect in coastal waters and estuaries before moving upstream, towards the spawning beds where, in the majority of cases, they have spent their own first few months of life. Fish can begin returning to the rivers up to 12 months before spawning commences, usually from October to January. Spawning takes place in suitable conditions, often in the tributaries of the main river. In order that the eggs have the best chance of survival they need to be laid in clean gravel of the correct size and depth with no silt, so that the river water is able to flow through the substrate as well as over it. The hen fish will then excavate a trench or 'redd' using her fins to displace gravel downstream. Once the redd is the correct size the male moves alongside the female and fertilizes the eggs as they are laid. All the eggs are not laid at once but in a succession of redds moving upstream, the material from the excavation of one redd covering the previous one downstream; the final redd contains very few eggs. Spawning is usually completed in 2 or 3 days but can take longer at lower temperatures. On average the female will produce about 1,200 eggs per kilogram bodyweight.

Development time for the egg varies according to water temperature. It takes approximately 500 degree-days (i.e. 50 days at 10 °C or 100 days at 5 °C) from newly fertilized (green) egg to hatch. The newly hatched fish, or alevin, at this stage continues to feed on the reserves on the yolk sac until it is fully absorbed, and until the mouth and digestive system complete their development. During this time the alevin remains among the gravel which provides it with support and protection. As the last of the yolk sac is absorbed the fish moves out of the gravel and begins to feed. Zooplankton now form the basis for the diet of the young fry but as the fish grows the diet changes to become almost exclusively aquatic insect larvae. The parr (see Figure 12.1) spend between 1 and 8 years in fresh water before undergoing physiological and behavioural changes prior to migration to the sea in May or June. These time differences are due in part to the supply of feed available for the developing young salmon. The average for fish in the British Isles would be 2 years with a survival rate of about 5–10% from egg to smolt.

Once the fish leave fresh water much less is known about where they go or on what they feed. It is probable that movements of the fish are to a large extent dependent on where the food species are, salmon having been caught along the edge of the Arctic pack ice and into the Labrador Sea. Some populations remain relatively close to home; for example the Swedish, Finnish and Russian stocks in rivers which drain into the Baltic tend to remain there. It is thought that initially they feed on shrimp and krill but, as they grow, fish are increasingly included in their diet, particularly the fattier species.

Salmon may return to spawn in their native river after only one winter at sea; most of these fish are male and known as grilse. The majority return after two or three winters at sea but can remain at sea for up to 5 years. During the spawning migration

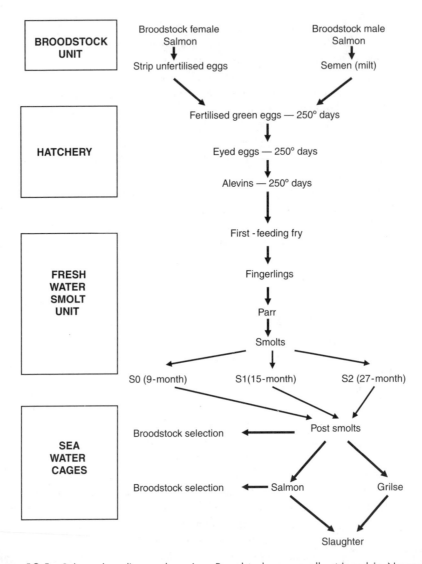

Figure 12.1 Salmon breeding and rearing. Broodstock are usually stripped in November/ December. However fish are now being photo-manipulated to produce 'out-of season' fish. This facilitates the production of S-zero smolts which are also photo-manipulated. This helps to reduce peaks and troughs in the production cycle.

to their home rivers the fish mobilize the fat reserves in their flesh for gonad development. During this development the pigment in the flesh is also redistributed and is used, particularly in egg production, resulting in a reduced colour in the flesh of the fish. The fish, particularly the male, undergo external changes when a large hooked lower jaw or kype develops. Once spawned, only about 5% of the fish will survive as kelts to spawn again on another occasion.

12.3.2 Atlantic salmon: on the farm

Atlantic salmon are now extensively cultivated in Norway, Chile, Canada, Scotland and Ireland where the colder water temperatures make it ideal for rearing this species. In order that this can be achieved profitably, a number of changes have been made to their natural life cycle, the fundamental change for farmed fish being that they are now confined within various tanks and pens. It is possible, with the correct feed and manipulation of their environment, to produce a fish of about 3 kg in 2 years (from egg to market) where it would have probably have taken 4 years at least to grow to this size in the wild.

Manipulation of the salmon begins as soon as the egg is stripped from the hen, with the selection of milt (sperm) used to fertilize it. The farmer can either use milt from his own stock or from sources outside his farm. As well as the selection of desirable production characteristics such as fast growth and low maturation, the overriding consideration for selection of gametes will always be sourcing them from disease-free parents.

A continuous production of optimally sized fish for market must be ensured. The farmer has to decide under what conditions to cultivate the eggs. Should they be heated or left to develop under ambient water conditions? This will determine when they hatch, so that it is possible to obtain batches of fry at different development points from the same eggs. As the fry grow and become parr it is also possible, once they have reached a critical size, to manipulate their photoperiod in order to induce early smoltification. Using this method smolts can be produced that are ready for transfer to sea in less than a year, traditionally known as S-zero smolts. Once smolted, the fish are transferred to seawater where they are on-grown on floating pens. Light manipulation during the first winter at sea is becoming increasingly common, to delay maturation. As well as being an advantage from a production perspective, this delay in maturation has welfare benefits as it will result in less grading, which always has the potential to damage fish.

Broodstock are usually selected either by line breeding or more commonly by mass selection. In mass selection the broodstock were often chosen by selecting the fastest-growing fish. Nowadays there is more interest in low-maturing and disease-resistant lines. Broodstock salmon receive no special attention other than that after selection they may be kept at a lower stocking density than market fish and at the onset of maturity receive a supplemented diet.

Survival rates in farmed stocks are much higher than those in the wild, with probably a 10% loss from egg to fry and a further 10% from fry to smolt. Survival at sea in farmed salmon is now in the region of 90–95% of the smolt input. There has been a significant improvement in survivability over the last few years, mainly due to the improved husbandry practices and the advent of vaccines against some of the major diseases that commonly afflict salmon in the seawater phase of the life cycle.

12.3.3 Rainbow trout

Rainbow trout are farmed over a wider geographical area than salmon, reflecting their greater tolerance to warmer water temperatures than salmon. Although there are strains of rainbow trout that naturally migrate to sea in North America as steelheads, the farming of these fish is usually confined to fresh water, grown to a market weight of about 500 g. (There are a few larger rainbow trout grown in the sea, especially in the brackish water of the Baltic.)

The life cycle is essentially similar to salmon with a high survival rate from egg to hatch, a reflection of the large egg size and plentiful yolk sac reserve.

12.3.4 Cod

The life cycle of the cod (*Gadus morhua*) takes place entirely in seawater. The egg incubation unit and hatchery will be land-based, with seawater pumped ashore. There have been encouraging developments in cod farming over the past few years especially, achieving more consistent results in the hatching and rearing of the juvenile stages. As the larger fish approach market size there can be some husbandry challenges often related to handling and crowding.

12.4 Feed and Nutrition

All fish farmers now use commercial 'dry' pelleted diets, formulated by large feed companies, tailored specifically for the fishes' needs throughout the production cycle. Much research and development has taken place in dry feed production, resulting in diets that now enable farmers to achieve rapid growth rates throughout the production cycle, at feed conversion rates that can be close to 1 : 1. (This often quoted ratio can be a little misleading as it relates to wet weight of fish in relation to the dry pellet.) Feed remains the largest variable cost to the farmer, thus fish farmers need to maintain the most efficient conversion rates to remain profitable. The feed is mainly derived from fish meal containing protein and oil. Most farmed fish are carnivorous and are not capable of digesting and metabolizing large amounts of carbohydrates. Fish meal is an expensive source of protein, and alternate sources are being investigated, especially the use of soya and other plant proteins. This is necessary work, as removing fish products from the sea to feed farm fish may not in the long term be sustainable. In the past, fish feed was supplemented with pig and poultry bloodmeal. This well-balanced and rich source of protein is no longer used due to perceptions (probably erroneous) of a risk to public health.

Oil levels from which the fish derive most of their energy source (high-energy diets) have risen over the last few years to up to 40% of the total diet. These oils have a protein-sparing effect, leaving the available proteins to be used for body growth rather than as an energy source. Rapid growth using high-energy diets does not seem to have consequences on flesh quality in market size fish, although the whole on-growing period must be evaluated to achieve good flesh quality, rather than just the last couple of weeks.

Although feeding by hand is still carried out, most salmon farms and even some larger trout farms are fed automatically, with the timing and amounts fed being controlled by a computer program. Often this system is connected to a sensor that will detect when the fish are satiated and the food is not being eaten. In other cases cameras are permanently in place to allow the stockpeople to view the feeding fish and can override the feeding regime if necessary. These technological innovations are very valuable to observe these farmed animals, often in a hostile and difficult three-dimensional environment.

It is usual to feed larger fish in 'meals' rather than continuously adding feed in small amounts. This method of introducing large numbers of pellets in a short time gives all the fish a chance to eat to get their share – rather than just the larger, more aggressive ones. This will help to reduce the size variation that can lead to an increasingly wide bimodal population resulting in increased aggression from the larger fish as well as the need for more grading with the potential for physical damage. Smaller fish, especially fry and first feeders, are usually fed *ad libitum* via automatic feeders.

12.4.1 Withholding feed

Fish may need to have their food withheld for a period of time for various reasons. Prior to a bath treatment (fish are bathed in a solution of medicine, usually to treat ectoparasites or superficial infections), handling or vaccination, fish may be given no food for 1 to 3 days (often depending on water temperature). This strategy helps to decrease the metabolic rate of the fish and reduce the bacterial loading from both food and faeces in the water. In addition, most fish will be starved to empty the gut prior to slaughter. This is necessary to ensure that there is minimal contamination of the flesh with gut contents. Gut emptying time will depend, like much else, on the metabolic activity of the fish, which in turn is related to the surrounding water temperature. In practice it will only be necessary to withhold food for 1 to 3 days to ensure gut emptying.

The old practice of withdrawing food for 2 to 3 weeks prior to slaughter in the hope of improving flesh quality has been shown to be fallacious, as well as having possible negative welfare implications. These animals have been accustomed to regular daily meals throughout their life. It would seem reasonable that withdrawal of food for a long period of time would have an adverse affect on welfare of the fish and indeed goes against one of the five freedoms, around which the cornerstone of all animal welfare is evaluated.

Some large salmon cages (Figure 12.2) may contain more fish than are destined to be harvested at one time. This can lead to the whole cage being starved for an extended period until all the fish are removed and killed. To some extent this has been addressed by the use of wellboats that have the ability to remove all fish from even the largest cages and thus transporting them to a harvest station/processing factory (see Section 12.9).

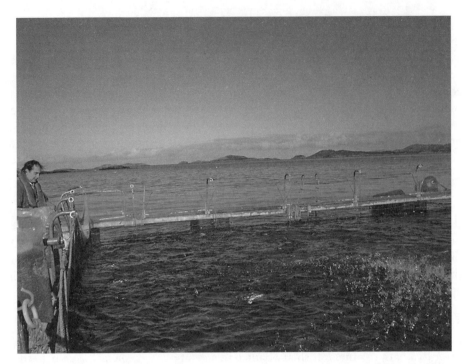

Figure 12.2 Salmon in sea cages being fed by hand. This method provides a good spread of feed and ensures that all fish get a ready supply of pellets. As cage sizes enlarge and the amount of feed that needs to be given every day increases, more farms are using automated feeding systems. This presents new challenges, especially ensuring that all fish are given an adequate ration and that the observation of the stocks is not neglected.

12.5 Environment

Most fish spend all their life in water. This has the advantage of providing the fish with support, making it relatively weightless. However, as the fish is so intimately surrounded by its environment any adverse changes in water quality can be much more serious than similar changes for terrestrial animals. These adverse changes may be caused by external factors such as pollution in the water body, or related to the fish farm itself. For example, water quality will deteriorate rapidly in the presence of excess food or faeces from the fish farming operation.

Some species of fish will tolerate poorer water quality than others. Typically carp can survive and grow well in water conditions that would kill most salmonid species. Similarly eels have the ability to grow well at much higher stocking densities than most other species of farmed fish, partly due to their tougher/thicker skin and also because of their ability to tolerate relatively poor water quality and lower oxygen levels. Individual parameters to measure water quality can rarely be made in isolation. Temperature, oxygen, ammonia, carbon dioxide, suspended solids and pH all modify each other in their effects on the fish.

12.5.1 Temperature

The body temperature of poikilothermic fish is about 1–2 °C higher than the water temperature. Any increase in water temperature will elevate the metabolic rate of the fish, which will in turn increase appetite (and excretory products), and so the demand for oxygen will be correspondingly greater. Conversely, at higher temperatures the oxygen-carrying capacity of the water decreases. This is exacerbated by the elevated levels of food and faeces, which will further increase the demand for oxygen (the biological oxygen demand). Achieving an optimal balance between high growth rate and good water quality, often at high temperatures, is a tightrope that the fish farmer must often walk. The problem can be highlighted in rainbow trout, which are much greedier than Atlantic salmon. Whereas Atlantic salmon will often naturally reduce their feeding levels at very high temperatures (usually over 19 °C), rainbow trout will eat to excess. At these high temperatures and low dissolved oxygen levels the increased demand for oxygen by the trout to metabolize this food cannot be met and death from anoxia may ensue.

12.5.2 Carbon dioxide

High levels of dissolved carbon dioxide (>10 ppm), especially at low pH, can cause problems with oxygen uptake. Elevated levels are often found in borehole water and some recirculation systems where the carbon dioxide is not blown off. Non-specific symptoms of poor growth in the fish can sometimes be the only clue to the problem. High levels of carbon dioxide in fresh water can lead to nephrocalcinosis where calcium carbonate formed by the disassociation of the gas in the water is deposited in the kidney.

12.5.3 Ammonia

The non-ionized form of ammonia is toxic, causing gill, liver and kidney damage. This toxicity is increased at higher temperatures and higher pH. The build-up of ammonia is more likely in recirculation systems, where the biological filtering may be inadequate and fails to convert the ammonia into the less toxic nitrite and nitrate. Ammonia can occasionally reach toxic levels from pollution of the incoming water, usually caused by agricultural run-off.

12.5.4 pH

Water that has been collected from peaty areas or run-off from snow melt will naturally have a low pH. The optimum pH for most species is between 6.0 and 8.5; outside this range, direct toxic effects can occur and stress levels will be high. Low, acidic pH can cause primary gill damage and is more common than excess alkalinity. In addition, acidic water can make some metals, especially aluminium, available to the fish in a more toxic form.

Table 12.1 Guidelines for acceptable water standards as specified by the RSPCA Freedom Food Scheme for farmed salmonids.

Parameter	Eggs	Alevins	Parr/Smolts	Seawater
Oxygen	7 mg/L	7 mg/L	7 mg/L	6 mg/L
Free ammonia	N/A	<0.025 mg/L	<0.025 mg/L	N/A
Carbon dioxide	N/A	<6 mg/L	<10 mg/L	N/A
Max. temperature (°C)	8	10	16	N/A
Minimum temperature (°C)	1	1	N/A	N/A
pH	5.5–8	5.5–8	5.5–8	N/A

Water quality parameters must not be evaluated in isolation. There is an intimate connection between temperature, dissolved oxygen, pH and ammonia and they all tend to modify each other. The condition of the water will largely determine the health or otherwise of the fish. Poor water quality associated with high levels of suspended solids can cause gill diseases, predisposing to other conditions such as bacterial and parasitic disease. Table 12.1 summarizes the guidelines for water quality set out by the RSPCA Freedom Food scheme. Although these standards are more demanding than those operating on many commercial units, they are realistically achievable.

12.5.5 Recirculation systems

In some freshwater systems the limiting factor for the biomass of fish produced is the volume of water available. However, it is possible to reuse water in a recirculation system using only 10% or less of new water from the outside source.

These systems involve mechanical filtration to remove gross particulate matter, biological filters to remove the nitrogenous waste as well as ultraviolet sterilization of the top-up incoming water. This system must be accompanied by a high level of stockmanship to avoid the build-up of pathogens and waste products. Such systems can make any chemical or antibacterial therapy problematic as this may destroy the bacteria necessary for proper functioning of the bacterial filter. Nevertheless, as water availability become increasingly fought over by conflicting interests, there are going to be more and more recirculation systems in land-based hatcheries, not only to maximize the use of water effectively but also to limit the environmental impact of the farm on the neighbouring water systems.

12.5.6 Oxygenation and aerators

Previously these systems were used mainly for emergencies such as when fish were crowded or there were water shortages, high temperatures, chemical treatments and during transport. Nowadays oxygen is routinely provided through micro-diffusers in many freshwater production systems. Aerators will provide some oxygen and will have the additional advantage of stripping both carbon dioxide and ammonia from the water, which is especially useful during transport.

12.5.7 Regulation

The biomass of fish, levels of food and faeces in the water as well as other environmental impacts are monitored routinely by the environmental protection agencies. These regulatory bodies control the discharge of effluent from a fish farm into the watercourse. They are also responsible for granting consents to discharge any medicines or chemicals that may be used for the treatment of the fish.

12.6 Fish-Keeping Systems

Aquaculture systems, compared with terrestrial ones, are usually three-dimensional. Fish do not just live side by side but above and below one another. This can make observation of fish stocks particularly difficult. Indeed it is quite possible that some fish in a large marine cage are never seen until slaughter.

12.6.1 Freshwater systems

12.6.1.1 Hatcheries

Salmon and trout eggs are usually reared in trays. The eggs are poured into these aluminium trays in a layer one to two deep. The trays have a perforated aluminium base through which the hatched fish, or alevins, can swim, ending up below the egg tray. These trays are usually stacked in layers, the water flowing over the eggs and down into the egg trays below. The eggs are kept in the dark or in very subdued lighting that will mimic the natural conditions found in the gravel redd in the river. As the tray can easily be removed for inspection, any dead eggs, which can be readily identified by their whitish opacity, can be picked out.

In larger hatcheries eggs may be incubated in large jars up to a metre high. The water is introduced at the bottom, rising through the column of eggs. While this method can save space and time, dead eggs cannot be removed, predisposing to fungal infections in the adjacent healthy eggs. The use of prophylactic antifungal agents was usually necessary to maintain this system but these are being used less and less because of increasing restrictions on use of some traditional antifungal remedies. Halibut, turbot and cod eggs are naturally planktonic (freely floating in the upper layer of the sea) and are incubated on the farm while suspended in the water column. Here, good water quality is very important; often this water is filtered and sterilized before being used again in a recirculation system.

12.6.1.2 First feed and fry rearing systems

The salmonid species produce large eggs which in turn produce large alevins. The development of these larvae is relatively uncomplicated. After swimming through the egg tray the alevins settle on the bottom of the tank, where they remain relatively immobile until most of the yolk sac is absorbed. Some substrate, either gravel or more usually a type of plastic imitation grass similar to Astroturf, is used to give these fish protection at this early stage. Once the fish have absorbed most of the yolk sac they will start to 'swim up' through the water column in search of food. The timing of the introduction of food to these fish is critical and requires a high level of stockmanship. Feed them too soon or too much and the waste food builds up, with a reduction of water quality, often leading to secondary gill disease. Start feeding too late and the fish do not have the energy to apprehend or metabolize the food – leading to emaciated 'pin heads' – typically a long thin body with a big head.

Cod, turbot and halibut larvae require live food as their first feed. Hatchery units usually include facilities for the culture of live food such as rotifers, artemia and copepods, which are themselves fed on algae specially grown in the hatchery. The rearing of the larvae is difficult and the techniques used are still being developed. Subdued lighting is essential at this stage to prevent aggression and cannibalism, especially in cod. The usual large losses that occurs in the eggs and larvae of these species is compensated for by the very large number of eggs produced by the female. However, there is still the potential welfare issue related to the loss of large numbers of small fish.

12.6.1.3 Fingerling and smolt systems

These systems can vary depending on the species involved as well as the type of water available. Most salmon and trout are reared from fingerling onwards in either circular tanks or freshwater cages. The tanks used vary in diameter from 2 m to 10 m, with a peripheral inlet of water. The angle of the inlet pipe can be varied to control the speed of water flow in the tank. The outlet is a screened central pipe where any dead fish can be collected. These tanks are usually shaded as most fish will naturally seek shade, but also to reduce the levels of stress associated with human beings, birds, and so on. The disadvantage to covering the tanks is that it can make observation of the fish more difficult. Such tanks can have a high capital cost compared with the alternative freshwater cages but offer the advantage of a more controlled environment. Observation of the fish is easier and both treatments and mortality removal are not as dependent on the weather as with freshwater cages. In addition, one of the biggest risks of freshwater cages is the possibility of spread of infection from wild fish in the same water body to the farmed fish.

Freshwater cages are used in smolt production, often for the 6 months before smolt transfer. Notwithstanding some of the difficulties of managing this system, these fish often grow extremely well and tend to adapt more quickly to the marine cages than their tank-reared counterparts.

Rainbow trout are usually on-grown in raceways or rectangular earth ponds. In both these systems water is introduced at one end, the outlet situated at the other, thereby operating a continuous flow-through system. (The use of static water systems does not produce a high enough water quality for salmonids – although a static system is often used for channel catfish and carp.) It can be difficult with raceways and earth ponds to get a good flushing effect. Failure to achieve this can result in an accumulation of faeces and uneaten rotting food. Raceways are often constructed of concrete, which can abrade the fins and skin. Earth ponds can provide a suitable habitat for some species of snail, which are the intermediate hosts of the brain parasite that causes whirling disease and eye fluke parasites. Fallowing these ponds or liming the empty pond may be necessary to break the cycle of infections. Generally earth ponds and raceways work well in growing rainbow trout. Rearing Atlantic salmon in similar conditions prior to seawater entry has given equivocal results and is rarely seen these days.

12.6.2 Marine systems

Marine systems for farming Atlantic salmon are similar to those developed for sea bass and bream in the Mediterranean and for cod in northern Europe. These systems rely on a floating walkway below which is suspended a bag-net enclosing the fish. These pens can be 12 m to 20 m square, octagonal or round. Square steel pens are usually grouped together with a central walkway, whereas round plastic, more flexible pens will be moored separately. The depth of the suspended net is variable but usually will vary from 5 m to 20 m deep. The total volume of water in one sea cage may be in excess of $10,000 \, m^3$. The mesh of the net is usually sufficiently open to allow a good water exchange without allowing fish to escape. The cages may be enclosed in another outer net – the predator net – which is used to prevent attacks from marine predators such as seals and diving birds. There is usually another predator net over the top of the cage to prevent herons, other birds, otters and mink removing or damaging the fish. The nets are individually weighted at the bottom corners to prevent distortion from the current, which would reduce the volume of the cage and the available space for the fish. The cages are moored to the seabed with anchors or large concrete blocks. Water exchange and hence water quality relies on tides and currents. This can be compromised if the net becomes heavily fouled with weed.

As already discussed, observation of fish in a sea cage will rely on the use of underwater cameras, sophisticated feeding systems indicating the feeding activity, as well as divers, who can be particularly useful to report any unusual behaviour. The experienced stockperson will rely on the behaviour of the fish visible near the surface to give an indication of the status of fish at deeper levels.

Mortality collection in sea cages is difficult, involving the need for divers, the use of removable internal baskets or nets situated at the bottom of the cage or, more recently, an air-lift system which lifts fish up to the surface from a pocket in the base of the cage (Figure 12.3). Mortality removal on a daily or very regular basis is essential to monitor the health of the stocks as well as to remove pathogenic organisms from the healthy fish (see Figure 12.4). This has become more and more necessary with the advent of some untreatable viral diseases.

12.7 Management of Particular Groups

12.7.1 Smolt transfer to seawater

Atlantic salmon smolts are traditionally transferred from fresh water to salt water in April or May, although photoperiod manipulation has now resulted in smolts going

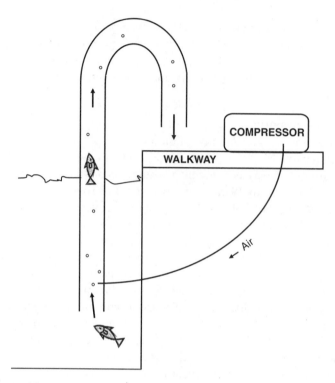

Figure 12.3 Air-lift system. This is used for moving live fish and, on some farms, for the retrieval of mortalities.

to sea at most times of the year. This dramatic osmoregulatory change from fresh to salt water is achieved more gradually in wild fish, where the fish will be able to adjust to the hypertonic seawater in the estuary.

Farmed fish, however, are transferred to seawater suddenly and so it is important that they are ready to adapt to this change. Generally it is more difficult to achieve complete seawater adaptation in all the out-of-season smolts (autumn and winter transfer) than the more natural S1 fish that will go to sea in the spring. Smolts that are ready for the sea will become more silvery, with black tips to their fins, and they will lose their parr marks. Analysis of the blood chloride levels of a few of the fish after they have been in full-strength seawater for 72 hours can be used to assess whether the majority of the population is ready for transfer. Blood samples are taken from anaesthetized fish or immediately after stunning. Blood is withdrawn into a syringe from the caudal vein between the anus and the tail. The use of vacuum blood collection tubes should be avoided since it will often collapse the blood vessels in a small fish. The large numbers of fish transferred at one time can mean that even a small percentage of non-adapted fish can result in a significant number of mortalities. Morphological and behavioural changes as well as blood chloride testing will help to

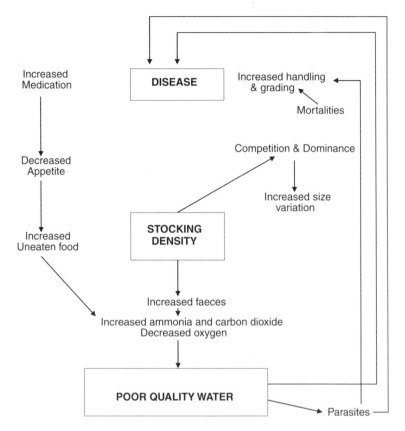

Figure 12.4 Pivotal relationship between water quality and disease.

assess the right timing for transfer and so reduce losses. These losses should be minimized not only for economic but also for welfare considerations.

12.7.2 Broodstock management

As the adult fish becomes sexually mature the appetite decreases and the pigment naturally occurring in the flesh is transferred to the egg. The fish becomes darker in colour, often with a reddening of the abdomen. Salmonid species produce relatively few eggs, whereas some flat fish such as turbot will yield over a million per kg bodyweight. Thus, relatively large numbers of salmon and trout will need to be kept as broodstock to ensure adequate numbers of eggs.

Selection of these broodstock fish cannot be made on fast growth alone as this method will tend to select for the larger males. Two to three times the number required for broodstock selection should be retained for potential use. This will give a cushion against too many early-maturing males, unexplained mortalities and some fish that fail to mature. Sex determination can now be carried out at a much earlier stage before the obvious morphological features by using ultrasound. This reduces the need to hold back too many fish. Later in the year, as the secondary sex characteristics become more apparent, this number can be reduced. Usually, to achieve adequate fertilization as well as maintain genetic diversity, one male is used to fertilize two females.

Fish are 'stripped' of the eggs or sperm (milt) under anaesthesia or immediately after stunning. This is usually done by manually squeezing the abdomen gently from head to tail. Other methods involve the use of gas introduced into the abdominal cavity, causing an increase in pressure, forcing out the eggs and sperm. This latter method should only performed in dead fish due to serious welfare implications that would occur in sentient fish. The milt is mixed with the eggs and any excess milt is washed off.

Most broodstock are very large fish and can be difficult to handle out of water. Generally speaking, manual removal of the gametes cannot be achieved in the unanaesthetized fish without causing damage and stress. The only licensed anaesthetic in the UK is tricaine mesilate (MS222; Pharmaq). The fish are immersed in a solution of this anaesthetic and are monitored to achieve the desired effect of sedation or anaesthesia whereupon they are removed from the bath. Usually the salmonid species are only stripped once and are then killed. The marine species such as halibut and cod, however, can be stripped on numerous occasions.

12.8 Grading and Handling

Grading fish is important to maintain uniformity of size in a population, otherwise the biggest, most aggressive feeding fish will eat most of the food. There is evidence to show that the smallest fish in a population are inhibited from feeding even in the presence of excess feed. In addition, freshwater parr can be very aggressive and will 'peck' or nip at the smaller fishes' fins and eyes. Ensuring a 'tight' size grade is important in the months leading to seawater transfer so that all the population will be ready at the same time. Grading and handling are especially necessary when fish are small and fast growing. At this time it can easily be achieved with the minimum of stress and damage. As fish become larger and heavier the physical effects of handling and grading can become more serious. These larger fish are more likely to suffer mucus loss, skin abrasions, bruising and eye damage, which may be routes of entry for systemic bacterial infections. Often the stressful effects of grading larger fish can lead to an outbreak of infection from a viral or bacterial disease.

Most systems growing larger fish, such as the seawater phase on salmon farms, will try to keep grading and handling of these fish to a minimum. To some extent photoperiod manipulation during the first winter at sea has reduced the necessity for grilse grading. However it may still be necessary to separate large numbers of sexually maturing grilse from the non-maturing salmon. This will be for commercial reasons (the flesh of a mature salmon is worth very little) and for welfare reasons, as this fish would naturally be seeking out a freshwater environment to allow spawning.

Size grading is carried out by pumping or netting fish out of the water over a series of adjustable bars through which the smaller fish will fall. Grilse grading entails manual selection of fish over a table with two or more chutes. The maturing grilse are separated into one pen for early slaughter – while the non-maturing salmon will be grown-on through the summer and autumn. Over the last few years more and more grading at sea has been carried out using well boats where the fish are pumped over a grading table on the decks before being returned to different cages depending on the size.

Any method of handling fish is potentially stressful and carries the risk of external damage to the fish. Small fish can be manually netted or pumped out of water without causing any damage. Care must be taken to limit the number of fish in a net. The fish at the bottom of a full net will be much more likely to be damaged than those at the top. Manually removing larger fish from the water by netting is not usually carried out these days, due to operator fatigue and the serious external damage that can occur to the fish. These bigger fish are usually handled by pumping systems or, more recently, using an air-lift system. These methods can be very efficient, causing minimal damage to the fish (Figure 12.3).

12.9 Transport

Fish are routinely transported by road in lorries, by air in helicopters and by sea in specially designed wellboats (Figure 12.5). The use of wellboats has become standard industry practice in the last 15 years for transferring smolts to sea cages and, more recently, moving larger fish to a killing and processing facility. To maintain good water quality the boat needs to be able to access fresh seawater and discharge some into the environment. This discharge can have a disease risk potential if the boat is passing neighbouring farms. When larger fish are being moved to slaughter, the water is often gradually chilled to ensure good water quality (the ability to hold more oxygen) as well as improving the flesh quality of the fish.

Irrespective of the method of transfer there are some basic principles that must be adhered to. The need to maintain good water quality is essential, with adequate dissolved oxygen, depending on the species, and low ammonia and carbon dioxide. Most fish are starved for 2 days prior to transport to reduce the biological loading from the presence of faeces and thus improve water quality.

All transport systems must have the ability to monitor both the fish as well as the quality of the water. Cameras as well as oxygen probes will be fitted into the tanks to give real-time information that can be viewed in the lorry cab or the wheelhouse.

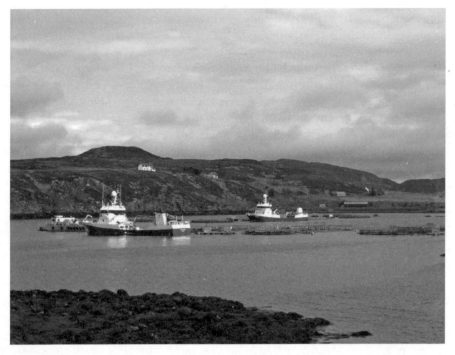

Figure 12.5 Two wellboats moving salmon from circular plastic cages to a processing facility for slaughter and processing.

Cleaning and disinfection of these systems must be thorough, usually involving a degreasing agent to remove the surface biofilm as well as a disinfection stage. Foaming agents incorporated in the disinfectant are often used to ensure adequate residence time on vertical walls and lids. From the author's experience one of the biggest biosecurity risks in wellboats is the discovery of a dead fish trapped in the boat's pumping system or jammed in the valves.

12.10 Slaughter

Prior to slaughter most fish will be starved for a period of time. It is only necessary to withhold food for the purposes of gut emptying. This is temperature dependent but in normal environmental conditions will be 1 to 3 days. During this time the gut contents will be eliminated, thus reducing the contamination to the carcass during processing and evisceration. There is very little evidence that withholding food for longer can improve the flesh quality and this practice is now discontinued. It is important that adequate training of personnel in slaughter techniques is carried out. (The Meat Training Council in the UK organizes a 2-day course on fish welfare which focuses on best slaughter practice.) Whatever method is used, it is important that the fish are rendered insensible as soon as possible and as efficiently as possible. The method used must be irreversible.

12.10.1 Salmon

12.10.1.1 Percussive stunning with exsanguination

A single hard blow or series of short sharp blows is delivered just behind the eyes. This method was traditionally carried out with a club, delivered manually, although automatic and semi-automatic methods are now commonly used. The bolt must deliver enough energy to cause shearing forces in the brain leading to irreversible damage and haemorrhage. The bolt must not penetrate the soft cartilaginous skull. Some of the most encouraging innovations involve persuading the fish to swim against the water current, then sliding down a chute to be automatically stunned. These fish are not handled and remain in water for the entire pre-stunning period. Stunning will be followed by cutting all four gill arches on one side to ensure rapid bleeding. This method is probably the best method to ensure good welfare and does not have a deleterious effect on flesh quality.

12.10.1.2 Carbon dioxide narcosis

The fish are placed in a bath of seawater previously saturated with gaseous carbon dioxide. This saturation can only be determined in practice by measuring the fall in pH. Narcosis is achieved after a delay of up to 5 minutes. There is a period of excitement and head shaking when the fish are first placed in the bath. In practice, the large number of fish being slaughtered at any one time on a commercial farm makes it difficult to maintain high levels of carbon dioxide. Often exhaustion and anoxia cause immobility rather than carbon dioxide narcosis and so the fish may be exsanguinated (gill cutting) while still sentient. If these fish are returned to seawater immediately after the carbon dioxide bath they will recover. For this reason, bleeding after carbon dioxide narcosis is essential. This method delivers poor welfare to the fish as well as poor flesh quality due to the massive muscular exertions. It is rarely used these days. However a variant of the carbon dioxide method is still commonly used where fish are chilled down over a period of 30 to 60 minutes in the same water. The carbon dioxide in this water will gradually increase due to the respiratory products of the fish until the fish emerging from this water exhibit the signs of carbon dioxide narcosis and anoxia. Sometimes these fish are often just bled out and not stunned. There are some real concerns over this method, both from a welfare and flesh quality point of view. The only claimed advantage is that it allows unskilled operatives to maintain the line with little monitoring necessary.

12.10.1.3 Electrocution

Killing salmon by this method is subject to the same constraints that apply to trout (see Section 12.10.2.1). In addition a much higher current is needed to kill fish in seawater. This method is still being investigated.

12.10.2 Trout

Most trout are killed at about 450 g and in very large numbers. There are inherent problems of humanely killing large numbers of small animals and this is typically seen in these small trout.

12.10.2.1 Electric shock

A pulse of direct electric current causes instantaneous immobilization of the fish and appears to be satisfactory from a humane point of view. However, until recently, this method has caused spinal fractures and haemorrhages into the muscle due to the massive muscular spasm. In the last few years there has been some impressive work done on modifying the voltage, current and waveform carried out in an enclosed chamber. The flesh quality is now much improved and this is probably the best method available. This enclosed system reduces the operator risk from electrocution.

12.10.2.2 Ice slurry

After the fish are removed from the water they are placed directly into an ice-and-water slurry at about 2 °C. These fish become torpid due to the cold and eventually death is by anoxia. This may take some time as the oxygen requirement at these temperatures is low. This commonly used method may give good flesh quality but there are serious concerns over the length of time these sentient fish may take to die (Humane Slaughter Association, 2005). This method is the industry standard method for killing bass and bream in the Mediterranean.

12.10.3 Flat fish

Methods used include:

- *Carbon dioxide narcosis*: See the concerns noted for salmon (section 12.10.1.2).
- *Stunning*: This is difficult without damaging or destroying the eyes although a specially adapted captive bolt gun has been developed that seems to address some of the concerns.
- *Severing the spinal cord*: This will not cause immediate insensibility as fish are tolerant to prolonged hypoxia and the brain may still be functional.

12.10.4 Emergency slaughter

From time to time, often as a result of a requirement for compulsory slaughter, large numbers of fish may need to be killed as soon as possible.

Some of the issues that will need to be considered are:

- humane killing;
- biosecurity;
- disposal of dead fish;
- speed of operation.

At the time of writing there are no published guidelines to ensure best practice. In addition it would be helpful to have a cadre of state veterinarians with sufficient knowledge to advise on these matters.

12.11 Health, Disease and Welfare

12.11.1 Health and welfare

The last few years have seen a considerable improvement in fish health in the UK – especially in Atlantic salmon. This has been brought about mainly by adopting sound principles of husbandry and hygiene well recognized in terrestrial farming. The advent of effective vaccines and other therapies has been vital in disease control, but they are not to be considered a prop that can be used against poor husbandry.

Most salmon farmers will now depopulate ('fallow') sea sites for up to 3 to 6 months before the introduction of new stock. Single year-classes of fish, hatched and grown at the same time, are also important industry standards, so further reducing the spread of disease from one group to another. These two measures have been largely responsible for the dramatic decline in bacterial, parasitic and viral diseases. New technologies, as described, have been developed that facilitate the removal of dead fish, especially from sea cages. This has helped to reduce the spread of disease.

High stocking densities can increase the risk of disease spread. New industry guidelines for stocking density are sufficiently low (usually a maximum of $20 \, kg/m^3$ compared to the RSPCA Freedom Food maximum of $15 \, kg/m^3$) to address concerns over overcrowding and disease spread. Low densities also decrease the need for thinning out and grading the fish later on – a stressful procedure that is likely to precipitate an outbreak of disease.

Rainbow trout farmed in fresh water are usually kept at much higher stocking densities than Atlantic salmon, often over $40 \, kg/m^3$. This species is better adapted to higher densities than salmon, with its tougher integument and greater resistance to surface abrasion. Even so, these high stocking levels are often reflected in poorer fin quality and scale loss, commonly seen in rainbow trout.

Most fish farmers have accepted the need for careful and patient observation of fish stocks. In the past they have had to be convinced that, like the shepherd leaning over the gate looking at his flock, time spent noting the behaviour and appearance of his fish is not a waste of time. As noted previously, the innovative methods of observing fish such as underwater cameras and looped back feeding systems have helped fish husbandry immeasurably.

Detailed records are necessary, not only to document any previous disease in the stocks, but also to record any treatments, changes in behaviour and weather conditions that may cause changes in water quality.

Consideration should be given to:

- the behaviour of the fish: opercular (respiratory) movements (are they lethargic, shoaling, swimming erratically, using the whole water column, crowding around the inlet or outlet pipes?);
- the external appearance of the fish: ragged fins, boils or furuncles, blindness and exophthalmos, unusual colour changes, excess mucus or fungus present, predator damage, spinal and jaw deformities;
- feeding response: vigorous, not at all, spitting out food.

Fish of varying sizes or a bimodal population may indicate faulty feeding, some metabolic disease or overcrowding.

12.11.2 Diseases

12.11.2.1 Bacterial infections

Furunculosis, enteric redmouth, vibriosis and rickettsia have been the main cause of large mortalities in farmed fish. Although effective vaccines are now available to control some of these diseases, the importance of good husbandry and hygiene is paramount. Overcrowded fish living in poor environmental conditions will often succumb to these infections even after vaccinations. These bacterial diseases can sometimes be controlled using oral antibiotics incorporated into the food. The build-up of bacterial resistance to these drugs has been very rapid in some cases, which is a cause for concern, especially as the number of antibiotics licensed for use in fish is limited.

Bacterial kidney disease (BKD) causes variable mortalities in both salmon and trout. This disease must be controlled, mainly by the production of disease-free stock. There is no vaccine available and the use of antibiotics is generally ineffective.

It is noteworthy that over the last 20 years the amount of antibiotic that is used to control bacterial disease in the UK has fallen by 90%. This is due to improved husbandry and biosecurity, low stocking density and the availability of effective vaccines.

12.11.2.2 Viral infections

Infectious pancreatic necrosis (IPN) virus can cause mortalities in first feeding and yolk sac fry in both salmon and trout. Salmon smolts entering the sea can succumb to IPN in large numbers but other causes such as inadequate smoltification, transport and handling damage must also be considered. Diagnosis is based on clinical signs, gross pathology, histology and serology. A vaccine is now available to help in the control of IPN.

Pancreas disease, caused by an Alpha virus, causes destruction of the exocrine pancreatic tissues, leading to anorexic moribund salmon. This disease is seen in the seawater phase. Losses are variable but the lack of an effective available vaccine or therapy, as well as no effective husbandry strategy, makes this a difficult and problematic condition. There is often a small proportion of fish which do not recover sufficiently to resume feeding. These fish should be removed and humanely disposed of.

12.11.2.3 Parasites

Newly hatched salmon and trout in fresh water are often parasitized with protozoal ectoparasites such as *Costia* and *Trichodina*. These are more common at higher temperatures and when the fish are overcrowded. Good hatchery management will incorporate regular microscopic investigations for these organisms before large numbers cause problems.

Lice are a major cause of loss of production and mortality in salmon in the sea. Infestation with large numbers can lead to skin and scale loss resulting in deep ulcerated areas round the head. This disease is probably the most important from a welfare and production point of view. Control will be based around bath treatments (pyrethroids and organophosphates) and in-feed medication (ememectin benzoate). As in other diseases, fallowing sites and separation of year groups has reduced the impact of this parasite.

12.11.3 Therapy

Fish may be treated orally using medication (usually antibiotic and sea lice treatment) incorporated into the feed pellet. Bath treatments (see above) are common for fungus and ectoparasitic infections. If adequate oxygenation is maintained, these bath treatments in fresh water are usually quite safe. Bath treatments in the sea, especially for sea lice, can be potentially dangerous as the fish may panic and burrow into the corners, causing large losses. This is especially risky with a high biomass and high summer water temperatures where supplying enough oxygen to the crowded fish can be challenging. Both salmon and trout are regularly vaccinated against the major bacterial and viral diseases. These vaccines are usually administered by intraperitoneal injection or by immersion.

The use of any medication for fish is restricted to those medicines for which the environmental authorities will grant a consent to discharge into the environment. So the fact that the veterinary surgeon or farmer may wish to use a certain licensed medicine will matter little if no discharge consent has been granted. This restriction is compounded by the fact that the number of licensed medicines available for use in fish is already very small. It is significant and worrying that there are no licensed ectoparasitic bath treatments available for use in fresh water. These constraints on being able to carry out effective treatments are a serious cause for concern and will continue to have a negative impact on both welfare and production.

12.12 The Way Ahead

The rapid growth in salmon and trout farming the UK seen in the last few decades may level off, possibly as a result of the lack availability of good sites. However, there will be progress in the farming of turbot, halibut, cod and other marine species. The general decline in wild fisheries will ensure a ready market for all these fish; the main challenge will be developing the technology for rearing and growing fish with such diverse life histories.

The use of high levels of fish meal in most fish feeds may not be sustainable in the long term. It makes little sense to feed marine protein from the sea to our farmed fish only for them in turn to be eaten by humans. Development of single-cell proteins from yeasts and bacteria as well as the use of modified plant proteins will be necessary to ensure sustainable and ready supplies of fish food. Perhaps farming herbivorous species such as carp and tilapia will become more common in the UK.

Finally, over the last 20 years there has been a gradual acceptance by farmers, scientists and veterinarians that fish kept on fish farms need to be treated in a humane and compassionate manner. As new technologies are developed and new species are farmed, so also do new welfare considerations arise, challenges which need to be constantly addressed.

References and Further Reading

Brown, L. (ed.) (1993) *Aquaculture for Veterinarians, Fish Husbandry and Medicine.* Pergamon Press: Oxford.

Bruno, D.W., Alderman, D.J. and Schlotfeldt, H.J. (1995) *What Should I do? The Practical Guide to the Marine Fish Farmer.* European Association of Fish Pathologists, Warwick Press, Weymouth, UK.

Code of Good Practice for Scottish Finfish Aquaculture (2006) Available at: http://www.scottishsalmon.co.uk.

Farm Animal Welfare Council (1996) *Report on the Welfare of Farmed Fish*, PB 2765 MAFF, London. Available at: http://www.fawc.org.uk.

Ferguson, H.W. (1989) *Systemic Pathology of Fish.* Iowa State University Press, Ames, IA.

Fish Veterinary Journal (Journal of the Fish Veterinary Society). Available at http://www.fishveterinarysociety.org.uk.

Humane Slaughter, Association (2005) *Humane Harvesting of Salmon and Trout.* Guidance Notes No. 5. Humane Slaughter Association, Wheathampstead, UK. Available at: http://www.hsa.org.uk.

RSPCA, Freedom Food (2007) *Welfare Standards for Farmed Atlantic Salmon.* Available at: http://www.rspca.org.uk.

South American Camelids

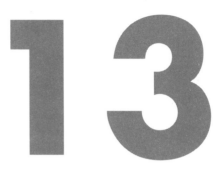

CRISTIAN BONACIC

13.1 Introduction

The members of the camelid family are among the principal large, herbivorous mammals of arid habitats; having evolved to cope with life in mountain areas, high plateaus, near-desert and desert conditions, they have made a crucial contribution to both human survival and development in these environments in Asia and South America. There are six types of camelid (Figure 13.1). The domesticated, one-humped dromedary of south-western Asia and north Africa, and the two-humped

Management and Welfare of Farm Animals: The UFAW Farm Handbook, 5th edition. John Webster
© 2011 by Universities Federation for Animal Welfare (UFAW)

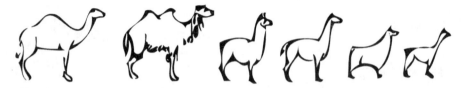

Figure 13.1 Camelid species, drawn to scale: from left, dromedary, Bactrian camel, llama, guanaco, alpaca, vicuna.

Bactrian camel, which is still found wild in the Mongolian steppes, are well-known, but four more species in the New World are also classed as camelids: the llama (*Lama glama*), alpaca (*Lama pacos*), guanaco (*Lama guanicoe*) and vicuña (*Vicugna vicugna*). The vicuña is the smallest representative of the South American camelids and the llama the largest. The vicuña and guanaco are both wild species and live in South America (Table 13.1). Guanacos are by nature the most adaptable, and thrive in a broad range of ecosystems from the Peruvian highlands to Chilean Patagonia. The range of the vicuña extends from a single site in Ecuador where it was reintroduced during the 1990s, through all the main Andean areas of Peru, extensive regions of the altiplano in Bolivia, the eastern side of the North Andean region of Argentina and the western slopes and altiplano in the north of Chile, all areas above 3,500 m. The guanaco is found today from Peru (8°S) southward to the central east and western slopes of the Andes, and across Patagonia, including Tierra del Fuego and Navarino Island (55°S). This species inhabits arid, semi-arid, hilly, mountain, steppe and temperate forest environments. In this wide variety of open habitats, four subspecies of *Lama guanicoe* are recognized (*L. g. cacsilensis*, *L. g. huanacus*, *L. g. guanicoe* and *L. g. voglii*).

Table 13.1 Original distribution of South American camelids.

Name	Order	Family	Genus	Species	Habitat
Llama	Artiodactyla	Camelidae	Lama	*Lama glama* Linnaeus 1758	Central Andes Peru, W Bolivia, NE Chile, NW Argentina
Guanaco	Artiodactyla	Camelidae	Lama	*Lama guanicoe* Muller 1776	Andean foothills of Peru, Chile, Argentina and Patagonia
Alpaca	Artiodactyla	Camelidae	Vicuña	*Vicugna pacos* Linnaeus 1758	Central Andes Peru to W Bolivia
Vicuña[1]	Artiodactyla	Camelidae	Vicuña	*Vicugna vicugna* Molina 1758	High Andes Central Peru, W Bolivia, NE Chile, NW Argentina

[1] Also recently classified as *Paco vicugna*.

Llamas and alpacas have been successfully domesticated by Andean cultures around Lake Titicaca (the highest lake in the world, 4,000 m) and became abundant and a key livestock herd for the expansion of the Inca Empire 500 years ago. The llama was among the world's earliest animals to be domesticated. While llamas are used mostly as a beast of burden in the Andes of Peru, Bolivia, Chile and Argentina, carrying things for the native herdsmen, they also provide local people with meat, wool, hides for shelter and manure pellets for fuel, and were used as sacrificial offerings to their gods.

Distinctive facial characteristics of the South American camelids (SACs) include prominent eyes and ears, and a lower lip with a central crevice. The feet are slender when compared to other members of the genus *Camelus* and present a soft pad instead of a hoof.

Wild animals within the genera *Lama* and *Vicugna* have persisted until the present, being represented by two species, the guanaco and vicuña, whereas llamas and alpacas originated from the domestication of their wild counterparts, a process which began approximately 7,000 years ago. Because the process of domestication is closely related to the cultural actions of humans with their livestock, the distribution and radiation of llamas and alpacas occurred in the Altiplano zones of the central Andes. Alpacas and llamas were domesticated several centuries before the beginning of the Inca Empire (fifteenth century) and played a major role in the success of the empire as pack and trade animals from the coast to the highlands. Under the Incas, the breeding of these animals was regulated as well as the use of their meat, hair and fur. In the sixteenth century, Europeans found millions of alpaca and a smaller number of llamas and other camelids in the Tahuantinsuyo (Titicaca Andean region). Beginning in 1539 these species were displaced towards marginal areas by sheep and cattle introduced by the Spanish conquerors. This process continued during colonial times and the republican era, so that the number of camelids was gradually reduced and remained mainly in the Peruvian and Bolivian highlands.

Llamas and alpacas currently reside in an area of 5 million hectares in the highest zones of Bolivia, Peru and border zones of the north of Chile and Argentina. These regions are mostly not suitable for intensive agriculture and traditional livestock production systems, but camelids are able to take advantage of the existing forages and survive in extremely dry and low productivity ecosystems. The rural population in the area under consideration is estimated at over 400,000 native Aymara and Quechua families, which depend mainly or entirely on raising alpacas or llamas and sheep for their subsistence because the climatic conditions allow no other alternative.

The origins of South America's domestic alpaca and llama remain controversial due to hybridization, near extirpation during the Spanish conquest and difficulties in archaeological interpretation. Traditionally, the ancestry of both forms is attributed to the guanaco, while the vicuña is assumed never to have been domesticated. Recent research has, however, linked the alpaca to the vicuña, dating domestication to 6,000 to 7,000 years ago in the Peruvian Andes.

South American camelids are considered an interesting new species for farming in the United Kingdom, Europe and elsewhere. Worldwide the alpaca population is estimated to be 3 million, with the majority in the South American regions of Peru, Chile and Bolivia. Today the alpaca is farmed not only in South America, but also in the United States, Canada, Australia and New Zealand. North American farmers have an estimated population of camelids close to 60,000, animals with Australia having a similar numbers. In the UK, current estimates are around 10,000 domestic camelids. Camelids are attractive, small and appealing because of their fine fibre and in some cases recreational uses (backpacking, exotic pets). Domestic South American camelids were introduced into different ecosystems of Chile during the 1980s, from Mediterranean to temperate rainforest areas and Patagonian grassland. Nowadays it is possible even to see small herds of llamas and alpacas side by side with wild guanacos in Southern Tierra del Fuego. South American camelids have been described as animals with the wool of a sheep, the strength of a horse and the brain of a dog. However, when contemplating South American camelids as potentially attractive species for hobby farming, we should not forget their origins and evolution. They all inhabit remotes areas of the Andes and Patagonia. Animal welfare recommendations should bear in mind the behaviour and natural adaptations of these four species that have developed in a region of the world where even the domesticated species are managed in an extensive way in open areas and have little contact with humans. South American camelids present a unique challenge for devising animal welfare criteria. These species have been historically interlinked with advanced ancient civilizations that developed sophisticated animal husbandry, practices domesticating the llama and alpaca and practising artificial selection before modern genetic knowledge. Alpaca mummies in archaeological sites shown fine fibre and colour variations that are not present in current herds. Also Andean cultures mastered sustainable ways of utilizing the vicuña, which was a sacred animal; every 4 years they were rounded up in a given region and brought into stone corrals for shearing and some for sacrifice. The finest wool in the world was considered a precious gift for the Inca and the four species of camelid played an important role in their traditions, trade and beliefs. Nowadays they still have an important place in their original distributional habitats, and also elsewhere. Different societies and individuals view South American camelids as pets, exotic animals, livestock animals, zoo animals and wild animals. Animal welfare recommendations need to recognize this variety of interactions between these species and humans and keep in mind that they can accomplish multiple roles rather than one single use by humans.

13.1.1 Origin and domestication

Camelids appeared in the late Eocene and were one of the first modern families of artiodactyls (even-toed ungulates), followed by pigs, peccaries and deer in the Oligocene, and giraffes, pronghorns and bovidae in the Miocene. The origin of camels, both those of South America and Asia/Africa, can be traced back to the ancestral camels of central North America. In fact, the camel family was entirely a North American group during most of the 40 to 45 million years of its evolution, with the critical dispersals to other continents occurring only 3 million years ago. The earliest camel (*Poebrotherium wilsoni*) stood only 30 cm at the shoulder and looked like a miniature, but slightly heavier-bodied, modern-day guanaco; this species of the upper Eocene period (40 million years before the present) had fours toes and a full set of 44 teeth with no gaps between them. From an ancestral Miocene form, evolutionary radiation in North America produced two important groups of advanced camelids. By the late Miocene (5–10 million years ago) the genus *Pliauchenia* had evolved, exhibiting many llama-like characteristics.

During the late Pliocene (3 million years ago), camelids first emigrated to Asia via the Beringia land bridge. When camelines (probably in the large Paracamelus form) reached the Old World, they spread rapidly west along the dry belt of Eurasia, reaching into East Africa and eastward across the Gobi Desert and into China. These Old World camels (camelines) eventually differentiated into the two present-day species – the two-humped Bactrian camel (*Camelus bactrianus*) of the Mongolian steppes and mountains and the one-humped dromedary or Arabian camel (*Camelus dromedarius*) of the southwestern Asian and North African deserts.

Meanwhile, the long-limbed *Hemiauchenia* was diversifying in central and southern latitudes of North America. Then, about 3 million years before the present day, the Panamanian land bridge gradually formed, linking the North and South American continents. Subsequently, one of the most spectacular and best-documented faunal interchanges took place, including the invasion of the llama-like *Hemiauchenia* into the Andes and onto the pampas of South America by the beginning of the Pleistocene. The centre and evolutionary origin for *Paleoloma* and modern *Lama* appears to have been the rugged Andean mountains, where their shorter legs provided better jumping ability and manouvrability in the rough terrain. The *Hemiauchenia* was a grazer, whereas the Andean *Paleoloma* became both a grazer and browser. *Lama* rapidly dispersed from its Andean homeland and extended eastward and southward over most of southern South America, overlapping extensively with the already established distribution of *Hemiauchenia*. While *Lama* expanded its range east and south, *Paleoloma* ranged west and north from its Andean origin (spreading as far north as Central America and the gulf coast of present-day Texas and Florida).

Toward the end of the Pleistocene Ice Age, 10,000 to 12,000 years ago, both genera of large llamas (*Paleoloma* and *Hemiauchenia*) became extinct. All other North American camelids also became extinct at about this time. The cause of the sudden demise of camels and other members of the American megafauna are debated, but current theories include climatic change, habitat change as a result of human activity, and overkill by an efficient and newly arrived predator, the human. However, the origin of the domestic species has been a matter of debate. Recent studies of variations in chromosome G banding patterns and in two mitochondrial gene sequences have shown similar patterns in chromosome G band structure in all four lamini species, and these in turn are similar to the bands described for camels, *Camelus bactrianus*. The combined analysis of chromosomal and molecular variation showed close genetic similarity between alpacas and vicuñas, as well as between llamas and guanacos. Current molecular biology research suggests that the llama would have derived from *Lama guanicoe* and the alpaca from *Vicugna vicugna*, supporting reclassification as *Vicugna pacos*.

13.1.2 Camelid species description

Today there are approximately 21.5 million camelids in the world, with around 7.7 million in South America (Macdonald, 2001). These comprise llamas (3.7 million), alpacas (3.3 million), guanacos (875,000) and vicuñas (250,000).

The llama is the largest of the South American camelids, has a slender shape, and may be found in up to 50 different colours. The llama has elongated legs, neck and face, and may reach as high as 1.5 to 2.0 metres from the ground to its head. Its long ears are erect and curve inward in a classic banana shape. Two breeds of llama are traditionally recognized – the woollier *Ch'aku* and those with less fibre on the neck and body, called *Q'ara*. Their fibre (technically it is 'fibre' and not 'wool') is less dense than that of alpacas, being an average of 26 microns on the undercoat and 70 microns on guard hair. Genetic selection produces distinctive fine fibre in llamas as it does in alpacas.

There are also two breeds of domestic alpaca distinguished by body size and wool characteristics. The more common *Huacaya* has shorter and more crimped and spongy fibre than the *Suri* with its long, straight or wavy wool fibers. The coat of Suri alpacas consists of long fibres with no crimp that hang down alongside the body in ringlets. Alpaca colouration varies from white to black with intermediate shades and combinations. The alpaca is the primary South American camelid fibre producer of the Andean highland. Alpaca wool (12–28 microns in diameter) is finer than that of the pack-carrying llama (20–80 microns) and body colour for both ranges from white to black, with some six intermediate shades of greys and browns. Dappled or spotty body colouration is more common in llamas than alpacas (Figure 13.2).

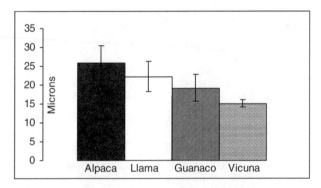

Figure 13.2 Comparison of fibre diameter (microns) between South American camelids. Error bars indicate standard deviation.

The vicuña is the smallest of the Andean camelids and has the finest fibre coat, the overall colour of the soft woolly coat is ochre, light cinnamon or reddish brown, with the under parts, insides of the legs, and underside of the head being dirty white. On the chest, at the base of the neck, is a peculiar, pompon-like 'mane' of silky white hairs which may be 20 to 30 cm (8 to 12 inches) in length. The vicuña is extremely slender, with long skinny limbs and neck. The head is small and wedge shaped, with small, triangular ears. Unique among living artiodactyls, the incisors of the vicuña are constantly growing, with enamel on only one side, to keep up with the wear caused by the tough grasses on which they feed. Vicuña fibre is the finest among all the animal fibres with an average diameter of 13–14 microns, but it is short, hardly reaching 3 cm. Its annual fleece can reach a maximum weight of 320 grams.

The guanaco has a similar silhouette to a llama, with a uniform colouration, with a dark brown upper body, neck and limbs; whitish fibre on the underside of the neck and belly; and greyish to black face. Guanaco fibre has a diameter of 18–24 microns.

13.2 Adaptation to the Environment

High altitudes, marked by intense solar radiation, extreme daily temperature variation, low oxygen concentrations and low quality of forages are the main environmental conditions to which South American camelids have adapted. The adaptive plasticity that camelids possess, due to their long evolution in arid climates, has made them very efficient in the use of vegetation present in marginal or low-productivity habitats (Box 13.1).

Box 13.1   Digestive physiology: main adaptations of the South American camelids

- Camelids are classified as functional ruminants. However, they have three compartments instead of four: C1 and C2 are equivalent to the rumen; the distal area of C3 contains secretory epithelium.
- The ability to select forage of high quality from natural pastures. This is based mainly on their feeding behaviour. Camelids have a highly diverse feeding niche from which they select on the basis of both availability and organoleptic forage quality.
- A high capacity to digest low-quality forage through prolonged particle retention time in the pseudo-rumen. The histological characteristics and motility of the digestive tract also differ from true ruminants.
- High efficiency in the use of water, especially when there is low consumption of feed.

- Larger foraging time than sheep and higher digestive efficiencies than goats in C4 when fed grass hay.
- Higher capacity to digest hemicellulose and more lignified grasses than other small ruminants.
- High nitrogen efficiency when recycling because of low renal excretion and high ruminal retention of the solid phase, allowing micro-organisms to process cell walls more efficiently.
- pH of the ruminal contents buffered by bicarbonate secretion from the first two compartments, closer to neutral, allowing more cellulotic digestion.
- Higher concentration of fatty acids in the first two compartments of the digestive system being available as energy source, compared to sheep and goat.
- Bloating is rare and all three ruminant compartments are glandular.
- Ulcers in the C3 are found in chronically stressed animals or after sudden stress episodes and in necropsies of stressed animals.

There are certain differences between South American camelids in terms of feeding behaviour. The guanaco and llama are considered to be grazers and browsers, while the vicuña and the alpaca are grazers only in their original habitats. This clarification is due to the fact that alpacas have developed browsing behaviour in more bushy environments, as has happened with individuals that have been transported from the Altiplano to the Mediterranean zone in central Chile. The camelids' diet varies during the year, depending upon forage availability and quality. Llamas and alpacas vary their diet in the Puna, depending on the dry and rainy seasons (winter and summer, respectively), and have also developed the capacity to select forage in all sorts of ecosystems, choosing rough forages when they have options.

Low oxygen availability in their natural high-altitude habitats has been a major natural selection force, reflected by specialized adaptations within the respiratory and circulatory system of South American camelids. Lung morphology is similar to that of the horse, but there are no lobules except for an accessory lobule in the right lung. The mediastinum is complete. Tidal volume of llamas is 0.5 L and dead space is 0.33 L, compared with human (0.30 L) and camel (0.25 L). High-altitude adaptation comprises anatomical, physiological and behavioural traits making South American camelids the best adapted farm animals to highland. For example, the oxygen haemoglobin curve is more efficient and the oxygen-carrying capacity of the blood is greater in South American camelids compared to other small ruminants. Erythrocytes number over 13 million per mm^3 of blood, haemoglobin between 13 and 15 g/100 mL, and packed red cell volume between 35% and 40%. Erythrocytes are ellipsoid in shape and have small size in comparison with other mammals (28–28.8 μm) that results in a relatively lower packed cell volume (PCV) and resultant low viscosity. Low oxygen at high altitudes is thought to have brought about specialized adaptations within the circulatory system in alpacas. The heart and vascular system as well as the respiratory system present some differences compared to other ruminants and mammals. For example, llamas maintained at 4,720 m above sea level did not show right ventricular hypertrophy, which indicates an adaptation to high altitude, suggesting that llamas and alpacas do not develop pulmonary hypertension.

The vicuña lives 3,000 to 4,600 metres above sea level and is well adapted to living in this harsh environment. It is clothed in a fleece of the finest known wool, one that has been valued and harvested since pre-Columbian times. This fleece protects the vicuña from the extreme cold and winds of the Puna, and also provides a cushion for its body when resting on the ground. In comparison to the Old World camels, the vicuña has more deeply cloven feet, which allow it to walk and run more adeptly on the rocky slopes, cliffs and rockslides that are common on the Puna. Another important adaptation is the vicuña's open-rooted, continuously growing incisor teeth that allow the animal to graze upon small forbs and perennial grass close to the ground. The vicuña's dental formula is 1/3, C 1/1, PM 2–3/1–2 × 2 = 20–22 (deciduous teeth) and I 1/3, C1/1, PM 1–2/1–2, M 3/3 × 2 = 30–32 (permanent dentition). The vicuña shows interesting similarities to the pronghorn antelope (*Antilocapra americana*) of North America. Although unrelated, both of these inhabitants of windswept grasslands are of similar size and extremely swift of foot, running at incredible speeds to escape danger. Both are also strongly inquisitive, walking toward any moving object that is partly hidden, as if to identify it by closer inspection. Vicuñas and other South American camelids defecate and urinate on communal dung piles. All individuals of a band, whether it is a family group or a male troop, use the same dung piles.

Many native highland plants are generally poor in quality due to high lignin concentration and low energy content. Indigestible lignin is an important component of a plant's defence against harmful ultraviolet radiation at high elevations. Animals grazing Andean pastures must be capable of extracting sufficient nutrients from coarse, heavily lignified material. Due to the distinct Andean 'wet' and 'dry' seasons, alpacas and llamas must cope with dry mature forage for over 6 months of the year. Such evidence that is available suggests that alpacas and llamas are more efficient digesters of this type of vegetation than either sheep or cattle. This is probably due to slower passage of ingesta through the alimentary tract, thereby allowing more time for fermentation. In consequence, South American camelids tend to consume less forage per kg bodyweight than sheep or cattle. Contrary to these animals' natural adaptations to rough forage, farmers in Europe and North America tend to overfeed camelids with protein and energy-rich forages and feedstuffs that contribute to obesity and can be an animal welfare problem.

Alpacas on the Andean high plateau reach 50 to 60% of adult weight by 6 months of age. In the adult alpaca, mean weights differ between animals at pasture with extensive traditional management and those fed intensively in stables. Experimental studies have shown guanacos to be extremely resistant to water deprivation, and even able to drink seawater or capture most of the water from mist deposited on plant leaves. However, llamas and alpacas in hot, wet ecosystems experience welfare problems when they are unshorn, and heat stress, dehydration and death are likely to follow. Domestic South American camelids living in hot, wet regions of the world are particularly vulnerable to these conditions and those planning transport must take into consideration water, ventilation and resting time.

Even during the wet season in the Andean region, strong winds keep the ground arid and the vegetation sparse. Ponds and more humid terrains are the exception rather than the rule in the Altiplano, and South American camelids are more adapted to intense solar radiation, cold weather at night and extremely dry air.

13.3 Reproduction and Social Organization

The South American camelids are social animals and in the wild form three basic social units during the breeding season: territorial family harems, non-reproductive male groups and solitary males. In captivity or on farms, juveniles and females are usually mixed together with crias (calves). Reproductive males are separated from herds and from each other to avoid fights and injuries. Guanacos and vicuñas are highly territorial but under extreme climatic conditions may displace to other areas.

South American camelids are naturally polygynous, meaning that an adult male defends a territory where females copulate with him. The guanaco or vicuña family group size in the wild ranges from 2 or 3 animals up to 13 (one leader male, five to seven females and yearlings). Males spend much time in active territorial defence against other males and drive their harem of females to more secure places and in the daily routine of grazing from resting places to grazing grounds. From the point of view of animal welfare, camelids are adapted to move in large open areas where visibility and group defence are closely interlinked.

In the wild, the reproductive cycle of birth, mating and early lactation coincides with the best environmental conditions during and after the rainy season. The timing of parturition varies with latitude. In the north of Peru, the offspring are born from April to June, while in Patagonia, births are delayed until between mid-November and the end of January. Guanacos in the Bolivian Chaco have their calving season earlier, between June and August, while on the arid coast of northern Chile it is possible to see neonates the whole year round, though births are more common between July and December. In the Andes of northern Chile, newborns begin to appear in August, but they are concentrated between November and February. In Torres del Paine National Park, female guanacos give birth between early December and January, with 49% of births occurring in early December. South of the park, guanacos in Tierra del Fuego give birth from mid-December to late February, with 85% of births occurring between mid-December and late January (Lichtenstein et al., 2008). Domestic camelids introduced in Patagonia closely resemble the natural annual cycle of the guanaco.

In South American camelids ovulation is induced by copulation. They deliver only one cria (calf) per year and females have no defined oestrous cycle but will ovulate 24–36 hours after copulation. Following copulation and subsequent ovulation, oestrus disappears within 8 days. If fertilization does not occur, follicles again become active and oestrus can be observed within 13 days. The absence of oestrus may be a diagnostic sign of ovulation or fertilization. Gestation period is approximately 11 months (340–350 days). This enables birth to occur when forage is green, nutritious and plentiful in early spring. Wild South American camelids shows a pregnancy rate between 50% and 60% and reabsortion and high juvenile mortality are the main constraints in the reproduction cycle. Llamas and alpacas in the Altiplano also show low fertility rate compared to other domestic species. Camelids tend to give birth during the day and guanacos show a synchrony with 78% of births being between 10:00 and 14:00 h. The concentration of births during the day, and in only a few weeks in the season, is an anti-predator strategy, producing an overabundance of prey during a very short period. Weight at birth is between 7 and 15 kg. Low weight at birth is related to high rates of mortality. Neonates have follower behaviour, being able to stand up as early as 5 to 76 minutes postpartum and mothers exhibit aggressive behaviour towards predators.

The newborn llama and alpaca depend on milk during the first months of life. Alpaca milk is lower in lactose and higher in protein, fat and ash than llama milk. Forage intake begins as early as 2 to 4 weeks of age in the wild in the case of guanacos and vicuñas. The response is a high growth rate during the first month of life with weight gain decreasing over time up to the following spring. The young stay with mothers for 1 year, with the juvenile males being expelled aggressively from adult male territories before the females, despite their submissive behaviour. The forced dispersal of juvenile guanacos and vicuñas by territorial males is due to competition for food resources on territories, while sex and time of dispersion are related to future reproductive performance. Females reach maturity at 2 years old, and males at 3 years old. The males are able to defend a territory only when fully grown, atr 3 to 4 years old, but many territorial males last only a few years defending a territory and the females in it.

In domestication, alpacas and llamas are not usually bred until they are 2 years old, although they are sexually receptive at 1 year. Breeding ratios are normally between 5 to 10 females per male. Reproductive parameters from other domestic species should not be considered a reference for South American camelids, given that they are considered closer to wild animals than to classic domestic and productive farm animals. Naturally, reproduction is limited by the extremely harsh conditions where they originally adapted.

Several factors contribute significantly to low fertility or birth rate under extensive conditions. These factors are associated with poor nutrition, harsh climatic conditions, rapid day/night changes in ambient temperatures, and possibly infectious and parasitic diseases. Inbreeding in small flocks may also contribute to the low reproductive rate. When South American camelids are kept outside their original distributional range and given excessive energy in the form of concentrate feeds, obesity may contribute to low reproductive success. In the wild, mortality during the first year may range from 50% to 90% in areas where harsh winter is combined with high predation rates by pumas and foxes. Under domestication, South American camelids are extremely sensitive to the presence of dogs, and even adult guanacos can be an easy prey for packs of feral dogs, and other carnivores. Any new farm that maintains llamas and alpacas in a new area should be extremely cautious about predation by dogs.

13.4 Attitudes Towards South American Camelids

People's attitude towards llamas and alpacas differ greatly between South America and Western countries, and this determines the kind of animal welfare problems that they have to endure. Llamas comprise extensive herds grazing in open and poor grasslands with extreme temperature variation between day and night in the Andes. Poor indigenous farmers developed a traditional way of farming llamas even before the Inca Empire. Welfare problems such as cold stress after shearing, predation, abandonment of crias, and outbreaks of infectious diseases such us enterotoxaemia, mange and rotavirus in crias cause large mortalities and losses in Andean herds. Shearing also causes deep skin cuts and infections due to the use of broken glass or rusted pieces of metal cans in places where shearing equipment is not available. In conclusion, hunger and cold stress are the main animal welfare concerns in South American llamas. At the other extreme, llama farming in North American llama herds presents problems of overfeeding, heat stress in hot, humid summers and behavioural problems in bottle-fed animals in close contact with humans. Moreover, isolation when llamas are used as pets can cause stress and abnormal behaviours. Deaths and stress caused by dogs is a common agent of poor welfare in the Andes as well as in new farms in Western countries. Alpacas are particularly susceptible to predation and injuries by dogs and feral dogs.

Premature cria should be treated like sick babies. They are not mature internally or externally, so cannot be expected to run or digest milk as other cria do, nor will they grow quickly. Interventions should only attempt to sustain life until the cria starts acting as a normal and healthy young animal. If possible *never separate* cria from the dam, even when you are responsible for feeding the cria. Cria should be encouraged to nurse from the dam and this can only be achieved by not overfeeding. Do not feed them during the night, 7 am till 11 pm is sufficient, unless they need more intensive care. Bottle feeding will not, or seldom, affect the willingness of the cria to feed from the dam and, where possible, it is better to encourage cria to suck than to adopt tube feeding. Some cria that are born to term can still have problems (difficult or prolonged birth) or be dysmature. If this is the case they should be treated like premature cria (see appendix).

Breeding of camelids, even in the most progressive farms in Bolivia, Chile and Peru, is at a very low technical level, because of the lack of knowledge on the biology of these animals and consequently of the management they require. Many problems of economic importance still remain unsolved. The problem of increased fertility and birth rate is likely of primary importance. On most of the alpaca and llama farms fertility or birth rate usually does not exceed 50%. This results in lower incomes and limits the selection possibilities. Most of the alpaca and llama farms are maintained without any definitive criteria of breed improvement. Neither qualitative nor quantitative selection for fibre, yield, animal weights and other economic features has been made. Little has been done in connection with nutrition; all food is derived from the natural high Andean pastures, most of which cannot be used for many other domesticated species. Pasture improvement and management are neglected practices and no systematic investigation has been achieved in this connection.

In the Andes, feeding practices are mainly extensive and involve low-contact management by farmers with no fenced areas and a daily routine of pastoralism and sometimes enclosure in stone corrals during the night. Aymara women and children drive animals from enclosures to wet and more productive patches of vegetation where animals roam freely during the day. The highland Aymara and Quechua human populations of South America are economically some of the poorest inhabitants of the continent, with a mean income of US$200 per family per year. Alpacas and llamas over much of their range suffer from disease, impaired hair production, low fertility and high mortality rates. These conditions are commonly attributed to poor nutrition due to overgrazing and improper herd management.

When domestic camelids are introduced into new ecosystems and are subjected to more close relationship with humans; rapid adaptation occurs involving significant physiological and behavioural adjustments. Captive-born animals reared under those conditions probably would not survive if returned to their original ecosystems. Therefore, animal welfare recommendations and husbandry procedures may differ dramatically for captive-born South American camelid in Europe or the USA compared to their original settlements in the high altitude plains of South America. South American camelids are fast learners and adapt rapidly to human influences. However, some basic needs rooted in their genes should be kept in mind to avoid forcing animals into a complete deprivation of natural and social behaviours.

13.5 Handling and Management

Old World camels and New World llamas and alpacas are domestic animals that have been important contributors to the culture and economies of their native countries for thousands of years. When accustomed to being handled, they are tractable, but like any other domestic animal, they must be tamed and trained. Camelids are commonly kept in zoos, and if the zoo's policy is a no-hands-on relationship with the keeper, a different type of restraint may be necessary. Guanacos and vicuñas are wild animals and may be difficult to handle. However, guanacos may be tamed and handled similarly to llamas if procedures are carried out slowly and quietly. Camelids may kick in any direction. This includes kicking with a sweeping forward and outward motion, as a cow kicks. Llamas and alpacas may also kick with a quick jab back, or jump with forelegs semiflexed to hit an opponent or a human. Guanacos in farms or bottle-fed animals can be extremely dangerous and even fatal to humans by kicking and biting. The padded foot lessens the sharpness of a kick, but the potential for injury from a large llama should not be underestimated.

Llamas may swing the head and hit a person in the face when an attempt is made to halter them. Alpacas are more prone to kick than llamas but with less strength due to their smaller size. Wild vicuñas handled for shearing are less aggressive and responsive to human handling than guanacos and tend to adopt a submissive behaviour often misdiagnosed as lack of stress response. While handling wild vicuñas for shearing the lack of response is indeed a stressful response that relates closely to handling time, visual contact with humans and restraint.

Llama males have sharp canines, but they are rarely employed against humans, except by behaviourally maladjusted males (too much human attention during early development or imprinted animals). In contrast to the males of most ungulate species, mature llama males may be safely handled by adults or children. The best restraint from an animal welfare point of view is no restraint. Replacement of restraint by careful observation, collection of non-invasive samples and careful interview of the owner should be a priority. Diagnosis and veterinary procedures in trained animals is easier, safer and causes less stress in the animals. Sometimes, veterinary restraint is necessary for a given protocol. Sampling techniques, facilities, previous experiences and the experience of the owner should be considered before any attempt to restrain an animal is made. Males tend to be more responsive and aggressive than females in all four species. Moreover males tend to be heavier, stronger and larger than females.

There are many ways to restrain a camelid depending on the farm and the way that farmers have trained or not trained their animals. If a camelid is being imported from South America to start a farm, veterinarians and farmers should be aware that restraint is not a regular activity for them, and more severe restraint should be used compared to an alpaca or llama born in captivity and reared in more direct contact with humans. Effective restraint requires understanding of camelid behaviour. All camelid species are social animals, which may be an advantage when driving the animal into a smaller enclosure for close observation or capture. Alpacas are more flock oriented than llamas and llamas more than camels. Vicuñas and guanacos are less flock oriented and their territoriality and family group structure makes it more difficult to mix groups of animals.

Well-trained animals do not require some of the techniques that follow. Use the least amount of restraint necessary to perform a task. Llamas may be herded into a narrow alleyway, or chute. Llamas may also be herded into a corner with ropes, poles or humans with outstretched arms. The arms should not be waved exuberantly, for this may alarm the animals. Only one person should signal the team to move forward or retreat. Boma-like visual barriers and swinging gates also help to drive wild camelids into a corral.

Two people may hold a rope (minimum length of 6 m) between them and even 10 to 15 people can drive wild vicuñas into a capture facility with a rope with colourful bits of plastic mimicking a barrier 1 m above the ground. Most farmed llamas will not challenge the rope, but a guanaco or vicuña might, and may sometimes even challenge people facing them with a rope. Occasionally, an individual will run under the rope or try to charge through it or, in the case of guanacos and vicuñas, may try to escape through wires and posts into the wild, fracturing their necks or legs. Zoo animals unaccustomed to being handled can be extremely dangerous to themselves their and handlers, and sometimes certain individuals should be handled only after sedation by darting. A handler may not be able to enter an enclosure housing an aggressive imprinted male, either domestic or wild. A South American camelid responds to 'earing' (pulling an animal from the ears) as does a horse, but it is contrary to good welfare. Also, holding a vicuña or guanaco by the tail is extremely stressful and undesirable. Ears and the tail are important in communication between camelids, and earing can cause damage and extreme pain. Ask the owner how each individual has been handled, before deciding on the most appropriate means of restraint. Optimal veterinary care of camelids requires suitable restraint facilities. Chutes and/or stocks should be provided so that work on the animals may be done safely and efficiently. Blood collection, diagnostic examination and, particularly, reproductive tract examination necessitate a chute or some degree of sedation. Rectal palpation can be traumatic in alpacas and llamas and repeated manipulation should be avoided. Many homemade chutes function admirably, as do commercially available chutes designed for deer or larger animals.

One may assess the docility of individual llamas by observing the ear set and tail position plus the intensity and frequency of vocalizations. The aggressive or agitated animal pulls the ears rearward over the neck, similar to an agitated horse. Although the alpaca has shorter ears, their position is the same. The body language of camelids involves the ear position, tail position and head position. Their long neck and agility to move makes them clearly an animal more close to a horse in terms of agility and speed than a sheep.

Camelids may vocalize during restraint procedures. Llamas may scream during restraint even when no pain is involved. Alpacas tend to be quieter and more submissive than llamas. Vicuñas are more like alpacas in behaviour; however, guanacos are the least tame and most dangerous of the four species. Angry llamas and male guanacos can jump and oppose human handling with great intensity, and always scream as if they were fighting between males.

South American camelids are also known for their spitting behaviour. An anti-disturbance police vehicle in Chile that has a water cannon is known as the guanaco. The actual spit is a regurgitated stomach content with a strong liquor odour and chewed grass consistency. South American camelids usually regurgitate their food close to midday when they lie and rest but in stressful situations they spit with great energy not only at other animals that cross their safe space but also at humans trying to handle them. Sometimes the spit of camelids distressed during handling can contain traces of blood due to lips cut by contact with capture facilities or pens. Traces of blood or obviously bleeding lips should be considered a sign of poor welfare during management, and corrections should be made to handling protocols, stock density during handling, time of the day and staff training.

The optimal method for initial capture is to drive camelids into a small catch pen or enclosure where animals are usually fed, hence accustomed to entering. The availability of water and food also helps when driving South American camelids into a handling area. Patience, training and careful handling allow safe and fast handling where animals show little stress. Camelids are extremely intelligent and learn routines quite quickly. Guanacos are perhaps the most intelligent and least docile, followed by vicuñas, llamas and alpacas. But all of them can learn to be handled and driven safely with little restraint and effort to handlers. In the Andes of South America they usually forage and move quite a lot during the day, and restraint and handling are rarely needed other than for shearing.

Camelids may be restricted by running them through chutes and narrow corridors with at least 1.8 m height (Figure 13.3). The walls of the chute should be solid to prevent the animal from sticking a foot through a space and fracturing a leg, and free of any sharp elements. Also no space or window of light should be allowed at the bottom to avoid them poking their heads through.

Clinical examination is easily carried out. Blood samples may be collected from the jugular vein. Venous distention is accomplished by digital pressure over the vein; male guanacos and llamas may tighten the muscles of the neck, making it more difficult to bleed them than an alpaca or vicuña. The lateral processes of the cervical vertebrae of camelids have an inverted U shape. The vital structures of the neck (trachea, vessels and nerves) are encased within the inverted U, protected from bites during aggressive encounters between individuals. The jugular vein can be easily hidden by a stressed animal and even the most experienced veterinarians may fail to bleed an animal that is stressed or aggressive. A technique that has been used for centuries is to restrain camelids in the sternal recumbent position with a rope made from llama wool placed as a loop around the front limb and rear limb, with a knot on the animal's back. The skin of the legs is extremely thin and prone to bruises, so tightening of the ropes should be done with care to avoid erosions and pain. Ropes

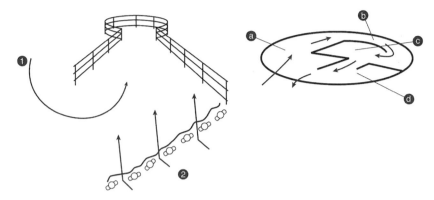

Figure 13.3 'The Chaku' handling facilities for camelids. 1 Funnel entrance. 2 People on foot driving vicunas into the corral; a, pre-handling corral; b, closed corridor and final enclosure; c, handling and shearing area; d, post handling corral.

around their body are not appropriate for restraint during shearing. In this case, hobbles, in the form of ropes in the carpal and tarsal areas, may achieve effective restraint. In the case of wild camelids, restraint can also be accompanied with a blindfold.

13.6 Camelid Welfare

13.6.1 Camelid community standards of care

A set of *Minimum Standards of Care for Llamas and Alpacas* has been developed (Box 13.2). These are the most basic requirements that all llamas and alpacas must have for physical welfare and, as such, define minimum requirements for animal control officers and government officials investigating questionable llama and alpaca care situations.

Box 13.2 Extract from Minimum Standards of Care for Llamas and Alpacas

1. *Water*: Animals should have continuous access to potable drinking water.
2. *Nutrition*: Animals should have nourishment adequate to sustain life and health.
3. *Shelter*: Animals should have natural or human-made shelter that enables them to find relief from extreme weather conditions. The sheltered area must allow the animals to stand, lie down, rest and reasonably move about.
4. *Mobility*: Animals should have a living area through which they can move freely and exercise independently.

---

5. *Neglect*: Animals should have a physical appearance free from signs of ambulation due to severely curled toenails, ingrown halters, or living conditions not meeting the minimums listed above.

6. *Safety*: Animals should be reasonably safeguarded from injury or death within their defined living environment and/or when travelling.

7. *Cruelty*: Animals should be reasonably safeguarded from cruel treatment and actions that endanger life or health or cause avoidable suffering.

8. *Socialization*: Llamas and alpacas are herd animals and should not live alone without a companion animal. A cria (a baby llama or alpaca under 6 months) should not be raised apart from other llamas or alpacas.

Source: Camelid Community Standards of Care Working Group © 2005.

Baseline values for a number of physiological parameters used to define welfare are given in Table 13.2.

13.6.2 Welfare of vicuñas and guanacos

Vicuñas and guanacos, which have no tradition of domestication, are managed now as zoo animals and as pets and are regularly captured and sheared in the wild in several South American countries. The so-called sustainable use programmes of capture for shearing wild camelids pay little attention to animal welfare standards, and a series of small enterprises are in place throughout the altiplano and

Table 13.2 Reference values for South American camelids relevant to animal welfare assessment. Source: Fowler (1998), Bonacic and Macdonald (2003) and Hoffman (2006).

Parameter	Llama	Alpaca	Guanaco	Vicuña
Bodyweight (kg)	100–200	55–90	100–120	45–55
Body temperature (°C)	37.5–38.5	37.5–38.5	37.2–38.8	37–38.9
Respiratory frequency (/min)	10–30	15–40	20–50	20–50
Heart rate frequency (/min)	50–90	60–90	60–90	60.90
Blood glucose (mg/dL)	74–164	90–141	75–111	90–110
Leukocytes/µL	7,500–21,000	8,000–21,000	9,000–15,000	7,300–13,000
Neutrophil/lymphocyte ratio	1–2.5	1–2.5	1.9–3.5	1.1–2.8
Cortisol (nmol/L)	20–40	20–40	30–50	29
Packed cell volume (%)	29–39	27–45	33–37	39.5
AST (IU/L)	128–450	128–450	68–227	60–246
Creatine kinase (IU/L)	29–39	27–45	33–37	39.5

Patagonia in Peru, Bolivia, Chile and Argentina for vicuñas and Argentina and Chile for guanaco. A special series of animal welfare considerations is necessary to ensure the welfare of these truly wild animals when brought into human contact. Both species offers challenges that are quite distinct compared to the domesticated cousins. Territoriality and group structure are both strong features in wild camelids. In order to handle them for shearing, large groups of vicuñas and guanacos are enclosed into corrals. This can cause social disruption, fights between males and crushing of crias while they wait to be handled. Accidents to humans are rare but can be fatal, particularly in the case of guanacos that can weight up to 120 kg.

Vicuña and guanacos have been captured, hunted, handled and shorn since the fifteenth century or before, when the Inca Empire conducted the 'chaku' throughout the Andes of South America for vicuñas, and South American tribes and hunters utilized the guanaco across many ecosystems where the species was abundant. The chaku consisted of herding thousands of vicuña into stone corrals for shearing. Local people surrounded vast areas and walked behind the animals, guiding them towards extensive corrals. Although large numbers of animals were shorn by this method, the associated morbidity and mortality probably had little effect on the population demographics because the process was conducted only once every 4 years in any given region. When Europeans arrived in South America, the traditional chaku was replaced by indiscriminate hunting. Current policies for vicuña and guanaco management include practices such as capture and shearing of wild animals, farming, ranching, and translocation and reintroduction. Little attention has been paid to the animal welfare implications of these interventions. It is reasonable to assume that both species become stressed by human contact in a similar way to other wild ungulates. The proposed sustainable use of vicuña and guanaco may result in an array of effects which could impact on their welfare: these include the introduction of new morbidity or mortality factors, increasing the risk of less efficient captures in the future, by affecting population dynamics, and the raising of concerns about the methods used to obtain the fleece, thus risking the economic viability of the programme. In the five South American countries there are estimated to be are more than 347,000 vicuñas, and more than 43 tonnes of fibre was sold at market in the last 10 years (McNeill et al., 2009). Guanacos are much more numerous and abundant in Patagonia, reaching more than 1 million (Argentina has the largest population of guanacos in the world). Many small enterprises are starting to capture animals for shearing and hunting quotas are allowed for guanacos in Tierra del Fuego (Chilean Patagonia).

The principles of the 'five freedoms' can be adapted to wild camelids as follows.

1. *Freedom from hunger and thirst*: Welfare could be compromised as a consequence of human action interfering with access to food, preventing access to watering points; or by limiting the access of the animals to those resources to which they are adapted.

2. *Freedom from discomfort and pain:* Discomfort and pain could be caused directly by humans due to the capture system, manipulation or captivity of a wild animal.

3. *Freedom from injury and disease*: Injury and disease could be directly attributable to humans as a consequence of hunting practices; due to an animal's exposure to an inadequate infrastructure, or an inappropriate management system; or by exposure, directly or indirectly, to contaminants or pathogens derived from domestic animals or humans. In addition, the close contact with conspecifics caused by confinement could also increase the risk of disease transmission and inter-animal aggression.

4. *Freedom to express their normal behaviour*: Animals should have adequate space and ecological niche resources that allow them to perform normal behaviours such as territorial defence, use of vantage points, sleeping and feeding sites, and so on.

5. *Freedom from fear and anxiety*: For a wild animal, this freedom implies that human contact must be kept to a minimum. There should be a protocol to assess any changes in the animal's behavioural and/or physiological expression as an indirect measure of potential suffering due to aversion, fear or anxiety during capture or captivity.

In general, capturing wild animals and placing them in captivity (either briefly in the case of wild harvesting or permanently when setting up a farm) exposes them to a variety of stressors grouped in three categories: physical, physiological and psychological. These stressors can result from the effects of capture, manipulation, restraint, drug immobilization, extreme temperatures, novel odours and noises, and so on. They might increase the risk of shock; capture myopathy and immunosuppression, among others. It is very important then to consider the current state of knowledge when a new species is going to be managed, for example: nutritional and habitat requirements, social organization, territorial behaviour, and so on. Neglecting these and failing to act upon them could cause high incidences of mortality during capture, disease post-capture and suffering during the entire process.

The impact of capture and restraint on animal welfare is influenced, to some extent, by the degree to which animals can adapt to human-designed environments, without experiencing any suffering. Since wild vicuña and guanaco are driven into human-made facilities, restrained, handled and shorn, it is reasonable to expect that animal welfare problems may occur. Vicuña management, both in the wild and in captivity, can produce immediate animal welfare problems including pain, injury, behavioural aversion, and other behavioural changes due to the effects of capture and manipulation. In captivity, there is the possibility of not having adequate access to food and water. There is also an increased risk of disease transmission from possible contact with domestic cattle and also through increased conspecific contact. Movement restrictions, limited ability to select habitat and changes in group composition due to human intervention also have the potential to impair welfare.

The stress of management, particularly shearing, has an exaggerated effect on the welfare and health of vicuñas by increasing the exposure to wind and low overnight temperatures in the extreme climate of the Puna ecosystem. The impact of capture and restraint on animal welfare is influenced, to some extent, by the degree of adaptation that animals can achieve in human-designed environments, without experiencing any suffering. Even when an animal has its basic needs fulfilled, such as food provision, and is physically healthy, the difficulty in adapting to captivity may be detrimental to its welfare and possibly affect aspects like reproduction that may indicate a long-term impairment. The opposite phenomenon also deserves attention: animals that adapt easily to the captive environment might not be able to cope in the wild again when released.

Whatever the chosen system of use for vicuñas and guanacos (shearing wild animals or farming them), the animals must be captured at some point. Studies with vicuña, conducted since 1995, have shown that five variables were affected by capture when compared with baseline values from captive animals. Rectal temperature, heart rate, respiratory rate, creatine kinase activity and plasma cortisol concentrations all increased as a result of capture, beyond the normal range described for vicuña and other South American camelids.

13.6.3 Animal welfare considerations and future challenges

The export of llamas and alpacas to various countries has only taken place to any extent since the early 1990s, and is still in the order of only a few hundreds per year. This spread of herds around the world presents unique challenges to those concerned for their welfare, not least because of the wide range of human attitudes to camelids. They are variously considered as wild animals to be hunted for sport, domestic animals to be farmed for fibre or even 'man's best friend'. The rediscovery of South American camelids as multipurpose species and the fact that interspecies breeding is possible open the discussion for what are the limits of human management. 'Cama', an interbreed species between camel and llama by artificial insemination, is the single case of species manipulation that generates a new life form. On the other hand, how far poaching associated to sustainable use of the vicuña and guanaco can severely affect welfare and even survival of the species in large areas is still unknown. Interbreeding alpacas and vicuñas for the paco-vicuña is also a matter for ethical discussion. The increased international expression of concern for animal welfare has extended to the South American camelids. It is clear, however, that much remains to be done to increase our understanding of their welfare and improve standards of husbandry for this group of species, unique in their physiology and behaviour and adapted to communal life in a unique habitat.

Appendix   Problems associated with premature births in camelid cria (calves).

Prematurity	Clinical signs	Complications	Actions
5–6 weeks	Weak, unable to stand, down on pastern, tremor in legs Sleepy, floppy ears, no teeth Sunken eyes, visually unaware Birth membrane attached to orifices (nose, mouth, anus) Raspy/wet/shallow breathing Body temp. <37 °C but *not* shivering, very short fleece	Systemic infection (mortality) risk Umbilical defect, herniation Respiratory infection No sucking reflex or unwilling to drink Retained meconium, constipation Overfeeding with bottle or tube No urine output	Keep cria on clean hay. Spray umbilical cord with iodine directly after birth. Wrap the cord in tissue and secure around belly with bandage until dry Monitor temp. daily: >39 °C can indicate infection Vitamin B complex injection Hold cria upside down to drain lungs Keep warm, rub body gently Stomach tube feeding colostrum Plama infusion when unable to suck Add liquid paraffin for constipation or give as enema Substitute glucose and electrolytes Monitor urine output (weigh dry and wet nappy)
3–4 weeks	As above but less extreme	Keep warm, monitor nursing Good chance of survival after 2 weeks old, but still at high risk	Expect slow weight gain only Inject vitamin B complex
>3 weeks	Floppy ears, can't straighten legs, shaky	Good chance of survival Check for full, round soft belly. After 3 weeks cria is out of immediate danger	Inject vitamin B complex
Term			Cria that look premature should be treated as premature

References and Further Reading

Alpaca World Magazine. Available at: http://www.alpacaworldmagazine.com/.

Bonacic, C. and Macdonald, D. (2003) The physiological impact of wool-harvesting procedures in vicuñas (*Vicugna vicugna*). *Animal Welfare* **12**, 387–402.

Bonacic, C., Feber, R.E. and Macdonald, D.W. (2006) Capture of the vicuña (*Vicugna vicugna*) for sustainable use: animal welfare implications. *Biological Conservation* **129**, 543–50.

Camelid Community Standards of Care Working Group (2005) *Minimum Standards of Care for Llamas and Alpacas*. Available at: http://www.camelidcare.info/MinimumStandards.htm.

Camelids Quarterly. Available at: http://www.llamas-alpacas.com/.

Fowler, Murray E. (1998) *Medicine and Surgery of South American Camelids: Llama, Alpaca, Vicuña, Guanaco*. Wiley-Blackwell, Oxford.

Fowler, Murray E. and Cubas, Zalmir S. (2001) *Biology, Medicine, and Surgery of South American Wild Animals*. Wiley-Blackwell, Oxford.

Hoffman, Eric (2006) *The Complete Alpaca Book*, 2nd edn. Bonny Doon Press, Santa Cruz, CA.

Lichtenstein, G., Baldi, R., Villaba, L., Hoces, D., Baiguin, R. and Laker, J. (2008) *Vicugna vicugna*. In *IUCN Red List of Theatened Species*. Version 2010.3. IUCN (2010). Available at: http://www.iucnredlist.org.

Macdonald, David (ed.) (2006) *The Encyclopedia of Mammals*, 2nd edn. Oxford University Press, Oxford.

McNeill, D., Lichtenstein, G. and Renaudeau d'Arc, N. (2009) International policies and national legislation concerning vicuña conservation and exploitation. In *The Vicuña: the Theory and Practice of Community-based Wildlife Management*, Gordon, I. (ed.), pp. 63–79. Springer, New York.

Manejo de Camelidos Silvestres (MACS). Available at: http://www.macs.puc.cl/.

Zapata, B., Fuentes, V., Bonacic, C., González, B., Villouta, G. and Bas, F. (2003) Haematological and clinical biochemistry findings in captive juvenile guanacos (*Lama guanicoe* Müller 1776) in central Chile. *Small Ruminant Research* **48**, 15–21.

Turkeys

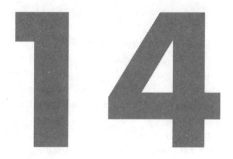

STEPHEN LISTER

Management and Welfare of Farm Animals: The UFAW Farm Handbook, 5th edition. John Webster
© 2011 by Universities Federation for Animal Welfare (UFAW)

14.1 Introduction

The current strains of turkey grown for meat production around the world are far removed from those which graced the table of the court of Emperor Montezuma. It was the Aztecs who first domesticated the turkey, prizing it for its decorative feathers as well as a source of meat. The turkey arrived in Europe in the sixteenth century, probably brought by merchants returning from the New World to Spain. From there, it found its way to the United Kingdom, into East Anglia, as the progenitors of the Norfolk Black, for many years remaining a speciality dish for high society. As domestication continued, strains were reintroduced to the New World and were bred with existing wild turkey strains there, giving rise to strains which survive today (e.g. the Narragansett from Rhode Island). A wide range of wild and 'domesticated' strains exist today, mainly for hobby breeders and showing. Some such as the Norfolk Black are bred commercially for niche sales in the commercial market, especially for seasonal whole bird production.

The vast majority of turkey meat consumed worldwide today comes from commercial broad-breasted hybrids derived from various white breeds, offering markets a wide range of weight of finished birds as whole oven-ready carcasses or those for butchering and further processing. There is marked sexual dimorphism with hens and stags (toms in the USA) usually being reared separately for specific weight band requirements.

Only a few primary breeding companies now supply most of the turkeys reared around the world, notably Aviagen Turkeys (incorporating British United Turkeys and Nicholas Turkeys) and Hybrid Turkeys (part of Hendrix Genetics). These companies maintain and develop genetic stock through pure line research and supply parent stock as poults or hatching eggs to breeder multipliers. Smaller breeders service the more specialist markets with strains used predominantly for free-range and seasonal production (e.g. KellyBronze, trademark name for Kelly Turkeys).

14.2 The UK Turkey Industry

There has been a considerable reduction in turkey meat production in the UK in recent years, poult placements dropping from around 45 million in 1997 to less than 20 million now, the lowest for 30 years. This reduction has been associated with a lack of increase in domestic meat consumption and increased levels of cheaper imports into the UK. During the same period, the number of turkeys reared specifically for the Christmas market has remained static at around 2 million per year. Therefore, although the traditional seasonal production is a significant market, the majority of sales are still associated with year-round production with volume sales of value-added products and portions greatly outstripping whole bird sales.

There are only a few relatively large companies involved in all-year-round turkey production, accounting for some 90% of total output. They are vertically integrated;

receiving day-old parent stock from the primary breeding companies for rearing and laying on company-controlled farms. Most operate their own hatcheries, hatching day-olds for growing on company or contract commercial farms to supply company slaughterhouses and processing facilities. Some independent breeders in the UK and mainland Europe supply day-old commercial stock to independent growing farms contracting to supply processors or butchery outlets for on-farm slaughter, processing and marketing.

14.2.1 Farm assurance and animal welfare standards

Most production in the UK is now monitored under a number of assurance schemes, established by the industry, retailers or other bodies. The largest is the industry-led Quality British Turkey (QBT) Agricultural and Animal Welfare Production Standards, now under the Assured Food Production umbrella scheme. Other standards exist, notably the RSPCA Freedom Foods Welfare Standards for Turkeys. These schemes set specific standards for production methods, environmental control and stockmanship and all participating premises are subject to regular and independent audit for compliance with these standards. Government also sets welfare standards in general animal welfare legislation and specifically in the DEFRA *Code of Recommendations for the Welfare of Livestock: Turkeys*. The last edition was published in 1987 and is in urgent need of updating to reflect current management practices and domestic and European recommendations (e.g. Council of Europe, 2001).

14.3 Reproductive Physiology

Modern breeders are brought into lay between 30 and 32 weeks of age for a laying cycle of up to 25 weeks. The onset of sexual maturity (semen production in stags and egg-laying in hens) is triggered by manipulation of daylength and, to a far lesser degree, point-of-lay bodyweight. Hens tend to be reared on 14 hours of light per day (minimum 60 lux) to about 18 weeks of age. They are then conditioned with a shorter daylength of about 7 hours of light, again at 60 lux. If accommodation has effective light-proofing, hens can be held at this photoperiod until onset of lay is required.

The onset of lay is triggered by rapidly increasing daylength to 14 hours at a minimum of 100 lux and this must be maintained throughout lay. Most accommodation for laying hens is in open pole barns, but to maintain good egg production natural sunlight must be supplemented with uniform artificial light to avoid the possibility of birds experiencing shortening daylength. Stags do not require the same initial conditioning but more simply commence semen production at sexual maturity on a daylength of 14 hours of light at a minimum of 50 lux. Reproductive performance varies depending on the strain of bird used, the weight of the hen at point of lay and consistency of bodyweight through the laying period. Modern strains aim for fertility rates in excess of 90%, peak egg production above 80% producing up to 120 eggs per hen at 25 weeks of lay, leading to around 95 poults per hen.

Due to significant sexual dimorphism in terms of bodyweight, breeding in commercial turkeys is by artificial insemination. Stags are milked (stimulated to release semen) usually twice a week to maintain semen quality and quantity. Semen from several males is pooled and then extended by being added to specific volumes of diluent prior to insemination of hens. The first insemination should usually be about 10 to 14 days after photo-stimulation, depending on the season, and should coincide with the first egg being laid. There should be three inseminations within the next 10 days, and then weekly throughout lay.

14.4 Nutrition

Turkeys are naturally omnivorous, feeding on plants, seeds, insects and worms. Commercially, nutrition is a major contributor to good performance and growth. Quality of raw materials, consistency of supply, presentation and physical appearance of feed are all important in ensuring health and performance. Specialist nutritional advice should always be sought and a planned programme for breeders and commercial stock should be established. Targets for weight gain in breeder birds and 'commercials' (meat birds) are given in Table 14.1.

14.4.1 Breeders

During rearing, feeding of breeders is aimed at increasing bodyweight in a controlled manner. This requires even, early growth to ensure the target growth curve is achieved but not exceeded. This is usually done by qualitative manipulation of

Table 14.1 Targets (kg) for growth in 'commercials' and breeding turkeys. The greater weights of the male breeding stock reflect extreme selection for weight gain. The commercial birds are hybrids between male lines selected for weight gain and female lines selected for their egg-laying ability.

Age (weeks)	Meat birds		Breeding stock	
	Stags	Hens	Stags	Hens
4	1.1	0.9	1.2	0.7
8	4.1	3.2	4.8	2.2
12	8.3	6.0	10.2	4.1
16	12.6	8.5	16.2	6.2
20	16.7	10.1	21.8	8.0
24	20.5		26.0	9.4
29			28.7	10.5
End of lay			33.3	10.2

energy and protein content of the ration rather than physical or quantitative restriction. Exceeding point-of-lay bodyweights for hens is likely to lead to poor laying performance as well as potential health issues. Quantitative restriction to prevent this tends to be far more problematic than for broiler breeders. Similarly, stags must reach target bodyweight to stimulate good semen production and this is usually achieved by *ad libitum* feeding until about 16 weeks of age. This enables good expression of genetic potential to aid selection. Following this, weight needs to be controlled to avoid overweight, mature stags whose semen output may be depressed and health can suffer. This weight control can be achieved by qualitative and/or quantitative restriction, although the latter requires specialist feeding equipment and adequate feeding space to avoid competition.

14.4.2 Commercials (meat birds)

The large weight range required for the market can govern target growth curves. Programmes for predicated growth rates must take account of these requirements in tandem with health and welfare requirements. Targets for metabolizable energy (ME), protein and amino acid (quality and quantity) and vitamin/mineral specifications must be agreed, with well-organized input from a specialist nutritionist taking account of the strain of turkey being grown to a specified slaughter weight at a specified age. Effective feed intake and performance will depend on adequate feeder space, feeder type, drinker availability and stocking density.

Most programmes start with a crumbed feed to 2 to 3 weeks of age, moving gradually to an increase in pellet size for later growing rations. Pellet quality is very important, as are all aspects of feed presentation and feeder space allowance, with a minimum of 3 cm trough space per bird or one tube or pan feeder for about 50 birds. Drinker availability is also significant to ensure adequate feed intake and a constant supply of fresh, clean water is essential. Closed nipple systems have the advantage of offering cleaner water but for older birds may supply insufficient flow to allow adequate intake, so open bell drinkers are more commonly used.

14.5 Environment

14.5.1 Controlled-environment housing

Conventional, enclosed, controlled-environment houses are usually windowless and power ventilated with control of heating, ventilation and lighting. Most have concrete floors for ease of cleansing and disinfection although some older units are based on compacted earth floors. Flock size can be up to 25,000 birds per house but is usually much smaller. No cages are currently used in the UK for turkey production. Birds are reared on litter, the substrate usually being shavings or straw. Most houses operate on an all-in, all-out basis but this may be on a multi-age site. Some companies use a brood-and-move system with specialist rearing houses to 6 weeks of age and then a move to pole barn or controlled-environment houses on the same site or on a separate growing site. It is usual to grow males and females separately. Stags are usually slaughtered between 21 and 24 weeks of age. Hens are slaughtered in relation to weight requirements and demand, often being processed between 9 and 16 weeks of age. Larger speciality and seasonal whole birds may be over 20 weeks of age at slaughter.

Stocking density is adjusted by placement stocking rates (i.e. the number of day-olds placed in a defined floor area per house) and subsequent moving of birds to fattening sheds, or later selections and thinning. The final stocking density for stags in controlled-environment housing may reach $60\,kg/m^2$, which for 21-week-old stags would equate to about three birds per square metre. Injurious pecking is controlled by reduced light intensity (around 10 lux) or through beak trimming (see section 14.7.2).

14.5.2 Pole barns
Most parent stock and some fattening birds, especially for the Christmas trade, are reared in open sided barns, mostly netted to avoid contact with wild birds. These sheds are naturally ventilated (Figure 14.1) with environmental control against

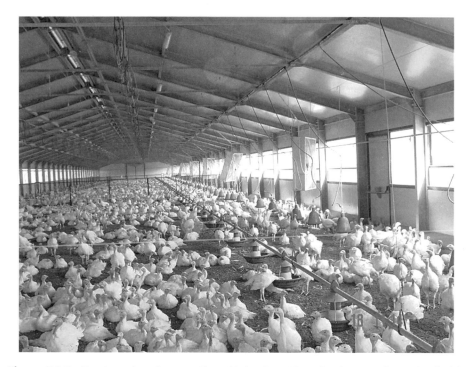

Figure 14.1 Rearing turkeys for meat. These birds, about 15 weeks of age, are housed on friable litter. The house is naturally ventilated and open sided with adjustable side curtains. Fans for circulation of air within the building hang from the roof.

the elements by the use of side panels or mechanically operated shutters, which may or may not be linked to an internal house thermostat. These birds may have been brooded in controlled-environment houses. The labour input is higher in naturally ventilated housing with the requirement for more regular littering down, usually with straw. Birds kept in such accommodation are usually routinely beak-trimmed. Maximum stocking densities vary from 25 kg/m^2 up to 38 kg/m^2.

14.5.3 Free range

There is an increasing interest in free range where pole barns or enclosed housing are used for overnight roosting but birds have access to range during daylight hours. Minimum requirements for stocking density, range access and slaughter age are outlined in the EU Poultrymeat Marketing Standards (Commission Regulation 2891/93E). Important considerations in encouraging good ranging behaviour include pasture management, land type and drainage, and provision of shelter.

14.6 Management

14.6.1 Young stock

Day-old poults must be placed in clean, dry accommodation supplying a comfortable thermal environment and free access to feed and water. Heat is usually supplied by gas brooders suspended over the birds at a height designed to give a concentrated spot heat directly underneath with a thermal gradient from the centre to the edge of the brooder ring. This allows poults to seek their own comfort zone. The behaviour and distribution of birds within the ring should be used to assess their state of comfort. Birds are initially placed in circular or oval surrounds constructed of a solid board or wire netting fence, depending on house design and layout. Between 300 and 500 poults are placed under each brooder and the brooder surround may be enlarged as the birds grow. A light is often hung next to the brooder heater to attract birds and illuminate feed and water. Feed is usually initially presented as crumb on trays to allow easy access and small font drinkers or disposable apple trays may be used to supply adequate water in the first few days. The young turkeys are usually released from the ring surrounds at 6 to 7 days of age and are then given access to the whole house, or the area allocated in the surround may be more gradually increased over a 3- to 4-week period. Feed is supplied from a variety of feeder types, most usually suspended circular feed pans or hoppers which are filled by tube or auger. Fresh clean water is essential and is most often supplied by bell-type drinkers, although various nipple and nipple/cup systems are available for younger birds.

Breeders are reared in a similar fashion but, prior to point of lay, are moved to specialist laying sites, usually of pole barn design. Hens and stags are housed or penned separately, both on floor systems, usually with straw as the litter substrate, although shavings may be preferred for stags. Hens are encouraged to lay in nest boxes placed around the pens. Trap nests are favoured which allow only one hen to enter a nest at any one time to allow privacy at egg-laying and reduce broodiness. The traps are usually hinged, such that the nest closes on entry, preventing a second bird entering, but then allows the bird in the nest to leave after egg-laying. Litter substrate for nests may be straw, sawdust or Astroturf. Automatic nest boxes are available which help to move birds off the nests at regular intervals, as a means of reducing the incidence of broodiness. In the case of manual nests, egg collectors will push hens off the nest at each egg collection, a minimum of six times per day. Any hens making repeated visits or spending long periods in nests can be identified as persistently broody (frequently soon after peak production). These may be removed from the flock and are then placed in a sparsely littered, cool and brightly lit broody pen until regular nesting and laying behaviour returns. Stags are penned in separate accommodation and may be placed on a feed restriction programme to help control excessive weight gain throughout their breeding life.

14.6.2 Environmental control

During the brooding period, heat is supplied to the day-old poults. After this period, house temperature is gradually reduced and for older birds management is designed to remove metabolic heat produced by the turkeys themselves. This can be achieved by adequate, natural ventilation or forced (mechanical) fans. Adequate ventilation is also essential to maintain a constant supply of fresh air and oxygen while removing excessive carbon dioxide, ammonia, dust and moisture. The efficiency of the ventilation system in achieving these goals will limit the stocking density that can be successfully and comfortably used. Any mechanical ventilation system must have an effective back-up generator or high temperature alarm. In hot weather, additional recirculation fans may be needed in the house to assist evaporative cooling. Well-managed ventilation also contributes to good litter quality. As birds spend their lives in contact with litter, it is essential to maintain the substrate in a dry, friable state. This will help to avoid painful conditions such as pododermatitis and breast blisters as well as reducing the likelihood of respiratory problems. Stocking rates and effective drinking management are important factors here. Drinkers should be set at the right height for the age and size of birds. The depth of water in each drinker should be sufficient to allow drinking without restriction but not overfilled, allowing spillage when knocked. There should be at least one drinker per 100 birds to avoid undue competition and, where possible, they should be movable to avoid litter under the drinkers becoming excessively wet or soiled.

Lighting is important to turkeys in terms of its intensity and quality as well as the photoperiod. It is clear that light intensity should be sufficient to allow birds to fully investigate their environment and undertake as many normal behaviours as possible. In brooder rings, a minimum of 25 lux is recommended.

The Council of Europe (2001) [Standing Committee of the European Convention for the Protection of Animals kept for farming purposes – recommendations concerning turkeys (*Meleagris gallopavo* spp)] recommended a minimum light intensity of 10 lux at bird eye level and, where possible, this should be supplied by natural light. With such light intensity, injurious pecking may be experienced and this may be controlled by reducing intensity to below 10 lux for short periods. The RSPCA Freedom Foods Standard requires a minimum of 20 lux across at least half of the available floor area. In some systems, beak trimming to prevent injurious pecking may be necessary if this level of light intensity is to be maintained, and informed decisions should be taken as to the necessity for trimming in specific circumstances. In breeder flocks, much higher light intensity (up to 100 lux) is required to maintain egg production, and in such situations beak trimming is regularly practised to avoid injurious pecking. A dark period in every 24 hours is considered advantageous for turkey health and welfare to allow birds to rest and sleep. Council of Europe (2001) suggests the need for an uninterrupted dark period of 8 hours as a guideline and recommends an absolute minimum of 4 hours.

Environmental enrichment is also important for floor-reared birds, allowing them to investigate and interact with their environment. The provision of low perches, straw bales and hanging toys or vegetation may be useful in promoting activity, which can avoid the likelihood of injurious pecking and improve leg strength and health.

14.6.3 Maintaining health and welfare

The importance of good stockmanship cannot be over-emphasized. Effective training and empathy for stock by all people involved with turkey breeding. rearing and slaughter are essential in ensuring the health and welfare of birds. All staff should be trained in all aspects of environmental control, management and husbandry. They should also be able to recognize the signs of health and ill health in the birds under their care. All stock should be inspected at least twice a day and preferably more often, taking time to walk within a metre of each bird in the house to assess general health of the flock as a whole as well as any problems with individual birds. Any sick or injured birds should be removed promptly and either placed in a hospital pen for treatment or, if recovery is considered unlikely, they should be promptly culled. Smaller birds may be culled by neck dislocation; but for these and for heavier birds the use of concussive humane killers is recommended as neck dislocation may not cause instant loss of consciousness.

Detailed records should be kept for mortality, culling and for all treatments. Where practical, recording of feed and water intake should be made, as this can give the first indications to stockpeople of ill health in a flock. Where flock problems are identified, prompt veterinary advice should be sought. Where there is significant mortality or sickness, accurate diagnosis is essential to ensure that effective and appropriate treatment can be given. Health issues in commercial turkeys are predominantly associated with enteric disease, respiratory disease and skeletal health or lameness.

As with all intensive rearing systems, prevention strategies and the use of available vaccines are essential to avoid harmful disease challenges. This is especially important since there is a paucity of medicines specifically licensed for turkeys in the UK and many parts of Europe, where turkeys are classified as a 'minor' species.

An effective written veterinary health and welfare plan and regular communication with a specialist veterinary surgeon is important in this process. An important part of this plan must be to set up an effective and workable biosecurity plan to help prevent the introduction of disease to a flock or site.

14.7 Welfare Problems

Commercial turkeys can grow to weights in excess of 20 kg and, as with all farmed animals, animal welfare considerations are important when such birds are used for meat production. Modern breeding programmes must take account of robustness and resistance to disease in developments for improved productivity. Programmes should be designed to avoid suffering or harm to parent stock and their progeny. At the farm level, the importance of effective stockmanship has already been stated. Historically, assessment of bird welfare has been based on welfare inputs (e.g. numbers of feeders/drinkers, stocking rates, and so on) whereas there is an increasing awareness that the best way to assess the suitability of any method of production for keeping of animals is better based on welfare outcomes. In turkeys, this may be assessed in terms of growth rates, feed efficiency, general health and mortality, although these may simply reflect how well a turkey is coping with its environment. There is a need to develop other factors on which to base this assessment. This may involve on-farm monitoring for pododermatitis, feather condition, injurious pecking or other signs and behaviours evident during rearing, factors identified at the processing plant such as the incidence of pododermatitis, injuries or other causes of condemnation or downgrading, which may enable an assessment of the quality of litter and environmental control as an indicator of general management and general stockmanship on-farm. There is a need for further research in these areas to establish and monitor robust and meaningful assessments of welfare outcomes. Some specific welfare issues that merit more detailed consideration are discussed below.

14.7.1 Stocking density

There is ample evidence in a variety of avian species of the importance of stocking rates and terminal stocking density in influencing bird welfare and expression of normal behaviour. The existing DEFRA *Code of Recommendations for the Welfare of Livestock: Turkeys* (1987) indicates a minimum floor area allowance of 260 cm^2/kg bodyweight. This equates to a stocking density maximum of 38 kg/m^2. The Council of Europe recommendations (2001) require a space allowance sufficient to allow turkeys to exhibit as wide a range of normal social behaviours as possible, but do not state specific maximum stocking rates or density. Commercial experience over the last 10 to 15 years has demonstrated that modern controlled-environment housing utilizing efficient forced ventilation systems can allow turkeys to grow to breed targets and expectations at stocking densities significantly above 38 kg/m^2 for older birds, without compromising welfare. In such situations, it may be appropriate to recalculate a stocking density for turkeys to recognize the growth characteristics of larger birds on a three-dimensional basis rather than a simple weight per floor area assessment. Farm Animal Welfare Council (FAWC, 1995) concluded when dealing with turkeys of different sizes, stocking densities should be scaled according to a two-thirds power of live-weight. On this basis, they established that it was possible for terminal stocking densities as high as 59 kg/m^2 to be justified for 20-week-old commercial stags in appropriate accommodation, equating to about three stags per square metre close to slaughter. Despite this theoretical approach, it is still necessary for individual farms to demonstrate that environmental control under practical conditions can ensure turkeys are able to exhibit as wide a range of normal behaviours as possible and not to suffer unduly from excessive extremes of temperature or significant health issues. For naturally ventilated houses, densities closer to 25 kg/m^2 are more suitable to prevent heat stress and maintain adequate litter quality. As indicated previously, welfare outcome assessments based on indices of performance: mortality rates, health and behaviour, and performed by a competent assessor, should reveal any harmful effects of overstocking in specific houses.

14.7.2 Beak trimming

Beak trimming is used in virtually all turkey breeding stock and a proportion of commercial meat birds to control injurious pecking. In controlled-environment housing using artificial lighting, coupled with effective light-proofing, behaviour likely to lead to pecking injuries may be controlled by reducing light intensity at specific ages. Beak trimming is currently an allowable mutilation in the UK for turkeys. A mutilation is a procedure resulting in damage to, or loss of, a sensitive part of the body, in this case up to a third of the upper mandible. Mutilations can cause pain and are considered by many to be an unnecessary welfare insult. Some production systems, e.g. free range at low stocking density and with certain breeds which appear to have a lower propensity to peck, obviate the need for such a procedure.

Within the EC, beak trimming is permitted in situations where it is considered that a failure to do so would be likely to give rise to far more severe welfare issues, notably, injurious pecking. Currently it is legal to beak-trim up to 21 days of age, preferably using a cold-cutting technique for the upper mandible only. It is generally believed that the insult to the bird may be less if done at a younger age, i.e. less than 10 days of age, but there is then a greater risk of subsequent regrowth. An interesting recent development is the use of infra-red beak treatment (e.g. NovaTech) which can be undertaken in the hatchery at 1 day of age. The bird's head is held gently on a carousel and the beak tip is exposed to an infra-red beam for about 5 seconds. The beam causes necrosis (death of cells) across the beak, the tip eventually falling off after 2 to 3 weeks, leaving a healed and altered (reduced) beak. This has the advantage of being performed in a controlled and consistent manner and no open wound is created.

Beak trimming or treatment may be considered a justifiable trade-off if it enables birds to be reared under significantly higher light intensity sufficient to enable turkeys to exhibit a wide range of investigating behaviours with a much reduced likelihood of injurious pecking.

14.7.3 Catching and transport

Turkeys should be caught and handled in a careful manner and only by trained, competent staff. Birds should be transported in containers appropriate for the size of bird, length of journey and expected weather conditions. Most transporters rely on natural ventilation to regulate the thermal environment for the birds. Problems may arise at high ambient temperatures, especially when vehicles are stationary. During inclement weather, side curtains can be used to prevent rain blowing in through the sides of perforated plastic crates.

Smaller turkeys should be picked up by placing a hand on either side of the body, holding the wings close to the bird's body. Turkeys should not be lifted by a single leg only. Larger turkeys may be carried by one leg and the diagonally opposite wing. In all cases, turkeys should be carried for the shortest period possible. They should then be transported without delay and be carried in crates at stocking densities appropriate to the size and age. Transport vehicles should be well ventilated and in any case journey times should be as short as is practical.

14.7.4 Slaughter

The processing of turkeys, especially large stags, requires careful handling of birds up to the point of slaughter. Transport to the processing plant and facilities at the lairage for birds awaiting slaughter should be designed and used to ensure the avoidance of injury or distress, and especially extremes of temperature. Lairage design and the use of trained personnel supervised by a dedicated poultry welfare officer throughout the time birds are present in the slaughterhouse are necessary to safeguard welfare. The live shackling of large stags as necessitated for electrical waterbath stunning methods is likely to cause pain in the shackled legs and a degree of distress to inverted birds. In such systems, turkeys should be handled carefully by well-trained staff and should be inverted for the shortest time possible prior to death. As a result of these concerns, the vast majority of turkeys in UK are now slaughtered using controlled-atmosphere killing. This procedure allows birds to remain in their transport crates without inversion and to be culled by introduction into gas mixtures sufficient to kill the birds *in situ*. This equipment requires constant monitoring and maintenance to ensure effective killing of all birds in the system.

14.8 Conclusions

Turkey production within the UK, although showing a decline in recent years, remains a significant industry, presenting a number of welfare and management challenges. High standards of stockmanship and the use of well-maintained and suitable accommodation can, with appropriate safeguards, ensure the welfare of birds reared in these systems. The challenge over the next few years is to establish welfare outcome assessments against which to monitor progress in all areas of the production process.

Further Reading

Council of Europe (2001) Standing Committee of the European Convention for the Protection of Animals kept for farming purposes – recommendations concerning turkeys (*Meleagris gallopavo* spp).

DEFRA (1987) *Code of Recommendations for the Welfare of Livestock: Turkeys*

FAWC (1995) *Farm Animal Welfare Council Report on the Welfare of Turkeys.*

Houghton Wallace, Janice (2007) *Not Just for Christmas: a Complete Guide to Raising Turkeys.* Farming Books and Videos Ltd, Preston, UK.

QBT (2006) *Quality British Turkey Standard for Agriculture and Animal Welfare.* Issue 2, revision 1, 2006.

RSPCA Freedom Foods (2007) *Welfare Standards for Turkeys.*

Ducks

15

KEITH GOODERHAM

Management and Welfare of Farm Animals: The UFAW Farm Handbook, 5th edition. John Webster
© 2011 by Universities Federation for Animal Welfare (UFAW)

15.1 Introduction

Commercial duck production forms a small fraction of the United Kingdom poultry industry. Carcasses are sold either as whole birds or are further processed into a range of fresh and cooked products. The major duck-producing countries of the world are China and other Southeast Asian countries which together account for over 90% of the annual world production of some 1,500 million head. The vast majority are 'Pekin' duck strains for meat production, these strains having been bred for rapid weight gain and high feed conversion efficiency. Some Muscovy ducks are produced as well as mule ducks, a cross between the two species. In some countries, native breeds are still used, but these do not have the commercial value of the modern Pekin hybrids. Again, mainly in Asian countries, strains of duck are reared for producing eggs for eating. For a more detailed description of domestic duck production, reference may be made to the book by Cherry and Morris (2008).

15.2 Biology and Natural History

Apart from the Muscovy (*Cairina moschata*), the ducks used for meat and egg production originate from the wild mallard (*Anas platyrhynchos*), a water bird of migratory habit. The bird is genetically adapted to life in environments as disparate as the Arctic Circle and the tropics, with all the variation of temperature, food types, light intensity and daylength that this produces. Selection for meat or egg production over the last 20 to 30 centuries has produced domesticated variants which are physically and physiologically better suited to modern commercial farming. Hybrids of various domestic and wild strains have been developed either for sustained egg production or for rapid growth and economic meat production.

15.3 General Management Considerations

The day-old duckling weighs approximately 50 g. It should appear lively and bright eyed. The navel should be well healed and show no prominent scab. Vent-sexing of day-olds can be done more easily than in the fowl or turkey. At day-old the male duckling has a distinct phallus which can be detected visually in the everted vent. In some eastern countries vent-sexing is carried out by sense of touch, the male phallus being palpated through the wall of the cloaca. From about 4 weeks of age the voice of each sex is distinctly different. The female utters a forceful 'quack', the male a more subdued 'squawk'. Further, the adult male shows some curled tail feathers.

The birds grow rapidly and, depending on genotype, exceed 700 g by 2 weeks of age. There is little sexual dimorphism although feather growth is slower in the male. Until about 3 weeks of age birds are usually kept in brooder houses. From that time they may be moved to field pens. The husbandry systems vary throughout the world and also within countries, from totally enclosed housing to open fields, with or without access to rivers or lakes. When the birds are first moved from brooding house to field, some protective shelter may be required for the first few days.

Potential breeder stock is often reared on a programme of controlled growth. For this reason, if the birds are to be field reared, the move is delayed until 5 or 6 weeks of age. By 6 weeks of age, meat birds will weigh approximately 3.0 to 3.5 kg although much depends on genotype and husbandry system. At about 8 weeks of age, new feather growth prevents clean plucking of carcasses. By sexual maturity the breeder duck should be about 80% of its *ad libitum* bodyweight. This results in best performance in terms of egg production, egg size, liveability and health. Published standards for husbandry and welfare of ducks have been produced by the British Poultry Council (2005), MAFF (1987), DEFRA (2009) and RSPCA Freedom Foods (2006).

15.4 Nutrition

Like the chicken and turkey, ducks have a simple alimentary system but they lack the 'crop' found in the other two species. The duck does, however, have a dilatable region of the oesophagus which is used for temporary food storage. In the wild, ducks are omnivorous. The timing of the breeding cycle is such that young ducklings have access to a plentiful supply of insect life as well as vegetable matter. In the domesticated state a complete formulated food must be provided for optimum effect, with a range of protein levels from about 20% for the very young duckling to 13% for a ration which will maintain a given bodyweight in breeding adults. When presented with a balanced diet, ducks will adjust their feed intake to maintain energy supply for maintenance, growth and reproduction, where maintenance requirement varies according to the prevailing environmental temperature. There is relatively little published research work on the nutrient requirements of the modern duck (but see Scott and Dean, (1991). Most of the current recommendations are based on

Table 15.1 Optimal nutrient composition of diets for ducks at different stages of development.

Ration	Starter	Grower	Finisher	Breeder	Developer[1]
Metabolizable energy (MJ/kg)	12.1	12.1	12.4	11.3	11.8
Crude protein (g/kg)	200	160	140	180	130
Methionine (g/kg)	4.4	3.3	3.3	10	6
Lysine (g/kg)	11	8.5	7.5	30	3
Calcium (g/kg)	10	8	6	3.5	5
Available phosphorus (g/kg)	4	3.5	3	5	
Salt (g/kg)	5	5	5		

[1] Young birds reared as breeding stock prior to the age of sexual maturity.

formulations which are found to be successful in commercial practice (Table 15.1). It is advised always to use feed manufactured specifically for ducks. Some additives in chicken or turkey feeds, e.g. anticoccidial drugs, are toxic for ducks. Other additives may not be licensed for use in ducks.

The starter feed should be given either as a crumb or small (e.g. 3 mm) pellet. Mash feeding is not advised. Pellets should be well formed and free from dust. Accumulation of dust in the feed hoppers can cause problems with meal build-up around the ducks' bills; it also leads to expensive feed wastage. Pellet size for birds over 2 weeks of age can be up to 4 mm in diameter. It is usual, commercially, to use a two- or three-stage feeding programme (i.e. starter, grower, finisher) to obtain optimum economic benefit and carcass quality. A similar approach is used in feeding birds intended for breeding: starter, developer and breeder formulations are common.

15.4.1 Feeding equipment

For growers, feed can be provided either via hoppers or tube feeders; either of these may be filled automatically from a feed bin. Hoppers are feed storage boxes with a trough below which fills as the feed is consumed. Tube feeders are similar, but the storage part is a metal or plastic tube. Again, the feed flows into a trough around the bottom of the tube. A minimum feeder space of 0.5 m per 100 birds should be allowed. It is not usual to keep meat ducks to more than about 7 weeks of age but, if this is done, the feeder space should be increased by 20%. For breeders on a controlled diet, floor feeding of measured quantities of food gives good control of weight gain and bird uniformity. In-lay feed may be offered either on a timed basis using flaps to limit access to the food trough or in measured quantities into the feeders. By whichever method food is offered, it is essential that there is opportunity for all birds to feed without undue competition.

15.4.2 Water

Water is an essential nutrient. Access to drinking water should be available at all times. A drinker space of 0.5 m per 100 birds should be allowed as a minimum with a 20% increase if birds older than about 7 or 8 weeks are to be kept. For starting ducklings, flat pans of water or drinking founts in addition to the normal drinker arrangements prove beneficial. Ducks take readily to drinking from nipple drinkers. This practice provides the birds with potable water as well as controlling the wetness of the litter. Better health and lower mortality rates are other noted benefits. Adult flocks producing eggs also benefit from nipple drinker provision, providing cleaner eggs without loss of fertility.

It is necessary, when placing ducklings, to ensure the birds find the watering facilities before the stockperson leaves the house. Water flow rates may require adjusting in very hot weather, as well as frequent 'bleeding' of warmed water from the ends of the water lines to provide cold water to the birds. Water troughs are frequently recommended and can work well for larger birds but it should be remembered that young ducks may drown in them.

In field rearing situations, it must be ensured that water lines do not freeze or that alternative watering facilities are readily available. Under field rearing conditions, drinkers may have to be moved daily to avoid the surrounding area becoming heavily fouled and muddy. The duck will dabble in such areas, causing drinkers to tip, with resultant flooding. In many tropical and subtropical areas, pond water is provided in which the birds can swim. This can help reduce the adverse effects of high ambient temperatures but creates a situation for potential helminth parasitism and bacterial and viral infections. In temperate climates swimming water is not generally provided for commercially reared birds; this may be considered a welfare disadvantage but has obvious health and management advantages.

Sufficient watering facilities must be provided to permit birds to perform their ablutions but there is no necessity for these to allow total immersion of the head as is sometimes argued. Such open drinking systems can create more problems of hygiene and welfare that they resolve and I am reluctant to advise them in the absence of top-quality stockmanship. Well-managed watering facilities will result in clean ducks. If watering facilities have to be altered for any reason, great care should be taken to introduce the ducks to the new system gradually and carefully. They may not readily find water presented in a fashion different from that to which they have become accustomed.

15.5 Housing

Up to 2 weeks of age $0.07\,\mathrm{m}^2$ per bird of floor space is desirable. At this time the birds will require some form of heating; the cost of this is minimized by providing well-insulated brooder accommodation. Gas brooders are commonly used. Duckling numbers per brooder should be about 66% of their suggested chick capacity, e.g. 1,300 ducklings per 2,000 chick brooder. Whole-house heating is often provided, but greater skill is needed to ensure an acceptable temperature is provided. Good stock observation is necessary to avoid overheating or underheating the ducklings. The temperature is right when the birds are seen to be comfortable. Sometimes, a perforated plastic flooring is used.

Over 3 weeks of age $0.13\,m^2$ per bird of floor space should be regarded as minimum for either wire/slatted floor houses or well-drained deep litter systems. Where drainage is poor, or drinker control inadequate, $0.18\,m^2$ per bird or even more may be necessary. Stocking density is dependent on litter management. During the grower phase, the requirement for good insulation is less important than in the brooding phase. Broiler type housing is commonly used but pole barn-style accommodation is equally suitable provided that protection from wind can be ensured.

Range rearing is common in some areas. The DEFRA Code of Recommendations (2009) suggests 2,500 grower birds per hectare. The actual area required will depend on the nature of the soil, particularly its drainage capabilities, and the nature of the ground cover. It will probably be necessary to move any frequently used equipment (e.g. feeders) regularly to prevent the land from becoming excessively poached. Drinkers will probably have to be moved daily. Protection from inclement weather may be required, particularly from high winds and rain but also from summer sun. Breeder birds during the lay period require a floor space of 0.4 to $0.5\,m^2$ per bird, depending on the ability to maintain dry litter.

One of the reasons for field rearing of growers and replacement breeders is to reduce housing costs. Another reason is the attempt, not always achieved, to improve duck welfare. Predator-proof fencing is expensive to erect and difficult to move when the ground becomes too fouled for continued use. The normal fencing required to retain the birds *in situ* is about 75 cm in height, which is no real obstacle to foxes or other predators. The use of electric fencing about 25 cm outside the duck perimeter fencing, and about the same height above ground, may be found a useful deterrent.

15.5.1 Litter

For birds up to about 10 days of age the use of wood shavings, sawdust or pelleted straw appears optimal but chopped straw can be substituted. In some parts of the world, other locally available material such as rice hulls might be used. Litter must be of good quality and as free as possible from *Aspergillus* and other moulds, to which duckling are highly susceptible. Long straw should be avoided for ducks at an early age. Because of the birds' high water use and intake, from about 2 weeks of age it will be necessary to spread fresh litter every day or every second day. It is advised to keep the feeders and drinkers well separated to try to spread the faecal loading on the litter. It does help the litter condition if the drinkers are placed over a wired or slatted area. The drawback of this is the disposal of the effluent so created. Feeders, drinkers and other pieces of equipment should be so arranged that ducklings cannot become caught in, under, or around them. All-in, all-out housing of ducks with end-of-crop litter removal, and with cleaning and disinfection of house and equipment, greatly help in the production of healthy ducks.

15.5.2 Temperature

The young duckling requires heat for the first 2 weeks or so of life, starting at about 32 °C. Using spot brooders it is easy for the stockperson to judge the birds' comfort. A brooder population in excess of 500 results in undue competition for heat, feed and water. The temperature should be decreased evenly, preferably no more than 0.5 °C each day but sufficient to avoid a temperature shock if birds are to be moved to ambient temperatures. For a fully feathered, well-grown or mature duck, the temperature for optimal productivity is around 17 °C.

15.5.3 Ventilation

The functions of fan ventilation in confinement houses are to provide an adequate supply of fresh air, and to remove heat, moisture, carbon dioxide and potentially toxic gases such as ammonia. The fan capacity should provide for minimal ventilation rates of 0.095 m^3/kg bodyweight per minute. In hot conditions these rates must be increased to remove heat and moisture either by a substantial increase in fan ventilation or by increasing the capacity for natural ventilation. For any given output of excreta, ammonia production is greater on straw than on shavings. The atmospheric ammonia level should not be allowed to rise above 10 ppm, although any smell of ammonia should instigate action. The upper legal limit for the stockperson is 25 ppm. Ducks will almost certainly suffer ammonia blindness at this level and a reduction in respiratory tract resistance to infection can be anticipated. The ventilation systems in use vary greatly, some taken over from, or modelled on, broiler growing farms. Totally fan-ventilated units as set up for broilers are adequate, but naturally ventilated units are cheaper to build, cheaper to run and do not require the provision of stand-by generators or other fail-safe devices. The effect of air movement over the birds should be taken into account when considering their comfort and welfare. Draughts can often precipitate outbreaks of infection, e.g. *Riemerella* septicaemia, especially when associated with a recent move.

15.5.4 Lighting

As with any species, light plays an important part in physiological development. The duck is essentially a migratory species and appears to tolerate anything from a 24-hour summer day in the Arctic Circle to an 8-hour winter daylength in temperate zones. For both grower birds and potential breeders, it appears to be advantageous to provide continuous light for the first 24- to 48-hour period. However, the DEFRA Code of Practice (1987) requires that a period of reduced illumination be given to accustom birds to accidental 'blackouts' due to power failure. For housed growers, a short period of darkness (about 30 minutes) must be provided to accustom the birds to the dark situation in case of such power failure. For breeders the normal step-down, step-up pattern of daylength (as for chickens) appears to be satisfactory both for the above purpose and for preparation for laying. Since the duck is a twilight feeder under normal conditions, its eyesight is geared to low light intensities. Growing birds do not discriminate, behaviourally, between 0.5 and 5 lux. This can be observed in free-range ducks at night when they may be actively moving and feeding in starlight. It is possible (but unproven) that some social interactions may demand a greater light intensity. Sufficient light intensity must be available, continuously or on demand, to enable proper inspection of the stock. Research has shown that, when given the choice, ducks show no preference in the range from 6 to 200 lux (Barber *et al.*, 2004). The light level for layers should probably be about 10 lux.

Since ducks can be grown for meat and eggs on range under tropical conditions there is clearly no upper light intensity limit under normal conditions. Ducks do not display feather pecking when faced with patches of bright lighting. For field-reared breeders it can prove beneficial to give the day's ration in the late evening when interference from wild birds is likely to be minimal.

15.6 Handling

Ducks should never be caught by their legs; they should always be caught by the neck, but avoid pressure on the trachea. They may be lifted until the weight can be supported by the other hand or by suitable equipment. Small birds may be restrained by placing a hand either over or under the body, care being taken not to press on the thorax or abdomen as excessive pressure in those regions could impair respiration. With larger birds, that is, once the flight feathers have started to develop, it is necessary to restrain the wings to prevent wing tip damage as well as injury to the handler.

Before handling ducks for any purpose, it must be remembered that, although food and water are provided *ad libitum*, ducks tend to eat communally. Recently ingested food is retained in the oesophagus from which regurgitation may occur if the bird is inverted or if the area is compressed. This is certainly stressful to the bird, and can cause death from inhalation of this material. It is good practice to remove food 1 hour prior to handling groups of birds as when moving them, vaccinating or blood sampling.

15.6.1 Vaccination

Subcutaneous injection is commonly used for vaccines and can also be used for the administration of antibiotics. The site of choice is the subcutaneous tissue at the base of the neck on the dorsal surface. Smaller birds should be held, with wings restrained, in the hand by one operator while the injector controls the head and neck with one hand, grasps the skin between forefinger and thumb and administers the inoculum into the thus 'tented' subcutaneous tissue at the base of the neck. Irrespective of the manner in which the bird is held, the vaccinator must ensure that the inoculum is not injected into the oesophagus or trachea, or into neck muscle where there is the potential for causing injury, particularly if oil adjuvant vaccines are in use.

Intramuscular injection may be used for either vaccination or antibiotic administration. The breast muscle or the thigh muscles posterior to the femur are suitable sites for injection. The inoculum should be delivered into the centre of the muscle mass.

Foot stab vaccination is almost totally confined to the application of duck viral hepatitis live vaccine to day-old ducklings. The vaccine is diluted according to the manufacturer's instructions. A needle with an eye at its point (such as a sewing machine needle) is dipped in the vaccine and then stabbed through the foot web of the bird, thus delivering a small amount of virus. Care should be taken to avoid the major blood vessels. The foot should be supported on a suitable pad to prevent blunting of the needle. Ensure that this pad has not been contaminated with disinfectant, which would destroy the vaccine virus.

15.6.2 Blood sampling

Blood sampling is usually carried out either to monitor efficiency of vaccinations or to monitor possible infectious disease contact. The normal sites for withdrawal of blood from the duck are the cutaneous ulnar vein or the metatarsal vein. The former location is to be preferred in birds once the wing has grown more or less to full size (around 35 days of age). In birds below this age the vein might be difficult to locate. For these younger birds, sampling from the metatarsal vein may be preferred.

15.7 Livestock Monitoring

It is now accepted practice that stock-keepers must inspect the stock and the equipment on which the stock depend at least twice daily. This should apply in both intensive and extensive production systems. With very young stock, inspections should be more frequent. In extensive systems, evaluation should be made of the additional risks to which the birds may be exposed. These may include the action of predators and the exposure to infectious conditions from wild birds. A necessary prerequisite of proper monitoring of stock for any signs of ill health or abnormal behaviour is a sound knowledge of what is the normal.

15.7.1 Normal behaviour

The duck is a strongly social creature. If birds are exposed to human presence regularly within the first few days of life they will become largely imprinted upon the stockperson and will allow a closer approach, showing less alarm than birds reared in greater isolation. Even in intensive units, birds may not be evenly spread. They will usually settle together in close contact in 'rafts' which may extend to several hundred birds. This does not imply that the birds are feeling cold or unwell. This normal tendency to gather together must not, however, be confused with huddling caused by chilling in very young ducklings.

Ducks over about 3 weeks of age are unlikely to suffer from low temperatures unless these are accompanied by wet and/or windy conditions. Sudden changes in temperature and/or air movement must still be avoided. Ducks which are subjected to high temperatures will attempt to increase heat loss by panting and radiating excess heat from feet, beak and underwing regions. Panting will be noted when the environment reaches 27 °C at a relative humidity of about 60% and at rather lower temperatures if the birds are very large or the relative humidity is high. Older ducks will keep cooler by wafting air using their wings.

Sometimes, birds lie with their legs stretched out behind them. In otherwise healthy ducks this is a sign of relaxed comfort, not to be confused with the postural abnormalities associated with bacterial infections (e.g. *Riemerella*, *Streptococcus* or clostridial enterotoxaemia). When disturbed or when moving for any other reason, ducks tend to move as a group. A bird separated from the group will show obvious distress, often making a plaintive noise until contact with other ducks is re-established. When inspecting a flock, all birds should be moved together without subdividing. Young ducklings tend to run rather than walk. Often, in the first few weeks of life, groups of birds will have a 'run around'. This results in a swirling mass of ducklings moving together, frequently in a circular path. The activity may change direction or cease as suddenly as it started. Sometimes small or weak birds may be bowled over during this activity. Birds so affected should be inspected and, if necessary, culled.

The 'critical distance' (i.e. how close they will allow a potential threat before taking evasive action) for domesticated ducks varies with their age and degree of human contact but it is usually in the region of 4 to 5 metres for birds over 1 week of age. Younger ducklings may well approach the stockperson, particularly if he/she stands still. Beyond the critical distance, healthy birds will show interest in and reaction to any movements the stockperson may make. Care must be taken to avoid frightening the birds, which will readily panic and possibly damage each other causing back-scratching and smothering.

Young ducks (3 to 6 weeks old) spent about 43% of their time sitting, 10% drinking, 17% preening and 2% feeding. Sieving the litter occupied about 15% of the time and standing and walking another 15%. Preening activity does not appear to differ significantly between birds kept on range or in intensive housing.

15.8 Breeding Strategy

Breeding stock will usually be purchased from specialist breeders, whose breeding programme selects lines optimizing the commercial performance. These breeders will advise on husbandry and nutrition to achieve the advertised performance standards. An alternative, less effective, practice is to breed from the farm's existing stock. If breeding selections are to be made, it will probably be necessary to identify the offspring of various parents or groups of parents from day-old. This can be done using wing tags to identify individuals, or by foot web notching; the latter is more often used for identifying groups of birds.

Genetic selection of elite breeding stock for meat bird traits should be made when they are reared to the usual slaughter age in order to identify those individuals showing the best performance. Several performance traits will usually be taken into account, including weight, feed conversion efficiency, amount of breast meat, leanness, mobility and general health. Reproductive capacity is largely a result of flock management in the rearing and laying programmes. Genetic selection for reproductive traits will involve trap-nesting in order to record which individual bird laid each egg, and pedigree hatching programmes.

15.8.1 Management of breeders

Birds selected for breeding at normal slaughter weights will probably be overweight for optimum lay performance. Some form of controlled feeding will be necessary to bring their bodyweight to that which experience of the strain has shown to be consistent with good reproduction. Birds purchased from a primary breeder should come with a firm set of recommendations with regard to the male and female growth curves. It is common to rear males and females together, or the two sexes within sight and sound of each other. Failure to do this may result in homosexual tendencies in some males and thus an effect on subsequent flock fertility. A mating ratio of one male to five females is usual for the parents of meat-producing birds but one to seven or eight for the lighter-bodied egg-laying strains.

Birds are usually brought into lay at about 24 weeks, later for larger strains, by increments in lighting period and feed. For birds intensively housed under controlled lighting this involves a reduction in daylength for the first 3 or 4 weeks of age to about 8 to 10 hours and then a step-up pattern of about $1/2$ hour a week from 15 weeks of age. In the case of birds reared on natural daylight, the reduction in natural daylength will have to be offset by the use of artificial light if flocks are to be brought into lay year-round. It is usual to bring birds into lay on daylengths of between 15 and 17 hours. At peak, daily egg production should exceed 90%. Broodiness is not a significant problem with ducks. Any marked deviation from the norm for the particular strain of duck usually implies an error in feed rates, light pattern or both. Egg size for any particular strain will have an optimum for the economic production of first-quality day-olds. Egg size can be held in heavy strains (e.g. at 88 g) by controlling the amount of feed provided but further attempts to reduce egg size can result in a reduction in egg numbers.

For optimum hatch results, eggs should be laid in specially prepared nests. Nests are most commonly kept to floor level with one cubicle for every five females in the flock. A nest size of 40 cm by 40 cm area with 40 cm high back and sides, with a 10 cm front lip but with no roof and no floor (but resting on the litter) appears to work well. The nest construction is traditionally of wood but other materials are satisfactory and may be easier to clean. Nest colour does not appear to matter. Nests should be introduced well before onset of lay to encourage birds to lay in them.

Nest material should be cheap (to permit frequent renewal), as contamination-free as possible and comfortable for the bird. Soft wood shavings are preferred. Nests should be kept as dry and clean as possible and changed regularly to reduce eggshell contamination. The recommended bird to nest ratio is lower than that for chickens but fewer nests will lead to floor laying and a resultant drop in egg hygiene. Moreover, ducks tend to bury their eggs. More than 95% of the eggs can be expected within 4 hours of the commencement of the 'day', thus once-daily egg collection is practised. The few eggs found during afternoon inspection should be picked up and held till the next day. The arrangement for provision of water should be planned to minimize carryover of water onto the litter as well as into the nest boxes. Segregation of groups of breeders can usually be achieved by the use of pen partitions of a height of about 75 cm. For the lighter, egg-laying strains, which may have a tendency for flight, clipping of the feathers of one wing is permitted and is effective. Surgical pinioning is not permitted.

A lay cycle of between 40 and 45 weeks is usual. It is possible to moult birds and bring them back to lay for a second season, if circumstances so demand. Ducks can be moulted by reducing their nutrient intake. It is helpful if daylength is simultaneously reduced to about 8 hours. Water should never be withheld.

15.8.2 Identification

Any mutilation of sensitive tissue or bone is not permitted in England. For the purposes of identification of ducks in breed improvement programmes, wing tagging, neck tagging and web notching are permitted (Mutilations (Permitted Procedures) (England) (Amendment) Regulations 2008). The 'pin type' wing tag can be inserted at day-old into the web of skin at the anterior aspect of the elbow. Care must be taken to pierce only the skin web. The main problems which may be met are:

- the tag becomes caught or the wing passes through the loop of the tag;
- the tag comes out (a tag in each wing is preferred);
- the puncture becomes infected. This is relatively uncommon when the tag is properly placed;
- the tags become outgrown and start to become embedded in the wing tissue.

Replacement of the first pin tags with larger tags may be necessary by 3 weeks of age. The birds should be checked a few days after tagging to ensure that mishaps have not occurred. For web notching, a small cut is made in the web between the toes of the day-old duckling. Using a sharp scalpel or sharp scissors, the cut is made, avoiding the obvious blood vessels.

15.9 Emergency Slaughter

However good the environment and health of the stock, there will be occasions when welfare or other considerations necessitate the culling of a small number of birds. This can be achieved by cervical dislocation although, because of doubts that this causes instantaneous loss of consciousness, other methods are recommended by the Humane Slaughter Association (2009). Cervical dislocation is done either by holding the bird by the legs at chest height in one hand and, with the other hand placed behind the skull at the back of the neck, pressing rapidly downwards while tilting the bird's head back, or by resting the bird's breast on the bent knee and then dislocating the neck as above. It may prove helpful to keep the arm straight and thrust down from the shoulder. Check that the operation has been successfully carried out by feeling for the gap in the vertebrae. For the largest birds (over 4 kg in weight) a captive bolt stunner is available.

15.10 Diseases

A detailed description of diseases, their recognition, treatment and control is beyond the scope of this chapter. For a fuller description see Gooderham (1993) and Pattison *et al.* (2008).

The duck is often regarded as the least prone of farmed poultry species to infectious diseases. This may reflect a lack of research into diseases of this species; it may also reflect less drive to intensification. However it is probably a myth. Under inappropriate management, loss from diseases, both infectious and non-infectious, can be considerable. Outbreaks of both infectious and non-infectious disease are most common on continuous production sites, or where management faults have arisen. Some of the more important diseases are briefly listed here.

15.10.1 Duck viral hepatitis-1

Duck viral hepatitis-1 (DVH) is an enterovirus infection of ducklings under about 4 weeks of age. Up to 95% mortality can occur. Older birds can be infected without showing obvious signs. They will, however, excrete virus. Control is by vaccination either of parents (to provide maternally derived immunity to their progeny) or of the day-old duckling itself. This condition is endemic on some farms, usually due to the vaccine virus readily reverting to pathogenicity.

15.10.2 Duck viral enteritis

Duck viral enteritis (DVE) is a herpes virus infection, especially of adult birds. Water is frequently involved in the spread of this infection, often being introduced by wild waterfowl. The risk is obviously greater when ducks are produced commercially in areas associated with open spaces of water. The disease can occur even in controlled-environment buildings, probably as a result of the virus being carried into the house on contaminated footwear. Mortality may be high. Falls in egg production occur. Vaccination is useful in control.

15.10.3 Riemerella anatipestifer infection

Riemerella anatipestifer infection is a septicaemic condition which may cause mortality and carcass condemnation in grower flocks. The disease is one which usually arises following stress or poor hygiene in grower birds, mostly between 2 and 6 weeks of age. Control is best effected by close attention to the birds' environment, avoiding drastic temperature or ventilation changes and avoiding high humidities. Treatment with amoxycillin may prove beneficial. Other useful treatments are available but usually unlicensed for commercially produced birds. Vaccines have been produced, both live, attenuated and inactivated. None of these is currently licensed.

15.10.4 *Escherichia coli* infection

Escherichia coli infection is a septicaemic disease similar to *R. anatipestifer* infection. It is considered as always being secondary to some other infection or to some managemental stress. Medication may prove helpful although there are frequently doubts as to the economic benefits of such action, unless the precipitating factor(s) can first be removed.

15.10.5 Streptococcal infection

A septicaemic condition, probably caused by *Streptococcus gallolyticus*, can occur, usually at about 10 days of age, the time when artificial heat has just been removed and the birds crowd together for warmth. Mortality is usually low. If treatment is considered necessary, amoxycillin proves effective.

15.10.6 *Pasteurella multocida* infection

Frequently a disease of adult flocks, *Pasteurella multocida* infection is seen as an acute septicaemia. Vaccination is useful for control where the disease is endemic.

15.10.7 *Erysipelothrix rhusiopathiae* infection

Erysipelothrix rhusiopathiae infection can occur in adult birds as well as younger stock. Vaccination may be considered on farms with a persistent problem.

15.10.8 *Aspergillus fumigatus* infection

Aspergillosis is a fungal infection of the respiratory tract. The term 'aspergillosis' is loosely used to describe all such fungal infections, some of which are caused by other fungi. The source of these infections is commonly mouldy litter which carries a heavy fungal spore burden. Mouldy feed, particularly in warmer climes, is another potential source of infection. The infection reflects a managemental problem: disease only results if spores are breathed in. Poor ventilation may also be a contributory factor.

15.10.9 Mycotoxicosis

Mycotoxicosis is a toxic condition associated with preformed fungal toxins in the feed. The duck is particularly susceptible to mycotoxins.

15.10.10 Amyloidosis

Amyloidosis is a disease in which amyloid is deposited, particularly in the liver. This results in an enlarged, sandy-coloured liver. The spleen is grossly enlarged and may rupture. Ascitic fluid may accumulate. Affected individuals may be seen with swollen abdomens before they die. The disease mostly affects individual birds and increases in incidence with age. Although the aetiology is uncertain it is commonly associated with chronic bacterial infection of heart valves or wounds of the integument.

15.11 The Future

Over recent decades, the development of the duck industry has resulted in larger populations of birds (both growers and breeders) being kept in controlled-environment houses or in naturally ventilated houses. Genetic selection for better carcass quality and improved feed efficiency is already making the duck a more affordable food for human consumption. Increasing public concerns in some countries about animal welfare in intensive systems may lead to an increase in the number of birds that are reared outdoors. The different husbandry systems demand different stockperson skills and different management approaches to ensure best bird welfare. The selection of one husbandry system does not of itself imply better welfare.

References and Further Reading

Barber, C.L., Prescott, N.B., Wathes, C.M., Le Sueur, C. and Perry, G.C. (2004) Preferences of growing duckling and turkey poults for illuminance. *Animal Welfare* 13, 211–24.

British Poultry Council (2005) *Duck Assurance Scheme*. BPC, London. Available at: http://www.poultry.uk.com.

Cherry, P. and Morris, T. (2008) *Domestic Duck Production: Science and Practice*. CABI Publishing, Wallingford.

DEFRA (2009) Codes of recommendations for the welfare of ducks. Available at: http://www.defra.gov.uk/foodfarm/farmanimal/welfare/onfarm/othersps/duckcode.htm#3.

Gooderham, K.R. (1993) Disease prevention and control in ducks. In: *The Health of Poultry*, Pattison, M. (ed.). Longman, Harlow, UK.

Humane Slaughter Association (2001) *Practical Slaughter of Poultry: A Guide for the Small Producer*. Humane Slaughter Association, Wheathampstead, UK.

Humane Slaughter Association (2009) Poultry Slaughter. Available at: http://www.hsa.
    org.uk/.
Ministry of Agriculture Fisheries and Food (1987) *Codes of Recommendations for the
    Welfare of Livestock: Ducks*. DEFRA Publications, London. Available at: http://www.
    defra.gov.uk/.
Pattison, M., McMullin, P., Bradbury, J. and Alexander, D. (eds) (2008) *Poultry Diseases*,
    6th edn. Elsevier Ltd, London.
RSPCA (2006) *RSPCA Welfare Standards for Ducks*. RSPCA, Horsham, UK.
Scott, M.L. and Dean, W.F. (1991) *Nutrition and Management of Ducks*. M.L. Scott,
    Ithaca, NY.

Game Birds

16

DAVID WELCHMAN

Key Concepts

16.1 Introduction

The term 'game birds' is broad and can be taken to include any bird shot for sport, whether wild or reared. This chapter will cover only those species that are commonly bred and reared for shooting, namely pheasants and red-legged and grey partridges. It will not cover species such as red grouse (*Lagopus lagopus*) (which are managed and

Management and Welfare of Farm Animals: The UFAW Farm Handbook, 5th edition. John Webster
© 2011 by Universities Federation for Animal Welfare (UFAW)

shot for sport but not reared artificially) and ducks (particularly mallard) which are sometimes bred and reared for game shooting but which are covered in Chapter 15.

The principal game bird reared for shooting in Britain is the common or ring-necked pheasant (*Phasianus colchicus*) which was originally introduced in the distant past (probably by the Romans), has been reared artificially at least since Victorian times, and which is common in the wild or semi-wild state. Its preferred habitat is woodland and woodland edges with ample cover of long grass and other undergrowth. Accurate figures are not available but it is estimated that 25 to 30 million pheasants are reared for shooting each year, an increase of 10 million since the late 1980s. There are several different strains of the common pheasant, broadly divided into the heavier types including French Black and Old English Black Neck and lighter types such as Fen, Scandinavian and Michigan Blue Back. Although proponents of individual strains claim various advantages, particularly in flying ability compared with other strains, all are bred and reared in a similar way.

The second most common game bird is the red-legged or French partridge (*Alectoris rufa*) of which an estimated 5 to 10 million are reared each year. This species is also found in the wild and semi-wild state and was first introduced in the eighteenth century from southern Europe. In Britain its habitat in the wild is open fields and downland and birds gather together in small family groups called coveys. The red-legged partridge was formerly often crossed with the chukar partridge (*Alectoris chukar*), a species not found in the wild in Britain, but the release of hybrid red-legged cross chukar partridges was discontinued in 1992.

The third species is the grey, English or common partridge (*Perdix perdix*) which is a native species of game bird whose numbers have been closely monitored in recent years as an example of a declining farmland species. Its natural habitat is fields and other open countryside with access to rough cover, and family parties stay together in coveys through the winter. Fewer than a million grey partridges, mainly of continental stock, are reared for shooting each year.

The purpose of game bird rearing in Britain is to produce a bird fit for release into the semi-wild for shooting in the autumn and winter. For pheasants the shooting season extends from 1 October to 1 February, and for partridges from 1 September to 1 February. The Game Act (1831) and other legislation enacted in the nineteenth century gives protection to birds during the closed season.

The rearing of game birds is essentially a seasonal activity which is still based on the natural seasonal life cycle of the birds in the wild state. The seasonal cycle comprises the selection of adult breeding stock in the spring, egg production, incubation and hatching, the rearing of young birds and their eventual release into a semi-wild state in the autumn. The large numbers of birds that are reared have necessitated the adoption of management and husbandry practices akin to those used in commercial poultry, for example for the incubation of eggs and the management of chicks during the critical first few days of life. The numbers of game birds bred and reared in this country are supplemented by imports, principally from France, and it is estimated that 40% of pheasants reared and 90% of red-legged partridges reared are imported, mostly as eggs or day-old chicks, with a smaller number of poults at a few weeks of age.

Game birds are bred and reared in a wide variety of enterprises. These include game farms which have their own breeding stock and hatchery, and which may rear tens of thousands of birds each year, and enterprises that buy in poults at a few weeks of age purely for release for shooting. As the number of game birds reared has increased, the methods used have become more intensive, along the lines of the poultry industry but with the important difference that the end result is required to be a bird which is able to survive in a semi-wild or wild state. The seasonal nature of game bird rearing means that the capital and labour costs involved have to be met over a much shorter period than in the poultry industry, and the level of investment, for example in hatcheries, is correspondingly lower except in the case of very large enterprises.

16.1.1 Welfare legislation and codes of practice

Codes of recommendations for the welfare of game birds reared for sporting purposes were published by DEFRA in 2010, under the Animal Welfare Act 2006. This builds on voluntary codes of practice, principally the *Code of Practice* produced in various editions since 1999 by the Game Farmers' Association (GFA) which lays down guidelines on good husbandry which must be conducted with all due consideration for the health and welfare of the birds concerned. However, in other respects game birds are covered up to their time of release into the wild by similar welfare legislation to poultry, including the Cruelty to Animals Act 1911, the Animal Welfare Act 2006, and the Welfare of Animals (Transport)(England) Order 2006 (and the equivalent legislation in Scotland, Wales and Northern Ireland). Game birds are also covered by notifiable disease legislation including the Avian Influenza (Preventative Measures) (England) Regulations 2006 (and equivalent legislation in Scotland, Wales and Northern Ireland) which requires premises with over 50 game birds to be registered in compliance with European Union requirements for the control of avian influenza.

16.2 Pheasant Breeding and Rearing

16.2.1 Breeding and egg production

The pheasant season starts in January and February when adult birds are selected for breeding. These are usually birds hatched the previous year and are either kept in large covered pens over the winter or are 'caught up' from the wild (that is, they are adult birds that were released the previous autumn, and spent the intervening winter period in a semi-wild state, often relatively close to their point of release). Good-quality, healthy that are free from injuries or evidence of disease birds should be selected for breeding. By the end of February the birds are placed into breeding pens which are usually on grass and of two general types:

- large group (flock) pens with up to several hundred females (hens) and an approximately 1 : 8 ratio of males (cocks);
- single harem pens containing eight to ten hens and one cock.

Flock pens on grass should have a space allowance of 4 to 5 m^2 per bird stocked, and egg production is generally better if flock size is less than 150 birds per pen. Flock pens should be arranged so that some cover is available to reduce aggression and fighting between the cocks and undue stress on the hens, poor egg production and infertility, and it is desirable that the pen should be subdivided into smaller areas to allow for the territorial nature of cocks. Perches should be provided for the birds, to allow for their natural roosting behaviour. Breeding pens are commonly enclosed with wire mesh sides up to approximately 1.5 m high. Single harem pens may be totally enclosed; if the breeding pens are open topped, the practice is to either clip the primary wing feathers of one wing or to fit an elastic 'braille' which prevents the bird stretching out one wing, in order to stop the birds flying out of the pen. Brailles should be removed when the birds leave the breeding pen. Adult breeding birds are sometimes fitted with 'spex' ('specs' or 'spectacles') which fit over the beak and are designed to obstruct forwards binocular vision to reduce aggression, cannibalism and egg pecking, but these can damage the nasal septum and should not be regarded as a substitute for good management. The space allowance required in single harem pens can be as low as 0.5 m^2 per bird. Single harem pens are more labour intensive and carry the obvious proviso that fertility should be monitored in the event of poor performance by the cock. During the breeding season the birds are fed a proprietary breeder ration with an 18% protein content (Table 16.1).

The first eggs are normally produced in early April and the laying season extends until June, by which time a hen pheasant will have laid up to 50 to 55 eggs. The layout of the pen should allow hens to have undisturbed access to nesting areas or nest boxes with nesting material such as straw, and it is important that this should be kept as dry as possible to reduce fungal and bacterial contamination of the egg shell. Eggs should be collected at least twice a day, in order to minimize the time the egg is left in the open. At least one collection should be made in the evening as the majority of eggs are laid in the afternoon and early evening. After collection, eggs should be sorted to discard any with cracked shells and other problems such as blue colouration of the shell (often associated with lower hatchability), and abnormally sized eggs; approximately 8 to 10% of eggs are discarded at this stage. The eggs should be washed (sanitized) promptly with a proprietary sanitizing agent following the manufacturer's instructions in order to prevent the entry into the egg of surface contaminants which may lead to death of the embryo. After sanitization and drying,

Table 16.1 Typical protein content (%) of commercial game bird feeds at different production stages.

Feed type	Purpose	Pheasants	Partridges
Pre-breeder pellets	From catching to 4 weeks pre-lay	15	15
Breeder pellets	From 4 weeks pre-lay and throughout lay	18	20
Chick starter crumbs	Chicks in first 2 weeks	26–29	26–29
Mini pellets	Chicks 3–4 weeks	24–29	24–29
Early grower pellets	Young birds 5–8 weeks Young birds 7–10 weeks	21–24	21–24
Grower/rearer pellets	Bought-in poults	19–21	19–21
Poult/partridge pellets	Poults/partridges 9–11 weeks	16–18	16–18
Maintenance pellets	For use during the shooting season and over winter	14	14

the eggs are stored at 10 to 16 °C before being set. However, there is a gradual loss of hatchability, reaching approximately 10% by 2 weeks.

Game bird eggs are universally set in artificial incubators, which vary considerably in size and design. The eggs are incubated at 37.6 °C and at approximately 50% relative humidity, to allow a target of 14% loss of weight over the incubation period for the airspace to develop. Large game farms and some smaller enterprises have access to their own incubators, but it is also common practice to send eggs away for incubation and receive an equivalent number of hatched chicks back afterwards, a practice known as 'custom hatching'. Custom hatching carries the risk of introducing disease from other sites. Eggs are often set twice weekly to achieve a compromise between management requirements and viability of the embryo. The principles of incubation and hatching, and the problems that can arise, are similar in game birds as in commercial poultry and outside the scope of this chapter, but further details can be found in references such as Game Conservancy Advisory Service (1993). The incubation time for pheasant and grey partridge eggs is 21 days, and for red-legged partridges 20 days, after which eggs are transferred to the hatcher. Hatching should be complete within a further 3 days. Under optimal conditions a hatchability of at least 70% should be attained for the season as a whole, although the method of calculating the figure depends on the numbers of 'help outs' (chicks that require help breaking out of their shell during hatching) that are included, which may comprise 10% of the total (Wise, 1993) but which may go on to rear as healthy chicks.

16.2.1.1 Alternative breeding systems

As an alternative to the grass-based system described above, it is also possible to house breeding pheasants in indoor flock or single harem pens, or to accommodate the birds in cages in the form of raised laying units. These birds can be stocked at higher densities than in outdoor pens but a minimum of $0.33\,m^2$ per bird is recommended by the GFA. Such systems require a particularly high standard of management to control aggression between the birds. Artificial lighting can be used to extend egg production earlier in the season.

16.2.2 Brooding and rearing

After hatching, the chicks are placed in chick boxes for transfer to the brooding site. It is important that chicks get a good start, particularly if they have a long journey from the hatchery to their destination brooding site, which can result in chicks becoming dehydrated and heat stressed. Chicks are traditionally placed in brooders as 'day-olds', but delays in the taking off of chicks in the hatchery and a long journey to their destination may mean that chicks are 2 or even 3 days old at the time of placement. This may be particularly significant if the chicks are derived from hatcheries in continental Europe. Initially the chicks are usually confined to a brooder ring approximately 2 m in diameter, within a permanent or temporary building. The brooder ring should be circular in shape to avoid the chicks becoming trapped and smothered in corners, and must be fully prepared in advance in terms of hygiene, bedding and ambient temperature. Scrupulous attention to hygiene is essential, particularly if the brooder accommodation is used for successive batches of chicks through the season, to minimize the transmission of disease such as rotavirus from one batch to the next or between different batches of chicks. Chicks are bedded at this stage on a variety of materials including wood shavings and shredded cardboard; sawdust should not be used because it creates dusty conditions and may be ingested by young chicks in mistake for feed. It is vital that the bedding materials are stored in a dry condition to prevent fungal growth which can result in outbreaks of aspergillosis in the birds. The background environmental temperature within the room must be carefully monitored and for the first 6 to 7 days should be at least $20\,°C$ throughout the day and night, and artificial heat is provided by gas brooders, or electrically powered heaters ('electric hens'; Figure 16.1) under which the chicks are brooded, and which need to be supplemented by a means of heating the entire air space such as infra-red heaters. The temperature underneath the heat source should not exceed $37\,°C$, with a gentle gradient out to the background temperature. The room should be well ventilated but draught free. Lighting should be controlled so that sufficient light is available for the chicks to move about and find feed but, if the light is too bright, wing pecking may occur. A ready supply of palatable feed should be made available on open trays on the floor, initially in the form of crumbs followed by a gradual transition to mini-pellets. Proprietary crumbs have a typical protein content of 26 to 29% (Table 16.1). Water is supplied either from floor drinkers or from overhead nipple drinkers which on many sites have replaced tray drinkers or bell drinkers. There should be a minimum of one drinker per 100 chicks placed. In the first few days of life chicks derive nourishment from their yolk sac but as this becomes utilized the chicks must start to find feed and water; failure to do so, or the ingestion

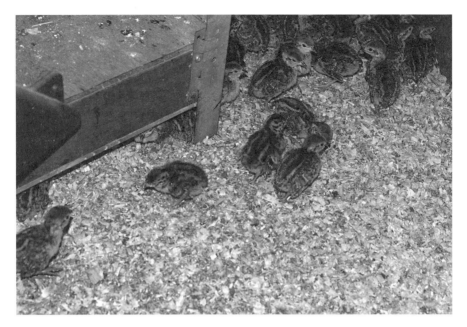

Figure 16.1   Young partridge chicks in a brooder ring. The chicks are bedded on wood shavings and can be seen emerging from beneath an `electric hen' heater.

of bedding material instead of feed, results in 'starve-out' and death in the first week of life. The principles of managing young chicks in the first few days of life are the same as with commercial, artificially reared chicks of any domesticated species, and attention to detail is very important.

Over the next 5 to 6 days the brooder surround is removed to give the chicks more floor space, and in warm weather conditions they are gradually given access through a pop-hole to a covered ark which is partly exposed to the weather conditions outside. The growing chicks are still allowed access to the brooder area at night but, depending on the weather conditions, increasingly are allowed to spend more time in the covered ark or night shelter, and then to a grass run with wire-netted sides and roof which adjoins the ark. During this time, the availability of background heating in the brooder house is gradually reduced, in general by keeping the heaters on by night but off by day. However, poults should not be released until they have been without artificial heat for at least 10 days. Drinkers and feeders are positioned for the poults in the outside run (Figures 16.2 and 16.3). This whole arrangement of brooder hut, night shelter and outside run is commonly referred to as the Burgate or Fordingbridge system, named after the Game Conservation and Wildlife Trust (formerly Game Conservancy Trust) headquarters in Fordingbridge, Hampshire. Chicks in this system can be stocked at 60 to 70/m^2 in the brooder hut and a minimum of 0.2 m^2 per bird should be allowed in the outside run. A recommended batch size is 250 birds, although up to 1,000 birds can sometimes be stocked; further

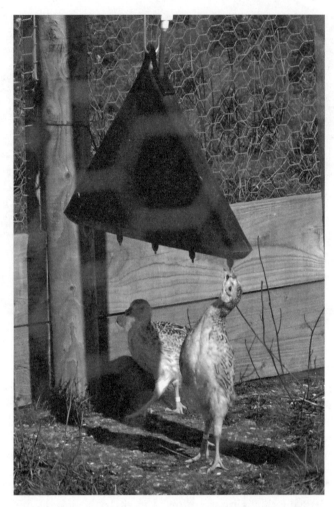

Figure 16.2 A pheasant poult drinking from a nipple drinker in an outside run. Note the correct height of the drinker above ground level.

details of the measurements and stocking density of birds are available (Game Conservancy Advisory Services, 2006). This type of accommodation is relatively easy to construct, can be used in both small and large enterprises and has the potential to be moved to alternative sites, which is important from a disease control point of view. Several brooder huts, night shelters and runs are generally set up side by side on the rearing field (Figure 16.4). There are also various alternatives to the Burgate system including the totally enclosed Sedgemoor house, systems using a permanent brooder house with access to an outdoor run and systems where chicks are reared on wire mesh. Wire mesh rearing systems have benefits in terms of disease control and in some cases are designed to minimize the handling of the birds. In all

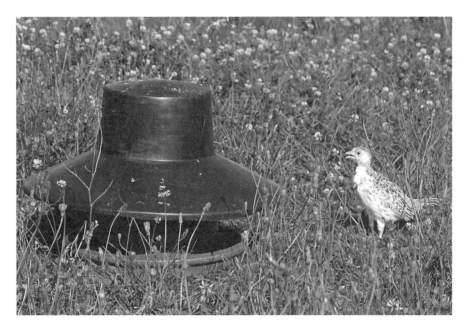

Figure 16.3 A covered feeder in an outside run. The photograph shows a good height of vegetation in the run which will help keep the birds occupied.

types of rearing accommodation, strict attention to hygiene is of critical importance, as without it infectious agents such as rotavirus can build up in the environment, leading to disease outbreaks in successive batches of birds passing through the accommodation.

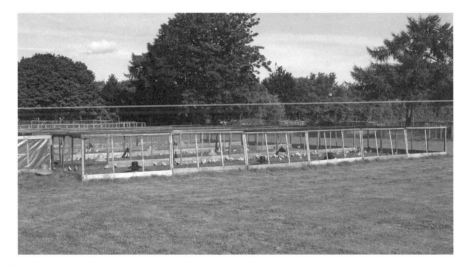

Figure 16.4 Overview of a pheasant rearing field showing the wire-netted runs.

While on the rearing field, the young pheasants ('poults') have to become adapted to outdoor life in preparation for entering release pens at 6 to 8 weeks of age. This process of adaptation is referred to as 'hardening off', and for successful release the poult must have a good covering of feathers. Feather growth appears to be stimulated particularly by wetting, either from natural rainfall or by artificial means, and from the resulting preening activity of the birds. However, the emerging feathers can easily become a target for feather pecking by other birds, leaving areas of bare skin over the back of the bird, resulting in poor protection and insulation in the event of adverse weather conditions in subsequent weeks. Such birds will often fare badly if released before the feathers have re-grown. Feather pecking can be reduced by good management, for example in the provision of stimulating surroundings with reasonably long (10 to 15 cm) vegetation and perches, to alleviate boredom. It has also been shown that increasing the stocking density in the first 6 weeks of life from 0.7 to 4.0 birds per m^2 in an aviary environment is associated with a significant adverse effect on plumage quality and increased skin damage (Kjaer, 2004). These are lower stocking densities than those used in commercial practice which may be up to 10 birds per m^2. It is also common for poults to be fitted with plastic 'bits' which clip into the nostrils and prevent feather pecking (Figure 16.5). The bits are fitted at approximately 3 weeks of age and initially can cause some difficulty in feeding, particularly if the pellet size is too large. It may therefore be preferable to keep the chicks on crumbs until 2 or 3 days after bitting before introducing mini-pellets unless the latter are of a very small size. Bits are usually removed when the poults are crated

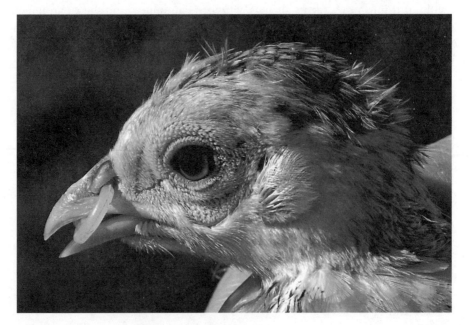

Figure 16.5   A plastic `bit' fitted to a pheasant poult.

up, prior to being moved to the release pen. They should be removed with clippers, rather than pulled out, to reduce the risk of damage to the mucous membranes of the nasal cavity. Different sizes of bits are available which can be used for different sizes of birds. Some pheasant rearers are, however, able to manage their birds successfully without the use of bits.

16.2.3 Pheasant release

At approximately 6 to 8 weeks of age the poults are caught and put into crates for transfer to the release pen. In many cases poults are reared by specialist game farmers and have to be transported over long distances for release. They can become subject to heat stress and dehydration if attention is not given to their welfare and management during the journey and on arrival at their destination. Pheasant release pens are normally set in woodland and are surrounded by wire mesh fencing to a height of approximately 1.8 m, which must be secured to the ground and protected with an electric fence or other means around the perimeter in order to exclude predators, particularly foxes. A low stocking density within the pen of 16 m^2 per bird is recommended. Feed and water is supplied to aid adaptation to this much more extensive existence. Proprietary feeds used in release pens have a protein content of 16 to 21% (Table 16.1) and are fed from hoppers, which should be shielded to prevent the feed getting wet. The poults are able to fly out of the pens and for the first few weeks can re-enter the pen for feeding through funnels in the fencing. Growth of the birds is not complete until 18 to 20 weeks of age, by which time (October to November) they spend most or all of their life outside the release pen, although supplementary feed is still provided for them, either in the form of proprietary pellets or wheat, or a combination of the two. The pheasant shooting season starts in October.

16.3 Partridge Breeding and Rearing

The principles of red-legged and grey partridge management are similar to those for pheasants, and the aim is likewise to produce fit birds for release into the semi-wild for subsequent shooting, but there are some differences including those summarized below. The breeding season for partridges extends from April to July, and potentially for longer in the red-legged partridge. The two species are expected to produce 45 (red-legged) and 60 to 65 eggs (grey) through the season. Breeding adults are overwintered from September in grass pens with the provision of additional cover for shelter and from January are paired off, and remain in pair boxes for the remainder of the breeding season, after which they are either released or retained for a second breeding season. Pair boxes are used because of aggression between males, and have been found to result in higher levels of egg production. The birds should preferably not be confined to the pair boxes for more than 6 months during a year, but in practice they are sometimes retained in pair boxes continually for up to three seasons.

The pair boxes are raised above the ground and comprise an enclosed nest box and a small covered exercise area with a floor of wire mesh and a feed area. The purpose of the wire mesh floor is to prevent the build-up of faecal material and enteric parasites, to which partridges are very susceptible. The box typically measures approximately 45 by 125 by 35 cm overall and a minimum floor area of $0.37\,\mathrm{m}^2$ is recommended by the GFA, or $0.65\,\mathrm{m}^2$ if partridges are retained in the boxes for longer than 6 months in any year. The bedding for the nest box is in the form of fine grit, sand or 'Astroturf'. The incubation of the eggs and management of the young birds through the brooder and rearing phases is similar to pheasants, except that the birds are transferred at 9 to 10 weeks of age into moveable wire-mesh release pens on grass and stocked at a typical density of $0.36\,\mathrm{m}^2$ per bird. After 1 to 2 weeks (during August and September) the birds are then released into a maize or similar cover crop, with feeders and drinkers placed in rides in the crop and in the release pens. Growth of the birds is complete at 14 weeks and the partridge shooting season starts in September.

16.4 Growth Rates of Game Birds

Table 16.2 gives a guide to the weights of the three game bird species at different ages, and is taken from Beer (1988). Growth rates of young game birds are affected by factors such as enteric disease and malabsorption, both of which are common, and the figures given should be taken only as approximate. There has been very little genetic selection of game birds, unlike in commercial chickens and turkeys, so the growth rates have changed little since the time they were originally published.

Table 16.2 Approximate weights (g) of game birds at different ages. Source: Beer (1988). Used with permission from the Game & Wildlife Conservation Trust (formerly The Game Conservancy Trust).

Age	Pheasant	Red-legged Partridge	Grey Partridge
Day-old	20	12	7
1 week	50	17	11
2 weeks	80	30	18
3 weeks	120	45	28
4 weeks	200	70	45
5 weeks	300	100	62
6 weeks	380	140	86
7 weeks	450	190	115
8 weeks	550	230	140
9 weeks	650	280	170
10 weeks	750	330	210
12 weeks	900	400	250
Adults: male	1400	540	390
female	1100	480	330

Table 16.3 Water intake (mL/day) of young pheasants. Source: Beer (1988). Used with permission from the Game & Wildlife Conservation Trust (formerly The Game Conservancy Trust).

Age	Water intake
A few days	10
3 weeks	28
4 weeks	41
5 weeks	57
6 weeks	62
7 weeks	67
8 weeks	72
9 weeks	74
12 weeks	77

16.5 Water Intake by Game Birds

A supply of clean and palatable water must be available at all times to game birds. Figures for water intake at different ages of pheasant have been published (Beer 1988) and are reproduced in Table 16.3. Figures such as these are useful in calculating the amounts of medication that should be added to the water should this need arise, but the calculations need to take into account intake from other sources such as dew. These figures should be used only as a guide, as water intake varies with the method of feeding; intake rises in hand-fed birds after the feeding period but is more evenly spread through the day in birds fed *ad libitum* (Wise and Connan, 1979). The physical consistency and water content of the feed may also affect water intake. There is little variation in water intake between ambient temperatures of 10 and 25 °C. Water consumption follows a diurnal pattern with peak intake in the early hours of the morning. There is an increasing tendency for water to be supplied via overhead nipple drinkers (Figure 16.2) which have the great benefit of being more hygienic than drinkers placed on the ground, and the supply pipes can be kept clean by periodically flushing with a biocide solution.

16.6 Nutrition

There has been very little empirical research into the nutrition of game birds to form a basis for commercially available rations. Several types of feed are used, varying in presentation and nutritional content according to the perceived needs of the birds. Examples of commercially available rations and their crude protein content are shown in Table 16.1. Feed is initially supplied in open trays to young chicks and then in covered feeders (Figure 16.3). Supplementary vitamins are commonly given via the water, particularly at times of potential stress such as transfer to release pens. Insoluble grit should be made available to birds that have access to grass and fibre, to reduce the risk of impaction of the gizzard with fibre. At all ages it is important that the feed should be stored and fed in a dry condition, as dampness can lead to fungal growth and outbreaks of aspergillosis in the birds.

16.7 Diseases of Game Birds

As with all livestock, good management and attention to detail are important in minimizing the effects of disease in game birds. Advances have been made over the last few years in the understanding of some of the common game bird diseases, but disease control is still hampered by the limited range of medicinal products available for treating birds. In this context, veterinarians usually have to use products licensed for use in poultry for treating disease problems in pheasants and partridges, and this may lead to suboptimal control of some diseases and parasites. In addition, the biosecurity standards of game bird enterprises often fall short of those in the poultry industry. Because of these and other factors it is unusual for the mortality rates between placing chicks as day-olds and transfer to release pens to be less than 5%. Readers are referred for further information on game bird diseases to reviews such as those of Pennycott (2001) and Welchman (2008). Some important game bird diseases are summarized below.

The role of hygiene has already been mentioned and nowhere is this more important than in the control of enteric diseases, especially rotavirus and salmonellosis in young chicks, coccidiosis in rearing birds (particularly partridges) and spironucleosis (hexamitosis) in rearing and release pen birds. Rotavirus commonly causes enteritis (diarrhoea, dehydration and death) in chicks from 7 days to approximately 3 weeks of age and survives well in the environment, so strict attention to cleanliness between batches is essential if the same brooder accommodation is used repeatedly through the season. No specific treatment is available to control the disease. *Salmonella* infections occasionally lead to outbreaks of disease, sometimes accompanied by high mortality, most often in young chicks. *Spironucleus* (or *Hexamita*) is a protozoan parasite associated with watery diarrhoea, ill thrift and death in growing birds between approximately 3 and 12 weeks of age, and is readily transmitted between birds in contaminated rearing accommodation. As with rotavirus, no specific treatment is available. Coccidia are also protozoan parasites which, unlike rotavirus and *Spironucleus*, are host specific and therefore cannot be transmitted between pheasants and partridges or vice versa, but can cause severe outbreaks of diarrhoea and mortality in partridges, in particular. The eggs (oocysts) produced by Coccidia are particularly resistant in the environment. Some measure of control can be achieved by the use of in-feed coccidiostat drugs but it goes without saying that the efficacy of the product relies on the birds eating the medicated feed. Outbreaks of coccidiosis can also be treated by in-water medication with products licensed for use in poultry for this purpose. All three of these diseases are essentially associated with poor hygiene and can build up in areas of heavy contamination such as around feeders and drinkers, but this build-up can be reduced by the use of overhead nipple drinkers.

A problem with using rearing fields and release pens for birds in successive years can be a build-up of parasitic worms (nematodes), of which the best known is the gapeworm, *Syngamus trachea*, which is a common parasite of the respiratory tract, particularly of pheasants. The eggs can survive for up to 9 months in the soil and for longer periods in transport hosts, which include earthworms and other invertebrates. Other nematode parasites include *Heterakis* species (the caecal worm) and *Capillaria* and related species, which parasitize the alimentary tract. Worm infections are routinely controlled by medication of the feed with anthelmintic products, and control programmes should include adult birds at the onset of the breeding season. *Heterakis* worms can carry the protozoan parasite *Histomonas* which is the cause of Blackhead (histomonosis), a disease occasionally encountered, particularly in partridges.

A commercially important disease of game birds is infectious sinusitis or myco-plasmosis, caused by *Mycoplasma gallisepticum* or mixed infections with this agent and other bacteria, or with viruses. Infection with this organism leads to a debil-itating disease characterized by swelling of the sinuses of the head, giving a 'bulgy eye' appearance. The disease is controlled via antibiotic medication of the water. *M. gallisepticum* can be transmitted from the breeding hen through the egg and it is therefore particularly important that breeding birds should as far as possible be free of the disease. Some veterinarians recommend blood testing of breeding stock for evidence of infection.

Game birds are susceptible to the notifiable diseases, Newcastle disease and avian influenza. Several outbreaks of Newcastle disease have been recorded in game birds in Britain, and outbreaks in captive game birds (i.e. prior to release into the wild) have been controlled under the statutory notifiable disease requirements in the same way as in poultry, with the valuation and compulsory slaughter of birds on infected premises if disease is confirmed. Game birds are also subject to the rules covering protection and surveillance zones that surround infected premises where Newcastle disease or H5 or H7 strains of avian influenza have been confirmed, including movement restrictions, requirements to house, and in some cases a ban on shooting. A lack of adequate biosecurity may be a particular problem on game premises in the event of notifiable disease outbreaks.

16.8 Game Bird Welfare

With the considerable increase in the numbers of game birds reared in the late twentieth and early twenty-first century, there has been a trend for increasing intensification particularly of the breeding, incubation, hatching, brooding and early rearing processes. This trend is largely driven by economic considerations and is likely to continue, and has raised concerns for the welfare of the birds which have been highlighted by the Farm Animal Welfare Council (FAWC, 2008). The *raison d'être* of game bird breeding and rearing is the release of birds able to survive in a wild or semi-wild environment, yet recent developments such as raised laying units with wire mesh floors for breeding pheasants have not been adequately researched with regard to the welfare of the birds, for example in allowing the expression of normal behaviour. However, the GFA has recommended minimum requirements in terms of floor area and other measurements for these units, and the provision of perches sufficient for all the birds to roost comfortably at one time. Research is needed on the provision of space and environmental enrichment to meet the physical and behavioural requirements of the birds in this system. Research is similarly needed to design improved accommodation for breeding partridges, bearing in mind that pair boxes have the benefit of reducing aggression and exposure to disease. In addition, many pheasants and the majority of partridges are derived from breeding units in continental Europe where intensive breeding systems have been more widely used than in Britain, and FAWC (2008) recommends that game owners should satisfy themselves that the health and welfare of the breeding stock meet the standards required in this country.

The use of particular types of management devices has also been highlighted by FAWC (2008). The requirement for specs in particular is not proven, and they inhibit the expression of normal behaviour and may lead to injury and discomfort by penetration of the nasal septum. Although less prone to cause injury, the use of 'bumpa-bits', which serve a similar purpose to specs in breeding pens, also requires justification. However, there appears to be some justification for the use of small conventional bits in controlling feather pecking in rearing birds. FAWC (2008) has recommended that the use of bits (and other devices) should be assessed on an individual site basis as part of a farm health and welfare plan developed in consultation with the owner's veterinary surgeon. There appears to be little justification for the use of beak trimming which is occasionally carried out as an alternative to, or in addition to, the use of bits.

Freedom from disease is an important component of animal welfare, and it is unfortunate that in the past relatively high mortality during the rearing period was accepted almost as the norm. However, with increasing intensification has come a greater appreciation of the importance of biosecurity and hygiene in minimizing the exposure of the birds to disease agents, with consequential benefit to bird welfare, and mortality in the best-managed rearing systems has considerably improved.

References and Further Reading

Beer, J.V. (1988) *Diseases of Gamebirds and Wildfowl*. Game Conservancy Trust Ltd, Fordingbridge, UK.

DEFRA (2010) Codes of recommendations for the welfare of gamebirds reared for sporting purposes. Available at: http://www.defra.gov.uk/foodfarm/farmanimal/documents/cop-welfaregamebirds100722.pdf

Farm Animal Welfare Council (2008) *Opinion on the Welfare of Farmed Gamebirds*. FAWC, London. Available at: http://www.fawc.org.uk.

Game Conservancy Advisory Service (1991) *Gamebird Releasing*. The Game Conservancy Ltd, Fordingbridge, UK.

Game Conservancy Advisory Service (1993) *Egg Production and Incubation*. The Game Conservancy Ltd, Fordingbridge, UK.

Game Conservancy Advisory Service (2006) *Gamebird Rearing*. The Game Conservancy Ltd, Fordingbridge, UK.

Game Farmers' Association (GFA) *Codes of Practice for the Welfare of Game Birds*. Available at: http://www.gfa.org.uk.

Kjaer, J.B. (2004) Effects of stocking density and group size on the condition of the skin and feathers of pheasant chicks. Veterinary Record **154**, 556–8.

Pennycott, T.W. (2001) Disease control in adult pheasants. *In Practice* **23**, 132–40.

Welchman, D. de B. (2008) Diseases in young pheasants. *In Practice* **30**, 144–9.

Wise, D.R. (1993) *Pheasant Health and Welfare*. Published by the author.

Wise, D.R. and Connan, R.M. (1979) Water consumption in growing pheasants. *Veterinary Record* **104**, 368–70.

Ostrich

17

FIONA BENSON

Management and Welfare of Farm Animals: The UFAW Farm Handbook, 5th edition. John Webster
© 2011 by Universities Federation for Animal Welfare (UFAW)

17.1 Introduction

17.1.1 The ostrich industry

While ostrich have been raised domestically in South Africa for nearly 200 years, ostrich production in the United Kingdom and the developed world is a relatively new industry that, at the time of writing, is transitioning from breeder markets to commercial production. Moreover it is only since the late 1980s that work was started on these birds' nutritional requirements and management systems to bring them in line with modern livestock production. Although South Africa market the meat, they have farmed ostrich primarily for their skins, with production measurements of performance, such as days taken to slaughter and improving feed conversion, not considered in their production methods or costs of production.

The World Ostrich Association, established in 2002, has steadily introduced guideline standards and grading systems to guide the industry through the transition from speculative breeder markets to commercial production. The transition to volume production will result in evolving systems as experience is gained and the association will ensure welfare standards are updated to keep in line with the latest developments. Currently there are very few meaningful ostrich production records, but there is now sufficient experience and knowledge to be able to establish achievable target production figures. Improvements in performance come as a result of a number of factors working together including, and in the following order: nutrition, feed management, farm management and genetics. A failure in any one of these sectors will impact on performance and profitability. The basic production principles required for commercial success are the same for small hobby farmers as they are for large-scale commercial production. The main differences are the economics that come with economies of scale.

When these factors are correctly in place, steady improvements will be seen year on year. The World Ostrich Association published production benchmark targets in 2006 to provide achievable goals when the correct management techniques are employed. These benchmark targets provide an excellent guide for farmers to know if their management and welfare standards are effective. Egg numbers from breeder birds, conversion of these eggs to chicks, chick mortality, days taken to slaughter and meat yield are all important measurements, with the most important being number of viable slaughter birds per hen.

The lack of records has resulted in much random crossbreeding and little knowledge of the genetics of the birds. Table 17.1 summarizes some essential features of eight breeds (or races) of ostrich. Missing from this list is the Australian Grey – a breed that evolved following the demise of the feather industry at the outbreak of World War I and the birds were allowed to go wild in Australia. It is our experience that, when raised in a well-managed domesticated environment, the live-weights listed are falling short of their genetic potential, but the differentials between the breeds are realistic. The number and type of ostrich kept and the stocking rate and/or housing density will depend on the suitability of the

Table 17.1 Summary of differences in features between the ostrich races. Source: from Brown et al. (1981) and Jarvis (1991).

Feature	N. African	Massai	Somali	Zimbabwe	Kalahari	Namib	W. Coast	Oudtshoorn
Crown (bald?)	Yes	No	Yes	No	No	No	No	Yes/No
Neck skin colour	Pink	Pink	Blue	Grey	Grey	Grey	Grey	Grey
Neck collar (white)	Wide	Thin	Nil	Thin	?	?	Thin	Variable
Neck bare	Yes	Yes	No	No	No	No	No	No
Eye colour	Brown	Brown	Blue	Brown	?	?	Brown	Brown
Body skin (male)	Pink	Pink	Blue	Grey/blue	Grey/blue	Grey/blue	Grey/blue	Grey/blue
Body skin (female)	Brown	Brown	Brown	Brown	Brown	Brown	Brown	Brown
Leg scutes (males)	Red	Red	Red & black	Red	Red	Red	Red	Red
Tail feathers (male)	White	Pale brown	White	Rusty	Pale brown	Pale brown	Pale brown	Rusty or white
Tail feathers (female)	Brown	Brown	Brown	Brown	Brown	Brown	Brown	Brown
Adult weight average (kg)	105	135	105	125	?	100	90	115

environment, the capacity of the farm, the competence of the stockperson and the time available to carry out their duties. Good stockmanship is of paramount importance in all systems of ostrich production.

17.1.2 Stockmanship

The most significant single influence on the welfare and performance of any flock is the stockperson. All stockpeople should be aware of the welfare needs of the stock under their care and be capable of safeguarding them under all foreseeable conditions before being given the responsibility for the flock. This requires the acquisition of specific stockmanship skills, through a combination of practical experience and training. Stockpeople should be trained in hooding, handling and restraint. Generally, at least two people are required to handle and move an adult ostrich safely. Stockpeople should know the signs of good health in ostrich of all ages. These include general alertness, free movement, active feeding, as well as absence of lameness, visible wounds, abscesses or injuries. The capabilities of the stockperson in charge of ostrich are a significant factor in determining the size of a flock. The unit should only be set up if the stockpeople have the skills necessary to safeguard the welfare of every animal in their charge and the infrastructure required to support them. The process of transition from small breeder units to larger commercial rearing units, developing the markets, and building sufficient volume to create a reliable supply for these markets requires a delicate balance.

17.2 Nutrition

Ostrich should be fed a wholesome diet that is appropriate to their species, their age and production group (Table 17.2) and this must be fed in sufficient quantity to maintain good health and satisfy their nutritional needs. Ostrich appear to have

Table 17.2 Production requirements for breeders and growers.

Ration	Production requirement
Breeders: off season	Replenishment of depleted nutrient reserves
	Build condition for the new breeder season
Breeders: in season	Good egg production
	Adequate nutrient transfer to ensure strong, healthy chicks at hatch
Baby chicks 0–2 months	Smooth transfer from yolk sac absorption to external feed intake
Grower birds	Optimum growth rates
	Optimum feed conversion
	Excellent muscle growth, meat and skin quality (slaughter birds)
	Good reproductive organ development (future breeders)
Pre-breeders	Continued reproductive organ development
	Early puberty

a low appetite relative to their bodyweight. This may reflect adaptation to a marginal existence in the wild. To ensure they have sufficient feed to support rates of growth and reproduction consistent with commercial production, they require rations that are nutrient dense and precisely formulated to achieve an optimal balance of energy, protein, minerals and vitamins.

For decades nutritional adequacy has been measured by the lack of symptoms of nutritional deficiencies, but today it is recognized that nutritional deficiencies do not have to show clinical symptoms to compromise a producer's return. In commercial terms they will be expressed as failure to meet their genetic potential measured in terms of growth and reproduction. Ostrich are most productive when fed precisely formulated, balanced rations as complete feeds to ensure accurate intake of all ingredients. Rations can be fed as ground meal or pelleted. A balanced ration must, of course, contain the right levels of water, protein, energy, vitamins and minerals. It must also be presented in a physical form that is appropriate to the feeding behaviour and digestive system of the birds. This requires a sound understanding of nutrition; sources, balance and interactions between nutrients. It also requires a sound knowledge of practical feeding. This involves both the chemical composition of the ingredients, ratios of ingredient type (forages, grains, protein and fat sources, vitamins and minerals) and their physical form (e.g. ratios of different particle sizes).

17.2.1 Ingredient types
A balanced production ration for ostrich should contain ingredients from the following types.

17.2.1.1 Forages
'High fibre, medium protein and energy' – quality lucerne (alfalfa) is an ideal forage for ostrich, being relatively higher in both digestible energy and protein than grass-based forages, feeding of which may result in loss of condition and reduced production. To rate as 'quality', lucerne should be fed dry (as hay or barn-dried) and have a protein concentration not less than 17%. Ostrich fail to thrive when fed fresh lucerne, or poorer-quality lucerne hay (more stemmy, protein <16%) (Table 17.3). An adequate supply of high-quality, appropriate fibre from a forage source is essential to sustain both optimal digestion and nutrient supply. All too often the word 'roughage' is used in a manner that indicates that it is fed 'over and above' the basic ration and simply there to 'aid' digestion. This is not true – the ration must include fibre at the right levels and from the right source. Remembering the very low daily feed intake of ostrich it is a challenge to pack all the required nutrients into a ration; therefore the forage (roughage) source must be highly digestible, containing the maximum nutrients possible.

17.2.1.2 Grains
'High in energy, low in protein and fibre' – grains utilized in ostrich rations should be quality, whole grain products, high in energy. High-fibre grains such as oats are not

Table 17.3 Productive values of the major ingredients.

Ingredient type	Productive	Use with caution	Non-productive
Forage	Quality lucerne – min 17% protein (dried/hay)	Grass and poor quality lucerne – <17% protein (dried/hay)	Fresh lucerne, fresh grass, straw, low-quality lucerne
Grains	Maize	Barley, wheat	Oats, milo/sorghum, rice, rye, triticale
Protein: oil seeds	Dehulled soya (Hi Pro) 47% protein, soya meal 44%	Full fat soya	Cottonseed, canola, rapeseed, peanut, sunflower, lupins
Protein: animal			Fishmeal, meat & bone meal, carcass meal. Any protein from an animal source
By-products		Distillers' dried grains, wheat middlings, wheat bran, corn gluten meal 60%	Hulls and husks, oat bran, corn cob fractions, mill screenings, brewers dried grains, peanut skins, grape residue, molasses, hominy chop, citrus pulp, corn gluten feed 20%, sugar beet (whole, pulp or peelings)

utilized well by ostrich. Maize is the best grain and a production ration requires at least 50% of the grain portion of the ration to be quality maize, as maize has certain characteristics that cannot be replaced by other grains. Grains should be fed ground to match the particle size of the other ingredients in the ration when the feed is not pelleted.

17.2.1.3 Protein

'High in protein, low in fibre and medium energy' – dehulled soya bean meal is an ideal protein source for ostrich, with the right amino acid structure. Most other oilseed protein feeds are less well balanced with respect to amino acids and may contain anti-nutrient substances, thus requiring higher inclusion levels, and can cause certain difficulties in achieving the correct ratios of protein feeds, grains and forages in the ration.

17.2.1.4 Major, minor and trace minerals

The highest grades of minerals have to be used for ostrich, as lower grades often contain many mineral contaminants that will interfere with other minerals in the rations. As productive ostrich rations are nutrient dense, these interferences are more pronounced and have to be watched carefully.

17.2.1.5 Vitamins

Vitamins are the nutrients that regulate the biochemical reactions by which energy and protein are used for health, growth, feed conversion and reproduction. Without vitamins these biochemical reactions will not occur. Vitamins are available from the major ingredients that are not subjected to heat treatment, but all vitamins require additional supplementation in the feed from quality sources.

17.2.1.6 Fat and oil

The major ingredients contain a certain level of fat. Additional fat must be supplied from a quality fat source. If animal fat is used it must be from a pure source, as poorly rendered fat sources could still contain some protein elements and risk of bovine spongiform encephalitis (BSE). There are many different fats on the market for use in livestock production, so care must be taken to ensure the source is of good quality and not recycled fats from supermarkets or restaurants or containing other additives that could interfere with other nutrients in the rations.

17.2.1.7 Other additives

These include additional amino acids, yeast culture, probiotics and similar natural ingredients, with the intention of supplementing nutrient supply and promoting healthy digestion. There is, at present, too little evidence to justify any definitive conclusions as to the benefits or justification for these supplements on grounds of health or economics.

17.2.2 Balance of ingredient type

It is important to maintain a balance of ingredient type without an excess of any one type. This can influence a number of utilization factors and the gut pH. This is particularly important with baby chicks in helping to establish a healthy bacterial population in the digestive tract. To help understand the productive characteristics of different ingredients in ostrich, one can classify ingredients as:'productive' and the best ingredients for ostrich; 'use with caution' – these ingredients can have a positive influence at controlled inclusion levels; 'non-productive' – these are ingredients that ostrich do not utilize well and their inclusion in ostrich rations will lead to loss of production at best and influence the overall health of the birds. Table 17.3 lists the ingredients that fall into these different categories.

It has been suggested that wheat bran can be used as a substitute for lucerne. This does not work as the type of fibre in bran is from a grain source and not a forage source. Moreover, wheat bran is seriously imbalanced with respect to calcium and phosphorus (see below). Grain also has different characteristics in the digestion process. Productive ostrich rations must contain fibre from an appropriate forage source, including chick rations. Using low-quality lucerne results in either reduced nutrient levels or incorrect ratios of forage, grains and protein ingredients.

17.2.3 Levels and ratios of amino acids

Proteins are complex compounds made up of a large number of amino acids, many of which are essential (e.g. lysine, methionine and tryptophan). Strictly speaking the nitrogen requirement of a non-ruminant animal, such as the ostrich, should be defined in terms of its specific requirement for these essential amino acids. That is why on occasion an 18% protein feed can work as well as or better than a 20% protein feed – because the amino acid profile is different between the two formulas. Since cereal grains (and lucerne) are deficient in certain essential amino acids it is important to supplement these ingredients to meet amino acid requirements, particularly during period of high demand, which include growth and egg production. It may be possible, and economically prudent, to provide these extra amino acids from a source of high-quality vegetable protein, such as soya bean meal. Alternatively these essential amino acids can be incorporated into pre-mixes that also provide supplementary vitamins and minerals. Because it is critical to balance nutrient supply to specific production requirements, it is an extremely dangerous practice to use a pre-mix designed by one nutritionist with another's ration formulations. Production premixes are designed to bind *all* the ingredients in the ration.

The major feed ingredients contain certain minerals in different proportions depending on plant type, local conditions and nutrients provided to the crop during the growing process. Additional mineral supplementation is also required and these are best added from inorganic sources. Animal protein products (APPs) can be rich in minerals and vitamins but they are likely to be unbalanced. Moreover, and fortunately, APPs are no longer allowed in many regions and should never be used for ostrich reared for meat because of concerns for human health. Apart from the negative nutritional aspects, this practice also compromises ostrich's greatest marketing tool, the perceived health attributes of the meat.

17.2.4 Ratios of particle sizes

There are many interrelationships between different nutrients, ratios of particle sizes being one. If a nutrient is provided in a form that can be absorbed into the bloodstream quickly and another nutrient is provided in a form that is absorbed slowly, then imbalances creating deficiencies and excesses will occur, even if the levels sample correctly in the ration. Another area where particle sizes are most important is the finished rations. If a ration is not pelleted it is most important that the finished ration contains all ingredients at a similar particle size to minimize the risks of the birds being selective in their feed intake. For example, grains should be ground and not included whole. Grazing grass or lucerne, feeding silage or any feed with high moisture content creates significant challenges to achieve balanced intake of all nutrients. Grazing not only changes in nutrient values depending on the season, from day to day and type of grazed material; it also varies considerably in moisture content, making it even more difficult to achieve uniformity in daily intake.

Practical example

Calcium is an excellent nutrient to illustrate the principles discussed above. The inorganic source for calcium will generally be limestone; however, there are many different grades of limestone. The lower grades have low levels of calcium and contain other mineral contaminants that will cause interferences with other minerals in the rations.

The major organic source is from lucerne. Soya meal and bone meal also supply a certain level of calcium. Bone meal is no longer allowed by many countries and, as discussed earlier, should *never* be used if we wish to ensure the 'clean and healthy' attributes of ostrich. When included as a source of calcium it has a very low absorption rate and results in very little of the calcium being utilized by the ostrich. Particle size is important as this also affects the rate of absorption. It is common knowledge that the calcium/phosphorus ratios are critical. However, if the calcium is from a source that is absorbed very slowly and the phosphorus from a source that is absorbed very quickly, they will not be in the digestive system together to work with each other, and deficiencies will occur. The ration will analyse correctly but the birds will show symptoms of deficiency. In order for the calcium and phosphorus to be utilized the ration must contain adequate levels of vitamin D to carry the calcium and phosphorus into the bloodstream. If the calcium and phosphorus levels, sources and ratios are correct, but there is a shortage of vitamin D, then deficiency symptoms will result.

17.2.5 Feed management

The nutrient requirements of ostrich, like any farmed animal, are defined by the needs for maintenance and production, where production includes growth, egg production, chick hatchability and survival through egg yolk nutrient transfer. A production ration must also take into account the need to replace lost body reserves in breeding stock after a long season of egg production. To achieve these, the nutritionist will be ensuring that birds achieve the correct intake of specific nutrients. This is done through the ration having the correct nutrient levels and being fed in controlled amounts.

There are two ways in which birds can be under- or overfed.

1. Variations in ingredient quality: A ration is made up of different ingredients, each of which provides a number of nutrients. One common error is to consider all lucerne as the same instead of sampling each batch and adjusting the formulas to allow for these changes. Soya meal is another ingredient that can come in different qualities. Incorrect ingredient quality results not only in over- or underfeeding (short feeding) of specific nutrients, it also results in rations becoming imbalanced as the nutrients are no longer in their correct proportions to each other.

2. Failure to weigh the feed accurately at feeding time: To underfeed an adult ostrich by just 100 grams is 5% of the total daily intake of an adult bird, very significant to ostrich, and short feeding by 5% will impact on performance.

The general rules of feed management come under six headings.

17.2.5.1 Know what you are feeding

Learn what to look for to ensure that rations have production potential and are not detrimental to bird health. Commercial feed labels will supply basic nutrient levels and the ingredients, but laws in different countries do influence the accuracy of this information. Learn how to identify from the feed label if the rations are put together with production potential in mind. Ostriches cannot tolerate changes in ingredients between batches of feed, and the practice of 'least cost' ingredient formulation can result in the birds 'going off feed' with loss of production and health. When mixing rations, it is important to ensure the use of correct ingredients, the vitamin and mineral pre-mix and rations provided are proven for ostrich. There are many rations published in the early to mid-1990s on the Internet and in some manuals that are now proven do not work for ostrich, but are, unfortunately, still available online.

17.2.5.2 Mixing accuracy

Accuracy of mixing is essential; ostrich are very sensitive to what may seem like minor errors or omissions in other species. Do not use pre-mixes designed for other species. If using a commercial mill, ensure that they use the ingredients in the amounts specified. To the mill, a minor alteration or substitution to the formula may seem insignificant, but to ostrich it will have a negative impact on their health and production. Always ensure the use of the highest-quality ingredients, and that everything is weighed accurately, mixed thoroughly and particle sizes are the same. Certain substances used for other species are toxic to ostrich, so great care is required to avoid any cross-contamination during the milling process.

17.2.5.3 Weighing

Determine how much should be fed of a particular ration and whether the ration should be limit fed or fed free choice.

Limit fed is a controlled, specific quantity per bird per day. The quantity fed at each feeding will depend on the number of times the birds are fed per day. It is essential that the birds are fed exactly the amount specified. Remember to allow for any potential loss from such factors as wind or wild birds. Watch the condition of the birds. Weigh all feed fed, do not feed by volume. Ostrich rations contain a high level of lucerne, which results in variations in ration density. The dangers from errors that can occur when feeding by volume cannot be overemphasized.

Free choice feeding allows the birds to eat as much as they like, as the birds are growing and increasing their intake daily as they grow. To feed free choice efficiently is an art. Just sufficient food should be placed in the troughs so that the feed troughs are emptied shortly before the next feed is due. Never put fresh food on top of the old.

Move the older food to one end of the trough and clean troughs every morning. Weigh any food taken away and monitor closely the total daily consumption. A drop in consumption is the first sign of impending problems – it could be an indication of a faulty batch of feed, reduced water intake or sickness. Food will deteriorate if exposed to air or to the sun and becomes less palatable very quickly. Ostrich are very sensitive to these changes, which may cause reduced feed intake. There will always be some birds that will consume at a faster rate than others, and one is at all times working to averages. The secret is to develop systems that will minimize this impact and always ensure all birds in the pen can eat at any one time.

17.2.5.4 Feeding times

Adult birds and growers over 3 months of age should be fed a minimum of twice per day. Young chicks require more frequent feeding. Notice the speed of deterioration of the feed colour – if it is rapid as a result of exposure to the sun, implement more frequent feeding times or take measures to protect the feed from the sun. Ostriches are very sensitive to aroma and colour; when this deteriorates their feed intake will be reduced.

17.2.5.5 Feeding troughs

Feed troughs must allow space for every bird in the pen to feed at any one time. The minimum requirement for adult birds is 0.5 metre per bird. This applies to birds that are fed on an *ad libitum* basis or on a rationed feed level. Feed troughs must be designed in such a manner that they are protected from the wind and rain.

17.2.5.6 Water

There must be a clean supply of fresh water freely available at all times for all ages of ostrich. Water should be sampled regularly to ensure that there are no abnormal mineral levels or other contaminants. Observe the daily water consumption to learn the 'norm'. Birds will slow down their drinking if the water is too cold or too hot. In cold climates, a proper water heater should be installed to keep water at 21 to 32 °C to maintain a steady consumption by the birds. Most common heaters only keep the water from freezing (around 4 to 7 °C) and that is too cold on wintry days, causing the water consumption to fall by 50% or more. When water consumption drops, feed utilization drops. There are special heaters available that will keep the water temperature at much higher levels. This will allow water consumption in winter to be nearly the same as summer water consumption and allows good growth and weight gains to continue through the winter months if the feed formula is correct.

Ensure that baby chicks have water available to them at all times.

17.2.5.7 Summary

Feed management is an art. Every operator has to work at it to eliminate errors and oversight. The 'skill' to feeding management is to put equal emphasis on all the details. A successful operation will be paying close attention to all the feed management details as best one can – and will have in place organized checkpoints to verify that all details are covered so some are not forgotten. The forgotten details can 'sneak up and bite'.

17.3 Environment, Management and Handling

Ostrich are maintained 'free range' with outdoor runs, with access to shelter, as appropriate for the climate. Ostrich should be given protection from adverse weather conditions, predators and have access to a well-drained lying area at all times.

Ostrich should only be held indoors for a period greater than 24 hours when weather conditions are such that it would be unsafe to allow them out, for example, extreme ice or flooding. Stocking density must ensure that under normal climatic conditions extreme muddy conditions do not affect their wing feathers. All fields and buildings should be kept clear of debris such as wire or plastic, which if ingested could be harmful to ostrich and all livestock. Ostrich can cope with a wide variety of climatic conditions if provided with suitable infrastructure.

Single breeding groups contain one male and one or more hens. Colonies contain more than one breeding group in the same pen. Ostrich use natural mating with breeding carried out in a free-range environment of single breeding groups or colonies. Artificial insemination is not currently in use with ostrich production. Breeding ostrich are encouraged to nest inside, thus a dry sand or earth flooring is required to enable the natural digging of a nest.

All ostrich farmers should have easily operated and efficient handling pens, to facilitate routine management and treatment, on a size and scale to suit the flock numbers (Figure 17.1). Pens and floors should be maintained in good repair and should not have any sharp edges or projections, which might injure the birds. Such handling should be kept to the minimum required to maintain optimum health. Well-designed collecting, loading and unloading facilities are required.

Fences and hedges should be well maintained so as to avoid injury to ostrich and prevent entanglement. Electric fences have not yet been tested with ostrich and, until this research is carried out, they are not recommended. Any fence must be highly visible. Hedges are suitable for ostrich, provided they are well maintained and gaps are filled. Barbed wire should never be used near ostrich. Fence height should be appropriate to the size of the birds being contained, with a minimum of 1.8 m for breeder birds, to prevent fighting across the fence. Alternatively breeding pens should be separated by a minimum of 2 m and minimum fence height of 1.5 m. Slaughter birds may be in pens with a minimum fence height of 1.5 m without pen separation. Any wire used should be installed in such a way to ensure the birds do not get their heads, necks or feet caught in the wire.

The plucking of feathers takes place after slaughter and is not permitted for commercial reasons by the World Ostrich Association while birds are alive. When the removal of feathers from a live animal is required for welfare reasons, care should be taken to cut the feather above the blood line.

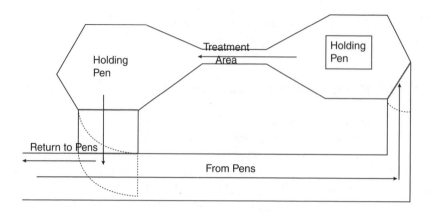

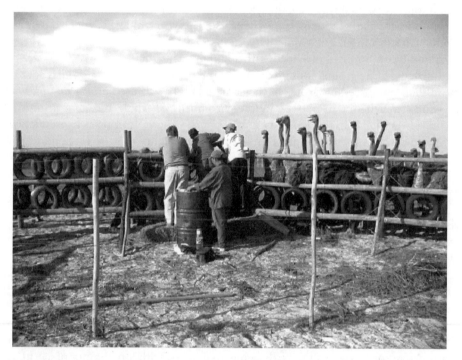

Figure 17.1   Handling facilities for ostrich. The photograph shows an ostrich being restrained in the treatment area.

Automatic handling systems at hatch are not currently in use with ostrich production. Any chicks that are deformed, sick or injured or that failed to hatch successfully should be removed immediately and destroyed humanely. Chicks should be handled with care during the transition process from hatching trays, to identification, sexing and despatch to rearing units and have access to feed and water as soon as possible after hatch. The design of transport boxes must ensure that there is adequate ventilation and air circulation to maintain an optimal temperature within the boxes during transportation. Holding facilities must maintain thermal comfort and ensure protection of chicks from any draughts, with a lighting level that ensures comfort.

During the first weeks baby chicks, especially while the yolk sac is still unabsorbed, must be kept warm and dry and not lie directly on the cold floor of the accommodation unit. Heated flooring or bedding in conjunction with overhead heating must be used to keep chicks warm and dry when night temperatures are likely to drop below 25 °C during the first month. Plastic or rubber matting that enables free movement of urine away from direct contact with the chicks may be used, and will discourage the baby chicks from eating bedding material that may be detrimental to their health. Chicks should be encouraged to have access to outdoor pens when the weather is suitable. Except when cleaning, chicks should have access to all areas of their pen 24 hours a day; the practice of shutting them out from their night quarters during the day is discouraged. Chicks for the first few weeks require a smaller area with freedom from draught with consistent night temperature. The number of weeks required is dependent on their rate of growth during this period. Table 17.4 illustrates the target weights. Studies have shown significant variablity from average live-weights with ranges of 2.5 to 6.0 kg at 30 days and 4.5 to 16 kg at 60 days.

Electric goads or striking with a stick should never be used for ostrich. Sticks and benign handling aids may be used as extensions of the arms. Loading facilities must minimize the incline of the ramp. When transporting, the vehicle should be suitable for the age group. Ostrich must be handled gently at all times during loading. Hooding is permitted during loading. Transport distances should be kept to a minimum. Ostrich transported for breeding purposes may require transport over longer distances. From a welfare/stress viewpoint, it is not advisable to offload

Table 17.4 Current benchmark targets for live-weight growth (caution: boneless meat yield is a better measure or performance).

Weeks	Days	Target weight (kg)
Week 4	28 days	6
Week 8	56 days	20
Week 13	90 days	35
Week 17	120 days	50
Week 21	145 days	70
Week 26	180 days	80
Week 30	210 days	95
Week 34	240 days	100
Week 39	270 days	110
Week 43	300 days	120

ostrich during transit. Floor space must be sufficient to allow each bird to rest and sleep without being trampled. Adequate stationary time and provision of food and water should be made available in the transport vehicle. When transporting ostrich it is important to remember they are a large animal with only two legs.

17.4 Health

Careful attention to nutrition, accompanied by high standards of feed and farm management, are the foundations for good health. Farm management includes such things as space requirement, buildings, stocking densities, pen design, biosecurity, farm records and disease prevention programmes. In most countries the regulations relating to health and welfare of animals require regular supervision of the livestock. Stockpeople should carry out inspections of the flock daily and pay particular attention to signs of injury, distress or illness, so that these conditions can be recognized and dealt with promptly.

Records should be maintained for any medicinal treatment given, and the number of mortalities. These records should be retained for a period as specified by legislation within the country of operation or assurance programme required by the markets served. It is advisable to have a written health and welfare programme. This should cover the annual production cycle, developed with appropriate veterinary and technical advice, reviewed and updated annually. The programme should include sufficient records to assess the basic output of the flock and should address, as a minimum, production performance, vaccination policy and timing and control of external and internal parasites. Particular attention should be paid to any stock introduced, including breeder hens, males, eggs or chicks, since diseases can easily be spread. At this time there are very few, if any, medications specifically developed and approved for ostrich in most countries. Therefore it is necessary to work closely with your veterinary surgeon to assess what is allowable in the country of operation. Because ostrich farming is a relatively new enterprise in most countries, there is, at present, little published evidence of problems arising from 'production diseases' (those attributable to breeding, feeding or management). However, leg problems (bow leg and rotation) in young chicks can be a major problem. In most cases they would appear to be nutritional in origin and can be ascribed to inadequacies in ration formulation.

17.4.1 Casualties

Any ostrich that appear to be ill or injured should be cared for appropriately without delay; and where they do not respond to care, veterinary advice shall be obtained as soon as possible. When necessary, sick or injured animals should be isolated in suitable accommodation with dry comfortable bedding as appropriate, remembering that ostrich do not like separation or change of location. Injured, ailing or distressed ostrich should be identified and treated without delay. Where the stockperson is able to identify the cause of ill health, he or she should take immediate remedial action. When in doubt, veterinary advice should be obtained as soon as possible.

If an unfit ostrich does not respond to treatment, it should be culled or humanely killed on-farm. In some countries it is an offence to cause, or to allow, unnecessary pain or unnecessary distress by leaving any animal to suffer. In an emergency, it may be necessary to kill an animal immediately to prevent suffering. In such cases, the bird should be destroyed in a humane manner and, where possible, by a person experienced and/or trained both in the techniques and the equipment used for killing ostrich. Usable methods are captive bolt, lethal injection or rifle, shot through the head if safe to do so.

If animals are killed or slaughtered on-farm, other than in an emergency, the operation may only be carried out using a permitted method and in accordance with current local welfare at slaughter legislation. An unfit ostrich may be transported only if it is being taken for veterinary diagnosis or treatment or is going to the nearest available place of slaughter, and then only provided it is transported in a way which is not going to cause it further suffering.

17.5 Economics

The commercial viability of a farm is critical to supporting high welfare standards. When the above management and nutrition standards are implemented the increased productivity brings about significant improvements in overall profitability. Egg production improves with increased hatchability and more chicks are reared to slaughter in fewer days.

Historically, skin has been the driving force for ostrich production. The market serviced was high end and low volume, dependent on fashion trends. There was little incentive to modernize production systems. A sustainable meat market offers the greatest potential for growth and commercial success of ostrich. Doubling meat yields and halving time taken to slaughter transforms the overall economics. As Figure 17.2 illustrates, the impact of increasing meat yields shows there will be increased meat revenue accompanied by a significant reduction in processing costs per kilogram of meat produced. Meat revenue should attract approximately 75% of revenue, with skins, fat and feathers adding valuable additional revenue.

17.5.1 Skins

The market available for skins is dependent on location and volume produced. Skins are sold under grading systems, which are required to set producer payment as well as finished leather prices. The following are the different options:

- Finished skins: used by tanneries or large producers tanning their own skins selling to manufacturers.

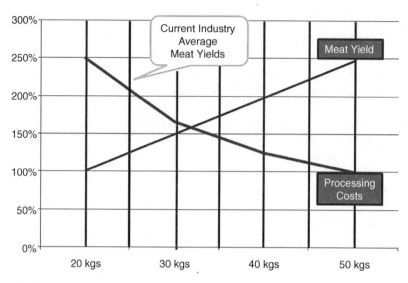

Figure 17.2 Influence of meat yield and processing costs.

- Crust: farmer payment, but requires delayed payment. Numbers are insufficient currently in the UK for this system to be incorporated, but is the fairest of all systems for farmer payment.
- Green: tannery to pay farmer or trader/dealer. Production levels are too small in the UK at this time to sell direct to tanneries.
- Green: trader/dealer payment to farmers. This is the main method of sale of skins in the UK at this time. A minimum number of skins are required and, when slaughtering low volumes per month, skins have to be stored until sufficient are available for the dealers to collect. Low volume carries with it high handling costs and therefore is the least attractive method of selling skins, but the only way for a producer while volumes are low.

Full details of the different grades and definitions are available at: http://www.world-ostrich.org/woaleather.htm.

17.6 Conclusion

Ostrich production is a new livestock production enterprise in the developed world, with significant commercial potential, provided the basic principles of livestock management, nutrition and welfare are incorporated in combination with strong market development. A strong market, with volume production, opens the door to genetic improvement to progressively improve the production potential of ostrich. Slaughter weight in less than 200 days, with a feed conversion of 2: 1, is achievable. However, care will be needed to ensure that welfare is not compromised.

References and Further Reading

Brown, L.H., Urban, E.K. and Newman, K. (1982) *The Birds of Africa*, Volume 1. Academic Press, London.

Jarvis, M.J.F. (1991) Regional differences between ostriches. *Ostrich Seminar*, 1–22.

World Ostrich Association. *Organic Standards*. Available at: http://www.world-ostrich.org/targets.htm.

World Ostrich Association. *Benchmark Targets*. Available at: http://www.world-ostrich.org/targets.htm.

World Ostrich Association. *Skin and Leather Grades*. Available at: http://www.world-ostrich.org/woaleather.htm.

Other reference sources

http://www.blue-mountain.net/research.htm – a number of studies, papers and articles.

http://www.blue-mountain.net/bulletins.htm – articles and papers on production and industry discussions.

Assessment, Implementation and Promotion of Farm Animal Welfare

18

DAVID MAIN AND JOHN WEBSTER

Management and Welfare of Farm Animals: The UFAW Farm Handbook, 5th edition. John Webster
© 2011 by Universities Federation for Animal Welfare (UFAW)

So far, this book has described, first in general terms and then on a species-by-species or group-by group basis, the principles and practice of good husbandry and its impact on the welfare of farm animals. In this final chapter we consider the broader picture: how to promote the cause of improved animal welfare through actions taken on the farm and within society at large. The steps in this process are:

1. Set high but realistic standards for husbandry and welfare on farms.
2. Establish robust protocols for monitoring husbandry and welfare on farms.
3. Implement and audit actions necessary to ensure overall welfare standards and address specific problems.
4. Provide incentives and rewards to farmers for complying with standards.
5. Promote public awareness and demand for food and other farm produce that demonstrably meets these standards.

18.1 Animal Welfare Standards

The aim of any set of standards for farm animal welfare is, of course, to ensure that the animals can sustain an acceptable quality of life, on-farm, in transit and at the point of slaughter, through the provision of adequate management and resources. Quality of life as perceived by the animals may be categorized and assessed in terms of paradigms such as the 'five freedoms' (Chapter 1). However, it is we humans who make the decisions as to the acceptability of specific practices (e.g. beak trimming of poultry, pregnancy stalls for sows) or the overall quality of life for the animals we use as sources of food and other utilities. Inevitably, therefore, it is our views of what constitutes good and bad welfare that determine how they live. Individuals from any background (farmers, veterinary surgeons, scientists, consumers and so on) would probably agree on broad descriptions of animals that were either clearly suffering or were obviously fit and well. However the situation can be less clear when describing the welfare implications of conventional husbandry systems or procedures. There is a clear diversity of views within public perceptions of animal welfare. Fraser (2008) has identified three 'world views' of animal welfare. Farmers and veterinarians may consider that health and productivity are most important (if not all-important). Ethologists may give highest priority to 'feelings', the emotional state of the animal. Those who consume meat, milk and eggs but have no direct contact with farm animals (i.e. the vast majority) may consider that good welfare can best be achieved by giving farm animals a 'natural' life. The increased demand for free-range eggs within affluent urban populations is a case in point. Acknowledgement of all three 'world views' can create useful frameworks for defining and assessing welfare as perceived by the animals. In practice, however, it is more relevant to our understanding of human attitudes to animal welfare, and the reasons why different individuals or organizations may come to different conclusions, especially in the context of setting standards for legislation and individual farm assurance schemes.

The simple definition of animal wellbeing as 'fit and happy' (Chapter 1) embraces the first two concepts but not the third. If the public is to buy into a high welfare/high price scheme for farm animals then the scheme will almost certainly need to be seen to provide the animals with sufficient elements of the 'natural' life.

18.1.1 Farm assurance schemes

It has been said that when a man has plenty to eat, he has many problems, when he has nothing to eat he has only one problem. Consumers who enjoy both spending power and the power of choice express a wide range of food concerns. These include provenance (country or even farm of origin), food safety, production methods (e.g. organic standards) and animal welfare. In response to these concerns producers, retailers and organizations such as the Royal Society for the Protection of Animals (RSPCA) have developed a series of farm assurance schemes that set, monitor and provide assurance with respect to standards in one or all of these areas of concern.

Farm assurance schemes have been developed for most livestock sectors in the UK and Europe (e.g. DEFRA, Assured Dairy Farms, RSPCA Freedom Foods). Different quality assurance (QA) schemes place different emphasis on food safety, animal welfare and the environment. For example, the Freedom Food scheme, set up by the RSPCA in 1994, is primarily designed to ensure high standards of animal welfare. Organic certification schemes, such as the Soil Association, have been primarily designed to ensure sustainability and environmental protection (Soil Association, 1999) although they too give strong emphasis to the provision of high standards for animal health and welfare. Every scheme depends, of course, upon agreement between interested parties (e.g. farmer and retailer). Both farmers and retailers are motivated by their legal obligations in the UK under the Food Safety Act 1990 to ensure 'due diligence' in producing safe food and by a desire to avoid adverse publicity (or obtain a marketing advantage) on issues such as animal welfare and the environment. Farmers and retailers, too, are motivated by the desire to do things well and to be seen to be doing things well.

Most current QA schemes are based on:

- A formal written standard that members are required to adhere to at all times.
- An assessment procedure for verifying that producers adhere to this standard.

Standards in animal welfare may be assessed according to the following criteria (Figure 18.1):

- *Resources* – provision of the facilities necessary to ensure proper feeding, housing and handling of animals;
- *Management* – provision of correct husbandry procedures and competent, sympathetic stockmanship;
- *Records* – written evidence of use of medicines, deaths and culls, incidence of disease and injury (etc.);

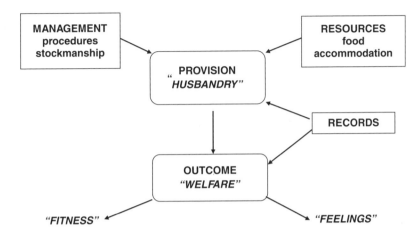

Figure 18.1 Elements necessary for assessment of the provision of good husbandry and welfare outcomes (from Webster, 2005). Used with permission of UFAW.

- *Welfare state* – evidence of physical fitness and mental wellbeing as perceived by the animals themselves.

It is important to recognize that the purpose of a QA assessment is to ensure compliance with the standards of the scheme and not to make some form of scientific evaluation of welfare. It is also easier to manage a QA assessment that is based on 'objective' observations of aspects of *provision* (management, resources and records) than one based on more 'subjective' assessment of the *outcome*, i.e. welfare state. Nevertheless, welfare state is ultimately what matters most to the consumers (and the animals themselves).

The following criteria are useful for assessing the effectiveness of the standards.

1. *Level of standards.* As a minimum, any QA scheme must include all legislation that is relevant to the stated objectives of the scheme. In the context of animal welfare and in the UK, these take as a baseline the DEFRA *Codes of Recommendation for the Welfare of Farm Animals*. However, the public appeal of a 'high-welfare' QA scheme, such as the RSPCA 'Freedom Foods', will also depend on the extent to which it is perceived to improve upon minimal standards, especially in regard to issues such as barren environments for laying hens or confinement of sows in farrowing crates. A scheme whose standards are designed to allow any farmer entry is not likely to impress the discerning customer. The standards should, however, be achievable.

2. *Scope of the standards.* The standards should include all resources and husbandry practices on a farm that could affect the welfare of any individual of the species covered by the scheme. This should include all types of stock. For example, QA on a dairy unit should incorporate calf rearing and the management of cull animals.

3. *Formulation of the standards.* The standards should be clearly definable, understandable and unambiguous. They should be regularly and frequently updated. They should be auditable and enforceable since a standard that cannot be verified on-farm is unhelpful and could lead to false claims by the scheme. Most aspects of animal husbandry (i.e. provisions for good welfare) can be assessed, provided the assessor has sufficient auditing and inspection skills. Welfare state is inherently more difficult to assess in a way that can be incorporated into clearly defined standards. Understandably, therefore, current standards have been based almost entirely on measures of provision rather than measures of outcome, although the trend within Europe is to place ever-increasing reliance on animal-based measures of welfare outcomes (e.g. the Welfare Quality® programme, www.welfarequality.com). These approaches are considered below.

18.2 On-Farm Assessment of Husbandry and Welfare

Any farm assurance scheme can only deliver an assurance to the consumer when there is a credible system for ensuring that the producer is complying with the requirements in the standard. Typically, there are three key stages to this process.

1. Farmers are required to be fully aware of the detailed requirements of the standard. The farmer should receive updated copies of the standards. Some schemes use a self-assessment system partly to draw the attention of the farmer to the standard requirements and partly to provide evidence that the farmer is complying with the standards since an external auditor can verify the accuracy of the self-assessment.
2. Advisers can assist the producer to comply with the standard. The veterinary surgeon is well suited to perform this task, ideally in association with regular consultations on herd health and preventive medicine.
3. A representative of the scheme (assessor) will usually need to visit the farm to verify compliance with the standard. In general terms the assessor is looking to gather evidence (visual, verbal or written) that verifies compliance with the standard. The assessor gathers this evidence from observation of records, resources and management, structured dialogue with stockpersons and, of course, observation of the animals in their environment.

The key aspects of the assessment procedure that may affect the effectiveness of the assessment include:

- *Robustness of the monitoring criteria.* The criteria used to assess husbandry and welfare need to be consistent, reproducible and not subject to observer bias. This is especially important in regard to animal-based measures of welfare outcomes, which are inevitably subjective. It is also important that observations made during visits by the assessor should, where possible, reflect long-term consequences of husbandry (e.g. body condition is a better measure of the adequacy of nutrition than presence of feed in the troughs at the time of the visit).

- *Competency of assessors.* This requires appropriate experience of the farming system under review and formal training in the conduct and report on the assessment.
- *Impartiality of the assessors.* is essential to the credibility of a scheme. This may be compromised if the assessor provides advice. It is necessary therefore to make a distinction between assessor and adviser.
- *Frequency and duration of visits.* Increasing the frequency and length of visits can increase the credibility of the assessment procedure. However, this obviously has a direct impact on the cost of the scheme. Assessors with suitable auditing and inspection skills (and suitable access to records) should be able to make some assessment of the management of the unit over a reasonable period such as one year prior to the visit. The assessments may need to be staggered to ensure that the farm is observed in different seasons.

Crucial to understanding welfare assessment is to first define the question that one is trying to address in such an assessment. For example, we could ask the following three questions when examining a novel husbandry system:

1. What is the impact of the husbandry system on the animals?
2. Are the actions of the owner managing the system acceptable according to legal requirements?
3. Is the welfare experienced by the animals within the system acceptable within the standards laid down by the QA scheme?

Each of these questions addresses a slightly different aspect of animal welfare and the answers that emerge are directed at a different audience. The first question requires consideration of the *welfare science* that might quantify the effect on the animal. The conclusions that emerge from this set of questions are likely to relate to specific aspects of welfare (e.g. lameness, behavioural problems) and to lead to specific recommendations directed to the farmer and his advisers. The second question judges the actions of the owner against the relevant *welfare legislation* and is likely to generate a 'pass or fail' decision that may be directed to regulatory authorities. The third question is a matter of *welfare ethics* as it addresses human perceptions as to the morality of the system. The conclusions will be more general and are likely to be directed at consumers, retailers and supervisory bodies (e.g. Soil Association, RSPCA Freedom Foods).

18.2.1 Animal-Based protocols for welfare monitoring

A structured approach to the animal-based monitoring of on-farm welfare has been developed within the pan-European Welfare Quality® Programme (www.welfarequality.com) (Table 18.1). It is designed to address the three questions posed above and to generate practical advice to farmers, ethical advice to consumers and

Table 18.1   The four principles and twelve criteria proposed by 'Welfare Quality' as elements of protocols for the direct, animal-based assessment of farm animal welfare (from Botreau *et al.*, 2007).

Welfare principles	Welfare criteria
Good feeding	Absence of prolonged hunger
	Absence of prolonged thirst
Good housing	Comfort around resting
	Thermal comfort
	Ease of movement
Good health	Absence of injuries
	Absence of disease
	Absence of pain induced by management procedures
Appropriate behaviour	Expression of social behaviours
	Expression of other behaviours
	Good human–animal relationship
	Absence of general fear

firm decisions on standards for legislators. It recognizes four principles of wellbeing: good feeding, good housing, good health and appropriate behaviour. These principles are, in essence, the same as those described by the 'five freedoms'. The four principles are defined according to 12 more specific criteria, each amenable to direct monitoring under farm conditions. For example, 'good housing' is defined by the criteria of comfort around resting, thermal comfort and ease of movement.

Figure 18.2 illustrates how this information may be directed to the various interested parties: producers, legislators and retailers. Standards defined by the 12 welfare criteria are derived from a larger range of observations and measures

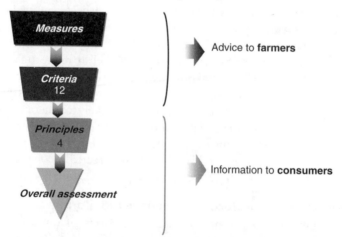

Figure 18.2   Characterization of measures and criteria used for the basis of on-farm monitoring of animal welfare and conveying information to farmers and consumers (adapted from Botreau *et al.*, 2007).

appropriate to the species and farming system under review. These would include proven robust measures of physical and mental state (e.g. body condition, prevalence of lameness, incidence of mastitis, evidence of feather pecking). A report based on the evaluation according to these standards and the measures upon which they were based forms the basis of a general conclusion as to the acceptability and quality of the farm and more specific advice to the farmer and his adviser.

While it can be relatively straightforward to define the adequacy or otherwise of husbandry provisions (resources, records and management) on a farm unit, it is inherently more difficult to make judgements with regard to overall welfare. Even when reduced to four categories (Table 18.1) conclusions as to welfare standards are unlikely to be clear-cut. Feeding may be good, health adequate but behaviour restricted (or any other combination of circumstances). Nevertheless, for the purposes of compliance with legislation or the standards of a particular QA scheme (e.g. as operated by a major retailer), it is necessary to give the assessment an overall mark. For legislative purposes this can simply be pass or fail. However, many retailers offer a range of products to allow their customers to make choices according to their own ethical beliefs as to the acceptability of different husbandry systems. Eggs may be sold as cage, barn or free range. Pork or farmed salmon may be simply labelled by country of origin or as produced according to RSPCA Freedom Food standards. This inevitably means that welfare standards on individual farms, however based on measures of husbandry provisions and welfare outcomes, need to be graded for quality.

Welfare Quality® has proposed that farms will be ranked on a four-point scale: unclassified, basal, good and excellent. This approach shows promise, but unresolved issues remain. Preliminary evidence would suggest that very few farms are likely to score 'excellent' according to all four principles. This poses several questions:

- How good is 'excellent'? Does it require evidence of positive welfare (e.g. happiness)?
- To what extent can excellence in one, two or three principles compensate for a score of basal or unclassified in another?
- Will retailers be prepared to accept a scheme whereby the majority of their produce is given a ranking lower than 'good'? It may be preferable to substitute a numerical ranking system (e.g. 0–3 stars).

The promotion of production and marketing systems that allow customers to express freedom of choice to decide what standard of welfare they wish to support is a matter for retailers, and falls outside the scope of this book. Different retailers, especially the major supermarket chains, compete with one another to attract customers into their stores. Price is one element of competition but so too is quality, and increasingly supermarkets are promoting their concern for animal welfare as a mark of quality and demonstrating their commitment through their quality assurance schemes. Since consumers (and individual retailers) cannot competently inspect every farm for themselves, they have to take on trust both the standards and the audit of these QA schemes. Readers of this book, however, are (by definition) those who have, or wish to develop, a direct and thorough interest in the management and welfare of farm animals. Our task is to develop the knowledge, skills and experience necessary to conduct a competent assessment of husbandry and welfare on farms and large production units, to make fair judgements as to standards, and (where appropriate) offer constructive advice as to actions necessary to promote and, where possible, improve welfare.

18.3 Welfare Monitoring Protocols

The exact details of an animal-based protocol for monitoring welfare will be governed by the species, the farming system, national legislation and the standards of value laid down by individual QA schemes. Many observations and measurements relevant to welfare monitoring for a particular farmed species have already been described in previous chapters. We shall not therefore attempt to present a comprehensive list of protocols but to illustrate an approach to the direct, animal-based assessment of welfare based on that adopted by the Bristol Welfare Assurance Programme (www.vetschool.bris.ac.uk/animalwelfare). These protocols for monitoring welfare under farm conditions are based on the five freedoms. In this chapter we highlight one example of a welfare outcome measure within each of the five freedoms that can be assessed during a farm visit. The examples are taken from our dairy cattle welfare assessment protocol (Whay *et al.*, 2003) and illustrate the information provided for each monitor. For each indicator of welfare within each welfare principle ('freedom'), we describe the criteria (what needs to be assessed) and the methodology (how the indicator should be assessed). This is followed by a brief explanation that can be used to explain the significance of each indicator to a farmer. Figures 18.3 to 18.6 present some of the illustrations that accompany these directions.

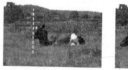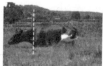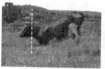

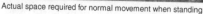
Normal movements when standing up and lying down

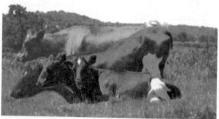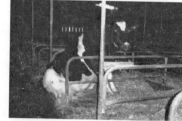

Actual space required for normal movement when standing

Dog sitting' posture indicating severe rising restriction

Figure 18.3 Freedom to express normal behaviour: example of assessment, standing up and lying down (source: www.vetschool.bris.ac.uk/animalwelfare).

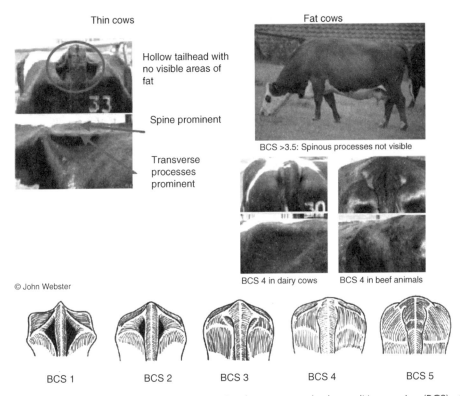

Figure 18.4 Freedom from hunger: example of assessment, body condition scoring (BCS) of cows.

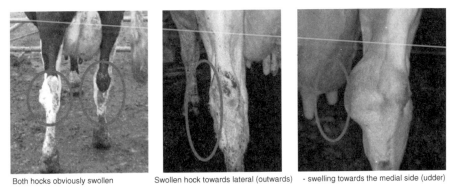

Figure 18.5 Freedom from discomfort: example of assessment, swollen hocks.

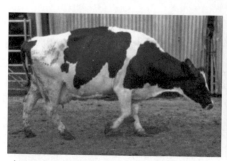 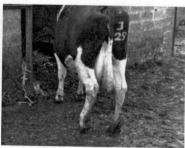

Lame cow: Walking with an uneven step rhythm, arched spine, nodding head and shortened stride length

Lame cow: reluctant to bear weight on left hind limb

Figure 18.6   Freedom from pain, injury and disease: example of assessment, lameness in dairy cows.

18.3.1 Freedom to express normal behaviour

Example: rising restriction during housing

Observation

A cow will normally rock in a forward lunge of 60 cm, then raise the rear end first, moving a front foot forward, finally lifting the shoulders and head, all in a single fluid movement (Figure 18.3a). Record if cows show severe rising restriction, e.g. performing behaviours such as rocking repeatedly, turning their heads sideways, dipping their heads as they stand, standing foot feet first, or hitting fittings during rising.

Methodology

If possible observe 10 animals standing up. Try to observe cows that rise voluntarily; do not force the animals to stand. If more than one group is involved, take a representative sample of animals from each group.

Farmer significance

Are cows having difficulty when rising or lying down? Cows are more likely to sustain injuries in areas such as the hips and ribs when they are too large for the cubicles. Severe restriction in the lying area may discourage cows from lying down. Reduced lying time is known to be a high risk for lameness, especially in heifers. Space restriction may be caused by factors such as cubicle design, yard design or stocking density.

18.3.2 Freedom from fear and stress

Example: flight distance

Observation and methodology

Ensure the cow is standing still in an area where she has sufficient room to move away from you. Ideally this should be in the animal's habitual environment (cubicle house or barn). Walk quietly and steadily towards the cow at right angles to her shoulder. Do not look into her eyes. Estimate how close you can approach before the cow turns her head away or takes the first step away. Record the result in metres. Make observations on at least 10 animals.

Farmer significance

How far (in metres) is the flight distance? A short avoidance distance reflects reduced fearfulness, makes daily inspections and handling procedures less stressful and is a good indicator for 'positive health'. The test can be influenced by a variety of factors (lameness, social/environment for testing, previous experience, unfamiliar/familiar test person) but reflects in general the quality and quantity of handling and stockmanship.

18.3.3 Freedom from hunger and thirst

Example: body condition

Methodology

Stand behind and beside the cow and assess body condition by vision only. Look especially at the tailhead, spine and transverse processes. Refer to DEFRA publications on condition scoring (www.defra.gov.uk/animalwelfare).

Recording – thin cows

Record cows with body condition score (BCS) < 2.0. The tailhead area is a deep cavity with no fatty tissue under the skin (Figure 18.4). Ths spine is prominent and the horizontal spinous processes (transverse processes) sharp.

Recording – fat cows

Record cows with BCS 4–5. The tailhead is completely filled with fat and folds and patches of fat are evident. The vertebral processes are not visible and the animal appears completely rounded.

Farmer significance

Body condition scoring is a technique for assessing the condition of livestock at regular intervals. The purpose of condition scoring is to achieve a balance between economic feeding, good production and welfare.

Does the animal have a BCS of < 2? If it does then it is excessively thin. Dairy cows are under considerable nutritional stress, and adequate feeding is essential to avoid excessive weight loss. These animals can suffer discomfort (especially in cubicles). At service, cows should not be in energy deficit as this may result in low fertility.

Does the animal have a BCS > 3.5? If it does then it is overweight. Cows should not be excessively fat, especially before and at calving. Fat cows may develop fatty liver disease or ketosis and are more prone to milk fever, mastitis, lameness, infertility and calving difficulties. It is also not economical to feed excessively.

18.3.4 Freedom from discomfort

Example: swollen hocks

Observation

Record if the cow has any obviously swollen hocks. This can be seen as an obvious increase in the hock diameter and may be caused by thickened skin, bursitis (hygromas) or increased fluid filling of the joints. The swelling can be seen on the lateral or medial side of the hindlimb (Figure 18.5).

Methodology

Assess both hindlimbs, standing behind and beside the animal, and include all swellings that are visible from a distance of 2 m. Compare to other animals in the herd and try to find a normal hock for comparison. In a normal hock all anatomical structures (bones, tendons) are visible.

Farmer significance

Does the animal have any swelling of the hock? This may indicate that the surface on which the cows are lying may not be comfortable. Swollen hocks are considered to be an indicator of discomfort in the lying area and are strongly associated with lameness.

18.3.5 Freedom from pain, injury and disease

Example: lameness

Observation

Record number of cows seen lame (limping). Do not include those who appear only to have tender feet, or slight abnormalities of locomotion. Lame cows may display an arched spine when walking or standing (Figure 18.6), shortened stride and obvious head nods when moving. One or more limbs may be only partially weight-bearing or rested when standing. Lame cows may be reluctant to stand or move. Note, heifers that are lame do not usually arch their spines. All animals observed to be lame should be included in the count. This should include mild cases since these are the cows that would benefit from early treatment before lameness becomes severe and expensive through loss of milk, fertility and time.

Methodology

When walking through the cows make a preliminary note of any animals that are lame. If the number of lame cows is a cause for concern then the whole herd must be assessed for lameness. The most convenient way is to observe all cows walking as they leave the milking parlour. Alternatively ask the farmer to walk the whole herd past you, a few cows at a time.

Farmer significance

Are there any lame animals? Early recognition, investigation and treatment of lame animals are essential to reduce pain and provide effective control of the problem. Increased levels of lameness are also expensive to the farmer through loss of milk, fertility and time.

18.3.6 Interpretation of observations

Figure 18.7 summarizes data from a survey of welfare on selected dairy farms in the UK (Whay *et al.*, 2003) to illustrate the prevalence (%) of four of the conditions described by the above examples. The herd distribution for these observations is presented in quintiles (i.e. best 20% in black, worst 20% uncoloured, with consistent patterns for the three middle quintiles). Figure 18.7 shows, for example, that for rising restriction, prevalence for the best quintile was below 10%; for the worst quintile it was 50–77%. For lameness, prevalence for the best quintile was below 14%; for the worst it was 30–50%. The figure also shows that there were no fat cows in the best 60% of herds.

The information gathered from this set of animal-based indices of welfare in dairy cows was circulated to 50 experts who were asked to indicate the herd prevalence (in these examples) which would indicate a welfare problem sufficiently serious to justify intervention at herd level, both for the sake of the animals and to ensure compliance with welfare standards laid down by QA schemes. A herd problem was defined as one where the prevalence or incidence was such that 75% of experts recommended intervention. In the case of thin cows, 75% considered that intervention was necessary for farms in bands D and E (i.e. 40% of herds in which prevalence was >21%). For lameness, intervention was recommended when prevalence was greater than 13% (bands B to E). Thus 75% of competent judges considered that lameness was a welfare problem that required attention in 80%

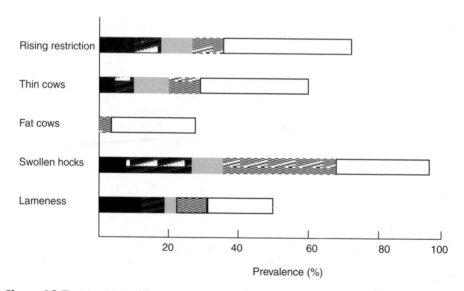

Figure 18.7 Prevalence of four indices of poor welfare in dairy cows (From Whay *et al.*, 2003). Each index is divided into quintiles indicating the prevalence of these conditions from the best 20% (in black) to the worst 20% (unshaded).

of the recorded herds! Overall lameness prevalence in this study was similar to that in other contemporary reports from Europe and the USA. This puts the spotlight on two very important messages. Lameness is the major welfare problem for high-performance dairy cows in the developed world (Chapter 3). A quality assurance programme that simply records the prevalence of a welfare problem such as lameness but does not lead to effective action is not providing the quality assurance it claims, either for the animals or for the public who are expected to put their trust in the system.

18.4 Implementation and Promotion of Good Welfare

So far, this chapter has described the principles and practice that should govern the assessment of the elements of animal welfare under farm conditions. This information can be used in several ways. It can be incorporated into a herd health and welfare plan tuned to the needs of the individual farmer. It can be used to set standards for QA schemes operated by producer groups, retailers or non-governmental organizations such as RSPCA. Finally, in extreme cases, it can be used to test compliance with national standards for legislative purposes. There is broad agreement that assessment procedures should incorporate both measures of the elements of good husbandry (e.g. resources, records and stockmanship) and direct animal-based assessment of the physical ('fit') and emotional ('feeling good') elements of welfare, based on sound foundations of animal welfare science.

The development of robust monitoring protocols for husbandry and welfare is an essential first element of welfare-based quality assurance. However, the scheme must also provide good evidence of quality *control*, namely, proof that the monitoring procedure leads to effective action designed both to ensure overall compliance with required standards, and to remedy specific areas where needs for improvement have been identified. Moreover, a market-led scheme that seeks to add value on the basis of assured standards of animal welfare that surpass the statutory minimum must ensure that this added value is recognized by both consumers and producers and properly apportioned through all links in the food chain. If customers are to pay more, they need to be aware of, and trust, the assurances provided by the scheme. If retailers are to reward their suppliers for their compliance with superior standards, they too need to promote the scheme to achieve financial reward through increased market share. If farmers are to invest increased time and resources to animal welfare they need a financial incentive, since most of them are doing the best they can with what they can currently afford. The farm animals, the objects of these good intentions, will only benefit if all three responsible parties can be persuaded to act together. Many of these schemes are still young and as yet there is little evidence from which to assess their impact. However such evidence as does exist (e.g. Figure 18.7) would suggest that they are not yet achieving the impact they would wish, either for the animals or for the general public. Possible reasons for this lack of impact include:

- inadequate monitoring procedures;
- failure to develop action plans based upon information gathered during the monitoring procedures;
- lack of financial incentive for farmers to implement action plans;
- lack of consumer demand for 'high-welfare' produce, arising from lack of aware-ness, trust, or perceived added quality of individual QA schemes.

If it is to succeed, a welfare-based QA scheme (or the animal welfare element of a broader scheme) needs to operate both on the farm and at the retail level; creating, in effect, two virtuous cycles of monitoring, action, review, reward and promotion, running together as elements of a single, continuous dynamic process. This has been described as a 'virtuous bicycle' (Webster, 2009). The design and development of this whimsical but conceptually sound model is illustrated in Figure 18.8. The right wheel of the bicycle illustrates action to progress the quality of husbandry and animal welfare on farm; the left wheel illustrates action to promote the market share for high-welfare products.

18.4.1 Implementation of good welfare: the producer cycle

Guaranteed quality assurance requires a continuous process of welfare assessment, action to address specific problems and review to address the effectiveness of the action. In the approach illustrated by the right wheel, the 'producer cycle' in Figure 18.8, each cycle begins with a formal written self-assessment carried out by the farm owner with inputs from stockpeople and veterinarians as appropriate. The self-assessment should be based on the standards of husbandry and provision set by the QA scheme and will include: housing and hygiene; records of feed provision, health, use of medicines, etc.; stockmanship and training; the existence and operation of a health and welfare plan. The farmer should also be required to outline any specific welfare concerns and priorities for action to address these concerns. The next stage of the cycle is the visit by the independent monitor, trained for and operating to the standards of the assurance scheme. The visit will include an interview with the farmer, to discuss and review the self-assessment, and an inspection of the animals to assess welfare according to the animal-based criteria and principles described in the previous section. The report of the monitor will provide an assessment of compliance with the overall standards and the four principles (Table 18.1) or five freedoms. It should identify and rank areas where it is desirable or necessary to improve welfare. The next step is to identify critical control points and prioritize an action plan designed to address these welfare issues. The extent to which the assessor may or may not act as an adviser at this stage is a matter for the directors of the scheme to decide. Having received the assessor's report, the farmer, probably after discussion with an inde-pendent adviser such as a veterinary surgeon, should produce a written response to the

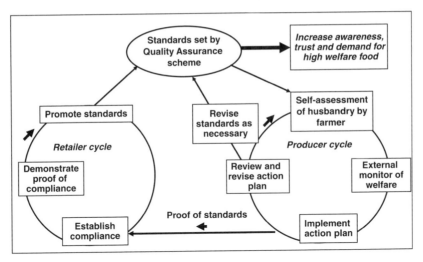

Figure 18.8 The 'virtuous bicycle': a vehicle designed to deliver improved animal welfare on-farm. The right wheel illustrates the process of self-assessment, external monitoring, action and review on-farm; the left wheel, the process of quality assurance and quality control at the retailer level (from Webster, 2009).

report to include comments on any areas of disagreement and a prioritized plan of action. Copies of both assessment and response should be submitted to the supervisors of the QA scheme. After an appropriate interval (e.g. one year), there is a further review of welfare in general and the effectiveness of specific prioritized actions. This should, once again, be based first on self-assessment, then independent monitoring.

The aim of this approach – self-assessment, independent monitoring, action and review – is to create a dynamic cycle of continuous improvement. The first benefit of starting with self-assessment is that the farmer can address elements of husbandry, provision and records in his/her own time, thus reducing the amount of work that has to be done at the time of the visit from the external assessor. It recognizes moreover that the farmer also knows most (if not necessarily best) the husbandry procedures that operate on his own farm and why they have evolved. The aim of the visit by the independent assessor is to mount a fair challenge to this self-assessment. While the first visit will have to be comprehensive, subsequent assessments can concentrate on the most important issues arising from previous assessments and the success or otherwise of the action plan.

The practical merits of this approach are as follows:

- Elements of husbandry, including records of actions to ensure welfare, are included in the self-assessment. This recognizes that much of the information necessary to assure the quality of welfare on farm must be obtained from evidence relating to the provision of resources and management on-farm, records of these provisions and records of outcomes, e.g. relating to animal health and use of medicines.

- Compliance with the standards of the scheme would not normally be based on the results of a single monitoring exercise but on the effectiveness of actions to promote welfare and address specific problems.
- Once the cycle of self-assessment, monitoring, action and review has been established it should be possible for farmers and assessors to focus on the most important issues, thereby avoiding bureaucratic and time-wasting repetition of all elements of the assessment protocol at every visit.
- A scheme where compliance (and/or star rating) is based not on the assessment protocol but on evidence of the effectiveness of actions designed to promote welfare is sympathetic to the farmer, since it reduces the risk of subjective bias in the assessor's report (and variation in standards between assessors). It is also more challenging to the farmer since it does not allow him to file away the assessor's report and forget about it until next year. He must provide evidence of effective action.

18.4.2 Promotion of good welfare: retailers and consumers

The left wheel of the virtuous bicycle (Figure 18.8) is designed to improve the public awareness of, and demand for, food and other animal products from farms operating to proven high welfare standards. The aim is to create an improved, sustained, verifiable process of information transfer to the public and retailers relating to welfare standards and actions to ensure welfare standards on farms operating within the QA scheme. The welfare standards necessary for compliance within the scheme (or ranking within the scheme) are stated at the outset and freely available to all both in outline and in detail. Entry to the scheme occurs when the farmer can establish compliance based on evidence that he has established the action plan for welfare. Subsequent cycles require continuous proof of compliance based on evidence of attention to welfare standards. Proof of compliance, supported by evidence, can then be used by the retailer to promote the scheme. The aim of the scheme, the direction of the bicycle, is towards increased awareness, trust and demand for high welfare food.

18.4.3 Delivery of good welfare

Welfare-based quality schemes are now a fact of life, and they are likely to become even more prominent in the future as results and strategies emerge from the Welfare Quality® programme. The tide of public opinion is in favour. However, if these schemes fail to deliver on their assurances through piecemeal approaches that fail to complete the revolution of both cycles of challenge, action, promotion and reward, then consumers could lose trust, retailers and farmers lose faith, and the cause of improved farm animal welfare could be set back for years.

The approach illustrated by the 'virtuous bicycle' is more time-consuming and potentially costly to both producers and retailers than most conventional QA schemes that tend to operate on the basis of an annual inspection, involving one day or less and the probability that, unless the farm actually fails the assessment, no action will be required until next year. It is therefore unrealistic to expect it to succeed unless it brings real reward to all stakeholders, namely consumers, retailers, farmers and the animals themselves, through proper recognition of the added value accruing through better attention to animal welfare. Thus produce bearing the logo of a value-added scheme should retail at a price higher than that for food (etc.) produced according to nationally approved (minimal) standards, and a fair proportion of this increased price should be passed to the producer. If it becomes pan-European policy to impose the monitoring standards and rating system proposed by Welfare Quality®, then it would be logical to equate 'unclassified' (or zero star) with compliance with minimum legal standards assessed at annual inspection and not, in this case, impose an action plan to promote improved welfare. Awards of one to three stars (or rankings of basal to excellent) would reward increments of quality in terms of animal welfare, with commensurate increments in the cash value of the produce.

The 'virtuous bicycle' is presented here only as one conceptual approach to the integration of quality control, promotion and delivery in the cause of high standards of animal welfare. It is, however, a concept that emerges from the awareness that current welfare-based quality assurance schemes have a long way to go to achieve their joint aims of significant improvement in animal welfare at farm level and significant increase in consumer demand for proven high-welfare food. For these things to occur in practice, a quality assurance scheme must be seen to bring rewards to all those involved in the process: consumers, retailers, farmers and, of course, the animals. Farmers are unlikely to buy into the scheme without the assurance that it will bring them rewards in the form of increased income and security of contract. Consumers are unlikely to pay more and retain faith in the scheme unless they can trust the evidence upon which the assurance is based. In short, the virtuous bicycle will only deliver when both wheels turn together. The success (or otherwise) of this and similar approaches to the promotion of good farm animal welfare will depend on how well they work in action.

References and Further Reading

Assured Dairy Farms (UK)*Farm Assurance Protocol*. Available at: http://www.ndfas.org.uk.

Botreau, R., Veissier, I., Butterworth, A., Bracke, M.B.M. and Keeling, L. (2007) Definition of criteria for overall assessment of animal welfare. *Animal Welfare* **16**, 225–8.

Bristol Welfare Assurance Programme. Available at: http://www.vetschool.bris.ac.uk/animalwelfare.

DEFRA. *Farm Assurance Schemes and Standards*. Available at: http://www.defra.gov.uk.

Fraser, D. (2008) *Understanding Animal Welfare: the Science in its Cultural Context*. Wiley-Blackwell, Oxford.

RSPCA Freedom Food. Available at: http://www.rspca.org.uk.

Soil Association Standards (UK)*Animal Welfare*. Available at: http://www.soilassociation.org.

US Department of Agriculture. *Animal welfare audits and certification programmes*. Available at: https://awic.usda.gov.

Webster, A.J.F. (2009) The Virtuous Bicycle: a delivery vehicle for improved farm animal welfare. *Animal Welfare* 18, 141–7.

Whay, H.R., Main, D.C.J., Green, L.E. and Webster, A.J.F. (2003) Assessment of the welfare of dairy cattle using animal-based measurements: direct observations and investigation of farm records. *Veterinary Record* 153, 197–202.

Index

Management and Welfare of Farm Animals: The UFAW Farm Handbook, 5th edition. John Webster
© 2011 by Universities Federation for Animal Welfare (UFAW)